How Essential is Fluoride?
What do the Experts Say?

By

Guy P. D. Armstrong, BSc.

The Nameless Publisher Tapui Limited

Thorndon, Wellington 6144, New Zealand

thenamelesspublisher@gmail.com

Editors: B. D. Armstrong & S. F. Moynihan

Book Design: B. D. Armstrong & G. P. D. Armstrong

Cover Design: coverover2020@gmail.com

ISBN 978-0-473-51018-3

First Edition (updated)

Contents

Introduction

In 2009 I was completing the final year in a biology degree at Victoria University, in my home town of Wellington, New Zealand. I had become very interested in studying evolution. One of the most important things I learned at university came from that course. I have thought back to it over the writing of this book, indeed I based much of my effort on the principle the following story illustrates.

Our professor told us that Charles Darwin spent twenty years studying barnacles. Darwin kept barnacles all through his home. He kept so many barnacles that when his son went to a friend's house, upon seeing the kitchen cupboards bare, he asked "where does *your* father keep all of *his* barnacles?" Darwin's son thought barnacles were part of the natural order of every cupboard. I understood that behind the story was a very important principle – one of patience and thoughtfulness. I remember in those moments feeling a far greater respect for Darwin. Thinking on it afterwards, I felt that in divisive topics what was or was not true was just as important as how much effort we put in to further our understanding. If we put in the time and patience that Darwin did, we'd understand some of the axioms and fundamentals involved and obtain a real grounding in our topic.

I share the story because I need to ask you to be patient in your perusal of this work.

As a teenager I had been interested in nutrition. This led me to university. After my degree, I needed a hobby. I remember reading my local newspaper one morning, and seeing the claim that fluorine was, or was not, a nutritional essential. A few days later I saw the opposite claim. Neither comment was made with any explanation. I began to think about it. What I knew then about fluorine's elemental properties you could fit into a thimble. Chlorine, sodium, potassium gates, G-proteins – we had spent hours looking at these, yet I wondered did fluorine have some role in the cell I knew nothing about? I had also not studied teeth at university, so I was doubly humbled.

I followed the topic casually for a few years, then became more serious about it. I became interested in Community Water Fluoridation (CWF). I began following the media, all the while looking for claims of a possible nutritional role, which sometimes seemed like a marginally important niche aspect, sometimes an all-encompassing pervasive substance like the air CWF would metaphorically breathe.

People argued back and forth. Often the same clichés and slogans were used on both sides. In all honesty, it was hard to tell clichés and slogans from solid scientific conclusions when these things appeared in media. I began to think that the impression of confidence from many people for and against CWF was harming the scientific aspects, purely because nobody wanted to appear weak in public. In the newspapers and the TV news, nobody really had enough time to flesh out an argument. Almost no-one (there were a few exceptions) who spoke publicly seemed able to say anything of any depth, anything with any real foundation to it. At best, largely due to space restrictions because editors are presumably under public pressure to show many points of view, letters to the editor could cite one review, one book, one handful of experts.

While my research began with a focus on the question of whether fluorine/fluoride is an essential nutrient, it soon became apparent that this issue is part of an immense and expansive debate that has lasted from the 1940s to the present day. Accordingly I came to look at the perceived role of fluoride in our lives, the contradictions evident in the written and spoken history, and how we came to be where we are today.

I compare three chronologies of information relating to this question: (1) what scientists have concluded in experiments, (2) what expert bodies like the American National Academy of Sciences, the World Health Organization and others have said, and (3) what experts have said in newspapers. I compare what these three groups have claimed over the past seventy or so years.

When I use the term "experts" here I take a narrow approach. I mean the people the media, universities, government and the like put forth to communicate the science behind Community Water Fluoridation to us. All of these experts are supporters of Community Water Fluoridation. The fact that I examine the statements of experts should not be taken as criticism or disrespect to people who oppose these programs. It is in *this* book that I use the term "experts" exclusively to mean supporters. Some of the statements of people who oppose fluoridation are given when required to provide context to expert statements.

One must understand that the question "is fluorine an essential nutrient" does not *always* have a *direct* relationship to Community Water Fluoridation. Regarding the experiments that are detailed in the first chapter, one will find they are invoked in books, arguments, documents, but seldom are *many* of them invoked at once. Seldom are contradictions, difficulties and the scientists' natural tendency towards hesitancy or their constant desire for more research, used to win arguments. Seldom are scientists' claims of weaknesses in their own conclusions invoked in the political arena. My work shines a light not only on the strengths of experiments, but on their weaknesses, and on the tug of war and the spin and selectivity that sometimes occurs in these obscure arguments. Every experiment is unique and different, and that's what I'm showing. I want to show you "each barnacle", so to speak.

One may ask the question why the experts (promoters of Community Water Fluoridation) are under the microscope, and not the people opposed to these programs. This is fair. One answer is that the experts present themselves, and are presented by journalists, as knowledgeable, objective, scientific, unbiased, progressive, and a whole host of other good things. Many of the people opposed on the other hand, may work full-time at a profession unrelated to CWF, may or may not have the technical qualifications the experts do, and are therefore not always considered "experts" by media, government, universities and other centres of power, prestige or influence.

The writings of people opposed to Community Water Fluoridation were harder to find because they were more obscure. Some articles read in citation lists were pamphlets that even librarians found difficult, sometimes impossible to track down. Some pamphlets I saw only in obscure archives, with no electronic acknowledgement. The work of the supporters was far more likely to be published in leading academic journals that were easily accessible.

This book is, then, not only an appraisal of a nutritional role for fluorine. It is also an appraisal of how this topic is treated, why different people at times have said it important or not important, and what it means not only to biochemistry but to dentistry and public health.

I wanted to provide something useful to the people of New Zealand and other countries that were having issues with dental health. My research then evolved into a greater focus on dental health. Teeth are made of, and need, many things. So this book elaborates on other nutritional and social factors important in dental health.

By way of introduction to the chapters, I note that I like the detailed fluoride experiments regarding dietary essentiality that I've discussed in chapter 1. They are not black and white. We go through each one – the introduction; the reasons why it was performed, the background of the experiment, then the approach, the methods; what was tried and why, what worked and what didn't, the results; what happened, then the conclusion, summary and discussion, and see what was deduced, what was learned, and what was left uncertain. It's less tribal and far more thought-provoking than a simple good/bad, black/white approach.

Experiments began around the 1930s but there were some from earlier. Community Water Fluoridation officially began in January of 1945 in America, and in the early 1950s here in New Zealand. I found little media discussion on this topic prior to the early 1950s.

I noticed patterns forming in two of the three chronologies, the timelines of information. This book is organized around these three categories, or chronologies. Chapter 2 lays out a selection of work from the National Academy of Sciences (NAS), the World Health Organization (WHO), other official expert bodies, and a few stragglers that may or may not be affiliated with any promoting agency. The charge of "semantics" is levelled at some. Chapter 3 takes a detour to some of the information regarding what New Zealand officials and experts had claimed in the past regarding a nutritional role for fluorine. I am a New Zealander and a patriot, and this chapter is of importance because the beginnings of fluoridation in this country are not well-discussed nowadays. Chapter 4 is about the abundance of fluorine. This chapter is appropriate because experts have claimed many times that water with less than 0.7 part per million fluorine is deficient – note these experts claim the *water* is deficient. Chapter 4 looks at the difficulties scientists mentioned in the first chapter had in creating fluorine-free diets. Also mentioned here are the National Academy of Sciences (NAS) and the World Health Organization (WHO) statements regarding levels of fluorine in foods.

Chapter 5 starts by examining the media, the results I obtained in my search of about 4,000 Australasian articles and between one and two thousand American articles. I was looking for claims of essentiality, or non-essentiality. I discuss the importance, and accusation of "semantics" – changing the meaning of words. Yet this is a returning theme, as the work of different experts needs appraisal when the work is mentioned, as the accusation of "semantics" rears its head a couple of times in Chapter 2. Another key theme we see in media and the more political aspects of Community Water Fluoridation is one of competition – the inevitable "both sides". I investigate how having two sides oppose each other affects a scientific issue, and look at the use of the term "propaganda".

Abuse is also examined. Arguments resorted to mud-slinging and smear tactics. This had a very powerful effect on media. Journalists and newspaper editors sometimes couldn't approach the subject without tempers flaring, regardless of what they wrote about it. Instead of becoming more involved which could have resulted in more clarity in at least some aspects, many of them withdrew. The issue suffered because of this. To my knowledge, the first book written on fluoridation by a journalist was published in 1986 in Australia, forty-one years after the programs began in America.

Money and the power it brings are influential factors. Money and media, money and universities, money and some of the corporations that funded a couple of the experiments mentioned in Chapter 1, as well as the sugar industry, are investigated. Are we undermining our own desires when every supermarket, every dairy, every petrol station sells cheap junk food, while the intellectuals desperately focus on the best science for public health? Does junk food advertising work? Does junk food harm children? How much? How does one measure 'harm'? How would you or I measure it? How would a junk food executive, or a lawyer measure it? How many generations does it take to see 'harm'? Chapter 5 ends with a return to New Zealand, and the town of Hastings. I share some documents from the New Zealand Health Department archives, and compare them with media statements and press releases from experts. This, too – the comparison of private, with public statements – is a recurring theme.

Chapter 6 looks at the dental health of New Zealand Māori and Australian Indigenous people before the influence of European and American nutrition.

Other questions are examined. How well can rodent experiments be applied to humans? How accurate can we be in the percentages of benefit CWF can give us when we don't examine individual diets? How much fluoride is an 'optimal amount' in the water? How much is an 'optimal amount' in a tooth? How much is too much? What are the effects of nutrients like calcium, iodine, iron, vitamins and protein on our dental health? And what is modern research showing us?

Our desire for equality, our compulsion to hear *both sides* has a very powerful, yet less visible effect: research in the middle gets ignored. Research that decisively concludes a substance or mode of action good or bad, right or wrong, too much or not enough, can be ridiculed and criticized by the side that doesn't like it, or championed by the side that does. Research that concludes that the substance we're for or against does nothing, research that is inconsistent in results, difficult to understand or explain in a 3-minute media segment, research fraught with complications, or that which might undermine *both* sides can be ignored for a simple reason: in a "both sides" debate it's useless to either side. It can be ignored, though it may be true.

Everybody wants "the latest research" which is understandable given the competitive market, but we fail to see our track record of ignoring the latest research when it doesn't suit. This is why an historical approach is important.

Political scientist John E. Mueller, writing in the **Western Political Quarterly**, wrote in 1964:

> "[Community Water Fluoridation] has transformed communities into laboratories of conflict, but the type of conflict is in many respects unique."[1]

I believe the "fluoridation controversy" as Mueller has called it, has had a significant impact on the evidence that reaches the public through media.

I do *not* examine social media in this investigation.

I have given a multitude of research and evidence in this work. I hope you will search out those things that either interest or placate you. We say "have a look yourself if you don't believe me" – we need to start saying "have a look even if you *do* believe me." Some of the statements people have made in this topic are *quite* outrageous. If you have a political or scientific bone in your body, I think you'll find this book somewhat enriching, maybe even entertaining.

Yet it is only sensible to take stock of *what* evidence we have, *how much* evidence we have, and its *quality*. From this, we are closer to seeing where truth lies. I have not seen a report or investigation that looks at the entire timeline of experiments, hence an historical approach is worthy. What happened decades ago influences our current understanding.

After a few years of data collection, I realised I'd obtained mostly American research. This appeared disconcerting at first as I didn't want to restrict myself any more than necessary. Then I realised it was in some ways a benefit: the New Zealand Health Department archives demonstrated that both supporters and detractors of fluoridation were in touch with their American counterparts. The arguments that played out in 1940s America were playing out all over again in this part of the world, in the 1950s. This appears to have repeated and repeated. Newspaper editors commented so many times on the repetitive nature, and lost interest. I often wonder how we would have approached fluoridation in this country without Uncle Sam's instruction and guidance, and how different the journalism could have been.

If the reader is a little flustered or intimidated by overly technical information, one need not worry. While it is difficult to focus on style in a technical document, I always approached this writing with an inclusive presentation of information in mind. Look to the essence of the work. For those who are detail-oriented, some experiments are readily available for perusal.

References are given in square brackets. Work that I quote will cite *other* work; these I often tracked down, if I didn't I put it in footnotes at the bottom of the page. References often contain extra information.

---

[1] Vol. 19, No. 1, p. 67.

Regarding terminology, fluorine with an 'n' refers to the element fluorine alone, fluoride with a 'd' refers to the element bonded to another element – usually sodium or calcium, but sometimes something else. When it's an important factor in someone's argument, it will be mentioned.

For documents, I went to the New Zealand Ministry of Health Library, and the Alexander Turnbull Library (also called The National Library). I sourced experiments through the Wellington City Library interloan department. There was simply no way of knowing who was telling the truth about fluorine's nutritional role until I went into the research, and even then, the topic was still contradictory until I had spent a lot of time on it. In the heat of debates, it seemed less important when compared with questions of safety, effectiveness, and cost.

For Australian media I used the database *Trove*, which is available through google. It was recommended to me by a librarian at Wellington's Alexander Turnbull Library. For New Zealand media, I used the search engines at Alexander Turnbull Library. I searched through about three thousand articles in total that came up with the words *fluorid* essential*. The asterisk denotes any word with the letters before it, so fluoride, fluorides, fluoridation, etc.

The National Library also contains other media which I used liberally; and I spent a day or so in the Fairfax Media building in Wellington going through their archive, and a few more days at Wellington Public Library looking through the archive of Wellington's biggest newspaper. Six months in the New Zealand Health Department archives yielded even more, as well as many letters to and from the Health Department.

For most American newspapers, I used the database Newspapers.com.

I am indebted to the hard-working archivists at Archives New Zealand, and the librarians and archivists at Alexander Turnbull Library. Of illimitable help were librarians at Wellington Central Library. This work would have been much the poorer without them. Jamie, Marilyn and Chloe, thank you again.

This book is lovingly dedicated to the people of New Zealand, Australia, Canada, the United Kingdom, and the United States of America.

Definitions

These definitions are from dictionaries I have found in my local libraries. A couple are online, included for international readers. I don't want the reader to think or feel that I am insisting on these definitions as perfectly appropriate or even *more* appropriate than others – quite the contrary. One of the things I want to demonstrate in this investigation is the pliability of words and terms. However, these definitions are typical, and helpful.

Nutrients:

Dictionary of Food and Nutrition by Lulu G. Graves and Clarence Wilbur Taber, 1938. - "Foods that supply the body with its necessary elements. Those containing carbon are *organic food nutrients*. Those which do not contain it are *inorganic food nutrients…*"

Dictionary of Nutrition and Food Technology, 4th Edition by Arnold E. Bender, 1975. - "Essential dietary factors such as vitamins, minerals, amino acids and fats. Sources of energy are not termed nutrients so that a commonly used phrase is "energy and nutrients" (calories and nutrients)."

Dictionary of Nutrition: A Consumer's Guide to the Facts of Food by Sheila Bingham, 1977. - "Substances, contained in foods, which provide energy and raw materials for the synthesis and maintenance of living matter. Human nutrients are protein, carbohydrate, fat, minerals and vitamins. Alcohol provides energy but is a drug rather than a nutrient. Those that cannot be made in sufficient quantities from raw materials in food in the body are called essential nutrients; vitamins, minerals, essential amino acids and linoleic acid. Lack of an essential nutrient results in a specific deficiency disease."

Stedman's Medical Dictionary for the Health Professions and Nursing, 5th Edition, by Thomas Lathrop Stedman, 2005. – "A constituent of food necessary for normal physiologic function."

Illustrated Medical Dictionary, British Medical Association, 2013. – "An essential dietary factor, including carbohydrates, proteins, certain fats, vitamins, and minerals."

Oxford Concise Medical Dictionary, 2015. – "A substance that must be consumed in order to provide the essential components needed for growth and the maintenance of life. Nutrients include carbohydrates, fats, proteins, minerals, and vitamins."

Essential Element:

The Concise Oxford Dictionary, 8th edition, by H. W. Fowler and F. G. Fowler, edited by R. E. Allen, 1990. - "Any of various elements required by living organisms for normal growth."

Stedman's Medical Dictionary for the Health Professions and Nursing, 5th Edition, by Thomas Lathrop Stedman, 2005. – "1. Necessary, indispensable (e.g. essential amino acids, essential fatty acids). 2. Characteristic of. 3. Determining. 4. Of unknown etiology. 5. Relating to an essence (e.g. essential oil). 6. SYN *intrinsic.*"

Essential Elements:

The Concise Oxford Dictionary, 8th edition, by H. W. Fowler and F. G. Fowler, edited by R. E. Allen, 1990. - "Any of various elements required by living organisms for normal growth."

Stedman's Medical Dictionary for the Health Professions and Nursing, 5th Edition, by Thomas Lathrop Stedman, 2005. – "Necessary, indispensable (e.g. essential amino acids, essential fatty acids). 2. Characteristic of. 3. Determining. 4. Of unknown etiology. 5. Relating to an essence (e.g. essential oil). 6. SYN *intrinsic.*"

Collins Dictionary of Biology, published in 2003. – "An element without which normal growth and reproduction cannot take place. In plants, there are seven major essential elements: nitrogen, phosphorus, sulphur, potassium, calcium, magnesium and iron. There are also **Trace Elements** required in much smaller quantities, for example, manganese, boron, chlorine. Animals also have requirements for elements, the list being quite similar to that for plants."

Source: W. G. Hale, BSc, PhD, DSc, FIBiol, V. A. Saunders, BSc, PhD, and J. P. Margham, BSc, DepAnGen, MIBiol, CBiol, *Collins Dictionary of Biology*, p. 316, 2003. At the time of publication Hale was Emeritus Professor of Animal Biology, Saunders was Professor of Microbial Genetics, and Margham was a principal lecturer and programme leader for biological degrees, all three at Liverpool John Moores University.

Essential Nutrients:

Oxford Dictionary of Food & Nutrition by David A. Bender, 2005. - "Those nutrients that are required by the body and cannot be synthesized in the body in adequate amounts to meet requirements, so must be provided by the diet: includes the essential amino acids and fatty acids, vitamins, and minerals. Really a tautology, since by definition nutrients are essential dietary constituents."

A Dictionary of Food and Nutrition 4th Edition, 2014. – "Those nutrients that are required by the body and cannot be synthesized in the body in adequate amounts to meet requirements, so must be provided by the diet: includes the essential amino acids and fatty acids, vitamins and minerals. Really a tautology, since nutrients are defined as essential dietary constituents."

Trace Elements:

Dictionary of Nutrition and Food Technology, 4th Edition by Arnold E. Bender, 1975. - "Refers to mineral salts needed by the body in very small amounts – iodine, copper manganese, magnesium, cobalt and zinc – as distinct from those required in relatively large amounts, such as sodium, potassium, calcium, phosphorus, sulphur and chlorine."

"Of these trace elements only iodine is of importance in the diet as the others are almost always in adequate supply. This is not true of domestic animals amongst which various mineral deficiencies occur in certain areas."

"Sixty minerals have been identified in plants, of which about one third have been shown to be essential to plant or animal nutrition."

Dictionary of Nutrition: A Consumer's Guide to the Facts of Food by Sheila Bingham, 1977. - "Minerals needed in tiny amounts in the diet for health. So called because older methods of analysis could detect only unmeasurable traces in food and living tissues. With modern methods of chemical analysis the needs for trace elements are becoming known more precisely, especially for animals, but accurate estimations of quantities in foods are still lacking. Ten trace elements are presently known to be essential nutrients for humans: iron, iodine, copper, zinc, manganese, cobalt, molybdenum, selenium, chromium, and vanadium. Silicon, tin, nickel and fluorine are essential nutrients for animals, but it is not known if they are necessary for humans."

A Dictionary of Diets, Slimming and Nutrition by Richard B. Fisher (Copyright © Richard B. Fisher, 1986. Reproduced by kind permission of AM Heath & Co Ltd.) - "Gases or minerals required for health in amounts below one ten-thousandth of a gram (0.00001) in the adult body. They include copper, cobalt, fluorine, manganese, molybdenum, vanadium and zinc."

"Like other nutrients, trace elements must be obtained from food. Vegetables are probably the best sources though fluorine, for example, may be taken from water."

"Not all functions performed by trace elements are understood. Fluorine stabilizes tooth enamel but may also play a role in bone. Copper is required for a few enzymes to function and for the proper formation of red blood cells. Manganese may also be a necessary part of certain enzymes. Cobalt forms part of vitamin B_{12}."

The Concise Oxford Dictionary, 8th edition, by H. W. Fowler and F. G. Fowler, edited by R. E. Allen, 1990. - "1. A chemical element occurring in minute amounts. 2. A chemical element required only in minute amounts by living organisms for normal growth."

Stedman's Medical Dictionary for the Health Professions and Nursing, 5th Edition, by Thomas Lathrop Stedman, 2005. – "Elements present in minute amounts in the body (e.g., Zn, Se, V, Ni, Mg, Mn), many of which are essential in metabolism or for the manufacture of essential compounds."

Black's Medical Dictionary 42nd Edition, 2010. – "Chemical elements that are distributed throughout the tissues of the body in very small amounts and are essential for the nutrition of the body. Nine such elements are now recognised: cobalt, copper, fluorine, iodine, iron, manganese, molybdenum, selenium and zinc."

Collins Dictionary of Biology, published in 2003. – "Any element that is necessary for the proper working of biological systems in concentrations less than 10^{-5}M. Absence can cause disease and death. For example, boron deficiency causes 'heart rot' in sugar beet, and cobalt deficiency causes 'coast disease' in Australian sheep and cattle."

Illustrated Medical Dictionary, British Medical Association, 2013. – "*Minerals* necessary in minute amounts in the diet to maintain health. Examples are *chromium, copper, magnesium, zinc,* and *selenium.*"

Oxford Concise Medical Dictionary, 2015. – "An element that is required in minute concentrations for normal growth and development; the body contains a total of <5 g of the element. Trace elements include fluoride, manganese, zinc, copper, iodine, cobalt, selenium, molybdenum, chromium, and silicon. They may serve as cofactors or as constituents of complex molecules (e.g. cobalt in vitamin B_{12})."

Encyclopaedia Britannica's website - "also called micronutrient - in <u>biology</u>, any <u>chemical element</u> required by living organisms in minute amounts (that is less than 0.1 percent by volume [1,000 parts per million])…"

Source: https://www.britannica.com/science/trace-element. Accessed 18th October, 2017.

From *Pearson: The Biology Place*'s website – "An element indispensable for life but required in extremely minute amounts."

Source: http://www.phschool.com/science/biology_place/glossary/t.html.

Micronutrient:

Oxford Dictionary of Food & Nutrition by David A. Bender, 2005. - "Vitamins and minerals, which are needed in very small amounts (micrograms or milligrams per day), as distinct from fats, carbohydrates, and proteins which are macronutrients, since they are needed in considerably greater amounts."

A Dictionary of Food and Nutrition 4th Edition, 2014. – "Those nutrients required in small amounts: vitamins and minerals."

Encyclopaedia Britannica's website – "as above for Trace Element."

Trace Mineral:

Oxford Dictionary of Food & Nutrition by David A. Bender, 2005. - "Those mineral salts present in the body, and required in the diet, in small amounts (part per million): copper, chromium, iodine, manganese, molybdenum, selenium; although required in larger amounts, zinc and iron are sometimes included with the trace minerals."

Ultra-Trace Mineral:

Oxford Dictionary of Food & Nutrition by David A. Bender, 2005. - "Those mineral salts present in the body, and required in the diet, in extremely small amounts (parts per thousand million or less); known to be dietary essentials, although rarely if ever a cause for concern since the amounts required are small and they are widely distributed in foods and water, e.g. cobalt, manganese, molybdenum, silicon, tin, vanadium."

Glossary

These are some of the terms and abbreviations used in this book.

Ppb – Part per billion

Ppm – Part per million

(Ppb and ppm will have both Ps lower case because they usually don't appear at the start of a sentence.)

Cation – a positively charged ion

Anion – a negatively charged ion

Public Relations – PR

Community Water Fluoridation – CWF

Abbreviations of Companies, Institutions and Qualifications

Aluminium Company of America – ALCOA or Alcoa

Doctorate of Dental Medicine – DMD

Doctorate of Dental Surgery – DDS

Indiana University – IU

Masters of Public Health – MPH

National Academy of Sciences – NAS

National Institute of Dental Research – NIDR

Procter & Gamble – P&G

Retired - Emeritus

United States Public Health Service - USPHS

World Health Organization – WHO

1. Is Fluorine/Fluoride an Essential Nutrient?

How do we test if something is an essential nutrient? Just what *is* an essential nutrient, anyway? This of course is a technical question, in that it means different things to different people, as you will see. I apologise if this is feels like an obtuse answer. Whether it should be something *necessary* or something *beneficial* is a cornerstone of this work. A far more important cornerstone of this work is how conclusions of necessity and benefit are treated in *public*, compared to how they are treated in scientific and more obscure and influential documents. Some definitions of common terms are given prior to Chapter 1.

How do we test if something is an essential nutrient? This question has been addressed by three people I will mention here. Full documentation and citations are given in the text.

On the 14th of October, 2013, an "expert panel from the University of Waikato" appeared on a Google Hangout. This is an online group discussion filmed with interaction from the public, who could ask questions through social media. I don't think it received much media attention; it may have been drowned out because this was near the time New Zealand's city of Hamilton, Waikato, was embroiled in fluoridation arguments.

A viewer asked if fluorine was "essential" or "beneficial". The experts discussed the question. Regarding specific criteria, Dr. Mucalo, Senior Lecturer in physical chemistry told viewers:

> "Yes, you need to design very careful experiments to specifically exclude fluoride from the diet before you could categorically prove whether it was or was not an essential element, and I think they've done that for things like silicon, where they've tried to prove whether it was essential for the diet but you'd have to do very excrutiatingly careful experiments to do that, so... at this stage I don't know whether anyone's done that yet."
> [1]

Many people have attempted such experiments.

Most of the experiments I have collected here have been cited in work like the American National Academy of Sciences and the World Health Organization, but also writings of people supportive of, and opposed to fluoridation.

In 2007, the National Academy of Sciences published a document which cited the 8th edition of a textbook called *Essentials of Medical Geology*, published in 2005. The sixth chapter is called *Biological Functions of the Elements*. It begins by looking at what constitutes an essential element. Author Ulf Lindh, Senior Researcher at the Biology Education Centre, Uppsala University in Sweden, says definitions have provoked much discussion, and that the earliest was borrowed from protein chemistry.

To paraphrase: the element should be present in living tissues in a reasonably constant concentration, it should cause problems – "anomalies in several species" when removed, and these anomalies should be corrected upon reinstatement of the element.

Lindh proposes the "current" (1998) definition:

> "An element is considered essential to an organism when reduction of its exposure below a certain limit results consistently in a reduction in a physiologically important function, or when the element is an integral part of an organic structure performing a vital function in the organism." [2]

Lindh notes problems associated with proving necessity and ascertaining exact requirements. Further into Chapter 1 we will see it is nearly impossible to completely remove fluorine from a diet. Reduction of *only one element* is difficult in food preparation - fluorine is apparently not the only element difficult to remove. Removal and reduction of one element may effect uptake of others leading to ambiguity of results.

Detection is also sometimes difficult. In terms of knowledge regarding necessary trace elements, we can be more certain about animal needs than human needs. Lindh doesn't say it, but this is probably true for toxic effects and upper limitations of tolerance as well. In a section called *The Functional Value of Trace Elements* he writes:

> "The paramount function is to be necessary for the structure and function of significant biomolecules, mainly enzymes."

All of the experiments in the first chapter have tested fluorine's essentiality on rodents. They have largely adhered to this criteria in terms of experimental design and intent, though some have used more or less imaginative, precise, and technological methods than others. This leads to the question of "how well can these be applied to humans?"

In Chapter 6, I discuss the 'for and against' arguments that have been given with regard to using conclusions of rodent experiments on humans, and look at some human experiments. Relevant here may be a sentence from the World Health Organization's 1970 monograph, *Fluoride and Human Health*:

> "Where fluoride data for man are unavailable, corollary studies on experimental animals are presented." [3]

Regarding experiments, I obtained almost every one I, or someone who had written on the subject, thought relevant. I also quoted from reviews that simply observed and critiqued experiments already in the literature. I feel we are quite lucky in this regard, because in cases of opposition or promotion, scientists seemed quite open about it, and none seemed set in stone regarding their conclusions, though a few were a little persistent. The reader will be pleased to note that there is almost no difference of opinion in terms of conclusion regarding *individual* experimentation in 'pro' or 'anti' literature with a couple of small exceptions, yet the *overall* conclusion – the 'yes, no or maybe' answer to the title of this chapter, is varied and nuanced, depending on the person to whom we go.

Different people have different criteria for what constitutes dietary essentiality. What I have quoted from Dr. Mucalo and Dr. Lindh is best termed "traditional," maybe even "standard" – I will introduce other criteria throughout, notably "prevention" and "benefit" have both been suggested.

Read through these experiments slowly and patiently. Some have concluded fluorine to be essential, while others have not.

These are mainly primary sources, meaning original experiments, though there are a couple of exceptions. I have avoided reviews for the most part until the next chapter, although if they have comments neglected by others that help enlighten understanding of experiments, these have been included.

I have kept to a reasonably chronological order. When a sequence of conclusions has been argued over for many years, for the sake of convenience I have given them breathing room before going back to the main stream of research. Please consider some disagreements take a long time to work through, some are argued about then forgotten, and some criticisms may simply be ignored.

Usually the researchers create diets that are as low as possible in fluoride, and add differing levels of fluoride to the rats' drinking water, or use foods with defined amounts.

Lindh's and Mucalo's discussions are very similar to what Drs. Messer, Armstrong and Singer from the University of Minneapolis wrote in a 1973 paper regarding two of their experiments that attempted the reduction of fluorine in the diets of mice.

> "A specific deficiency state should be produced by a diet lacking the element in question, but which is otherwise adequate and satisfactory."
>
> "The deficiency should be prevented or cured by addition to the diet of that element alone." [4]

This is what I will call "Messer's first criterion". I don't know if the words originated in *his* mind, but I will attribute it to him because another scientist did so in a 1974 presentation. In the text I will refer to the set of four papers in the early 1970s by this group as being by either Messer *et al.* or Armstrong *et al.*

The statement quoted is from 1973. I will introduce many experiments before that year, but it should be understood that this criterion is what all of these experiments have aimed for, though they had different ways of doing so.

Because of nuances in methods, one cannot simply "count the number of times a particular conclusion appears" and claim "one conclusion wins". This is shortsighted and presumptuous, as will be shown.

Obviously conclusive strength depends on a myriad of factors. I will discuss individual aims, methods, results and conclusions of each experiment. Chapter 1.2 will elaborate on some of these, and introduce more.

As far back as the 1800s researchers were considering the question of fluoride's essentiality. Dr. Gerald Cox, writing in a 1952 National Academy of Sciences publication, pointed out that before the year 1933, accuracy regarding analysis of fluoride was poor. In his words "little reliance can be placed on any quantitative analyses for fluorine reported" [5] before Willard and Winter's 1933 method of isolation by distillation. I point this out because I show a couple of experiments and papers before this date, and I do not want you to feel that the conclusions of an experiment done almost a century ago should be set in stone. Each experiment should be viewed in and of itself. Some yield plenty of information on their own, others more when compared with the rest.

1.1 What Do Scientists Who Performed Animal Experiments Say?

In 1933, the **Journal of Nutrition** published an experiment [6] by George Sharpless and E. V. McCollum from the School of Hygiene and Public Health, at the Johns Hopkins University of Baltimore. They stated at the beginning of their experiment that the question of fluoride's essentiality was unanswered. The purpose of their experiment was to test if nutritional requirements can be satisfied with diets containing as little fluoride as possible. Ten rats, five of each gender, were fed a low fluoride ration, while another three of each gender were fed the same but with 0.001 percent (10 parts per million, abbreviated to "ppm") fluoride added. Once per week iodine was added to (distilled) drinking water in order to avoid iodine deficiency. Rats were kept in a room where no roach powder was used, and when females became pregnant they were taken to individual cages, and given filter paper clippings (fluoride free) in which to nest. Offspring did not live long; Sharpless and McCollum attribute this to neither the absence or presence of fluoride, but noted that the results on reproduction seemed to favour low fluoride.

Sharpless and McCollum state their diet was

"very low in fluorine but not quite free."

"The rats on the low fluorine diet looked very well, were quite fat and on the whole appeared normal."

There were no notable differences between the control rats (10 ppm) and the rats on the low fluorine diet, except the rats on the low fluorine diet had hair that was "a little coarser" but this did not appear "striking". Both groups of animals had incisors that were a deep orange.

"The teeth showed no caries and from gross appearances seemed to be perfect."

Regarding a necessity for fluoride in teeth, Sharpless and McCollum claimed there was no detectable fluorine in the teeth of rats on the low fluorine ration.

"Thus, if fluorine is present as a factor in the consolidation of the tooth, abnormalities should appear in the histological[2] picture. There is, however, no marked abnormality in the structure. The teeth seem to be excellent, no indication of caries, and seemingly perfect calcification."

The scientists claimed that fluorine could be removed from teeth until only between six and twenty-five ppm remained, with no defect, though of course perfect determination in the 1930s was difficult. There were no structural issues, nor were there any noticed changes in the calcium to phosphorous ratio in bone caused by the low fluorine diet. Quantities of fluorine were measured in the bones and teeth of the rats. The scientists wrote a lot on the preparation and accuracy of their method, it follows a "colorimetric determination". Reported accuracy by duplicating determinations of values is shown (**Table 1**).

While they had a difficult time preventing the death of rats while young, the low fluoride groups reproduced more. They suggested some unexplained factor may have caused early deaths in young rats. Two tables from this experiment are reproduced (**Table 2 & 3**).

---

[2] Histology is the study of microscopic anatomy.

FLUORINE DETERMINATIONS TO SHOW ABILITY TO DUPLICATE VALUES

Sample	Wt. Sample	Dilution	% Fluorine
11	0.4172	5.0	0.0059 (59 ppm)
11	0.6779	5.0	0.0054
8	0.2218	10.0	0.0834 (834 ppm)
8	0.1438	5.0	0.0766

Table 1. Fluorine determinations to show ability to duplicate values. Source: Sharpless and McCollum, 1933 [6].

REPRODUCTION RECORD (TOTAL LITTERS)

	Second Generation			Third Generation		
	Number of Litters	Number of Rats	Number of Rats that Lived	Number of Litters	Number of Rats	Number of Rats that Lived
Low Fluoride	8	64	24	9	63	5
Control (10 ppm Fluorine)	5	46	7	5	30	0

Table 2. Reproduction Record (Total Litters). Source: Sharpless and McCollum, 1933 [6].

REPRODUCTION RECORD (FIRST LITTERS)

	Second Generation			Third Generation		
	Number of Litters	Number of Rats	Number of Rats that Lived	Number of Litters	Number of Rats	Number of Rats that Lived
Low Fluoride	5	43	12	8	58	0
Control (10 ppm Fluorine)	3	27	0	5	30	0

Table 3. Reproduction Record (First Litters). Source: Sharpless and McCollum, 1933 [6].

While some scientists have claimed that fluoride is a requirement for reproduction in the rat, Sharpless and McCollum concluded otherwise:

"Rats grow normally on a diet low in fluorine. A diet low in fluorine does not affect reproduction in any way."[6]

Floyd DeEds was Senior Toxicologist at the Bureau of Chemistry and Soils, U.S Dept. of Agriculture, and lectured at the Department of Pharmacology at Stanford University School of Medicine in San Francisco. In 1933 the journal **Medicine** published his 60-page review [7] of the literature on fluoride from the previous fifty years. His review serves as perhaps the first of its kind. He looked at over one hundred experiments, that he noted had been "largely uncorrelated". I believe he wanted to take stock of what did and did not need to be studied in future.

I include the review by DeEds here because it contains information that was relevant in the past. It may no longer be relevant to an appraisal of a requirement for fluoride in human nutrition, but it has certainly shaped the research and serves as an interesting benchmark of our understanding. While the title of the review suggests a toxicological appraisal, I will remind the reader that (obviously) *anything* in excess is almost always harmful, and keep strictly to the study of essentiality/non-essentiality, or what DeEds called a "biological role of fluorine".

DeEds discussed work by a scientist named Gautier in 1914. Gautier proposed that fluorine's role is in helping to "assure the fixation of phosphorous in the organism and of the soft nitrogenous organic matter." Gautier looked at the ratio of fluorine to phosphorous in animal tissues used for ornamentation, protection and defense (hair, feathers, nails etc), found them to be close to the ratio existing in mineral fluoro-phosphates (about one part fluorine to five parts phosphorous). For less active tissues like bone, tendon and cartilage, Gautier suggested the ratio was one part fluorine to between one hundred and thirty and one hundred and eighty times its weight of phosphorous. I think Gautier believed that in the shedding of these tissues, unwanted or unnecessary fluorine could be removed from the body.

DeEds disagreed with Gautier's conclusion, and mentioned the 1933 Sharpless and McCollum study, wherein the fluorine content of bones could

> "be reduced to between six and twenty-five ppm, and could be eliminated from the teeth, without showing any gross deleterious effect." [7]

He mentioned four scientists who had found fluoride in all tissues examined. This was around the end of the nineteenth century. He wrote:

> "... the constant occurrence of fluorine in tissues does not constitute proof that fluorine has a biological role. In view of the widespread distribution of fluorine in soils, waters, and plants, it is entirely possible that the presence of fluorine in animal tissues is an expression of the inevitable tendency to establish a chemical equilibrium between the organism and its environment."

Like others, DeEds believed one would have to minimize fluorine and create a deficiency in a population with definite symptoms of that deficiency, before claiming a necessity for the element.

Three scientists from the University of Wisconsin, two of whom were from the Department of Agricultural Chemistry and the third from the Department of Animal Husbandry performed an experiment five years in length culminating in late 1933 [8]. The experiment was published in 1934 in the **Journal of Biological Chemistry**. Doctors Phillips, Hart and Bohstedt wanted to determine if fluorine in mineral supplements for dairy cattle would increase fluorine content of milk to harmful levels.

The authors claimed the food used in the experiment contained ample amounts of other nutrients. They divided the cows into six groups, which were fed grain, corn silage, and hay, with differing ratios of bone meal and rock phosphate. Seven groups of rats (one control, then one for each lot of cows) were fed milk from cows within the six groups. Milks were mineralized with iron, copper and manganese. Rats were sacrificed after 140 days on the diet then fluorine body ash determined.

Phillips' team noted that

> "our results are interesting in view of the concept that fluorine has an essential role in the animal body because small graded amounts of fluorine in the diet did not visibly increase growth in these rats."

They suggested that renal (meaning kidney) mechanisms influenced the ability of the rats to dispel an excess of fluorine, and while they encountered toxic levels of fluorine in the cows, they did not in the rats. This is evidence that mammalian milk is low in fluorine. The last sentence of their experiment is relevant to our purposes:

"It is apparent from these data that fluorine in concentrations greater than 1 part in 10,000,000 in the diet has no essential function in the metabolism of the rat."

One part in ten million is 0.1 ppm. With regard to teeth, Phillips' team wrote "no evidence of typical fluorine toxicosis was apparent". By "typical fluorine toxicosis" I am assuming they meant dental fluorosis, because the next sentence reads "the characteristic bleaching effect upon the incisor teeth was entirely absent..."

Paul Phillips, a biochemist mentioned in the previous, 1934 experiment, and Robert Evans, a Moorman Manufacturing Company fellow, used milk mineralized with iron, copper and manganese in an experiment to test fluoride's necessity in the skeleton, growth and reproduction of rats. Their experiment was published in 1939, also in the **Journal of Nutrition** [9].

One male and three females were used in each lot. There were eight different diets. The additions of aluminium and percomorph oil (a fish oil containing vitamins A and D) were to test if either of these substances in excess would inhibit the effects of the higher levels of fluoride. (**Table 4**)

AVERAGE SKELETAL FLUORINE CONTENT (IN PPM) OF ADULT RATS

Generation	Age in Months	Lot 1 Basal	Lot 2 Basal + 0.1 ppm F	Lot 3 Basal + 1.0 ppm F	Lot 4 Basal + 10 ppm F
F	4	16	72	297	1639
F1	7	16	44	355	2781
F2	4	16	54	265	1729
F2	7	8	54	341	2695
F3	4	10	71	265	1573
F Intake (mg/kilo/day)		0.05-0.06	0.075-0.082	0.3-0.42	2.5-3.2

Generation	Lot 5 Basal + 20 ppm F	Lot 6 Basal + 20 ppm Al	Lot 7 Basal + 20 ppm F + 20 ppm Al	Lot 8 Basal + 20 ppm F + Percomorph Oil
F	2562	71	2339	2335
F1	4522	42	4067	4527
F2	--	--	--	3065
F2	--	--	--	4063
F3	--	--	--	2992
F Intake (mg/kilo/day)	5.05	0.05	5.05	4.9-6.3

Table 4. Average skeletal fluorine content (in ppm) of adult rats. Source: R. J. Evans and P. H. Phillips, 1939 [9]. 'mg/kilo/day' refers to milligrams per kilogram of body weight, daily.

Evans and Phillips wrote that

"In general the levels of fluorine administered had no beneficial or adverse effect upon reproduction."

However lots five, six and seven all failed to reproduce beyond the first generation. There was no real explanation given for this, although excess fluorine and aluminium seems probable at first glance. To quote:

"Fluorine is not necessary for the rat in amounts larger than the 0.1 to 0.2 ppm found in milk... Food consumption records showed that only 0.05 to 0.06 mg. of fluorine per kilogram of body weight were ingested per day [basal diet]. It is plainly evident that in this species, which can on occasion withstand relatively large quantities of fluorine, very little fluorine is necessary."

They claimed that fifty micrograms of fluorine per kilogram of body weight per day is enough for growth and general wellbeing in rats. The rats weighed 40 gram each. Adding 0.1 to 20.0 ppm did not give any "measurable improvement".

Phillips and Evans also claimed that bleaching of teeth occurred above an intake of 3.0 mg of fluorine per kilogram of body weight per day. Difficulties can arise in the appraisal of these measurements – mg of fluorine per kilogram of body weight per day is different to total daily intake, or mg of fluorine per day.

The work of the 1930s is mentioned in early American scientific literature, but not often discussed in detail beyond a simple acceptance of conclusion. It is also mentioned in some of the World Health Organizaton (WHO) documents discussed in Chapter 2.3.

In 1945, H. H. Mitchell and Marjorie Edman from the Division of Animal Nutrition in the University of Illinois, Urbana, wrote a paper for the journal **Soil Science** that contained a section called *Dispensability of Fluorine in Animal Nutrition* [10]. They wrote,

> "Though various essential functions of fluorine in the animal body have been proposed, convincing evidence of their reality has not been forthcoming."
>
> "Attempts to raise laboratory animals (rats) on rations containing extremely low concentrations of fluorine have been uniformly successful."

They discussed an unpublished experiment by Lawrenz in which 14 pairs of albino rats were fed diets with 0.47 and 2.5 ppm fluorine for 207 days. These rats were produced by mothers that had lived on a low fluorine diet (exact amount unspecified, presumably the 0.47 ppm diet). These rats contained 0.8 ppm fluorine, compared with rats containing 5 to 7 ppm raised on a diet of "natural foods". After 207 days there were no differences in growth rate, or dry weights of skeleton or teeth. Retained were averages of 0.210 mg and 1.648 mg for the low and high fluorine diets respectively (see **Table 5**).

RETENTION OF FLUORINE – UNPUBLISHED DATA FROM LAWRENZ

	Average Total Fluorine Retained (mg)	**Average Fluorine Concentration (ppm)**		
		In Skeleton	**In Teeth**	**In Soft Tissues (fresh condition, not dry)**
Basal diet (0.47 ppm fluorine)	0.210	15	15	0.12
Supplemented diet (2.5 ppm fluorine)	1.648	117	80	0.25

Table 5. Retention of fluorine – unpublished data from Lawrenz. Source: Mitchell and Edman, 1945 [10].

Mitchell and Edman wrote that the teeth of four rats on the basal diet (0.47 ppm fluorine) were examined by Dr. Isaac Schour, a dental histologist of Illinois University's College of Dentistry. Though the teeth were "not fixed in formalin as soon after death as they should have been for the most effective examination", Dr. Schour detected no abnormalities in them. No amount of time was given from death to fixation and there is no year mentioned for this experiment.

Mitchell and Edman said the rats on the low fluorine diet received a total of 0.88 milligrams of fluorine over 207 days, "equivalent to 27 microgram per kilogram of body weight daily" with "no signs of malnutrition".

I haven't seen this work discussed except for a couple of mentions.

None of the above experiments showed problems with a low fluoride diet.

However, a study that concluded fluorine to be essential appeared in the **American Journal of Medical Science**, in May, 1945 [11]. It was performed by Jesse Francis McClendon and Wm. C. Foster, from the Hahnemann Medical College Department of Physiology, and aided by a grant from ALCOA, the Aluminum Company of America. An abstract was published in The American Institute of Nutrition's **Federation Proceedings** in 1944.

There are three experiments I have found in which McClendon concluded fluorine a dietary essential in rats. In all three his method was similar. He performed the experiments on a farm to minimize exposure of rats to fluoride particles from city air.

The experiment did not discuss previous experiments relating to the topic of fluorine's essentiality at all. If he knew of these experiments, they are not mentioned in the work attributed to him here. In the 1953 and 1954 experiments (discussed below) he mostly cited his own work.

Regarding the 1944/1945 experiment, I have seen the abstract cited more frequently than the full experiment, which is only slightly longer.

The diet McClendon used was half corn, thirty percent glucose, and the rest beans, bean and corn leaves, salt, yeast and oils. In the 1945 experiment McClendon mentioned that the plants were grown hydroponically as a way to produce "fluorine-free" plants. No amount or concentration was given regarding the fluorine levels in these plants, or that of any other compound or element.

Two rats were put on a diet at the age of twenty-one days. Their mother's diet contained 0.3 ppm fluoride (the 1939 experiment by Phillips and Evans [9] claimed fluoride is transferred through the placenta, therefore these rats would have retained some). One of the rats starved to death after forty-eight days - its teeth had decayed such that it could not chew. The other rat was "saved from starvation" with "milk containing 1 microgram of fluorine, but died of starvation in 70 days."

McClendon wrote that

> "The crowns of the 12 molar teeth of each rat were practically removed by caries except that the caries of the 3rd molars (which are of little use in chewing) was less extensive. This is the most extensive caries seen in any rat on any diet for any number of days."

Also,

> "Fluorine is passed from mother to offspring and the less fluorine in the mother's diet, the fewer young are born and the less is the milk supply of the mother. All these rats had extensive decay of the molar teeth; in some cases all of the crowns were lost."

The first statement is from his study in the **Federation Proceedings** and the second is from the **American Journal of Medical Science**. In the abstract McClendon compared these results of 12 carious teeth per rat in 48 and 70 days with 0.3 carious teeth per rat in 75 days on a diet

> "... which was apparently not superior except that it contained 0.3 ppm fluorine, and no caries in 75 days when 10 ppm fluorine was added to the drinking water."

His article ends with the statement:

> "fluorine is necessary in a diet that has to be chewed." [11]

His experiment used very small sample sizes (three sets of two rats), but results were consistent.

McClendon created a fluorine-free diet using water-culture crops designed specifically for studying deficiencies in animals. This is discussed in his 1953 experiment [12] with Jacob Gershon-Cohen, from the Albert Einstein Medical Center in Philadelphia. This experiment was published in the **Journal of Agricultural and Food Chemistry**. The two men went into a lot of detail with the preparations, their previous and following experiments did not focus so much on method. They used rain water (with 0.002 to 0.004 ppm fluorine) that ran off an aluminium roof at the experimental farm twenty-five miles from Philadelphia. The rain water was passed through ion exchange resins to remove halogens and sodium, before being used for the growth of plants in 200-litre tanks. No figure was given for fluorine in rain water after halogen removal, but one could assume extremely low. Nutrient solutions were added to this, daily additions of iron and manganese were given, and salts added once a month. They took frequent measurements of the solution in which the plants grew. They used salts of reagent purity.

The tanks were covered with aluminium foil, except for holes cut where plants could grow through. Of the health of the plants, the researchers wrote:

> "The best crop yields were obtained from sunflowers. Corn was not always well pollinated. Legumes produced lower yields and rice did not head in the short season." [12]

The rats used were litter-mates, 21 days old at the beginning of the experiment. Diets contained corn, sunflower seed and leaves, and ten percent each yeast and sucrose. One group of 19 rats were fed the food grown in the fluorine-free water-culture, with added distilled water.

> "The controls were either on the same diet with the missing elements added or on a diet of the same proportions made from the same varieties of plants but grown in soil."
>
> "Normally grown crops comprised the diet of the control rats, whose drinking water contained 20 ppm of fluorine." [12]

The words "missing elements" refer to either fluorine or iodine. The water-grown plants were deficient in iodine. This experiment [12] was also looking at need for iodine. In the fluorine-free group, obviously iodine was added. I am not reproducing the results of the iodine-related work here. A research grant was given from the Chilean Iodine Educational Bureau. There is no mention of research grants or funding from any other persons or organizations in this experiment.

McClendon and Gershon-Cohen wanted to use yeast with which to supplement rat food, but couldn't find a halogen-free variety. Instead, a long-winded method of juicing halogen-free corn and sunflower stalks followed. The stalks and juice were boiled, with fructose and sucrose, ammonium nitrate, potassium dihydrogen phosphate, *l*-aspartic acid, and inositol added. When the mixture cooled, bacteria (*Saccharomyces cerevisiae* or *Torulopsis utilis*) were added. Calcium, boron, vitamins and transition metals were supplied by this mixture.

One may inquire what ratio of soil-grown to water-culture plants were used in the controls. This is not mentioned. The control rats were fed 20 ppm fluorine in water. The following pictures (**Figure 1**) are x-rays of one rat jaw from each group.

ROENTGENOGRAMS OF LOWER JAW OF RAT

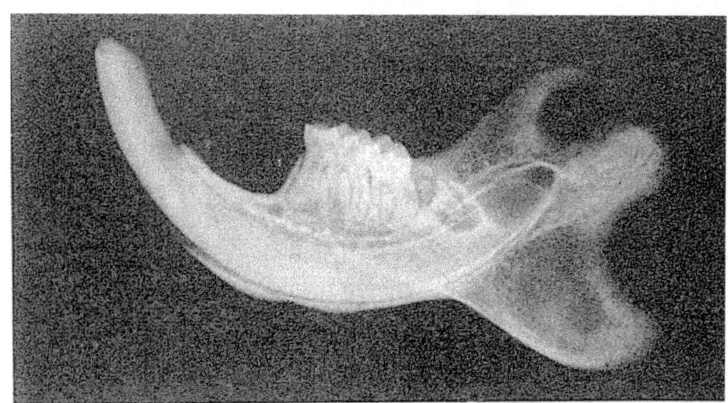

Figure 1. *Roentgenograms of lower jaw of rat.* Upper: Healthy molars in control rat on water-grown and soil-grown ("normal") diet containing 20 ppm of fluorine in water. Lower: Extensive caries of molars in litter mate rat in fluorine-free water-grown diet. McClendon and Gershon-Cohen, 1953 [12].

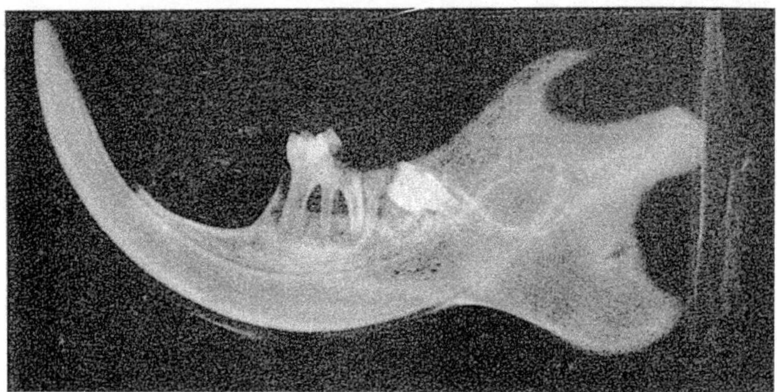

After two months on the experiment, soft tissues, teeth and bones were studied.

This experiment found a lot of difference between the growth of rats on control diets and fluorine-free diets, shown below (**Table 6**).

EFFECT OF FLUORINE-FREE WATER-GROWN DIET ON WEIGHT AND DENTAL CARIES IN RATS

	Number of Rats	Average Weight in Grams at 22 Days	Average Weight in Grams at 88 Days	Number of Carious Molars per Rat
Controls	18	41.2	128.1	0.5
Fluorine-Free Diet	19	40.8	51.2	10.2

Table 6. *Effect of fluorine-free water-grown diet on weight and dental caries in rats. Source: McClendon, 1953 [12].*

Discussing their results, McClendon and Gershon-Cohen in 1953 [12] said:

"A number of female rats fed a fluorine-free diet and mated to normal males did not produce viable offspring. Therefore we suspect that fluorine is necessary in the diet of the rat."

In 1954, McClendon and Gershon-Cohen repeated their water-culture experiment, using 16 rats. Again, 21-day-old rats at weaning were used. The water-culture method was justified:

"In attempts to extract halogens from natural foodstuffs, two difficulties arise: (1) complete extraction is impossible, and (2) when extraction is done, other essential nutrients are also removed. To obviate these difficulties, foodstuffs might be grown lacking these nutrients."

Of the diets, they wrote:

"The water-cultured diets were made up of yellow corn, sunflower seeds, leaves and yeast, all grown in fluorine-free water, with additions of fluorine-free chemicals: glucose, corn oil, cod liver oil (containing 9 ppm iodine), and sodium chloride." [13]

The rats on the diets lower in fluorine did not grow well. They were given methionine, cystine and lysine when their growth was especially slow. The purest quality reagent calcium citrate was added to the others fed the low-fluorine food, though this did result in an extra 0.004 ppm fluorine to the diet.

They did not discuss the health or vitality of the plants in this experiment, therefore it is probably safe to assume not much had changed from the previous experiment published the year before. Results are shown in **Table 7**.

DENTAL CARIES IN RATS FED VARYING CONCENTRATIONS OF FLUORINE IN FOOD AND WATER

	Number of Rats	Number of Carious Molars	Percentage of Carious Molars	Percentage of Fluorine in Molars
Water-culture fluorine-free diet and fluorine-free water	6	65	84	0.01
Fluorine-free diet and water containing 10 ppm fluorine	3	2	6	0.03
Fluorine-free diet supplemented with 10 cc. milk containing 1 mg. fluorine	3	9	25	0.02
Soil-grown foods and fluorine-free water	4	11	23	0.02

Table 7. Dental caries in rats fed varying concentrations of fluorine in food and water. Source: McClendon and Gershon-Cohen, 1954 [13].

The scientists wrote:

"Animals fed on water-cultured fluorine-free foods tended to die within two to three months and this premature death could be partially delayed by a feeding of 10 cc [cubic centimeter] milk containing 1 mg of fluorine." [13]

This experiment also made the statement that female rats fed fluorine-free diets did not produce "viable offspring". From this, and for dental reasons, the scientists suspected fluorine is necessary in rat nutrition. McClendon said that no fluorine was found in the faeces or urine of fluorine-free rats, which was indicative of retention from parents.

The scientists noted that their experiments indicated that foods low in fluorine uniformly produced periodontoclasia.

"Therefore we suspect that fluorine is necessary in the diet of the rat."

At no point did the scientists cite any of the previous experiments beyond their own, regarding fluorine as a necessity. This is true for all three of the McClendon experiments here. Regarding the length of this 1954 experiment, I believe it lasted for only one generation. They wrote:

"If the element is transmitted from the mother through the placenta and milk, it would be desirable to continue the diet through two generations."

"The teeth of our rats on a fluorine-free diet contained some fluorine inherited from the mother. Since the chemical tests showed a lower concentration of fluorine in the dentine of these animals, and since no excretion of fluorine was noted in the urine or feces, this small concentration of maternally derived fluorine seems to be fixed or retained."

Research grants were given for this 1954 experiment from Lever Brothers, a toothpaste manufacturer, and from the Aluminum Company of America (ALCOA). Some scientists have expressed ideas on these experiments, which are discussed in the next chapter.

Assistant Professor of Chemistry Joseph Muhler was a man who spent many years studying fluorides. He worked in the Department of Chemistry at Indiana University. Countless boxes of his research exist today in storage. His PhD thesis published in 1951 [14] has been cited in much of the literature. According to the **New York Times** (15):

"He received his D.D.S. in 1948 from Indiana University, followed by a doctorate in chemistry in 1951, the year he joined the faculty as an assistant professor of chemistry. In 1972 he was named a research professor of dental science and director of the School of Dentistry's Dental Research Institute." [15]

In 1954, Muhler performed an experiment in which he attempted to create a diet completely free of fluoride [16]. It was published in America's **Journal of Nutrition**. Muhler looked at weight, growth and reproduction, as well as fluoride levels in femurs of male and female rats.

He stated that the criterion for dietary use of fluorine is the uptake of fluorine by the skeleton. He used four diets with fluoride concentrations in ppm of 3.1, 2.2, 1.8, and less than 0.1. Muhler concentrated largely on storage of fluoride but pointed out very little real difference in rats fed different diets. One of his objectives, necessary for testing the essentiality of fluoride, was to make a diet completely free of the element, however this could not be done (obviously this was the reason McClendon grew his crops in water-culture). Muhler stated that

"even with exceptionally careful purification the diet still contained traces." [16]

By 'traces' he meant less than 0.1 microgram per gram (0.1 ppm). He knew there were traces due to its presence in the skeleton. For this reason, Muhler wrote that this experiment could not conclude anything definite about fluoride's essentiality.

"The most common finding was related to the difficulty of obtaining young from rats receiving the highly purified diet. After many attempts to obtain second generation rats, a different diet had to be used. Attempts to determine if this was due to the highly purified nature of the diet or to the lack of fluorine were inconclusive…"

In 1957, Dr. Richard Maurer and Professor Harry Day (a mentor of Joseph Mulher's), from the Department of Chemistry, Indiana University in Bloomington, performed an experiment which they introduced with the recognition that while fluorine was of "practical significance" in the protection of teeth from decay, studies were inconclusive regarding its essentiality.

The experiment was supported by the Medical Research and Development Board, Office of the Surgeon General, Department of the Army and published in the **Journal of Nutrition**. It was a smaller part of a thesis submitted as part of Richard Maurer's Doctor of Philosophy degree. Mentioning the conclusions of experiments (see above) done by Sharpless and McCollum (1933), Phillips, Hart and Bohstedt (1934), and Evans and Phillips (1939) [6, 8, 9], Maurer and Day concluded that under the conditions used in these experiments fluorine had not been proved necessary in nutrition.

They also noted that McClendon (1944) and McClendon and Gershon-Cohen (1953) [11, 12] had concluded that fluorine was essential, based on rats fed a diet of mainly corn and sunflowers grown in rain water between 0.002 and 0.004 ppm fluorine (although "no data were given on the fluorine content of either the diet or the animals"). They also mentioned McClendon and Gershon-Cohen's 1954 conclusion that periodontoclasia was a symptom of fluorine deficiency [13].

Maurer and Day spend three pages discussing their own methods, which to some may seem overly precise. For example, each individual animal was housed in a stainless steel cage, fabricated without using any fluorine in the welding or soldering fluxes.

The diet used had casein, corn oil, salts and corn starch as its primary components. Supplements like vitamins were added.

After purification, the diet contained no more than 0.007 ppm fluorine. Maurer and Day wrote:

"Under the extremely rigorous conditions of this study fluorine was not found to have any influence on the growth and well-being of rats.

Thus it is justifiable to conclude that under some conditions fluorine may not have any value in nutrition or even in the maintenance of dental health." [17]

They commented on the animals with the low fluorine diet having sleek coats and appearing in good condition, indistinguishable from the animals that were given fluorine. Animal teeth were examined with a dental probe. They found no dental defects.

"The diet was not conducive to impaction and it contained no fermentable sugar; thus the results indicate that fluorine is dispensable in the maintenance of sound teeth if cariogenic factors such as high concentrations of sugar are not operative." [17]

With regard to reproduction, this experiment found the element unnecessary. Four generations, 110 animals were raised. All females had a successful pregnancy, giving birth to live young.

The experiment ended with the conclusion that fluorine was not a dietary essential. Maurer and Day described their experimental conditions as "rigorous". The final sentence of their experiment says fluorine's value is:

> "... apparently limited to the promotion of resistance to dental caries."

This experiment did not find any dental difference between the two groups of rats.

In 1959, the research of R. E. Wuthier and Paul Phillips from the Department of Biochemistry at the University of Wisconsin was published in the April issue of the **Journal of Nutrition** [18]. They performed an experiment which was designed to examine the long-term effects of differing levels of food and water-borne fluoride on rats over a two-year period.

They noted that

> "no demonstration of absolute essentiality"

had been made for fluoride. They cited experiments by Maurer and Day [17] from Indiana University, and Evans and Phillips [9] from the University of Wisconsin, but suggested more existed.

Funds for this experiment were supplied partially by the Research Committee of the Graduate School from funds supplied by the Wisconsin Alumni Research Foundation. Merck and Co. supplied vitamins (of which no details were given).

Wuthier and Phillips used seven groups of twenty-five litter-mates, fed a "semi-natural cariogenic diet" for a year. They planned to remove three rats from each group at 3, 6, 12 and 18 months, and the rest at two years for testing. They would look at fluoride femur levels, dental caries incidence and severity, wear of molars, general health, reproduction, growth rate, number and weight of litters and weanlings. Unfortunately, due to respiratory and glandular infections causing death among rats, the experiment could only last one year.

The main constituents of the diet fed to the rats were ground oat groats, soybean oil, sucrose and dry skim milk powder. Corn and halibut liver oils were added, as were calcium, salt, and iodine. The diet contained approximately 0.5 ppm fluoride.

Of the seven groups of twenty-five rats each, one was given the basal diet with distilled water, and had only the fluoride that occurred in the food (0.5 ppm). All rats had the same diet, although three groups (given distilled water) had differing levels of fluoride added to food – 1.2, 3.2 and 7.2 ppm. Two groups had 1.2 and 3.2 ppm added to distilled water instead of food, and one group had city water (1.0 ppm) instead of distilled.

The scientists wrote:

> "The severity of dental caries, molar wear, and periodontal effects increased progressively with time. Fluoridation of either water or food at these low levels did not alter the pattern of these changes."

> "No significant protective effect against dental caries was observed from any of these fluoride levels studied."

> "Growth rates, mature weights, reproduction, and lactation were all normal and reflected no effect due to fluoride."

"After the fourth month the general health of this strain of rats was poor, but again, no effect attributable to fluoride was indicated." [18]

The only places I have ever seen this experiment mentioned are a 1974 National Academy of Sciences publication, **Effects of Fluorides in Animals**, and Eric Underwood's textbook *Trace Elements in Human and Animal Nutrition.* These are discussed a little in Chapter 2.

In 1963, five scientists from the Departments of Agricultural Biochemistry, Botany and Poultry Science at the University of Arizona, Tuscon, carried out an experiment with a goal similar to those mentioned here. They discussed previous attempts to show an essential role for fluoride. Their study [19] was abstracted in a 1963 volume of **Federation Proceedings** and published in full in the **Journal of Experimental Biology and Medicine** in 1964. It was supported partially by the USPHS (United States Public Health Service).

Doberenz and co-workers pointed to the minimal diets produced by Sharpless and McCollum (1933), Phillips, Hart and Bohstedt (1934), Evans and Phillips (1939), Lawrenz (1945) and Maurer and Day (1957) [6, 8, 9, 10, 17]. They cited five of the experiments mentioned here previously to conclude that

"in no case has an indication of an essential function for fluoride been noted."

They did point out the 1953 experiment by McClendon and Gershon-Cohen [12] as an exception to this trend, mentioning the reduced growth rate and dental caries on the rats fed the fluorine-free diet. However, they also pointed to a lack of information regarding levels of fluorine in the tissues of the animals.

Doberenz and co-workers cultured soybean and grain sorghum in a greenhouse built for the purpose of minimizing fluorine in hydroponically grown crops. The greenhouse was fitted with

"evaporative coolers with microfilters to minimize dust." [19]

Silica sand was used as potting medium, after treatment to remove fluorides. Water was double distilled, deionized, and purity was checked throughout.

Chemicals used contained less than 0.01 ppm fluoride. The nutrient solution contained less than 0.001 ppm fluoride. The details involved in minimizing the fluoride levels in the food ingredients were quite particular. The main constituent of the diet was soybeans (55%). The rest included grain sorghum (23%), sucrose (10%), and minor constituents vitamin mix, salts and corn oil. Sodium bromide was also added. Doberenz and co-workers said the diet

"was supplemented with vitamins and minerals adequately to satisfy the requirements for these micronutrients."

They claimed the diet contained less than 0.005 ppm fluoride.

This was fed to the first group (no added fluoride), and also to the second group (2.0 ppm fluoride added). A third group was fed field-grown sorghum and soybean, which contained 2.67 ppm fluoride.

Nine rats were used in each group, in a ten-week experimental time. An average carcass fluoride analysis was 0.72 ppm (fresh weight). After the ten weeks, average tibiae content of the first group (less than 0.005 ppm) of fluoride was 2.92 ppm. The second and third groups had 34.63 ppm and 12.54 ppm fluoride in tibiae respectively.

While starting weights were near identical, the rats with the added sodium fluoride had final weights less than the others. Doberenz and co-workers wrote in their summary that the only significant differences in enzyme activity were "an increase in serum isocitric dehydrogenase and a decrease of this enzyme in the liver." This work has been cited frequently in the literature of the United States National Academy of Sciences before 1990.

Reproduced in **Table 8** are the starting and final weights, and the fluoride storage in tibiae.

MINIMAL FLUORIDE DIET EFFECT ON RAT GROWTH AND FLUORIDE BONE DEPOSITION

Diet	Mean Starting Weight	Mean Final Weight	Mean ppm Fluoride in Tibiae at 91 Days Old
Minimal Fluoride (less than 0.005 ppm)	36.3	267.8	2.92 (5 rats)
Minimal Fluoride with 2.0 ppm Fluoride added	36.2	251.4	34.63 (4 rats)
Field-grown (2.67 ppm Fluoride)	36.1	277.7	12.54 (4 rats)

Table 8. *Minimal fluoride diet effect on rat growth and fluoride bone deposition. Source: Doberenz et al., 1964 [19].*

In 1972, the journal **Bioinorganic Chemistry** published an experiment by Dr. Klaus Schwarz and David Milne from the Veterans Administration Hospital in Long Beach, California.

Schwarz and Milne claimed that:

> "fluorine, supplied as potassium fluoride, is essential for optimal growth in rats which are fed highly purified amino acid diets and kept in trace element controlled isolators." [20]

A trace element controlled isolator is a plastic housing for animals which inhibits movement of breathable particles with a couple of filters.

Schwarz and Milne used

> "highly purified, chemically defined amino acid diets"

that varied in fluoride levels, as low as below 0.04 ppm, however some control diets contained 0.21-0.46 ppm. Like other scientists, they found it very difficult to keep fluoride levels minimal. To these diets they added 1.0, 2.5, and 7.5 ppm fluorine.

The authors claimed that an added 1.0 ppm caused a 17% increase in average growth rate (17 rats used), 2.5 ppm caused a 31% increase in average growth rate (17 rats used), and 7.5 ppm caused a 28% increase in average growth rate (19 rats used).

Rats on a second basal diet with 2.5 ppm added grew 20% better than controls. They said:

> "Rats receiving fluoride were generally better developed, as evident from their dimensions and from x-ray pictures of their skeletons."

According to Schwarz and Milne, growth is "the most sensitive indicator of an existing deficiency" in a trace element isolator[3]. However, other problems occurred in almost all animals, such as shaggy fur, loss of hair and seborrhoea (an over-activity of oil-producing glands on skin), which were apparently "not affected by fluorine additions". It is not mentioned whether these things were caused by dietary or other factors.

They suggested a level of 1.5-2.5 ppm fluorine as essential for rats, and said the same is appropriate for humans. They also mentioned the Messer, Armstrong, and Singer experiment [28] (via personal communication, it had yet to be published) as another proof that mice fed diets with low levels of fluoride had impaired fertility, and that 50 ppm fluoride added to drinking water prevented small litter sizes.

Schwarz would state publicly that his work applied to humans (discussed in Chapter 5.2). In this experiment he claimed:

> "The metabolism of fluorine in mammals presents several features which support the concept that it is essential." [20]

This remark is made with citations to three textbooks – *Fluorine Chemistry Volumes 3 and 4* edited by J. J. Simons (1965), *Fluorides and Human Health* by the World Health Organization (1970), and *Pharmacology of Fluorides* by Smith (1966).

Fluorine Chemistry Volume 3 by Harold C. Hodge, Frank Smith and Phillip S. Chen, focussed a lot on excess fluorine, with chapters on fluoroacetate, phosphofluoridates, and organic fluorine compounds [21]. I found nothing on the topic of a nutritional role.

Volume 4 by Harold C. Hodge and Frank Smith, published in 1965, contained some interesting observations, but concluded:

> "At present there is no generally accepted demonstration of the essentiality of fluorine in the diet of man or animals using growth or reproduction as indices. In the diet of civilized man, traces of fluoride (1 ppm fluoride in the drinking water) confer such notable improvement in tooth health that one is tempted to describe this role as essential." [22]

This book is discussed a little more in Chapter 1.2.

The 1970 World Health Organization monograph is discussed in detail in Chapter 2.3. The sections on essentiality in the second and sixth chapters of the monograph looked only at experiments on rodents and claimed more research was needed before a conclusion of essentiality for fluorine could be reached, though the introduction of the monograph, written by a different author and without recourse to experiments, claimed fluorine essential. Schwarz and Milne also cite page 183 of this 1970 document at the start of their experiment which is where the sixth chapter's discussion on essentiality begins.

The 1966 textbook by Smith *et al.* is highly technical and goes into great detail regarding the chemistry of elemental fluorine [23]. Regarding essentiality, we are referred to work by Muhler [24] and Underwood [25]

---

[3] Schwarz and Milne claimed to have used this method to demonstrate the essentiality of vanadium and tin [20].

(both are discussed in the following chapter as neither are original experiments but summaries of others' work), as well as the 1965 book edited by Simons [22].

The following is Frank A. Smith's conclusion:

> "Suffice it to say that unequivocal evidence that fluoride is required for growth, reproduction, or skeletal development, has not yet been forthcoming. Unquestionably, fluoride does improve dental health and in its absence this condition is impaired; however, the animal does not die in the absence of this optimal dentition. On the basis of present knowledge, fluoride is classed as essential by Muhler and as probably essential by Underwood." [23]

Schwarz and Milne presented their findings on the 28th of December, 1971 at the 138th meeting of the American Association for the Advancement of Science in Philadelphia, and again on the 10th of April, 1972 at the International Atomic Energy Agency Symposium on Nuclear Activation Techniques in the Life Sciences in Bled, Yugoslavia.

On the 20th of April 1973, Dr. Schwarz presented his research at the 57th Annual Meeting of the Federation of American Societies for Experimental Biology in Atlantic City, New Jersey. He was the sole author of a paper on fluorine and other elements. He cited his previous work [20] as one demonstration of fluoride's essentiality in the written version of this paper on fluorine and silicon, chromium, vanadium and tin, published in **Federation Proceedings** in 1974.

Again, Schwarz suggested a level of 1.5-2.5 ppm fluorine in water to yield optimal growth for rats, with varying levels for humans. Note that this is a *concentration in water, not a dose or defined amount.* He wrote:

> "Compared to the amount of fluorine found in the earth's crust, the dietary requirement for fluoride appears very small."
>
> "Rats in the trace element sterile isolator fail to develop normal incisor pigmentation." [26]

He believed that tooth pigmentation was improved by fluoride, if compromised by a lack of vitamins E, D, and A, or deficiencies in calcium, phosphorous, magnesium and iron. In 1973 two people wrote of Dr. Schwarz's work. Nielsen and Sandstead, a Research Chemist and a Director from the United States Department of Agriculture's Agricultural Research Service, presented a review on nickel, vanadium, silicon, fluorine and tin at the Annual Meeting of the Institute of Food Technologists in Miami. The paper was published in 1974, in **The American Journal of Clinical Nutrition** [27].

With regard to work on the dental and skeletal benefits of fluorine since the 1930s, they quoted Dr. Mark Hegsted:

> "If an essential element were defined as one which has a beneficial effect in health and well-being, under the usual conditions in which individuals live, then in the light of the above evidence, fluorine would be considered an essential element in human nutrition."

(Dr. Hegsted's work is discussed in the next chapter.)

Nielsen and Sandstead also looked at the claim by Messer and Armstrong, that fluoride was required for growth and reproduction (see below). They didn't go into details, but their conclusion indicates their disagreement:

"At present, a requirement for fluorine cannot be estimated."

Their review also contains the criticism/caution of Schwarz's experiments using the trace element isolators:

"This observation must, until confirmed, be viewed with reservation for the following reasons: 1) The control rats experienced suboptimal growth, even though they were supplemented with fluoride. 2) Although significant, the differences in weight gain between the deficient and the control animals were small, approximately 6 g over 26 days, even though the diet contained all known essential elements including vanadium, silicon, and tin. 3) Others have not been able to confirm this finding even though they have fed diets containing less fluorine. Clearly more research will be necessary before it can be stated that fluorine is essential for growth." [27]

The article concluded in a summary by saying that fluorine and tin had not been shown essential for humans, although it seemed probable that they were needed somewhere in the human metabolism, and therefore in nutrition.

Here, a rat suffering suboptimal growth is compared with a normal rat. These photos (**Figure 2** a and b) are taken from Schwarz's 1974 paper. The sick rat is explained by Schwarz's statement that

"… chemicals needed in diets to produce trace element deficiencies… must be of a degree of purity which greatly exceeds that normally encountered in chemistry."

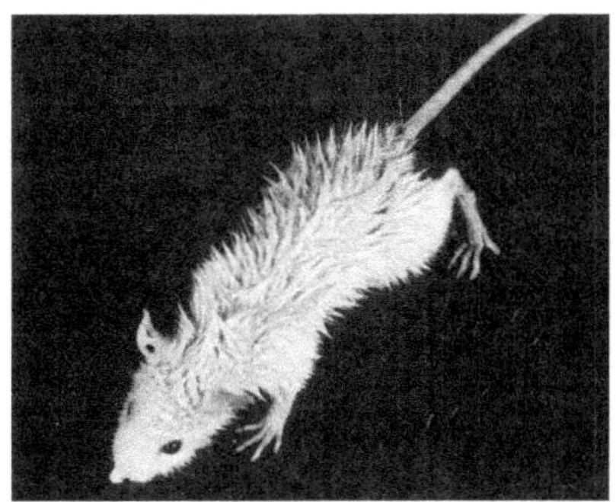
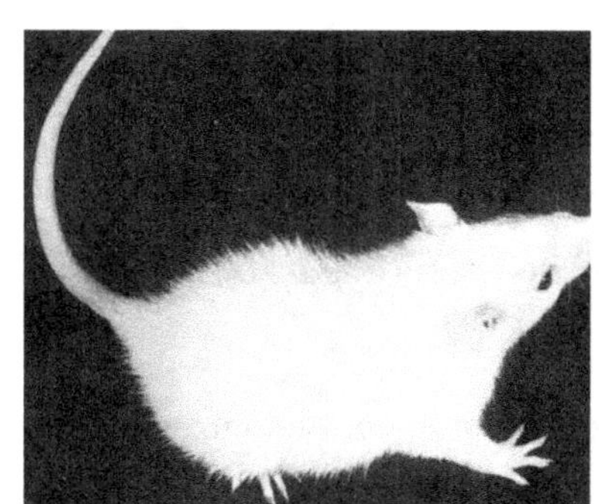

Figure 2. Both animals were on the same diet. The animal on the left (a) was typical of animals kept for 20 days in the trace element sterile environment system. The animal on the right (b) was an "outside control, kept under conventional conditions on a purified diet." Schwarz, 1974 [26].

Dr. Schwarz pointed out in his second paper that previous researchers, notably Maurer and Day, and Doberenz (both of whose means he described as "rather sophisticated"), had found a much lower amount of fluorine necessary than what he had. Schwarz said the reason for this was not clear to him.

"It is well known, however, that the fluoride requirement is influenced by the levels of calcium, phosphorus, magnesium, and various other constituents of the diet."

"In our experiments, these were contained in adequate but balanced amounts in an amino acid diet which was completely defined. The fluoride supplement was added to the diet while most other investigators supplied it in the drinking water."

Schwarz believed that the absorption (he used the word 'utilization') of fluoride in water was different to that in foods; this is something believed today. Ions of fluorine floating freely in water are obviously absorbed in greater amounts than fluorine bound to food. He also claimed that silicates could interfere with fluoride use in the body, 50 mg/100 ml sodium metasilicate inhibited the effect on growth.

> "The level of fluoride required to produce growth is approximately 2.5 ppm. This amount is physiological; it occurs normally in foods and feeds, including average human diets." [26]

Dr. Schwarz did not go into detail in either of these papers about why he thought earlier work was "useless" – due to its inadequate methods. Experiments discussed here in 1939, 1945, 1954 and 1959 would perhaps demonstrate his "discrepancy" – they didn't all use fluoride in water, they used it in food, and as Nielsen and Sandstead pointed out, at levels below what he used. Perhaps he considered McClendon and Gershon-Cohen's approach extreme, but said nothing in the two papers mentioned here.

Schwarz did not elaborate on his claim that a need for fluorine was influencd by other minerals. His work made headlines (discussed in Chapter 5.2).

In September 1972, the journal **Science** published the work of Drs. Messer, Armstrong and Singer, working in the Biochemistry Department (Health Sciences) of the University of Minnesota, Minneapolis.

This is the first of four of their papers I will discuss here. As noted previously I will refer to these papers throughout this book as being authored by either Messer *et al.* or Armstrong *et al.* They introduced this experiment by drawing attention to the fact that

> "satisfactory evidence of a deficiency state with respect to fluorine has not been demonstrated despite several investigations with this purpose." [28]

In support of this statement, they cited experiments by Muhler (1954), Maurer and Day (1957), and Doberenz *et al.* (1963) [16, 17, 19].

Female mice were put in two groups and given deionized water (58 mice) or deionized water with 50 ppm fluoride as sodium fluoride added (55 mice). Both of these groups were fed a diet containing from 0.1 to 0.3 ppm fluoride. They were grouped four females to one male for 25 weeks. The dietary effects were exclusive to the females, the males were fed normal laboratory rodent food and swapped between the low and high fluoride animals. Armstrong and co-workers wrote:

> "Litter production was observed over the 25-week period to a maximum of four litters. Each litter was reduced to six pups and all pups were removed at 5 days of age to promote a rapid breeding rate."
>
> "Mice in the low fluoride group showed a progressive impairment in reproductive capacity."

All of the first generation animals gave birth. Below half the mice produced four litters. The second-generation mice on the low-fluoride diet suffered a

> "... progressive decline in litter production."

Twenty percent of this group did not produce even one litter, over half did not produce four litters. Regarding earlier experiments that concluded there was no need for fluoride in reproduction, Armstrong and co-workers wrote that

"The failure of previous studies to demonstrate a role of fluoride in reproduction may be attributed to the small numbers of animals involved and the short duration of the studies, since in this work the infertility developed slowly in each generation." [28]

This is an inaccurate comment, as the Maurer and Day study, cited by Armstrong, Messer and Singer, went on for four generations. Armstrong *et al.* did not mention this. Maurer and Day observed most animals for 150 days, but kept two pairs, one with and one without fluorine, on their diet for 325 days [17].

The Doberenz study was ten weeks long [19].

Armstrong and his co-workers mated their mice at eight weeks.

The Wuthier experiment (no effect from low fluoride) lasted for a year, but Armstrong, Messer and Singer didn't mention it. It was not a popular experiment. They also didn't mention the five-year 1934 study, which claimed to have kept rats on the diet for 140 days [8]. This was mentioned in the 1957 experiment, but not acknowledged by Armstrong *et al.* This was possibly not considered long enough, which I think from their point of view, is justified.

They did point out that they had no definite basis for infertility, no physiological or molecular reason why low fluoride should cause restrictions in reproduction. They suggested that infertility was common in nutritional deficiencies, so infertility caused by low fluoride intake,

"...may represent, at least in part, a nonspecific response to the stress of a nutritional deficiency." [28]

They also investigated if additions of fluoride could restore fertility to fertility-impaired mice. Female mice were kept on the low fluoride diet and mated after 8 weeks as before, and put into two groups. Half the animals were given added fluoride (50 ppm), and both groups were re-mated after one week away from males, then their litter production was monitored over the following 20 weeks.

Results were as expected: only 40 to 50 percent of mice on the low fluoride intake produced four litters, while 85 to 90 percent of mice on the high fluoride intake produced four litters. Armstrong and co-workers wrote:

"This study demonstrates that fluorine satisfies the major criteria for an essential trace element: (i) A deficiency state, characterized by a delayed production of the first litter and a progressive infertility, has been produced in mice on a diet low in fluoride. (ii) The deficiency is prevented and cured by addition of fluoride alone to the diet. (iii) The deficiency correlates well with low tissue (bone) levels of fluoride. Thus, there is good evidence that fluorine is an essential element, at least in the diet of the mouse." [28]

In this experiment Armstrong and his co-workers wrote that after they had sent their experiment to be printed, they received word from Schwarz and Milne, claiming that fluorine added to highly purified diets "significantly enhanced" growth in young mice and improved the pigmentation of the incisors. They claimed the amount used was relevant to amounts in human diets.

In December 1972, **Nature New Biology** published an experiment by H. H. Messer, K. Wong, M. Wegner, L. Singer, and W. D. Armstrong, again from the same university. [29]

The experiment suggested that diets for mice low in fluoride (commercial rodent food contained between 40 and 60 ppm) "interfered markedly with haemopoiesis" – the formation of platelets and blood cells. Recognising again that there was no definite conclusion of fluoride's essentiality, they wrote:

> "Many attempts to demonstrate the dietary essentiality of fluoride have yielded equivocal results and none of the studies have connected fluoride to a specific metabolic deficiency (refs. 1–5 and personal communication from K. Schwarz)."

The 'attempts' cited were four that have been discussed – Sharpless and McCollum (1933), Phillips, Hart and Bohstedt (1934), McClendon and Gershon-Cohen (1953), Maurer and Day (1957) [6, 8, 12, 17] – and one other with researchers from the Department of Physiology at the Dartmouth Medical School in Hanover, New Hampshire, and the Battleboro Memorial Hospital in Vermont. It was published in 1968 in the **Journal of Nutrition** [30].

In this 1968 experiment the diet used was 60% seed rye flour, 30% skim milk, 9% corn oil, 1% sodium chloride, with ferrous sulphate and vitamins added.

Regarding the water used, the scientists wrote:

> "The basic drinking water contained, as soluble salts: (ppm element) zinc, 50; manganese, 10; copper, 5; chromium, 1; cobalt, 1; and molybdenum, 1. The water was obtained from a spring and was doubly deionized."

To this water, 10 ppm sodium fluoride was added for one set of female, and one set of male mice. There were 54 animals in each sample, males and females each given fluorine, and males and females not given fluorine.

Females who received fluorine experienced "enhanced growth" after one and a half years of age, such that their average weights exceeded males by 2.1 and 5.2 grams.

> "According to measured life spans, male mice fed fluorine lived longer than their controls by 29 to 60 days at 3 intervals, whereas females did not." [30]

Fluorine in soft tissues was not found in fluorine-fed mice, nor their controls, in this experiment. Bone was not analysed.

Longevity was defined as "the mean age at death of the oldest 10%." For males, this was 830 ± 28.3 days on fluorine vs 806 ± 34.3 for controls, females 838 ± 14.5 vs 855 ± 29.3 for controls.

This experiment also looked at zirconium, niobium and antimony. Of these, antimony and fluorine were not detected in the diet. The other two elements were, at 2.66 micrograms per gram zirconium and 1.62 microgram per gram niobium. The researchers calculated fluorine intake by the "assumption" that mature mice ingest 7 grams of water and 6 grams of food per 100 grams of body weight per day. From this, they concluded that the control mice ingested 0.6 microgram per 100 grams of body weight daily (6 micrograms per kilogram), and the fluorine-fed mice 70 micrograms per 100 grams of body weight daily (700 micrograms per kilogram).

Dr. Armstrong and co-workers suggested that many experiments had not gone on long enough to demonstrate fluoride's essential nature. In the previously mentioned, 1968 experiment the rats had lived until natural death, but the researchers were not looking at blood formation or reproductive ability.

Due to animals having a store of nutrients, an animal deprived of a key nutrient may function without exhibiting signs of deficiency for an amount of time, until what is stored in their bones/organs runs out. This is pointed out in Dr. Schwarz's solo paper [26] and implied in others, like *this* one [29] – Armstrong *et al.* are basically suggesting that scientists like Maurer and Day [17] could raise rats on a fluorine-deficient diet, because the animals had a store of fluorine since birth.

Maurer and Day raised their first set of animals on a diet with 0.6 ppm fluorine, upon sexual maturity, those animals were bred and their litters fed the purified diet of 0.007 ppm.

Armstrong and co-workers designed an experiment [29] in which milk and cereals were fed to mice. They used 58% whole wheat flour and 21.6% skim milk in their diet. Deionized water was given to twenty mice, and deionized water with 50 ppm sodium fluoride was given to sixteen mice. Blood was taken from tails 2 days prior to mating (which occurred after 10 weeks) and 5, 10, 15 and 19 days after mating, red cell volumes measured after centrifugation.

Body weight before mating, body weight 19 days after mating, general appearance of health, and litter size were not influenced by maternal fluoride intake.

The mice had haematocrit examined at ten, twenty and sixty days of age.

The authors claimed that addition of fluoride to the diet prevented this interference with the rats' normal function of blood cell creation. They also claimed that the mice on the low fluoride diet developed anaemia; iron deficiency.

In 1973, the **Journal of Nutrition** published a summary [4] of the previous two studies [28, 29] by Messer, Singer and Armstrong that claimed to have found a fluoride deficiency in mice. This study was supported by the National Institute of Dental Research (NIDR). The scientists presented their work at the 50th Annual Meeting of the International Association for Dental Research at Las Vegas, Nevada, March 1972. It was lengthier and included investigations on weight.

Typical of rodent diets, wheat flour, skimmed milk powder, vegetable fat, casein, vitamins and salt were used. At least fifty animals were used in each group. All were fed the low fluoride diet (0.1-0.3 ppm - "growth rates of mice and rats fed this diet were found to be at least equal to those of animals fed a standard laboratory ration"). Animals were given water containing 0, 50, 100 or 200 ppm fluoride (sodium fluoride to deionized water).

Messer and his co-workers noted that animals fed very low amounts of fluoride had grown perfectly fine in certain experiments - he cited the 1933, 1957 and 1964 experiments [6, 17, 19]. They also cited the experiments by Schroeder *et al.* [30] and Schwarz and Milne, [20] and the previous experiment suggesting fluoride supported normal growth and reproduction [29].

Messer and co-workers claimed:

"Mice with a low fluoride intake developed signs of fluorine deficiency, with a progressive development of infertility in two successive generations… the percentage of mice producing litters was lower." [4]

They noted that infertility and anaemia are common in nutritional deficiencies. Anaemia of course relates to iron, and Messer and co-workers said fluoride increases iron absorption, and may contribute to absorption of other nutrients.

Concluding, the authors stated:

> "The only criterion of essentiality for which at least partial evidence is lacking with respect to fluoride is the identification of a specific biochemical role for fluoride. Apart from this, there is now strong evidence that fluoride is required in the diet, at least of mice." [4]

This conclusion of essentiality was in many newspapers (discussed in Chapter 5).

Another write-up [31] of this data by Messer *et al.* appeared in the journal **Trace Element Metabolism in Animals-2**, in 1974. It is abundant in citations for such a short document, I feel. A discussion section between other scientists appeared at the end. Their 1974 write-up was a little different to the previous one, and they wrote:

> "The demonstration of a deficiency state, and its prevention and cure by fluorine alone, justify the tentative inclusion of fluorine in the list of essential trace elements."

Sometimes I wonder why certain facts are left out of experiments. Not mentioned in *any* of the previous experiments from Messer *et al.*, [4, 28, 29] but mentioned in the discussion of the 1974 summary, Dr. Messer declared that his diet

> "… contains about 25 ppm of iron which is somewhat marginal. I don't recall the exact concentration of copper but it is also marginal." [31]

Copper and iron are both essential nutrients (using "requirement" as a criterion for essentiality).

Therefore Dr. Messer has violated his first criterion: that to demonstrate a deficiency of a certain element, a diet should be adequate in other respects. Why this was not mentioned in the previous experiments [4, 28, 29] is exasperating for the thorough researcher, especially when Messer and co-workers cited in two of their previous papers [4, 28] a study from the **British Journal of Nutrition** called *The Effect of Copper Deficiency on Reproduction in the Female Rat* [32].

Above, I discussed the Nielsen and Sandstead review [27] that defined essentiality as being simply beneficial. It is interesting to discover that different scientists have different definitions of the word "essential".

In their 1973 summary, [4] Messer and co-workers gave criteria for what constitutes the creation of a deficiency condition, when testing for essentiality:

> "A specific deficiency state should be produced by a diet lacking the element in question, but which is otherwise adequate and satisfactory."

> "The deficiency should be prevented or cured by addition to the diet of that element alone."

Thus, for fluoride to be essential (according to Messer's definition) it should not be substituting for another, lacking element. For example, in a hypothetical case of "element X" deficiency, "element Y" may step in to replace X, perhaps improving a compromised bodily function somewhat. This would not constitute Y's essentiality, even though Y would have done something beneficial in this hypothetical instance.

With this in mind, please consider the differences between the terms "essential" and "beneficial" with regard to function and criteria of classification.

Dr. Klaus Schwarz is quoted in this discussion as saying:

> "I must say I have some misgivings, to put it mildly, with the first criterion of essentiality mentioned by Dr. Messer. If we were to stick to that, neither riboflavin, pantothenic acid, vitamin B_6, or vitamin A would be recognized, because the discovery of these certainly was made with diets which did not contain all of the essential ingredients. This criteria of essentiality is, in my book, absurd." [31]

I would certainly not accuse a single one of these gentlemen of any deliberate misleading or deception. We can see differences lie in the fact that some have a more relaxed definition of terms. Dr. Schwarz believed Messer's rule too strict.

Dr. Suttie, a researcher from Madison, Wisconsin (an organizer of the symposium and an editor of the book compiled from the presentations), suggested that an experiment testing for essentiality using an incomplete diet may be of some help at first, however eventually one would have to use a complete diet in order to produce a deficiency condition that was definite. (I agree with this.) Suttie said:

> "There certainly has been a number of people who have produced diets which are probably somewhere between 0.1 and 0.3 ppm fluoride and have not obtained any response from additional fluoride. Because of this, I think it is premature to call fluoride essential at this time."

After this point, a scientist named Klevay from Grand Forks, Michigan, suggested that perhaps fluoride had a substituting effect, or could be replaced by something else. Dr. Schwarz half-addressed this:

> "I don't think any of the other agents which we have tested will substitute for fluoride. Therefore from that point of view, I think the criterion of essentiality is fulfilled."

Schwarz did not mention the possibility that fluoride was substituting for, or aiding the incorporation of some other component, a relevant point in light of two experiments performed in 1976 that will be discussed.

Klevay's point of view on fluoride's essentiality echoed DeEds' [7]: discussing the ratio of water to needed Vitamin B_{12} during normal temperatures (10^8 ratio) and high temperatures (10^9 ratio), requiring in the latter case ten times as much water for the same amount of Vitamin B_{12}, he stated

> "I don't believe you can tell anything about essentiality of a material by considering how much of that material is present in the diet." [31]

The conversation ended with a *very* relevant comment from Dr. Schwarz relating to definitions of the word "essential":

> "However, I can probably repeat what I said in Atlantic City: at the moment, essentiality, just like beauty, is pretty much in the eyes of the beholder." [31]

I have often wondered about the exact meaning of such a statement. Schwarz did a lot of work on the roles of other elements in nutrition.

In 1976 the experiments by Dr. Messer and his co-workers [28, 29] were repeated with a few minor changes by two scientists; S. Tao and J. W. Suttie (mentioned previously in the 1974 discussion), from the University of Wisconsin. The work was published in the **Journal of Nutrition**. Funding is discussed in **Table 9**.

They used "the same basal diet", however claimed a fluoride level of 0.2-0.5 ppm, and added 2 and 100 ppm to the other two groups. They found no difference in growth, reproduction or litter size (however the group fed 100 ppm had slightly lower copper in liver and kidneys). The diet contained 7.5 ppm copper and 144 ppm iron (compare this with Messer's "marginal" copper and 25 ppm iron).

The authors concluded:

> "Although fluoride may yet be shown to be essential for some physiological process, sound evidence for a claim of essentiality of fluoride for reproduction is still lacking."

> "The results of this study have failed to confirm an earlier report that fluoride in the maternal diet is essential for reproduction in the mouse." [33]

In support of this statement they cited three of Dr Messer and Dr. Armstrong's papers they believed their work had refuted [4, 28, 29]. Tao and Suttie did not find any relation of haematocrit levels to fluoride levels. They performed femur analyses which they considered of more accuracy than diet analyses. The femur analyses showed lower amounts of fluoride (76 and 90 ppm) than Armstrong and co-workers showed in *their* mouse femurs (100 and 90 ppm). This was proof that the diet used by Tao and Suttie contained either less or the same amount of fluoride as that used by Armstrong *et al.*

This experiment suggested that

> "relatively high levels of fluoride are able to exert a beneficial pharmacological effect on the utilization of iron when suboptimal concentrations of iron are present in the diet." [33]

In October of 1976, an experiment looking at the relationship between iron and fluorine was published in **Proceedings of the Society for Experimental Biology and Medicine** [34]. This experiment was supported by a Public Health Service research grant from the National Institute of Dental Research, and authored by Wegner, Singer, Ophaug and Magil, again from the Department of Biochemistry at the University of Minnesota Medical School in Minneapolis. Wegner and Singer had appeared before in experiments with Armstrong and Messer. Looking at the diet used in the studies on anaemia, they agreed that it was below marginal in copper with 2.7 ppm (they claimed 5 ppm was a requirement).

The diet used was almost sixty percent whole wheat flour, which they claimed contained phytic acid. This can interfere with intestinal absorption of iron and copper. Skim milk (twenty percent) was also used, presumably vitamins, minerals and oils were added to this. The amount of fluoride in the diet was probably near-identical to those used in the experiments featuring Wegner and Singer, with Armstrong and Messer [28, 29, 31].

These scientists experimented with three groups of rats – two groups were used to reproduce the conditions of the previous experiments that dealt with iron levels in fluoride-high (50 ppm) and fluoride-low (deionized water only) mice. Both groups were supplemented with 195 ppm iron chloride ($FeCl_3 \cdot 6H_2O$). The third group of mice were fed commercial rat food with 200 ppm iron, 8 ppm copper, and between 20 and 60 ppm fluoride.

The water used for this group was tap water with 1.0 ppm fluoride. In other work with copper supplementation, copper did not appear to affect anaemia levels.

Mice were uniformly weaned at 20 days (to eliminate non-uniform amounts of iron in mother's milk) and mated at 8 weeks. Milk is the only source of iron to young before weaning. These researchers claimed that the fluoride content of rodent milk was unknown, but suggested it would be "extremely low". This was based on their knowledge of fluoride levels in milk of other species.

Dams (female mice) were kept on the diet for a year, then sacrificed. Iron did not appear to influence fluoride storage in the skeleton. Pups born to these mice had average haematocrit levels, with iron supplements yielding an increase. Weights at birth were "similar for all groups." However the high-fluoride animals at 15 days of age were less anaemic than the low-fluoride animals. The results of this investigation indicate that the control group, fed iron in food, had greater absorption and retention of iron than experimental groups. That a "beneficial effect on the haematocrit" occurred in the young because of the iron supplementation, is obvious. Higher levels of fluoride helped increase iron absorption when iron levels in the diet were low. One is reminded of the idea of Gautier in 1913, who suggested fluorine's use was one of transporting other nutritional essentials in the body. In this experiment, the possibility of a classification for fluorine as 'essential' or 'non-essential' was not mentioned.

The study concluded that higher fluorine increased the iron content of the milk. I am unsure if recent research has been done to verify or refute the 1976 experiments discussed here. In Chapter 2.1 you will see I have looked in much of the National Academy of Sciences literature, and these two experiments are mentioned on occasion. In more public literature the pickings are even slimmer; I never saw these experiments mentioned once in any newspaper. I have never seen a refutation of their conclusions.

In June of 1973, two scientists from the Department of Poultry Science, College of Agriculture, at the University of Arizona presented their work at the Second International Symposium on Trace Element Metabolism in Animals, held in Madison, Wisconsin. It was published in the same 1974 document as the previous study by Messer *et al.* [35]. They had performed an experiment which looked at the possibility of an essential requirement for fluoride in mice. Using soybean and sorghum, Weber and Reid created a "low-fluoride" (0.2 ppm) diet. To this they added 6 ppm fluoride. To serve as a control diet they used field-grown ingredients.

Weber and Reid looked at body weights, femur fluoride, femur citric acid, and small intestine lipase levels. They found the mice on the high fluoride diet had more than ten times the femur fluoride levels as the mice on the low fluoride diet (267 and 22 ppm respectively). They did not conclude that fluoride was essential for growth. Food intake and body weight between the three sets of mice had no significant difference.

The final sentence of their experiment sums up:

"No significant differences were observed between the low-fluoride and 6 ppm fluoride-treated mice through six generations." [35]

The Messer *et al.* experiments mentioned the possibility that stored fluorine took so long to be used up that experiments lasting less than theirs in length were basically invalidated. Consider: the Schwarz and Milne paper [20] was made up of ten, four-week experiments. The 1974 Weber and Reid experiment [35] used females fed for 120 days, and achieved six generations on a diet of 0.2 ppm. The 1976 experiment [33] by Tao and Suttie went on for 33 weeks (231 days) at 0.1 ppm (the same or less than the amount in Armstrong and co-workers' experiment on haematocrit levels, this found by bone analysis). The 1976 experiment [34] by Wegner *et al.* on iron and fluoride levels and anaemia, went on for a year. The table below may help your consideration of these experiments.

Table 9. SUMMARY OF ANIMAL EXPERIMENTAL DATA AND CONCLUSIONS

Length of Time and *Number of Subjects* refers only to those given lowest fluoride levels, unless otherwise indicated. See individual experiments for more details.

Year	Researcher/s, and Funded by	Length of Time	Lowest Amount of Fluoride	Number of Subjects	Conclusion
1933	McCollum, Sharpless [6]	4 months	"very low but not quite free"	10 rats	Fluoride not essential for reproduction or dentition (but found in bones)[1]
1934	Phillips, Hart, Bohstedt [8], *Ruhm Phosphate and Chemical Company*	140 days	0.1 ppm	4 rats per group (many groups)	More than 0.1 ppm not essential for rats
1939	Evans and Phillips [9], *Works Progress Administration*	4 months or 7 months, up to 4 generations, see experiment	0.05-0.06 ppm	4 rats, see experiment	More than 0.1 ppm not essential for rats. Less than 50 microgram per kilogram of body weight required daily, if there is a requirement
1945	Lawrenz [10]	207 days	0.47 ppm	14 pairsof rats	Non-essential. No signs of malnutrition on less than 27 microgram per kilogram of body weight daily
1944 (abs.), 1945	McClendon and Foster [11], *Aluminum Company of America*	48-75 days, see experiment	0.3 ppm in mothers, unknown amount in diet, but plants grown in 0.002-0.004 ppm rain water run through resin to remove halogens	3 sets of 2 rats	Fluoride essential for dentition in rats
1953	McClendon and Gershon-Cohen [12], *Chilean Iodine Educational Bureau*	88 days	Unknown, plants grown in 0.002-0.004 ppm rain water run through resin to remove halogens	19 rats	Fluoride suspected necessary for reproduction and dentition in rats
1954	McClendon and Gershon-Cohen [13], *Aluminum Company of America and Lever Brothers*	Animals died between two and three months	Unknown, plants grown in 0.002-0.004 ppm rain water run through resin to remove halogens	6 rats	Fluoride suspected necessary for reproduction and dentition in rats. Premature death prevented by fluoridated milk
1954	Muhler [16], *Medical Research Development Board of U.S. Army*	240 days	Less than 0.1 ppm	27 rats	Inconclusive using bone retention as a criterion

Year	Researchers/Funding	Duration	Fluoride level	Subjects	Conclusion
1957	Maurer and Day [17], *Medical Research Development Board of U.S. Army*	325 days, four generations of rats	Approximately 0.007 ppm	110 rats total	Fluorine is not a dietary essential, "dispensable"
1958	Wuthier and Phillips [18], *Wisconsin Animal Research Foundation (Merck provided vitamins used)*	One year	Approximately 0.5 ppm, added 1.0 ppm city tap water	25 rats	Fluorine is not a dietary essential
1963 (abs.), 1964	Doberenz, Kurnick, Kurtz, Kemmerer and Reid [19], *United States Public Health Service*	10 weeks	Less than 0.005 ppm	9 rats	Fluorine is not a dietary essential
1972	Schwarz and Milne [20], *United States Public Health Service grant from National Institute of Arthritis and Metabolic Diseases*	10 four-week experiments	Basal diet varied between 0.04 to 0.46 ppm, added 1.0 ppm	Eight or six rats per isolator	Fluoride is essential[2]
1973	Schwarz [26], *National Institutes of Health*	28 days	Basal diet varied between 0.04 to 0.46 ppm, none added	19 rats	Fluoride is essential[2]
1972	Armstrong, Messer and Singer [28]	25 weeks	0.1 ppm	55 mice	"Fluorine satisfies the major criteria for an essential trace element"[3]
1972	Messer, Wong, Wegner, Singer and Armstrong [29]	60 days	0.1 ppm	Ten mice	Low-fluoride mice developed severe anaemia[3]
1974	Messer, Armstrong and Singer [31], *National Institute of Dental Research*	25 weeks	0.1 ppm	55 mice	(This was a summary of previous research.) "Strong evidence fluoride is required", "tentative inclusion" in trace element category[3]
1976	Tao and Suttie [33], see note 3 below for funding	33 weeks	0.1 ppm	10-13 average mice litter size	Fluoride is not an essential nutrient[3]
1976	Wegner, Singer, Ophaug and Magil [34], *Public Health Service Research Grant from the National Institute of Dental Research*	One year	0.1 ppm	27	Higher levels of fluoride helped increase iron absorption when iron levels in the diet were low
1974	Weber and Reid [35], *supported in part by USPHS Grant*	Females fed for 120 days, six generations raised, see experiment	0.2 ppm	Five female mice, see experiment	"No significant differences" in enzyme levels and body weights (6 ppm added)

1) Six ppm was the lowest concentration found in bone. To conclude 6 ppm was the lowest fluoride diet fed to the animals would be foolish because fluoride accumulates in bone. Evans and Phillips in 1939 found a range of 1 to 31 ppm in bone on a diet of 1.6 ppm. Takao Suzuki from the Department of Hygiene, Tokyo Dental College, in 1969 fed rats only 0.45 ppm but found around 14 ppm in bone (his work discussed in the next section).

2) This claim was criticised by Nielsen and Sandstead in 1974, for three reasons: control rats grew suboptimally, there were only small differences in weight gain between control and deficient animals (6 grams), and other researchers prior were unable to replicate Schwarz's claims of a fluoride deficiency even with less fluoride. Schwarz probably also used a more relaxed definition of essentiality.

3) The 1974 document is a summary of the team's previous research, not a new experiment of its own. In this presentation Dr. Messer admitted this diet was marginal in iron and copper, which violated his own first criterion for essentiality: that a diet should be adequate in all other respects. In 1976 Drs. Tao and Suttie repeated this experiment with abundant iron and copper, and concluded fluoride had had a pharmacological effect (e.g. drug-like, rather than correcting a physiological or metabolic effect caused from a deficiency) resulting in increased iron absorption in these experiments. The experiment by Tao and Suttie boasts a huge string of supporters: the College of Agricultural and Life Sciences, University of Wisconsin in Madison. Research grant from the Aluminum Company of America, Aluminum Company of Canada, Kennecott Copper Corporation, Monsanto Chemical Company, Ormet Corporation [4], Eastalco Aluminum Company, Stauffer Chemical Company, Reynolds Metals Company, Kaiser Aluminum and Chemical Corporation, Anaconda Aluminum Company, Martin Marietta [5], U.S. Steel Corporation, Intalco Aluminum Corporation, National Southwire Aluminum Company, and in part by a grant from the USPHS.

I have not given my opinions on these experiments in this first chapter. This is for the same reason I quote heavily: I want the reader to receive purely what the scientists who performed the experiments have said, without causing potential confusion between their remarks and my own.

Please do not think the subject – even as far as the experiments are concerned, ends here.

Some experiments from outside the United States, as well as comments and criticisms of these and previous experiments made by people in the same field, follow.

---

[4] An aluminium corporation (previously Harvey Aluminum).

[5] An aerospace and defence corporation.

1.2 What Do Other Scientists Involved Say?

"... essentiality, just like beauty, is pretty much in the eyes of the beholder."

- Dr. Klaus Schwarz of the Veteran's Administration Hospital, California, quoted in (Discussion) **Trace Element Metabolism in Animals-2**, p. 437, 1974 [31].

I'd like to open this section with a statement that may elaborate a little on Dr. Klaus Schwarz's, above. It's one of Dr. Joseph Muhler's, from a book he co-authored that was published in 1960. This is the third sentence of a chapter Muhler wrote, entitled *Is Fluorine a Dietary Essential?*

> "Perhaps one of the most troublesome aspects of this question is not the technical problems of the investigations, even though they are quite difficult to resolve, but rather the uncertainty about the term "dietary essential" itself. The words have quite different meanings to different people, depending very often on which field of investigation the research worker belongs to." [24]

Muhler wanted to emphasize the fact that people attribute different meanings to the term. He gave a few dictionary definitions, yet claimed he did not want to limit its use.

This chapter focusses on what scientists have said about the experiments mentioned previously. Relevant statements from other researchers who contributed to the discussion have been included. Much of this work is behind the scenes in the sense of it being quite technical, not casual or reader-friendly. I'll also include some other experiments that may be of interest. Here I am more concerned with experiments rather than definition of terms, however it is wise to consider the statements of Schwarz and Muhler with regard to criteria used.

The 1933 Sharpless and McCollum experiment [6] has not been discussed much in the literature, beyond what is obvious. That the Willard and Winter method of fluorine determination was unknown to them justified their own method of determination; duplications were included to demonstrate this method's accuracy.

Evans and Phillips concluded in 1939 that if there is a requirement for fluorine in the rat, it would be less than 50 micrograms per kilogram of body weight daily [9].

Neither this, nor the 1934 experiment [8], were discussed much beyond a simple acceptance of their existence and conclusion. This is possibly because they were carried out before Community Water Fluoridation (CWF) began, though there may be other reasons.

The experiment by McClendon and Foster [11], abstracted in 1944 and published full in 1945, also came out around the time CWF began.

McClendon's full write-up is not much bigger than the abstract, at barely a page. As has been mentioned, no details were given on levels of fluoride in food or what was retained in the bodies of rats. That only three sets of two rats were used has (to my knowledge) gone unmentioned, unnoticed by so many, although there was definitely scepticism of McClendon's work in the scientific community. In fact the most favourable statements I've found regarding it, other than Joseph Muhler's, is that it is suggestive, or there was not quite enough information to make definite claims.

A paper in the 1947 **New Zealand Dental Journal** by Muriel Bell and Marion Harrison looked at various dietary substances, and mentioned the 1945 McClendon and Foster experiment in a positive light, but said it was

"too early to make pronouncements on studies of this type". [36]

The 1965 textbook edited by Simons was more favourable to McClendon's research. Calling it

"... a single, unconfirmed report that gives one, if not the only, hint of fluoride essentiality." [22] (page 119)

Regarding low fluoride diets, the authors also looked at experiments by Muhler [16], Sharpless and McCollum [6], Evans and Phillips [9], and Maurer and Day [17].

Three of McClendon's experiments [11, 12, 13] concluded fluorine a necessity. Only the 1954 experiment was most definite, when both sets of rats were given the water-culture food.

It has been argued that the problems with teeth and growth occurred because McClendon gave poor quality vegetables grown in his water-culture tanks to the fluoride-free rats. That he sometimes gave different, soil-grown food to control rats *with* fluoride in the 1953 experiment, was criticized by an anonymous article in the May, 1954 issue of the journal **Nutrition Reviews**.

That the two groups were fed completely different diets, was called

"an obvious departure from sound experimental procedure." [37]

This is a fair criticism, as both sets of rats should have been fed only the water-culture diet, with added fluorine for one group.

McClendon's conclusion of fluorine's essentiality is based upon the belief that the water-culture diet was complete in all other dietary essentials. This is questionable when one set of rats was fed soil-grown food and was healthier.

For example: if the water-culture crops were calcium deficient, McClendon would have seen poor teeth and growth rate, and attributed this to lack of fluorine. Given he was looking at teeth, it would have been only more difficult for him to define a difference between deficiencies in calcium and deficiencies in fluorine. Perhaps a similar case could be made for phosphorous. This becomes an even more valid point when we see previous experiments had minimized fluorine levels, and McClendon never discussed levels of fluorine in diet or carcasses.

This anonymous author also wrote:

"The extremely slow growth of the control rats was not commented upon. The average gain of 10 g per week among the controls is so far below the usual growth rate of 85 g per week that these rats must have been deficient in one of more nutritional essentials."

I will remind the reader that the rats in the 1954 experiment died quickly on the water-grown crops; this was obviated by milk with added fluorine [13].

No information was given on the amount of nutrients in the plants, nor in the carcasses of rats, nor on the growth of rats in the 1954 experiment, however there were fertility problems on the fluorine-free rats fed the water-culture diet. McClendon did not discuss the **Nutrition Reviews** article, presumably his report, published a month after his own 1954 work had already been submitted.

The following point is made by **Nutrition Reviews** with regard to the plants needing or not needing fluorine:

> "The growth of a foodstuff devoid of any element must depend on whether that element is essential to the plant."

> "Certainly, on the basis of the studies by McClendon and Gershon-Cohen… we have no right to accept the essentiality of fluorides for rat growth nor the toxicity of comparable low amounts of fluorides in the second generation. Studies of both the above types lend themselves to misinterpretation and misrepresentation of the facts and may easily serve to obscure well-substantiated data obtained from more carefully planned and conducted experiments." [37]

McClendon's work was also criticized for never discussing levels of fluorine in diet or carcasses. Maurer and Day wrote,

> "no data were given on the fluorine content of either the diet or the animals." [17]

Doberenz and co-workers wrote,

> "… no data were presented on the fluoride content of the tissues of the animals at the beginning or end of the experimental period…" [19]

That this can occur in four of his write-ups (three papers and one abstract) over ten years of experimentation is perhaps one reason why his experiments are hardly mentioned, even by those who support fluoridation. His work is seemingly only mentioned in scientific documents, only once discussed in American media [38], and when mentioned by fluoridation advocates like Mitchell and Edman, Harrison and Bell, it is mentioned in passing with no real detail. About a month after the first draft of this book I eventually found a couple of very brief articles touching on his work in New Zealand archives. These are mentioned in Chapter 3.2.

The reason such absent analyses were important is explained: at the *beginning* of the experiment, it is wise to check that the rats' store of fluorine is low, otherwise even those fed a diet very low or absent in the element being tested can use the "stock" of it that they have in their body, and at the *end* of the experiment, it is to see how much of this element (and others if relevant – we're looking at teeth, so calcium and phosphorous levels would also be important) remains. Instead, McClendon measured fluorine levels in urine and faeces of rats fed his fluorine-free diet, claiming there was none, therefore any fluorine in the rats fed the water-culture crops would have been there since birth. Given fluorine's proclivity for bones and teeth, it is not surprising he found none. There is something else we must consider: fluorine ions in water are more absorbed than food fluorine. This probably explains why he saw none. This may lead us closer to a conclusion of essentiality at first glance, if one considers retention a demonstration of necessity. Yet retention on its own is a not a demonstration of necessity if a specific purpose cannot be identified. Put in layman's terms, just because it's there, does not mean it's doing anything.

McClendon's results on their own are impressive in the 1954 experiment, yet the method and information presented are lacking in detail.

In McClendon's experiments the rats on the fluoride-free diets were fed plants grown in altered rain water. As much water comes from below the earth, plants with deep roots will not be sucking up rain water until it has passed through soil, probably influencing its mineral content.

In addition, soil bacteria helps plants utilize beneficial compounds in the earth: there is a symbiotic relationship between plants and soil inhabitants that is not reproducible in the method McClendon and his co-workers have used. For these reasons I think his conclusion of essentiality is weakened or compromised.

McClendon had his own doubts: he said toward the end of his experiment

"... furthermore, there is doubt as to whether all essential food components are known." [12]

He means known *to science* or to human knowledge. He's putting his own experiment in a bigger picture context with this statement. I believe he is suggesting his water-culture crops may have been deficient in potential unknown necessities.

In the previous chapter I pointed out that McClendon and Gershon-Cohen wrote:

"The best crop yields were obtained from sunflowers. Corn was not always well pollinated. Legumes produced lower yields and rice did not head in the short season." [12]

Processed foods and purified chemicals do not create healthy offspring. One is led to wonder whether his all-plant diet was protein deficient, with no dairy or meat. They did use yeast, important for some amino acids, yet the two could not find a halogen-free variety. In 1972 Armstrong *et al.* pointed out that fertility problems are often associated with nutritional deficiencies – it's obvious that he meant animals, but I would suggest there is a possibility it applies to plants, based on increased levels of mutation in DNA replication in the absence of transition metals available during replication [39, 40].

The "rice not head[ing]" refers to a reproductive stage in rice growth.

"Rice is said to be at the 'heading' stage when the panicle is fully visible. Flowering begins a day after heading has completed. As the flowers open they shed their pollen on each other so that pollination can occur." [41]

Perhaps the growth issues of the plants were simply a reaction of the water-culture crops to their unnatural growth medium: filtered rainwater and purified chemicals. Even though the chemicals were basically nutrients, calcium etc, the incredible variety yielded from natural soil is bypassed.

Maurer and Day used casein in their diet, a milk protein with phosphorous and calcium (both very important components of teeth). They used the word "dispensable" to describe fluorine.

"There was no indication of difference between the fluorine-deficient and fluorine-supplemented males." [17]

McClendon gave his rats fluoridated milk and kept them alive longer; he didn't discuss the effects of his diet's lack of dairy on the rat. Milk also contains proteins and fats which may have helped the rats' lifespan. However, note the massive reduction in carious molars in the rats with the use of fluorine in water in the 1954 experiment [13].

I believe it can be suggested easily that McClendon's fluoride-free rats have suffered deficiencies of other nutrients. In 1941 Professor McCollum had found potassium important for development of rats [42].

There isn't enough detail in the 1944 and 1945 writings [11] to suggest the same thing is happening there – although this in itself can be criticized. In the 1953 experiment, McClendon and Gershon-Cohen wrote that their water-culture technique had evolved over nine years [12].

McClendon's experimental design itself, is an argument *for* the abundance of fluorine, and an argument *against* the realistic possibility of a fluorine deficiency occurring under normal conditions.

In the application of these experiments to humans, every city's water supply is probably different, none (or very few) of us drink distilled, or deionized water, which is what is often used in laboratory conditions. It is possibly *this*, more so than differences between humans and rats, that potentially disqualifies rat experiments.

From an experimental perspective, the fact that McClendon had to go to such fastidious lengths to minimize fluorine levels may render the conclusion of essentiality less effective, due to the probable nutritional deficiencies created in the rats fed water-culture crops. It may also inspire a renunciation of a belief in the possibility of fluorine deficiencies.

Then again, perhaps this can be turned around: from an evolutionary perspective, one may argue that since we have evolved with this element in such abundance, perhaps its essentiality is more elusive. For instance Gautier's idea [7] regarding the fluorine to phosphorous ratio may become more worthy in light of McClendon's effort. Or perhaps there were a lot of volcanic explosions tens of thousands of years ago, and we're slowly adapting to the fluorine that was emitted [43].

The worst thing about McClendon's conclusion of essentiality was that he ignored the conclusions of the experiments carried out in the 1930s [6, 8, 9]. His opinion of them would have been worth including. Surely these early experiments were relevant if he was working in the 1940s and 1950s? Is it enough to publish results that contradict the findings of previous studies without considering the possible reasons?

Regarding fluorine's essentiality in plants: in 1945 Mitchell and Edman wrote that there was no evidence to suggest fluorine essential for plants [10]. McClendon claimed in 1954 that plants grow without halogens or sodium [13]. In 1971 the National Academy of Sciences (discussed in Chapter 2.1) pointed to one study suggesting fluorine essential for corn as a lone contender, but not plants in general.

Turning to the issue of dental health, in 1953, Mitchell and Edman would cite McClendon's 1944 abstract, along with a 1950 experiment by O. Rygh [44] in reference to the statement,

"... it [fluorine] may be essential to the formation of a normal tooth." [45]

They didn't cite any of the other experiments I have shown at the beginning of Chapter 1.1.

The paper by Rygh concluded fluorine and calcium both very important for enamel; neither worked without the other. Rygh suggested that the fluorine content of enamel was higher than the inner osseous layer of the tooth underneath it, which contained a lot of calcium, and that fluorine would do nothing to strengthen enamel if calcium underneath it was insufficient. (Although strontium and vanadium could excite the action of calcium; barium, zinc and thallium could affect ossification by removing it. Fluorine, beryllium and silicon had no effect *here* according to Rygh). The enamel would turn transparent, and eventually break with poor calcification underneath. Rygh claimed there were three experiments looking at calcium salts in osseous tissues – I believe he meant dentin. This made a fourth. He claimed fluorine had no effect on these tissues (the layer beneath enamel).

No details on diet were given beyond the facts that the animals were rats and guinea pigs, and the experiment went for ninety days. While Rygh found fluorine was not required for the inner part of teeth, he wrote of enamel,

> "The enamel of the teeth needs fluorine for its proper formation." [44]

He claimed it was necessary for fluorine to be available when the enamel is forming, pre-eruption.

> "The fluorine must be supplied before or during the enamelling of teeth. At other periods a fluorine supply is not so useful…" [44]

Rygh cited his own work published the year before, wherein he claimed to have

> "… succeeded in producing an experimental diet absolutely free from all traces of inorganic nutritive microelements and suitable for experiments with rats and guinea pigs." [46]

He claimed it impossible for the animals to live longer than four weeks on this diet, however with the addition of salts

> "of nutritive micro-elements compounded on the model of seaweed ash are added to this basic diet, the animals live as long as reasonably required and are even capable of reproduction."

Seaweed of course, is high in minerals. Rygh concluded that strontium and barium were of "vital importance" using a stock of more than 500 animals. He called strontium "indispensable." He wrote that without adequate strontium and/or vanadium dental caries appeared in the animals, even though the diet contained calcium, phosphorous and Vitamin D in "sufficient quantities".

I have not researched strontium or vanadium in teeth in much depth, but Underwood's early work followed this a little [25]. The third edition of his very detailed textbook *Trace Elements in Human and Animal Nutrition* claimed the work of Rygh was "unconfirmed" in 1971.

Biochemist Frank McClure from the (US) National Institute of Dental Research would cite the paper by Mitchell and Edman in a book he published after his retirement in 1970. He cited this to conclude that fluorine does not have the dimensions of a nutrient. I don't know why he looked at their paper regarding this topic as their comment on essentiality seemed made in passing. His attitude to fluorine's essentiality [47] is discussed in more depth in the next chapter.

In 1954, Joseph Muhler wrote, in his experiment on low-fluorine (0.1 ppm), "purified" diets:

> "The most common finding was related to the difficulty of obtaining young from rats receiving the highly purified diet. After many attempts to obtain second generation rats, a different diet had to be used. Attempts to determine if this was due to the highly purified nature of the diet or to the lack of fluorine were inconclusive…" [16]

In 1958, Dr. Muhler concluded that fluorine was an essential nutrient. An abstract of his paper that focussed on previous experiments was published in the **Journal of the American College of Dentists**. He mentioned:

> "carefully conducted animal studies, the first of which was published in 1933" [48]

Presumably here he meant the Sharpless and McCollum experiment. He claimed these did not demonstrate fluorine's essentiality, when growth was used as the primary criterion.

He said that studies done at Indiana University resulted in "inconclusive results" regarding fluorine's ability to improve growth and reproduction, although he said there were "repeated suggestions" that a case may be made for such a claim.

He claimed McClendon's results

> "demonstrate the necessity for fluorine in order to maintain growth and to promote resistance to dental decay."

Muhler wrote:

> "Based upon these latter experiments [by McClendon] and upon extensive human data showing statistically significant reductions in dental decay in areas where fluorine is present in the water, one must conclude that fluorine is an essential dietary factor. It may be classified as 'essential' as a result of its proven effect on resistance to dental caries, in the same manner as many other nutrients are essential for promoting optimal health for only one physiological function of the body." [48]

In 1959 Muhler co-edited the book with M. K. Hine, which contained the chapter Muhler had written entitled *Is Fluorine A Dietary Essential?* (The 1958 abstract mentioned previously is taken from this work.) This book was cited in support of fluorine's essentiality, along with the second edition of Underwood's textbook [25] by Frank Smith in 1966 [21].

Muhler introduced this chapter with the statement quoted earlier:

> "Perhaps one of the most troublesome aspects of this question is not the technical problems of the investigations, even though they are quite difficult to resolve, but rather the uncertainty about the term 'dietary essential' itself. The words have quite different meanings to different people, depending very often on which field of investigation the research worker belongs to." [24]

Dr. Schwarz will serve as a splendid example of this (also quoted at the beginning of this chapter, and see Chapter 1.1).

In the same document Muhler wrote,

> "Perhaps future scientists will recognize the concept that fluorine is essential to the "normal" development of sound teeth, and that this fact in itself is sufficient to put fluorine in the category 'essential'. Certainly, the status of present evidence condemns the concept that it is 'nonessential.'"

Citing a paper by Schulz and Lamb from 1925, Muhler quoted

> "It is quite generally considered as being one of the inorganic elements essential in [human] nutrition, which is necessary in small amounts only, although there is no evidence of its necessity except its occurrence in the animal body." [50] (The word 'human' added by Muhler).

As well as this study, Muhler looked at the work of Sharpless and McCollum 1933, Evans and Phillips 1939, McClendon 1944, 1953 and 1954, the anonymous entry in the May 1954 **Nutrition Reviews**, the Maurer and Day experiment of 1957, his own 1954 study, his Ph.D. thesis [14], and a few others I didn't think relevant to include.

He pointed out that most studies evaluating fluorine deficiencies had done so by looking at amounts in the skeleton; I haven't studied these beyond his 1954 experiment and what little else I've mentioned in chapter one.

(Fluorine accumulates in the skeleton. Human research is discussed in Chapter 6. Takao Suzuki, whose work is discussed below, found 14 ppm in the bone of rats fed food containing less than 0.5 ppm. Evans and Phillips found 54 ppm in bone after 7 months on food containing 0.1 ppm [9]. The 1965 text by Smith and Hodge mentioned a study by Smith, Hodge and another that looked at the ash of ribs and vertebrae of newborn humans that contained 50 to 60 ppm. The mothers ate food containing 0.06 ppm fluoride [22]. Charles Weber writes about a 1937 experiment by Marcovitch, Shuey and Stanley that fed rats rice and milk with 0.6 ppm added for 35 days. Bone fluoride analysis showed 50 ppm. Other rats were fed cryolite with 4 ppm and yielded 117 ppm in bone, those fed 7 ppm yielded 239 ppm [51]).

Muhler suggested that studies focussing on weight and reproduction "have not contributed significantly to our knowledge."

> "The promotion of resistance to dental caries would seem sufficient reason to classify fluorine as an essential element, especially if repeated human studies and experimental studies similar to those of McClendon and Gershon-Cohen continue to show the need for fluorine. On the basis of these studies, many of which required several years to conduct, it is still not possible to state unequivocally whether fluorine is essential for growth in human nutrition." [49]

Muhler pointed out that no diet has been completely empty of fluorine, and that those diets used by McClendon and Gershon-Cohen had an unknown amount of fluorine (noticed by others). He also stated that purification of diets may affect growth and reproduction (obviously other factors too) simply by the purification process itself. This is because in removing fluorine, other nutritional components are removed as well.

> "Attempts to add fluorine alone to improve such diets result in inconclusive information."

> "It can be stated with certainty that there is strong suggestive evidence from the studies of McClendon and Gershon-Cohen, as well as from human studies in natural and artificial fluoride communal fluoride areas, that fluorine is essential for dental health. This in itself should classify fluorine as an essential element." [49]

Fluorine's abundance had defied the creation of a deficiency, yet the necessity was apparent from the benefits.

He then states that fluorine's role in the calcification process needs "much further study", perhaps being of "physiological significance."

In 1970 Muhler would change his mind and write in a World Health Organization monograph that more research was needed on the subject of fluorine's essentiality. This is discussed in more detail in the next chapter. Without being able to access his archives or interview him, it is difficult to follow his reasoning on what is probably to many, a minor issue. Perhaps an American researcher will find an answer.

McClendon did not demonstrate that the water-culture crops were sufficient in terms of calcium, iron, protein, fats and other nutrients required (recall Dr. Messer's first criterion), but some may argue he didn't need to, because his 1954 results show 10 mg fluorine (added to water) was required to prevent cavities in all but 6% of molars. That 1 mg added to milk – something with known, necessary nutrients – did not prevent as many cavities (25% carious molars) is certainly indicative of at least, a beneficial effect solely attributable to fluorine, at most, a conclusion of essentiality. I believe the latter is what Muhler took from this experiment.

At the end of the chapter, Muhler states that fluorine can be classified essential because of its role in caries reduction, and that studies on rats with extremely low fluorine diets (for example the Maurer and Day experiment using 0.007 ppm) and perfectly functional teeth don't qualify it to be non-essential.

An experiment [52] discussed in Charles Weber's 1966 PhD thesis [53] didn't help: A whole-milk powder was used as a diet for rats in 1925. The animals lost the ability to reproduce, until sodium fluoride and potassium iodide were added. Weber claimed that no information was available regarding the content of protein or other dietary essentials. The beneficial effects of the compounds added could not be attributed accurately, as the compounds were added together. This meant that the researchers were unable to conclude whether it was sodium, fluorine, potassium, or iodine that had helped repair the reproductive capacity, or a combination of those four, or one or more of those four in concert with already available dietary ingredients.

Weber also discussed a 1929 study from Argentina that found quicker growth with 50 mg fluorine per kg of body weight daily in rats [54]. After three or four months the growth of the rats was depressed and after six months their weight was 20 percent less than the control rats, without added fluorine. This escalation, then depression of activity is perhaps similar to the effect of a stimulating drug: an increase of activity (hy*per*-activity), followed by a decrease of activity (hy*po*-activity). The female reproductive cycle of these rats given added fluorine was also impaired.

Of McClendon's work, Weber wrote,

> "No data for dietary or carcass fluoride levels were presented in any of the three papers by McClendon and associates."

Phillips, Hart and Bohstedt said *if* there was a need for fluorine, 100 microgram per day was enough for the rat [8]. Phillips and Evans said *if* there was a need for fluorine, 50 microgram per kilogram of body weight was enough for the rat [9]. Mitchell and Edman concluded 27 microgram per kilogram of body weight enough [10].

According to a 1925 experiment by Professor McCollum, rats' teeth grow 2.5 millimetres per week, on average [55].

Looking at the experiments performed by Sharpless and McCollum, Evans and Phillips, Muhler, Maurer and Day, Doberenz *et al.*, [6, 9, 16, 17, 19], Charles Weber wrote in 1966,

> "... effects of fluoride on reproduction is questionable and there is a good chance that dietary factors other than fluoride have been involved in the results. The purification of diets to remove the fluoride raises the question of what else may have been removed in the process." [53]

In 1938, Dr. Wallace D. Armstrong[6] investigated the average fluorine content of enamel in sound (non-decayed) and carious (decayed) teeth. He concluded that carious teeth contained less fluorine than sound teeth. He conducted a little over eighty analyses, and concluded that these results,

> "being due to chance alone is somewhat greater than 5,000,000 to 1, a probability so remote as to demonstrate that the difference is certain." [56]

Funnily enough, he claimed a cautious attitude, with a willingness to change the implications of the data, were different information to come to light. After suggesting his certainty, he wrote:

> "The low fluorine content of enamel of carious teeth, most probably not being secondary to the carious process, must therefore, *if associated with the condition in any manner,* bear a causal relationship." (His emphasis.)

Put simply, he was suggesting low fluorine content causes caries. He was also claiming it improbable that caries cause low fluorine.

> "The fact that teeth exhibiting severe degrees of mottled enamel and containing a considerably increased amount of fluorine may become carious does not argue against the hypothesis set forth above."

(Why would decay not diffuse over an entire surface of a tooth, instead of being confined to one or more particular spots or places? Armstrong explains there are factors which induce caries such as food residue and certain geometric aspects of teeth, for instance places of attrition where teeth meet in chewing, as well as gum margins.)

In 1963, Dr. Armstrong performed a reinvestigation of his 1938 research, and reversed his position. He concluded that,

> "No difference in fluoride content of enamel of sound teeth from that of the sound enamel of carious teeth was found with teeth of persons in the same decade of life. The results demonstrated that an increase in fluoride content of the whole sound enamel of carious and non-carious teeth occurred with increasing age. These findings invalidated a correlation, with caries status..." [57]

He cited two experiments, one that agreed, and one that disagreed (by Frank McClure) with his 1938 investigation. He cited four experiments that looked at fluorine content of teeth increasing with age. These led him to consider that age should be a factor in a reinvestigation.

The age of individuals was not mentioned in the 1938 investigation,

> "because age, as a factor in enamel fluoride content, was not then appreciated." [57]

He believed this reinvestigation "confirmed and extended" the work of others who had looked at fluorine content of teeth increasing with age. I did not find the 1938 experiment cited in either of Joseph Muhler's papers, though I would be surprised if he did not know of it.

All of the experiments discussed in this and the previous chapter suffer for one perhaps subtle reason: they are looking at diets that have had the ratio of fluorine to other elements reduced.

---

[6] The same Dr. Armstrong featuring in the experiments of the early 1970s with Dr. Messer and Dr. Singer discussed in Chapter 1.1.

The conclusive strength of *all* these experiments is weakened by the fact that the *ability* of an element to function is possibly influenced not only by the amount of *that* element, but of others. Elements interact with each other. Consider the 1976 experiments demonstrating fluorine's pharmacological effect on iron absorption [33, 34].

Essential fatty acids are one example of ratios being important in nutrition. Omega-3 (alpha-linolenic acid, ALNA) and omega-6 (linoleic acid, LA) are substances used in the building of cell membranes and other cellular components and architecture. They're also very important in metabolism, oxygenation of tissues, and numerous other functions. The ratio of omega-6 to omega-3 in many people is about 20:1, yet a healthy ratio is about 3:1 [58].

Recall that DeEds quoted Gautier as saying the fluorine to phosphorous ratio was one to five, in minerals and in the human body [7]. In teeth, some may argue it's about the same. One of Armstrong's papers from 1946 put phosphorous levels in teeth at a little over 17% [59], one of his earlier papers put fluorine at between zero and 3.5%, using seven studies. To quote:

> "The analyses made since McClure's [1803-1933] review have indicated a lower fluorine content of teeth and teeth structures than had been found by the older investigators." [60]

McClendon and Gershon-Cohen claimed the teeth of their rats were saved from decay with 20 ppm of fluorine in water. Consider that Phillips and Evans in 1939 claimed 10 ppm is where dental fluorosis begins in a rat ("the borderline zone for bleaching of the teeth occurred at a level of 10 ppm". This was between 2.5 and 3.0 mg fluorine per kilo of body weight per day, above 3.0 mg, bleaching of teeth always occurred. "Neither aluminum at the level fed here nor the percomorph oil prevented bleaching of the incisors.") Perhaps this was due to the rats in the 1939 experiment having a better diet all-round[7].

This 1939 experiment fed 20 ppm fluorine, aluminium, and the two elements together, only to experience failure in reproduction, though this was not the case for those rats given the oil. I would suggest the percomorph (fish liver) oil, with Vitamins D and A, may have helped counteract the effects of excess aluminium and fluoride [62].

Do experiments "cancel each other out"? The 1954 experiment by McClendon and Gershon-Cohen [13] had additions of 0.004 ppm in the fluorine-free rats, yet their teeth were still carious. Doberenz *et al.* in 1963 managed to grow rats in 0.005 ppm fluorine – hardly a huge difference – with no stunted growth, and no problems in teeth mentioned [19]. I'm amazed this wasn't discussed by more people involved, for it suggests more than just fluorine may affect our teeth. How important is fluorine compared to calcium? Less important? More important? What about when compared with phosphorous and magnesium and other building blocks of teeth? These questions are discussed more throughout Chapter 6.

---

[7] McClendon and Gershon-Cohen used albino rats, well known for their reaction to fluorine [61]. Evans and Phillips, in this experiment gave no more details than "young rats, weighing 40 gm each."

Another man who had an influence on this question of a nutritional role for fluorine was Dr. Mark Hegsted. Mark (he liked a first name basis) earned a Ph.D. in 1940 from the University of Wisconsin, and worked for the famous Dr. Fredrick Stare (who recruited four other alumni also from the University of Wisconsin) at the Department of Nutrition in the Harvard School of Public health until 1978, when he went to work at the U.S. Department of Agriculture.

In 1967, Mark wrote:

> "The time has come to consider whether or not fluoride should be classified as an essential nutrient. Although many people consider an essential nutrient as one which must be provided in the diet in order to permit survival, this definition is not adequate."

> "Numerous examples may be provided where this is not true." [63]

His examples were that vitamin D can be obtained from sunlight, vitamin K and other vitamins can be obtained from gut microflora. He said the amino acid arginine is considered essential for the young rat. Due to difficulty in its synthesis, it is not quick enough "to permit normal growth."

Mark wrote:

> "Thus, it would appear more suitable to define an essential nutrient as one which is ordinarily required for normal growth and development under the usual conditions in which people live."

> "... It is proved beyond doubt that maximal resistance to dental caries requires the consumption of fluoride even though the flora of the mouth and the kind of diet consumed may be important." [63]

He was elected to the National Academy of Sciences (NAS) in 1973, however this does not seem to have changed the NAS' point of view on fluorine's essentiality (see the next chapter), which was mostly negative when animal experiments were used. He was the recipient of many awards and honours, and the author of over 400 papers [64].

In 1969, Takao Suzuki from the Department of Hygiene, Tokyo Dental College, performed an experiment over three generations of rats,

> "to elucidate the essentiality or non-essentiality of minute fluoride..." [65]

The rats were fed a diet of 0.45 ppm fluoride, (he claimed about one hundredth the usual amount in commercial rat food), with doses of water with fluoride concentrations of 0.0, 0.5, 1.0, 10 and 50 ppm. Suzuki wrote that blood examinations showed no significant differences in "erythrocytes and leucocytes count, hematocrit, ALP[8] and GOT[9]." His experiment is written mostly in Japanese, but bullet-pointed in English.

In the introduction I have discussed how I had read newspapers quoting experts from "both sides" of the fluoridation debate regarding a necessity for the element. Publicly, there were very few deviations from the general pattern of those who wanted it added to the municipal water supply believing it an essential nutrient,

---

[8] Alkaline Phosphatase, an enzyme used to test a variety of liver and bone disorders.
[9] Glutamic-oxaloacetic Transaminase, an enzyme that can indicate liver damage in excessive quantities.

and those that didn't want it added, believing it non-essential. The subject was not mentioned often in the newspapers.

One can see a flexibility in definition and criteria.

Dr. Hegsted and Dr. Muhler have claimed a widened definition of the term "essential" – the word can be stretched to include, or encompass other words like "beneficial." Sometimes 'essentiality' (or 'necessity') means 'benefit and/or necessity', and sometimes 'essential' means only benefit, and no longer means 'essential' at all. Hegsted's words have been quoted by Nielsen and Sandstead [27] from the U.S. Department of Agriculture, and Australian researcher Eric J. Underwood [25].

In my opinion there are more politicians on the fluoridation-supporting side; possibly this helps with the pliability of precise terms and the changing of definitions. I've *only once* seen pliability of definitions discussed in media with regard to fluorine's essentiality, yet as you can see the topic *is* discussed in the scientific literature.

Those opposed to fluoridation obviously look to the animal experiments – those of Maurer and Day, Phillips, Weber, etc, and claim the element non-essential, for the reason that no real, definable deficiency state has been shown to exist. Advocates of CWF have cited these in technical documents but not in public, though they were happy to champion the Schwarz and Messer *et al.* studies. This coupled with the fact that no diet ever had absolutely zero fluoride, making the exercise in testing difficult, suggests there is enough of the element in basic diets to go around.

That rodent teeth were perfectly functional with no apparent problems, suggests that maybe fluorine is *not always* needed to confer maximum resistance against caries. Or that if it is needed, it is needed in such tiny amounts as to be almost negligible.

Those opposed to CWF also point to the fact that research from the early 1970s was refuted, and obviously take a stricter definition of the word "essential."

The important factor we must consider is one of honesty and accuracy: have the people writing articles in newspapers and the like been open and honest about telling the public that definitions have changed?

Or has a semi-misleading picture been presented publicly? Ideally, we should *at minimum* be completely transparent about what criteria we are using, assuming we are discussing this in public. This is obviously based on the assumption that we want the public to know the truth as best they can.

1.3 Discussion

After looking through literally thousands of media articles, my impression is that the public has been given almost no knowledge whatsoever that criteria for fluorine's essentiality may be compromised to include benefit, or may be as subjective and relaxed to the point where it's "in the eye of the beholder".

This imprecision can result in an inflation or exaggeration of fluorine's necessity or importance. This is discussed in more detail in chapters 4 and 5.

I have not found recent American, physical, experimental research that looks into this topic of essentiality in much depth, even though there is disagreement, seldom discussed. The experimental work I have collected is very dated, and has possibly suffered from a lack of technology's precision. However I have not found recent research from any other country on this topic, if I had I would have included it here.

More recent statements from experts are made in following chapters.

The primitive nature of the early experiments may have led to diets far more in natural compatibility with animal biology. Heavily purified and refined food may be representative of laboratory conditions. Fluorine occurs widely and has a tendency to increase in calcified structures over time.

It is sensible of the reader to inquire about the stances of the scientists quoted here regarding Community Water Fluoridation (CWF). Dr. Wallace Armstrong and Dr. Joseph Muhler were both promoters of CWF and very public about it. Dr. John Suttie became an official member of the National Academy of Sciences in 1996, a group (discussed in the next chapter) that has consistently endorsed CWF. Suttie co-authored a 1971 document for the NAS on air pollution. I did not find any instance of him recommending or cautioning against CWF openly in media. He investigated the effects of fluorine pollution on humans and animals for the aluminium industry in the 1960s and 1970s, this is discussed briefly in Chapter 5.6.

Dr. Isaac Schour, the dental histologist of Illinois University's College of Dentistry, had examined the teeth in the unpublished Lawrenz experiment prior to 1945, the year CWF began. According to Donald McNeil (author of *The Fight for Fluoridation*), Schour was a friend of Dr. E. L. Sevringhaus, the committee chairman who was investigating the fluoridation of Madison, Wisconsin in 1946. According to McNeil, Schour said

> "... that unless Madison was prepared to spend several thousand dollars annually for 'careful studies', the city should wait ten to fifteen years until experiments elsewhere were completed." [66]

No reason for Schour wanting to wait is given by McNeil. This hardly puts Schour in the same boat as others who were openly opposed to CWF. Schour was described by McNeil as a "firm opponent of mass fluoridation" by 1947. It is difficult to believe these things would have influenced Schour's appraisal of Lawrenz's pre-1945 research, and this is hard to tell given that no year is mentioned [10], but I will stand corrected should I see evidence. Though I have no problem believing McNeil, I've never seen evidence of Schour's opposition, and McNeil presents no reasons for it. In my years of research, I've only seen his name appear in McNeil's book, in relation to the Lawrenz work, and in a 1952 study I quote from briefly in Chapter 6.4. In the January, 1956 issue of the **Journal of the American Dental Association**, an article discussed Schour's winning of the Columbia Alumni Medal for "outstanding contribution in dental research."

Dr. Paul Phillips' name is prominent in research on fluorine, but I have never come across an article in which he himself recommends or opposes CWF.

It was impossible for researchers to create a diet with absolutely zero fluorine/fluoride, due to the abundance of fluoride compounds[10]. Some may argue that this makes it difficult to say for certain that fluoride is *definitely not* a trace element – something required[11] in less than a concentration of 10^{-5}M (this is going from a 2003 definition – see the list at the beginning of this book). Yet we have no "fluorine deficiency" to point toward, which would help categorize it as a trace element.

However, the fact that diets extremely low in fluoride, yet abundant in other elements and compounds, have yielded animals with no problems in health, make it very easy to say that fluoride is *definitely not* an essential nutrient, this is using a definition meaning it is required in amounts of *more* than 10^{-5} M. It has been suggested that in removing fluoride from a diet, other elements and compounds that are definitely important or essential are sometimes removed; this can sometimes explain why some animals in laboratory conditions suffered. Animal experiments and human experiments are both appropriate and problematic in their relation to public health and human nutrition in some ways. Scientists have tested many different diets on animals to see where nutritional limits are.

Rat incisors (the two sets of two teeth at the front of the mouth) grow approximately 2.5 millimetres every week, are worn down by attrition (grinding against each other during chewing), thus a low-fluoride diet in a rat with perfectly fine teeth is a good indication of fluoride's *complete* non-essentiality, and an indicator of the importance of other nutritional and possibly even lifestyle factors. It's easier to scrutinize the near-exact composition of diets, even over generations, in animal experiments. To do this in humans is problematic – humans live long enough to make multi-generational experiments impractical and expensive. Short experiments can suffer in precision because humans eat different foods on holidays and eat foods imported from different countries. Trade and political arrangements may affect foods brought into various countries, scientists may be unable to measure the nutritional worth of their subjects' parents' diets, which would have affected the subjects 'stores' of certain nutrients in bone and organs.

Essential nutrients and trace elements are called such because they are *required*, not because they are simply beneficial (but see the previous footnote). Community Water Fluoridation's benefits have been used as a criterion for fluorine's nutritional essentiality. I have found almost no examples of the changing of definition debated or contested within public (media) literature, though in some instances in the scientific literature the experts are forthright in stating benefit is the criterion used to demonstrate essentiality. The examples I have found are recent.

Nor have I found examples of other elements or compounds wherein benefit is a criterion for necessity.

---

[10] There is only one exception to this, the 1968 experiment discussed in Chapter 1.1. There is no remark or comment made by the scientists who make the claim - clearly they thought it insignificant. When compared with other experiments, such a finding is clearly not.

[11] I have yet to see a definition of the term 'trace element' that is 'useful but not required' though some possibly exist, and some people use the term as though this is what it means, without defining it. All dictionary definitions that *I* have seen claim that a trace element is necessary in some very small amount.

2.   What Do Experts Say about a Nutritional Role for Fluorine/Fluoride?

"At the end of the day we're guided by the experts."

- Dr. Rob Beaglehole, Spokesman for the New Zealand Dental Association on Water Fluoridation, quoted in **The Nelson Mail** (New Zealand), 16th May 2015. [67]

In this chapter I will present what various experts have written throughout the years about the necessity for fluorine or fluorides. Note that this is in *some* ways *separate* to a necessity for *Community Water Fluoridation*. This becomes a little difficult when we see the topics overlap. That this has occurred should be obvious, and often serves to make the subject more daunting.

This chapter differs from the previous chapter in that these writings are more public, and while some contain references and citations to experiments, very few *are* experiments. I consider this kind of work "halfway between experiments and newspapers" – if it could be put into a more casual context. These reviews summarize and comment on experiments, and they're available to the general public, but with a little more effort than that needed to obtain a newspaper.

American research has influenced the understanding of the rest of the world hugely, so an American origin is a very important thing to present. I will begin with the American National Academy of Sciences (NAS), as they represent a prestigious, well-respected group, often of senior scientists. Their work on *necessity* for fluorine has been, in many instances, consistently evidence-based, this is at least how it appeared to me at the beginning of my investigation.

What the NAS says about benefit from fluorides and fluoridation is available for others to investigate; I have not looked at more than what has overlapped the subject of what the group says about fluorine's essentiality.

However, the NAS' stand on Community Water Fluoridation (CWF) is similar to that of many governments and dental groups around the world: that it is a safe, effective way of preventing dental decay.

It appears to me that they have maintained this stance since the introduction of CWF. In this investigation they will serve as a worthy benchmark of understanding. This is because they have an evidence-based approach, they represent a prestigious position among United States science, and they are a non-profit organization. This at least, was my impression going into the study.

2.1 What Does the U.S. National Academy of Sciences Say?

The United States National Academy of Sciences (NAS) was established in 1863 as a "private, nongovernmental institution to advise the nation on issues related to science and technology", according to their website [68]. Nowadays about 6,000 experts work for the NAS writing and investigating topics that are of importance to America.

The majority of the following publications are freely available on the NAS website, www.nasonline.org, though they can also be found in libraries in New Zealand, and presumably around the world. I can only encourage readers to obtain the publications.

In compiling this research, I decided to observe if and how professional opinions of experts have changed over the decades. In case of the NAS this has been very worthwhile, and somewhat tragic. The most thorough investigations that the NAS have done on fluoride's essentiality that I have found were carried out in 1971, which looked at five experiments [69], and in 1974, which cited eight experiments, yet was only half as long in explanation [70]. In the late seventies and early eighties, the NAS did not worry so much about fluoride's essentiality, and in their publications kept it included in chapters on nutrition. They acknowledged for the most part that there was no real necessity for fluorine, thus no RDI (Recommended Daily Intake – one would have this for elements that *are* essential) so instead spoke of 'optimum/optimal' amounts.

The NAS have basically accepted the animal experiments regarding essentiality. They have applied these to animals and humans with little to discriminate between the two, however some NAS publications deal with only animals, this being evidenced by publication titles (most publications here deal with fluoridation of *human* drinking water). Using animals for experimentation makes sense from a methodological standpoint – it is easier for animal experiments to be performed according to Dr. Messer's first criterion: that a diet used for testing fluorine's essentiality should have all other necessities in abundance (so that we don't end up calling an iron deficiency a fluoride deficiency, as Messer *et al.* did).

> "A specific deficiency state should be produced by a diet lacking the element in question, but which is otherwise adequate and satisfactory." [4]

This is obviously very difficult to do in a huge city with millions of people. Consider that in order to come close to *exactly* fulfilling this criterion one would have to monitor each participant's intake of not only fluorine, but of *all* nutritional components, *and* consider the amount of fluorine already stored in individuals at the beginning of the experiment. If such an experiment *did* occur, it would probably be compromised by the amount of estimation.

I have not found any NAS publication discussing the benefits or drawbacks of the use of Community Water Fluoridation (CWF) experiments in cities as a test for fluorine's essentiality. I have looked through at least thirty-six NAS publications, a small number considering there are eight thousand freely available on their website, and probably more that are not online. I'm unaware how many of these eight thousand deal specifically with fluorine or fluoridation.

While the excerpts of the documents here are looking at fluoride's essentiality, most of them claim it is beneficial in the prevention of dental caries. Where benefit has been claimed as a criterion for essentiality I will point this out. The NAS are believers in 1.5 to 4 mg as an adequate amount per day (for adults) and ardent advocates of CWF as a means of achieving this [71]. These figures are taken from a 1997 document which is cited in a 2017 document [72].

To give an example, in 1968 the Food and Nutrition Board of the Nutrition Research Council (NRC – a subgroup of specialists from the NAS) called fluoridation "a very important nutritional public health measure…" and mentioned the "nutritional advantages that result from fluoridation of the water supply."[73]

The National Research Council of the NAS in 1951 wrote that,

> "Under normal conditions of living, fluorine is a trace element in human nutrition. A variable and important source is drinking water. Many of the public water supplies in the United States are deficient in this element."
> [74]

In a paper submitted in 1846 to the *Royal Society of Edinburgh*, George Wilson M.D. carried out a review on the chemistry of fluoride in animal bone and plants [75]. Worldwide, many chemists before him had found contradictions regarding fluoride content of animal bones, with some always claiming a presence, and others claiming none whatsoever. Given the poor technology and lack of methodological uniformity at the time, this is understandable. Wilson's own experimentation used fluorine from bone to etch glass. His conclusion was quite philosophical. The following statement from Wilson is cited by Dr. Gerald Cox in a NAS publication, dated 1952:

> "… physiologists will doubtless now be tempted to speculate on the possibility of fluorine performing some essential function in living animals. Its occasional absence from their bones would not disprove that it may be necessary for the perfection of certain organs, though not for all.
>
> "Quantitative analyses appear already to have indicated that the enamel of teeth contains more fluorine than any other part of the body. If that result shall be confirmed, we may suppose that, if fluorine be furnished when the development of the teeth is proceeding, it may be wanting at other periods, without injury to the animal; just as chloride of sodium must be considered as essential to the healthy life of most creatures, though they may be deprived of it for long intervals, without death ensuing.
>
> "The small quantity of fluorine found in living structures can be counted no argument against its occasional or constant importance. Quantity, is at best, but a rude measure of the value of an ingredient, in relation to the necessities of an organism. The law of final causes, in truth, would indicate that only a minute proportion of fluorine should occur in any organ; for it would be perilous to an animal to introduce into its system a large quantity of fluorides, which can so readily be changed into the deadly hydrofluoric acid. Such speculations, however, are premature. It will be time enough, when many qualitative, but especially quantitative, researches have been prosecuted, as to the presence of fluorine in animal structures, to consider of what service it is to them; if it be of any." [76]

Fluoride's effects have been considered pharmacological in nature. The NAS wrote in 1971 regarding rodent experiments:

"if fluoride is a dietary essential for the species studied, its requirement must be extraordinarily low. Indications that fluoride might be essential for any other species are also lacking, and the beneficial effects of fluoride on dental health or bone metabolism should be considered as pharmacologic responses, and not as a cure of pre-existing deficiency condition. [69]

Please bear in mind this was *before* the Tao and Suttie experiment in 1976 which claimed,

"The results of the present study suggest that the apparent essentiality of fluoride previously observed [in the Messer *et al.* experiments] was due to a pharmacological effect of fluoride in improving iron utilization in a diet marginally sufficient in iron." (page 1115)

"It seems more likely that relatively high levels of fluoride (50 ppm in the drinking water) are able to exert a beneficial pharmacological effect on the utilization of iron when suboptimal concentrations of iron are present in the diet." [33] (page 1121)

This 1971 document [69] cited the second (1962) edition of Underwood's classic [25], a study on osteoporosis from Harvard that they said was not relevant to the issue of essentiality (basically reflecting the argument "just because it does something, doesn't make it essential"), the chapter from the book by Muhler and Hine [24]. This differs to what the NAS wrote over a decade later, that fluoride's beneficial effect,

"...in itself is no indication of fluorine essentiality, inasmuch as caries incidence depends on many factors, and many persons with perfectly sound dentition have only had minimal exposure to fluoride."[69]

Here, the NAS are not using benefit as a criterion for essentiality as Muhler was in 1959. I have looked through two others I have cited in the previous chapter [17, 53], and a couple of studies testing fluorine's effect on plants, which they claimed were 'unconvincing'.

Rats have a much higher tolerance for fluoride than humans. Remember this beneficial pharmacological effect was seen in rats; I have seen no discussion on whether the same has been demonstrated in humans.

This 1971 document, like the two published the year before (see below, McClure and the World Health Organization), was a little ambivalent about fluorine's essentiality. The authors wrote:

"It cannot definitely be concluded from these experiments that fluoride is nonessential for the nutrition of these species." [69]

In 1974, in **Effects of Fluorides on Animals**, the NAS wrote,

"... it has not been possible for most investigators, until recently, to prepare nutritionally adequate diets that are either wholly devoid of fluoride or sufficiently low to demonstrate conclusively that it is or is not required."

In support of this statement they cited experiments by Evans and Phillips [9], Wuthier and Phillips [18], and Joseph Muhler's Ph.D. [14]. Discussing experiments of McClendon and Gershon-Cohen (1953 [12]), Messer *et al.* (1972 [28, 29]) and Schwarz and Milne (1972 [20]), the NAS wrote,

"These findings suggest a deficiency state that is specific for fluoride. Although the question of whether fluoride is an essential nutrient has not been completely resolved..." [70]

The NAS did not mention the criticism of the 1953 work (see Chapter 1.2), nor Nielsen and Sandstead's criticism of Schwarz's work (see Chapter 1.1).

In 1979 the NAS wrote in **Nutrient Requirements of Swine**, that fluorine was "required by one or more species, probably are also required by the pig but at such low levels that their dietary essentiality has not been demonstrated." [77]

The 1974 study by Dr. Messer *et al.* mentioned Walter E. Brown, Ph.D., as claiming that between 0.0002 and 0.002 ppm fluoride "should be sufficient to promote apatite formation *in vitro*." [78]

"The widespread occurrence of F may prevent its complete elimination from animal systems, and thus preclude a convincing demonstration of its requirement in calcification." [31] (page 428)

The NAS **Drinking Water and Health** volumes 1 and 2 did not discuss a nutritional role for fluorine in any real depth.

NAS **Drinking Water and Health** volume 3, published in 1983, referred to fluoride as a nutrient at first (p. 4). In the Executive Summary they state:

"When the intake of a particular nutrient by the general population or a particular group is marginal, the contribution by water may be important in preventing deficiency and ill health. This may be the case for magnesium, fluoride, iron, copper, zinc, vanadium, and chromium."

But later on (p266) the authors introduce a slight uncertainty about putting fluoride in the category:

"... decided against including an in-depth review because of its uncertainty concerning fluoride's essentiality to nutrition. However, in view of the contribution of fluoride to overall dental health and, through this, its effect on total health, some discussion of fluoride has been included." [79]

With regard to deficiency, the NAS told us in this report (p. 281) that fluoride's benefit was demonstrated in humans, and that low-fluoride diets were associated with dental caries.

Then in a chapter titled "Toxicity Versus Essential Levels", under the subheading "Deficiency" the NAS told us:

"Fluoride has not been shown unequivocally to be an essential element for human nutrition, except for its effectiveness in reducing the incidence of dental caries."

And:

"The fluoride concentration in drinking water is not critical for caries protection."

They cite research from Schwarz and Milne (1972 [20]), Messer *et al.,* (1972 [28], 1973 [4]), Tao and Suttie (1976 [33]), and Wegner *et al.,* (1976 [34]). They followed this eventually with a sub-chapter titled "Contribution of Drinking Water to Fluoride Nutrition" (p. 282).

The 1989 **Diet and Health: Implications for Reducing Disease Risk** called fluoride "an integral part of the food chain" but did not define this in greater detail [80].

Also in 1989, the NAS published the tenth edition of **Recommended Dietary Allowances**, in which they looked at some of the research relating to fluorine's role in nutrition (Schwarz and Milne 1972, Weber and Reid 1974, Messer *et al.* 1973, Tao and Suttie 1976), and wrote,

"These contradictory results do not justify a classification of fluorine as an essential element, according to accepted standards." [81]

However, the NAS put fluoride in the category 'Trace elements'. Trace elements are often defined as required, see the definitions provided.

Citing this work, the 1991 NAS publication **Nutrition During Lactation** told us "… fluoride is not considered to be an essential nutrient…"

However, it was considered beneficial. They also noted that caries is a "multifactorial disease."

"The subcommittee found no studies that directly assessed the relationship between the mode of feeding in infancy and the incidence of caries." [82]

The 1993 publication, **Health Effects of Ingested Fluorides**, told us that

"although fluoride is no longer considered an essential factor for human growth and development[12], many believe that there is an optimal dose of systemic fluoride for maximal benefit against caries." [83]

This statement is made over ten years after the most recent known American research, and fluoride was still considered non-essential. However, this would change.

In 1997 the NAS introduced the term "Dietary Reference Intakes" (DRIs) which

"replace[d] the periodic revisions of the Recommended Dietary Allowances (RDAs),"

used since 1941.

"DRIs encompass the Estimated Average Requirement (EAR), the Recommended Dietary Allowance (RDA), the Adequate Intake (AI), and the Tolerable Upper Intake Level (UL)." [71]

The differences in these terms are explained below, in the 2008 document.

1997's **Dietary Reference Intakes for Calcium, Phosphorous, Magnesium, Vitamin D and Fluoride** includes fluoride as a nutrient, but not essential (I didn't know this was a category when I read this) [71]. There is much written on reasons why an Estimated Average Requirement (EAR) cannot be used, so pages and pages are written on Adequate Intakes (AI), which is based on an amount the NAS claims is most beneficial in caries reduction.

It was reading this 1997 document that I began to see something strange in the writings of the NAS. I'd already seen a 2007 document (mentioned in a letter to an editor discussed in Chapter 5.1) that put fluoride in the essential category with selenium, calcium and the rest, and I think it was here that I saw them moving closer and closer to this conclusion of essentiality without actually formalizing it with research or reason for a change in criteria. Possibly by this time of course, the research carried out on animals in the 1950s and 1970s was considered not quite as relevant as it used to be, and there were more than enough studies concluding beneficial effects from CWF to warrant an essential status.

Fluorine's abundance had defied the creation of a deficiency, yet the necessity was apparent from the benefits.

As far as children in fluoridated communities with bad teeth were concerned, the element almost *had* to be essential… possibly (?)… probably (?)… because of the amount of junk food children were eating. (One of the NZ Minister of Health's letters claimed New Zealanders would continue to suffer serious tooth decay "unless we could eliminate all sugary foods…"discussed in Chapter 3.)

---

[12] Here they cite the work of the National Research Council from 1989 [81].

This is where we find an overlap – childhood tooth decay is a painful, seemingly malicious thing inflicted upon the young, sensitive and innocent. Why would it even matter if fluorine was in some nutritional category?

How could CWF *not* be essential? If it could prevent even a tenth of the suffering it's supposed to, *anyone* would be in favour of it.

You can see that this is where we step away from the question "is *fluorine* an essential nutrient?" and ask, "is *Community Water Fluoridation* an essential step in preventing cavities in children?"

These are two separate questions and it is easy to see how the specific division between them may blur with imprecise or non-specific definitions of words, or in emotional arguments.

Protecting children's teeth was paramount, drawing lines between different classifications of nutrients could take a back seat to suffering children. This mentality is a *good* thing. It comes from a good intention, or at least a practical intention – that helping children is more important than classifying data.

It seemed a foregone conclusion. The NAS spent so much time with studies claiming a benefit from CWF, it just about had to be a necessity. At first glance I couldn't blame them for changing their conclusion, what with previous documents tracing deprivation experiments with stricter controls back to the 1970s (or the 1930s and earlier if one spent a little more time). If you've ever read a newspaper article on fluoridation, or seen it discussed on social media, you may believe there's no middle ground. This must make it difficult for the NAS (or anyone) to be neutral about it. They had written of animal experiments as authoritative for so long, yet human experiments seemed to demonstrate so much benefit from fluoridation, this must have affected their decision.

I believe that the late nineties is when the NAS began to change their tune, albeit without even knowing it. There is variance in the authorship of these documents, but still I noticed a flow toward fluoride becoming more and more a requirement for good nutrition, with experimentation regarding concrete proof of a demonstrable necessity or a deficiency state less and less relevant.

One is led to consider the number of people involved in these committees, and how often they may move and change, as well as committees simultaneously carrying out investigations, each committee with different study goals.

In 2001, the NAS publication **Nutrient Requirements of Dairy Cattle** included fluorine as a "perhaps" in the category of trace mineral, to be required in milligram or microgram amounts. They devoted half a page to fluorine and summarized:

> "Although fluorine in very small amounts can increase the strength of bones and teeth, it is generally not regarded as an essential dietary component." [84]

In 2006, the NAS published **Dietary Reference Intakes: The Essential Guide to Nutrient Requirements**. I think it demonstrated that the NAS was one step from finally calling fluorine essential. In a chapter called "Criteria for Determining Fluoride Requirements, by Life Stage Group," they looked at Adequate Intake (AI), a value based on the prevention of dental caries. That fluorine was "vital for the health of teeth and bones" was evidenced by a sub-chapter entitled "Inadequate Intake and Deficiency" [85]. It appears that this document was heavily influenced by the 1997 document mentioned previously.

In 2007, the NAS published **Earth Materials and Health: Research Priorities for Earth Science and Public Health**, a document that included fluorine as a trace element among "mineral elements currently considered essential for human health and metabolism" in the trace elements section, along with phosphorous and iodine [86].

Work by the NAS only six years previous had been outright contradicted with no acknowledgement or explanation given for this. It is relevant that the 2001 work looked at cattle and the 2006 and 2007 work looked at humans.

The citation given for fluorine's essentiality was a 1979 paper by E. J. Moynahan, published in the Philosophical Transactions of the Royal Society of London. Moynahan's opening comment was sensible – what we see with regard to deficiency states in animals we should see in humans. Though this had only been proven in five elements – iron, copper, iodine, cobalt and zinc. Most of his paper focusses on these. He claims "there is no precise definition of a trace element" – the term itself was used when analyses were not accurate enough to measure the tiny amounts of certain elements in body tissues. Moynahan posits the same requirements as Lindh for an element to be considered essential, mentioning the name Cotzias.

Moynahan listed fluorine under the heading "Essential Trace Element Deficiencies Awaiting Confirmation in Man". This is quite incredible given the huge number of pre-1979 claims made by experts in newspapers that fluorine was a trace element in which our teeth, soil and water were all deficient (see Appendix 1). He claimed it appeared essential, saying this was evidenced by the way in which it prevents decay when added to water in CWF. Personally I would consider this a case of "benefit as a criterion for essentiality". He believed it was unclear at this time whether fluorine affected microbes on the tooth, or incorporated into the enamel. He cited none of the experiments I've mentioned in Chapter 1 beyond Underwood's 1977 work and the 1974 symposium (this document in regard to zinc).

Turning to page 39 in the 2007 NAS document, we see two diagrams – one the typical bell-shaped curve with deficiency, normal, then toxic effects as consumption goes from lesser to greater in essential elements; and a horizontal line that veers off into "toxic" then lethal effects as consumption increases in non-essential elements – no "deficiency" state exists in this second diagram.

In 2007 the NAS misread or misquoted the 1979 paper which claimed deficiency should be demonstrable and "specific". In my opinion there is only one reason why they did not quote Moynahan's categorization word for word. Fluorine would be considered non-essential.

Relevant also is a 2005 textbook called *Essentials of Medical Geology* [87]. Pages 161-177 are cited by the NAS [86] regarding the abundance of various elements. This is Chapter 7, written by Gerald F. Combs, Jr. of the US Department of Agriculture's Agricultural Research Service. On page 162 we see a table with three columns: *Accepted essentials, Suspected essentials,* and *Known or implicated functions.* Fluorine is in the *Accepted essentials* table and its known function is "protects against dental caries". Combs looks at many elements – iron, potassium, chlorine, magnesium, phosphorous and more. On page 167 Combs tells us that fluorine can stimulate new bone formation and reduce acid production from plaque bacteria. This, along with "enhanced remineralization of dental enamel" is considered a cariostatic (inhibits dental caries) effect. Combs tells us that people drinking water concentrations of at least 0.7 mg per litre would have between 40 and 60% less dental caries. He states that while dental fluorosis is "a largely cosmetic effect", skeletal fluorosis can lead to stiffness of joints and other bone problems. In his summary, Combs tells us that fluorides are required, just like calcium, phosphorous and magnesium.

Regarding the reduced acid from bacteria, a 1990 study from Chow is cited [88], as well as a textbook, the *Handbook of Nutritionally Essential Mineral Elements* by Boyd O'Dell and Roger Sunde, both of the University of Missouri [89]. I'm sure fluorine's property as enzyme inhibitor is believed useful in thwarting the proliferation of bacterial acids.

The study from Chow observes work performed on cariostatic effects of tooth-bound fluoride in "recent" (before 1990) literature. It suggests topical application may be aided by including a "dicalcium-phosphate-dihydrate-forming treatment" to aid further fluoride incorporation into the tooth.

The textbook by O'Dell and Sunde is very detailed and lengthy. Combs cites the twentieth chapter, authored by Florian L. Cerklewski of the Department of Nutrition and Food Management of Oregon State University, who casually claimed fluorine was a nutrient in his first paragraph, yet later on expressed that this was not definite. Due to time and other factors, I am only showing a small number of his claims here, future editions of my work will include more.

After a small focus on the history and basic properties of fluorine, Cerklewski concluded his first paragraph by claiming presence and benefit as criteria for essentiality:

> "Fluoride is classified as a trace element because the total body content of fluoride is less than 5 g and it is beneficial when consumed at levels much less than 100 mg per day." [89] (page 583)

Compare this with the definitions of trace element provided at the start of this book, noting the difference between "beneficial" and "required". He opened his second paragraph by pointing to H. Trendly Dean's 1938 study on mottled enamel[13]. He then suggested (with some ambiguity) that Dean believed or claimed fluorine to be a nutrient:

> "The observation by Dean, however, demonstrated that, like other nutrients, fluoride can have either a positive or a negative effect on metabolism, depending on the level of intake."

---

[13] H. T. Dean, *Endemic Fluorosis and its Relation to Dental Caries*, **Public Health Reports**, Vol. 53, No. 33, pp. 1443-1452, 1938.

In the study cited that was authored by Dean[13], there was no claim that fluorine should or should not be considered a nutrient. In fact Dean actually expressed more of a curious or quizzical attitude, asking (on page 1451) if the higher fluoride content of mottled enamel was the "immunity-producing factor" and whether fluorine's role as enzyme inhibitor was responsible. Dean then claimed that:

> "... the possibility should not be overlooked that other [non-F] elements of comparatively rare occurrence in water or ordinary constituents of drinking water present in unusually large concentration may directly or through a synergistic action with the fluoride, produce the observed effects. For this reason, it appears essential to obtain as complete chemical analyses as possible of the domestic water of communities which are under investigation for dental caries." (see footnote)

If Dean had claimed fluorine was a nutrient in other work (and he quite possibly had), Cerklewski did not cite or discuss it. I don't think there's anything dishonest about Cerklewski's words here, I think they simply demonstrate that essentiality is presupposed much of the time. Dean pointed to the possibility of other elements influencing decay; this is almost never done in any detail in much promotional work on fluoride.

The sixth section of Cerklewski's chapter is one paragraph entitled *Pathology of Fluoride Deficiency*. I will discuss this more in future editions due to time and publishing constraints (I am currently still working on obtaining and reading many of these experiments). He cited seven experiments here, three of which he claimed showed an inhibition of kidney calcification, saying:

> "It is likely that the mechanism of this effect involves fluoride's affinity for calcium, but definitive data in this regard are lacking." [89] (page 591)

He cited a paper[14] by Donald Taves, which concluded there were lower rates of coronary heart disease in fluoridated versus non-fluoridated cities. He then pointed to three experiments looking at fluorine's relationship to blood, claiming two[15] [34] showed it lessened the effects of iron deficiency in haemoglobin and haematocrit, and claiming the other did not [33]. All of the experiments he cited in this section except for the work of Taves were carried out on rodents. He also looked at fluorine's relationship with osteoporosis. This topic is discussed in my work a little in Chapter 6.2, though I have left out Cerklewski's research.

Cerklewski's final statement on requirement for fluorine cited a report by Walter Mertz (of the U.S. Department of Agriculture, and Temporary Adviser to the 1973 WHO Technical Report Series 532):

> "Although fluoride can only be classified as an essential element if a broad definition is used [16]..." [89] (page 593)

---

[14] D. R. Taves, *Fluoridation and Mortality Due to Heart Disease*, **Nature**, Vol. 272, pp. 361-362, 1978 (Taves of the University of Rochester's School of Medicine and Dentistry). Taves' study contained data from thirty-five cities. Not included in Cerklewski's one hundred and thirty citations was another study published the same year in the **American Journal of Epidemiology** that contained heart disease data from four hundred and seventy-three cities and concluded there was "no consistent relation between fluoridation and observed changes in mortality" (Vol. 107, No. 2, pp. 104-112). Both studies looked at a 20-year period.

[15] F. L. Cerklewski, J. W. Ridlington, *Influence of Zinc and Iron on Dietary Fluoride Utilization in the Rat*, **Journal of Nutrition**, Vol. 115, p. 1162-1167, 1985.

[16] Walter Mertz, *The Essential Trace Elements*, **Science**, Vol. 213, pp. 1332-1338, 18th September, 1981.

If this is true, then we should not consistently read in media (see Chapter 5) that fluorine is like iodine, like selenium, and other nutritional factors (see Chapter 5). It appears to me that most experts likening fluorine to iodine and selenium, and claiming us, our waters and soils are all deficient in it, are unaware or unconcerned of the weaknesses upon which the claims of deficiency rest.

Mertz's criteria:

> "An element is essential when a deficient intake consistently results in an impairment of a function from optimal to suboptimal and when supplementation with physiological levels of this element, but not of others, prevents or cures this impairment [See figure 2]. Essentiality is generally acknowledged when it has been demonstrated by more than one independent investigator and in more than one animal species." [16] (page 1332)

He then lists a group of elements "considered essential in animals" – iodine and selenium are present, fluorine is not. Then of fluorine, he wrote:

> "Growth depression resulting from deficiency of fluorine and tin and growth stimulation following supplementation with these elements have been reported, but not yet confirmed."[16]

He cited a presentation of Dr. Schwarz, published in a 1977 book[17]. From the one sentence Mertz provided, this appears no different to what Dr. Schwarz had claimed in the early 1970s.

> "Nevertheless, fluorine can be considered essential on the basis of its demonstrated effect on dental health."

Here, Mertz cited page 364 of the 1970 WHO document *Fluorides and Human Health*. Strangely, he did not mention its contradictions regarding fluorine's essentiality (discussed in Chapter 2.3). My copy of this document only goes up to page 354, following this is the index, so perhaps this is a typographical error, or he intended to cite the concluding remarks: that fluoride had an "outstanding ability" to prevent decay, though the exact mechanism was unknown.

In the statement quoted ("Nevertheless…") Mertz also pointed to Figure 1 of his article – a picture of the periodic table with fluorine and other elements considered essential shaded in. It's relevant to the primary claim of expert exaggeration I make that he did not point to Figure 2 of his article – a bell-shaped curve typical of trace elements, with death, deficiency and marginal states at one end, optimal in the middle[18], then marginal, toxicity and death from excess at the other.

When Mertz discussed what constituted a trace element, he pointed to this curve. When he discussed fluorine, he pointed to the periodic table with fluorine and other elements highlighted. Bear in mind Mertz knew a thing or two about trace elements. There's a very important disparity here that I believe he saw – "death" in his curve as a result of a deficiency state, and no death from lack of fluorine. In the textbook featuring Cerklewski, there are discussions on death from lack of iodine, death from lack of potassium, death from lack of selenium. Death

---

[17] K. Schwarz, in *Clinical Chemistry and Chemical Toxicology of Metals*, by S. S. Brown, Ed. (Elsevier/North-Holland, Amsterdam, 1977), pp. 3-22.
[18] Note that this is "optimal concentration of an element in tissue" and should *never* be confused with "optimal amount of fluorine in water".

from lack of fluorine is not discussed. I have seen it mentioned only once beyond the few refuted rodent experiments in Chapter 1, in a newspaper article discussed in Chapter 5.2.

On page 1335 of his article he has a table in which he claims the "deficiency signs" in animals are "caries, possibly growth depression" and in humans; "Increased incidence of caries; possibly risk factor for osteoporosis" – summarizing with "Deficiency and excess known."

These of course should be considered along with the rest of the claims and evidence presented; I also refer the reader to Chapter 2.3.

Cerklewski continued:

> "... if a broad definition is used [here is the citation to Mertz], its valuable effects on dental health have been recognized by the statement of a provisional recommended dietary allowance."

Here he cites pages 235-240 of the tenth edition of the National Academy's **Recommended Dietary Allowances**.

The first paragraph of page 235 discussed fluoride's abundance in food, water and soil, and its excretion from the human body. Quoting the second paragraph:

> "The status of fluorine as an essential nutrient has been debated. Several studies in rodents have provided conflicting results." [81]

Five of the rodent studies I discussed in Chapter 1 are quickly summarized in this paragraph, then the NAS conclude the contradictions do not warrant the inclusion of fluorine in elements considered to be essential "according to accepted standards", however they claim it is still beneficial to humans.

I am tempted to jest that Cerklewski did not read this paragraph, though this is unlikely given that he presented the further claims on "estimated safe and adequate intake" that the NAS explained on pages 237-239. I do not know why he would leave it out of his sixth paragraph given that he had accepted other rodent experiments, including the Wegner *et al.* experiment. He possibly thought it unnecessary.

Cerklewski finished his chapter by looking at future (post 1997) research. He pointed to the benefits, though claimed that "the exact mechanism" by which the benefits accrue, "remains unclear."

His work is similar to other work, in that he began by claiming fluorine essential, then later admitted this is only true if definitions are broadened.

In their introduction, O'Dell and Sunde [89] point to four methodologies used in discovery of essential function: purified diets, parenteral nutrition ("intravenous infusion of highly purified nutrients"), the study of mammals living in environments thought to be deficient in certain elements, and fourthly, "the determination of the basis of certain genetic diseases." Gene mutations may occur if DNA is not replicated accurately. Without cations like magnesium, DNA polymerase enzymes come off the DNA strand, which can lead to mutations [40].

O'Dell and Sunde claim that the most important of these is the purified diet. One can see why the experiments in Chapter 1 are cited by prestigious scientists in the WHO and the NAS. O'Dell and Sunde claim the parenteral nutrition methods an extension of these dietary purification experiments. They write that deficiencies were discovered accidentally, presumably a researcher would observe a lack of function in a life form and then measure concentrations of elements in soil and water. A possible complication in these experiments is noted; that an essential element may be abundant or optimal in diet, yet obscured or inhibited in its use by another element or compound. The next section of their introduction is called *Definition of Essentiality*. They claim that an element is essential if it is required to support growth, reproduction and health throughout the organism's life. The obvious question is *how much* of these things are adequate – where does one draw the line?

> "Under normal circumstances, an element is clearly essential if a distinct pathology results when it is omitted from the diet." [89]

Consider this statement with regard to the experiments mentioned in Chapter 1.

They claim essentiality is less definable in a changing environment, with small changes in growth or microbe-infected animals.

As a "pertinent observation that led to the discovery of the essential element" the 1938 work of Dean is cited for fluoride (see footnote previously). The authors note it is not the only relevant study. One page over, fluoride is in the category *Essentiality suggested by physiologic impairment*. They note that some of the elements in this category are expected to be placed in the other category, *Essentiality confirmed by biochemical mechanism(s)*, along with calcium, phosphorous and others.

The next section of their work looks at roles of biological elements: *structural*, *catalytic*, and *signal transduction*. They discuss how elements like phosphorous, sodium, potassium and chloride are important in protein structure and nerve function. They discuss the catalytic functions of iron, iodine, copper, manganese and zinc. Cobalt only functions as a part of Vitamin B_{12}, yet there was no necessity for cobalt as an ion. They discuss molybdenum and selenium deficiency.

The following section of their work is called *Mechanisms by Which Mineral Elements Exert Function*.

> "Fluoride is probably unique among the essential micro elements in the sense that its function appears to be more protective than catalytic. Low fluoride intake often results in dental caries, but it is not essential to prevent caries under all conditions."

> "Fluoride is a structural component of bones and teeth, but there is no evidence that it exerts a specific biochemical function." [89]

They also claim sugar has a large role to play in development of caries.

Also of relevance here are the sixth and twelfth chapters of *Essentials of Medical Geology* [87] (this was cited by the 2007 NAS document mentioned previously [86]). The sixth chapter is called *Biological Functions of the Elements*. I quoted this at the beginning of Chapter 1.1. It begins by looking at what constitutes an essential element. Author Ulf Lindh [19] says definitions have provoked much discussion, and that the earliest was borrowed from protein chemistry.

---

[19] Lindh is Senior Researcher at the Biology Education Centre, Uppsala University, Sweden.

The element should be present in living tissues in a reasonably constant concentration, it should cause problems – "anomalies in several species" when removed, and these anomalies should be corrected upon reinstatement of the element.

This is very similar to what Messer *et al.* wrote in 1973 [4]. Lindh proposes the "current" (1998) definition:

> "An element is considered essential to an organism when reduction of its exposure below a certain limit results consistently in a reduction in a physiologically important function, or when the element is an integral part of an organic structure performing a vital function in the organism."[20] (page 115)

Lindh notes problems associated with proving necessity and ascertaining exact requirements. Much of this has to do with what has been said previously, namely reduction of *only one element* is difficult in food preparation. Removal and reduction of one element may effect uptake of others, and this of course leads to ambiguity of results.

Detection is also sometimes difficult. In terms of knowledge regarding necessary trace elements, we can be more certain about animal needs than human needs. Lindh doesn't say it, but this is probably true for toxic effects and upper limitations of tolerance as well. He takes us through roles and properties of magnesium, calcium, nitrogen, sodium, potassium and chlorine.

When he comes to a section called *The Functional Value of Trace Elements* he writes:

> "The paramount function is to be necessary for the structure and function of significant biomolecules, mainly enzymes." [87] (page 125)

Enzymes are made of amino acids; to my knowledge fluorine is not a necessary component of any amino acid. This is concluded from two textbooks I used throughout my time studying [90]. I do not believe it is required in enzyme activation. When I studied DNA replication, this was done with cations like magnesium.

He writes that most trace elements are transition elements, and in the fourth row of the periodic table. He goes on to discuss vanadium, cobalt and nickel, then chromium, molybdenum and tungsten. Then manganese, iron, copper, zinc, selenium and iodine. He discusses in great detail these elements and their relationships with gene expression and proteins, and some practical applications of this knowledge.

The twelfth chapter of *Essentials of Medical Geology* contains three statements regarding fluorine deficiency:

> "Fluorine is an essential element in the human diet. Deficiency in fluorine has long been linked to the incidence of dental caries, and the use of fluoride toothpastes…" (p. 301)[21]

> "In the early studies, a strong link between caries and low-fluoride water emerged and this led, as early to 1945, to the fluoridation of fluoride-deficient water supplies in Grand Rapids, Michigan." (pp. 302-303)

A 1950 study from Maier is cited [91], no experiments or contradictions in literature were mentioned beyond this. The third statement from *Essentials of Medical Geology* is:

---

[20] Lindh cites *Review of the Scientific Basis for Establishing the Essentiality of Trace Elements*, **Biological Trace Element Research**. "An expert panel" of the WHO/Food and Agricultural Organization/International Atomic Energy Agency (Mertz, 1998).

[21] Chapter 12 authored by Professor Mike Edmunds and Dr. Pauline Smedley, both hydrogeochemists of the British Geological Survey, NERC.

"Surface waters rarely have fluoride concentrations sufficiently high to be detrimental to health and if fluoride-related health problems exist, they are more likely to be linked to deficiency." (page 325) [87]

The paper by Maier did not go into any detail regarding deficiency, though it acknowledged that there was a sixty percent reduction in dental caries in people whose water was fluoridated at 1 ppm, when compared with people whose water was not (note this is a concentration, not a dose). Much of this article focused on costs and availability of various compounds used in CWF, and of companies that supplied feeding equipment.

Maier wrote early in the paper:

"That the removal of fluorides from water will prevent one disease, while their addition to water will prevent another, entirely different defect from developing, is one of the most curious reversals in the history of water supply engineering." [91]

He means the causing of dental fluorosis and the prevention of tooth decay. He went on to discuss fluorosis a little, claiming it would occur in children drinking water with over 1.5 ppm.

This (1.5 ppm) is currently the WHO guideline, according to a 2004 WHO document [92], and the British Geological Survey's website [93].

I do not know if, or how much the Maier paper influenced this guideline, the WHO website does not give the bibliography of the 3rd edition of this document, and the 4th edition does not directly cite Maier's paper [94].

Deficiency was mentioned three times in Chapter 12 of this textbook [87], with no real desire to address the actual definite creation of a deficiency, even though many experiments had looked at this. Maier seemed to take fluorine deficiency as factual and real, and he did not give a citation to further evidence after his statement quoted above.

In 2008, the NAS again looked at an AI for fluoride, based on the following reasoning:

"The Estimated Average Requirement (EAR) is the level of intake for which the risk of inadequacy would be 50 percent. The RDA (Recommended Dietary Allowance) is two standard deviations (SDs) above the EAR, covering 97 percent of the population. The Adequate Intake (AI) as a reference value was not envisioned until the lack of dose–response data precluded study committees from determining the level at which the risk of inadequacy would be 50 percent. This was often exacerbated by a lack of longitudinal studies[22]. As a result, AIs were generally set when an EAR could not be established. These include calcium, vitamin D, chloride, chromium, fluoride, potassium, manganese, sodium, and vitamin K." [95]

I should point out to the reader that there have been literally thousands of studies carried out on the differences between fluoridated and non-fluoridated cities, and in many instances the NAS has used *none* of these as a worthwhile test for the question "is fluorine an essential nutrient?"

The NAS had sometimes included fluorine with elements known to be necessary based on its benefit. Essentiality was implied because of benefit. It seems that when the animal studies (see Chapter 1) were

---

[22] An explanation of longitudinal studies can be found on the **British Medical Journal** website, *Epidemiology for the Uninitiated*: "In a longitudinal study subjects are followed over time with continuous or repeated monitoring of risk factors or health outcomes, or both." [96]

discussed, they were treated as having authority regarding the issue of essentiality in NAS publications. (I must also mention a 1958 document from the NAS discussed in Chapter 5.2 that uses benefit as a criterion.)

The format of this 2008 investigation allowed the public to ask questions of the experts. Dr. Sanford Miller was invited at one point to contribute to the discussion by Dr. Coates, who "noted Dr. Miller's considerable experience with DRI development." Miller suggested that AIs were,

> "developed primarily as 'placeholders' because no other data were available to allow a recommendation to be made."

Miller explained that in cases where no value has been supplied at all, there is an implication that any amount of an element is safe, a belief potentially leading to negligence, thus the need to give *some* numbers to at least hopefully keep things sensible.

These publications seem to have a huge amount of information but I question the practicality of memorizing how much of every element or compound we need daily, and counting or adding up each item to ensure we're in the 'enough' part of the spectrum, in between 'deficient' and 'excess'. Common sense and convenience cry out for a simpler way.

In this summary of 14 samples, I have marked 3 for essential, 7 for non-essential, and 4 for maybe or undecided.

I have not included Walter Brown's experiment in this sample. I have included the document **Nutrient Requirements of Swine** as a maybe or undecided, and the 2006 DRI document as essential, and I have not included the 1958 document. I believe it is more relevant in the chapter on media, although it would go in the essential pile if you wanted to add it (taking the sample size up to 15).

Sometimes it's good to state the obvious, just so we're all equally grounded in our understanding, and are less prone to hyperbole and exaggeration. People authoring the NAS documents change, which inevitably has an effect on content. It is worth noting that when the NAS consider more research, in the form of studies that test for essentiality, they seem to be more likely to come to a conclusion of non-essentiality [69, 70, 79, 83].

In the literature that claims fluorine essential, the NAS have either used benefit as a criterion for essentiality, assumed essentiality but noted that fluorine's abundance defied the creation of a deficiency, or looked at almost no studies that have to do with essentiality [77, 80, 85, 86].

2.2 U.S. Government Literature

A 1956 New York City Health Department document prepared by Dr. Norman Jolliffe gives the definition:

> "Whether fluorides are to be considered a "nutrient", a "medication" or "poison" depends on the amount entering the body." [97]

Would this mean titanium could be a nutrient if only a trace entered the body? Implied in Joliffe's statement is the bell-shaped curve typically seen when one discusses trace elements, yet Joliffe does not mention any deficiency state. Joliffe then goes on to compare fluorine with Vitamin D.

In 1991, the United States Public Health Service (USPHS) published a document that claimed to be a "comprehensive review and evaluation of the public health benefits and risks of fluoride in drinking water and other sources."

Regarding a necessity for fluoride, the authors wrote,

"Although fluoride compounds occur naturally, both in the environment and in most constituents of the body, there is no conclusive evidence that fluorine or any of the fluoride compounds are essential for human homeostasis or growth[23]. Researchers have found that, depending upon the level of exposure and the mechanism involved, fluoride produces beneficial or adverse effects." (page 7) [98]

I have not found anything to suggest these experiments mentioned by the USPHS have concluded an essential role for fluorine.

"In summary, it is not yet clear whether fluoride is essential for reproductive performance."

(This sentence under the heading "Human Studies".)

A document from the US Department of Health and Human Services dated 2003 states that,

"the human database mostly consists of epidemiology studies designed to assess whether consumption of fluoridated water is associated with adverse health effects, particularly skeletal effects and cancer."

"Most of these studies are community-based and do not provide data on individual exposure levels or the particular fluoride compound." [99]

It said that fluorosilicic acid and sodium hexafluorosilicate were the "primary" compounds used in Community Water Fluoridation (CWF) programs, however monofluorophosphate and others used in dental treatments would contribute to total fluoride exposure.

I believe (and I'll stand corrected if I'm wrong) a lack of "individual exposure levels" have allowed a relaxation of criteria surrounding what constitutes an essential nutrient. Dr. Messer's first criterion has slowly become less relevant, the untold benefits of fluoridation have pushed it aside.

"Conflicting results have been obtained from animal experiments addressing whether fluorine is an essential element. Much of this conflict appears to result from the great difficulty in preparing an animal diet that has negligible amounts of fluoride, but otherwise allows normal animal growth and development." [99]

The authors noted that experiments by Messer *et al.* in 1973, and Tao and Suttie in 1976 demonstrated a benefit in iron absorption through the intestine. They also pointed to the 1957 Maurer and Day experiment which demonstrated almost no need (<0.007 mg/day) at all for fluoride.

This document also cited the WHO 2002 document (see below).

"The World Health Organization (WHO) considers fluoride to be 'essential' because it considered 'resistance to dental caries to be a physiologically important function' (WHO 2002)." [99] (p. 74)

---

[23] Here the USPHS cite McIvor ME, Cummings CC, *et al.*, *The Manipulation of Potassium Efflux During Fluoride Intoxication: Implications for Therapy*, **Toxicology** 37(3-4):233-40, 1985.

2.3 What Does the World Health Organization Say?

The World Health Organization (WHO) was founded in 1948 when diplomats in 1945 came together to create the United Nations. There are approximately 7000 people working worldwide with/for the WHO [100].

The reader may be offended at the absence of a more detailed investigation into what the WHO have said about fluorine's status as essential or non-essential – why should *they* not be in the position I have put the National Academy of Sciences (NAS)?

I believe that American research has influenced the behavior of New Zealand's experts more than the WHO, at least around the 1950s, when Community Water Fluoridation began in New Zealand. Dr. Muriel Bell, a New Zealander, was a co-contributor on the 1970 WHO monograph, discussed below. Dr. Bell was heavily influenced by American researchers.

This 1970 World Health Organization monograph – note the word '*World*' – meaning *the whole sphere* – has two sections on fluorine's essentiality/non-essentiality that are written by Dr. Joseph Muhler, an American, and Dr. P. Venkateswarlu, an Indian based in Minnesota, America. Both authors used *only* experiments from America, with no discussion on lack or abundance of experiments featured in overseas literature pertaining specifically to the creation of a deficiency.

This 1970 WHO document was reviewed by experts all over the world. If there was a study of great relevance to Muhler's or Venkateswarlu's topic – for instance a *human* study that kept strictly – or as strictly as one could – to Messer's first criterion, one can assume that a reviewer would have told them, and that they would have been receptive to it. This explains why I did not pursue non-American literature too extensively: when I *did* find some, it pointed straight back to American literature.

At the beginning of the 1996 WHO document cited below, we see that the document was written under the supervision of Dr. Walter Mertz, Director of the United States Department of Agriculture's Human Nutrition Research Center in Beltsville, Maryland.

This study is about comparing the published and public statements, mainly of American and Australasian experts, with American experimental evidence and thought. However, this chapter does contain statements from international literature.

A study comparing the WHO statements with more complete international research may have greater relevance to the international community than this study. In Chapter 1.2 I've mentioned French, Argentine and Japanese work, for example. Thus, the WHO is not a primary recipient of my observation, though I have looked. I have also included research from the WHO about the *abundance* of fluorine, as this seems relevant (see Chapter 4).

A paper from the Department of Biophysics, Panjab University in Chandigarh, India, told us that fluoride

"is an essential trace-element having unique physiological properties." [101]

The citation supporting this statement is:

"Ericsson, Y. (1970) In Fluoride in Human Health, Chapter 1, p. 59, World Health Organization Monograph Series."

The article ending on page 59 is sub-titled *Miscellaneous fluorine-containing drugs*; there is no mention of fluoride's essentiality or lack of it. Citing page 59 is obviously a typographical error, because this is *monograph number 59*. The next section on the same page is called *Inhalation from dust or vapours*, again there is nothing about the element's essentiality or lack of it.

Ericsson's introduction begins on page 13, and on page 14 he claims:

"The question 'is fluorine an essential element?' has naturally been raised. It has not been possible to find a definite answer owing to the difficulty of producing a diet for animal experimentation that is fluorine-free but adequate in every other respect. However, there are indications that traces of fluorine are necessary for normal mineralization, and possibly also for normal reproduction. For the formation of a caries-resistant enamel, a certain fluoride supply is evidently essential." [102]

How much has our modern world – junk food, depression, stress, unemployment, pollution etc, contributed to our tooth decay rates, and how has this impacted our understanding of fluorine's essentiality? I ask this because WHO documents and others consistently state that caries is a problem of the developing world. The following statement is also from Ericsson's introduction:

"... since water fluoridation is at present limited to waterworks of a certain technical standard and thus will leave out large population groups, particularly in developing countries, whence unanimous reports indicate a rapid, often alarming, rise of the caries rate." (page 15)

None of the documents I have read that suggest water fluoridation be a policy for developing countries also suggest limiting the amount of processed or extremely sweet foods for sale as a policy, though many claim CWF to be *not* the only step forward. Development, it seems, demands processed, nutrient-irrelevant food, and the advertising that helps to sell it.

The 1971 National Academy of Sciences publication quoted previously suggested fluorine was non-essential, but was open to changing this in light of subsequent work.

We have two documents, each from a prestigious organization full of experts (neither of which are anywhere near the dissident fringe, both organizations support CWF), only a year apart, claiming opposite things – if we look *only* at Ericsson's introduction of the WHO monograph. This is complicated by Dr. Muhler's writing in the second chapter, and Dr. Venkateswarlu's writing in the sixth chapter of the WHO monograph.

Ericsson authored the introduction of the 1970 WHO document. The second chapter was authored by Muriel Bell, Joseph Muhler, E. J. Largent, T. G. Ludwig and G. K. Stookey.

In 1971, Dr. T. W. Cutress of the Dental Unit of New Zealand's National Health and Medical Research Council in Wellington reviewed the 1970 WHO document in the **New Zealand Dental Journal**. His review was complimentary, describing the review as objective and impartial, until one small paragraph:

"Professor Y. Ericcson, special consultant and editor, introduces the monograph with a short but comprehensive and interesting introduction. I found his statement (page 14), 'For the formation of a caries-

> resistant enamel, a certain fluoride supply is evidently essential', provocative on two accounts, and not proven on the evidence supplied by the contributors to this volume." [103]

Joseph Muhler's work in the 1970 WHO monograph largely eliminates any contradiction between this and the 1971 NAS document. However, I'll point out that what we see when we look closely (Muhler's or Venkateswarlu's detailed investigation here) is in many ways contrary to what we get in a simplified expression (Ericsson's introduction and most newspaper articles mentioning a nutritional role, for example).

Discussing his own 1954 experiment [16], Muhler wrote,

> "Weight gain and reproduction in the animals receiving the highly purified low-fluorine diet were definitely affected. However, considerable caution must be exercised in relating this observation to the low fluorine content of the diet."

Muhler's discussion is more reserved than Ericsson's. He began by commenting on the abundance of fluorine in water, plants, animals, and air, and the difficulty that arose in making diets low in the element, then wrote:

> "Moreover, the analytical difficulties encountered in accurately measuring such microquantities of fluorine as occur in many foods add to our vague interpretation of the element's position in nutrition and physiology."
>
> "... since only trace amounts of the element are required by the organism and since almost every food, as well as air and water, contains some fluorine, animals and human beings are probably very seldom in acute need of it."
>
> "It is also possible that our present state of knowledge concerning optimal levels and essential functions may be quite inadequate, and with additional investigations it might well be demonstrated that the microquantities normally present in most commonly eaten mixed diets and water supplies are not fully 'adequate'." [102]

After looking at experiments (discussed here in Chapter 1) by Sharpless and McCollum (1933), McClendon (1944), McClendon and Gershon-Cohen (1953), his own work (1954), Maurer and Day (1957), and Doberenz *et al.* (1964), Muhler states:

> "Further study, with the use of diets lower in fluorine content than those reported here, concerning the essentiality of fluorine is needed, especially in regard to the effects on cellular enzyme systems, on normal and pathological calcification processes and on reproduction and initial growth responses."

This is also in slight contradiction with what he had written years before, in 1958 and in 1960 [48, 24].

Possibly his view had changed to include soft tissues and a wider definition with regard to the essential elements, yet there was also a narrowing of his definition to not include what he had included in 1960:

> "... strong suggestive evidence ... from human studies in natural and artificial fluoride communal fluoride areas, that fluorine is essential for dental health." [24]

He did not suggest any reason why his view on fluorine's essentiality had changed from including human experiments. In 1960, he looked at nine experiments (that *I* cited – or eight plus his Ph.D., which I've never read), in 1970 he looked at six. In this 1970 WHO document, he discussed only animal experiments which had attempted to create a deficiency, and did not discuss whether these findings would also apply to humans. Perhaps (and I can *only* speculate) he had decided the basic criterion of minimizing fluorine levels in human diets, while ensuring abundance of other nutritional factors, was an extremely difficult thing to create and maintain in cities with tens of thousands of people, with differing dietary habits.

Obviously one would be hard-pressed to find a 'deficiency state' in such a setting, though one may certainly see a reduction in dental caries, supposing this is fluorine's effect. Perhaps Muhler had at the time of writing this, a more well-defined idea of what constitutes 'essential' compared with what constitutes 'beneficial'.

The sixth chapter of this monograph was authored by G. N. Jenkins, P. Venkateswarlu and I. Zipkin, with the section on essentiality solely written by Venkateswarlu [102][24]. He acknowledged fluorine's beneficial role as a controller of dental caries in human and animals. He then discussed much of the work Muhler had in the second chapter, looking at studies by Sharpless and McCollum [6], the unpublished work of Lawrenz [10], McClendon [11] and McClendon and Gershon-Cohen [12, 13], Maurer and Day [17] and Doberenz [19].

There is very little more that needs to be said on these beyond the fact that he pointed out Maurer and Day's work was sensitive to no less than 1.0 microgram fluorine, whereas the method used in his own work from 1962 was capable of detecting as little as 0.1-0.2 micrograms.

Venkateswarlu's work used what he called "a diet extremely low in fluoride" without specifying an exact amount. This diet was fed to both groups of rats, with one group also receiving double-distilled water, and the other group receiving water containing 10 ppm fluorine. He wrote:

> "There was a slight suggestion that the reproductive capacity of the animals in the low-F group was less than that of those in the other group. However, the difference between the two groups may have been only a chance result."

Venkateswarlu wanted to observe the rats through 3 to 5 generations, but had to abandon the experiment because "few animals reproduced beyond the third generation..." Those that did have offspring did not nurse them adequately.

> "The cause of these unexpected developments may perhaps be traced to the artificial diet. Either some unknown deficiency was inadvertently created, or some toxic factor was produced in the preparation and storage of the diet in the refrigerator."

He looked at Joseph Muhler's PhD thesis, claiming Muhler also abandoned his experiment,

> "because the purified diet would not sustain reproduction."

He finished by discussing the rest of the chapter his co-authors had written, and looking to the future:

> "... some hypotheses on the role of F in the formation and maintenance of apatitic structures are described. If these can be confirmed in experimental animals raised on fluoride-free diets, the essential nature of F for the development of calcified tissues would appear to be established." [102]

Neither Muhler's nor Venkateswarlu's writing in the 1970 monograph came to a definite conclusion on fluorine's essentiality.

---

[24] Department of Biochemistry, University of Minnesota, Minneapolis, Minnesota, USA.

An hypothesis regarding an "essential role of fluoride in calcification" was suggested. Fluorapatite is the most stable of the apatites[25]. Realising this, two researchers[26] suggested the "provocative" idea that the formation of apatitic structures would not be possible without the presence of fluoride.

The WHO in 2002 wrote:

"An expert consultation of the WHO on trace elements in human nutrition and health (WHO, 1996c) categorized fluoride among 'potentially toxic elements, some of which may nevertheless have some essential functions at low levels.' Fluoride was regarded as 'essential,' since the consultation 'considered resistance to dental caries to be a physiologically important function.'" [104]

This was based on a 1996 "expert consultation of the WHO on trace elements". This 1996 document claimed:

"The complex and frequently indirect relationships between low fluoride intakes and increased susceptibility to dental caries have been reviewed elsewhere[27]. Fluoride is reported to be required for the transformation of osteocalcium phosphate to apatite, the chief mineral component of skeletal tissue." [105] (page 187)

Note the word "required". They point to the work of Schwarz and Milne [20] regarding the concluded growth requirement for rats (see Chapter 1.1), without mentioning any of the criticisms, not even the fact that others had used less fluoride to breed healthier animals. The WHO also pointed to a study on goats:

"Diets low in fluoride content (< 0.3 mg of fluoride/kg dry matter) offered to goats during pregnancy and lactation and to the kids during postnatal growth reduced by 16% the 4-year life expectancy of the latter. This effect was not apparent if dietary fluoride was in the range 1.5-2.5 mg/kg.[28]" [105] (page 188)

This 1996 document was the only place I have ever seen this experiment mentioned. The experiment on goats was from the textbook *Trace Elements in Man and Animals*, Volume 7, published in 1991. I have ordered a copy of this publication but have yet to obtain it to get more details. You will note that Volume 10, published in 2000, does *not* include fluorine as a trace element.

Quoting the WHO:

"Although fluoride should probably be regarded as essential, there is no evidence so far from human studies that overt clinical signs of fluoride deficiency exist. No specifically diagnostic clinical or biochemical parameters have been related to fluoride inadequacy. The Expert Consultation was therefore unable to specify a minimum desirable intake. However, in view of the toxicity associated with excessive fluoride ingestion from a variety of sources, recommendations for maximum safe intakes are required. For this purpose, dental mottling may be taken as a definitive indication of toxicity." [105] (page 192)

The NAS use the phrase 'Adequate Intake' which implies the existence of an '*in*adequate intake'. Yet in the above quote the WHO tells us no such thing exists. This is contradictory, and something I have never seen discussed.

---

[25] According to W. E. Brown, **Clin. Orthop.**, Vol. 44, pp. 205-220, 1966; and Newesely, **Dtsch. Zahnärztl. Z.**, Vol. 20, pp. 753-766, 1965.

[26] H. Newelsey, **Archives of Oral Biology**, Vol. 6, pp. 174-180 (Special Supplement: Proceedings of 8th ORCA Congress, London, July, 1961) and W. G. Perdok, In: *Advances in Fluorine Research and Dental Caries Prevention*, Oxford, Pergamon, Vol. 1, pp. 85-93 and **Archives of Oral Biology**, Vol. 8, (Special Supplement, pp. 85-93, Proceedings of the 9th ORCA Congress, Paris, June 1962).

[27] Murray JJ, Rugg-Gunn AJ, Jenkin GN. *Fluoride in caries prevention,* 3rd ed. London, Butterworth-Heinemann, 1991 is cited here.

[28] Anke M, Groppel B, Krause U. *Fluorine deficiency in goats.* In: Momcilovic B, ed. *Trace elements in man and animals-TEMA7.* Zagreb, University of Zagreb, 1991: 26-28.

There is no elaboration on regarding fluoride as essential even though no evidence of a deficiency state in humans exists. The first sentence is a contradiction if we consider that deficiency is a criterion for essentiality.

The WHO did not point out that in conventional trace element research a deficiency state should be demonstrated in order for an element or compound to be considered essential, nor did they point to any other criteria, such as replicability in many species or restoration of function when the element in question is reintroduced. None of the other studies discussed in Chapter 1 were mentioned beyond the Schwarz and Milne work.

The example given here is illustrative of the contradictory nature found within literature looking at fluorine's role. It also serves to demonstrate how seemingly unimportant the topic of essentiality is to many experts (in technical literature).

A report from the Office of the New Zealand Prime Minister's Science Advisor was released in August of 2014 [106]. The report's conclusions and recommendations are not being examined here. This will serve as an interesting insight into who the experts go to for advice.

One of the many reports the 2014 report looked at was a 2002 report from the US Institute of Medicine (IOM), a group established in 1970 by the NAS. This IOM report, **Evolution of Evidence for Selected Nutrient and Disease Relationships**, concluded that since 1997, the evidence of a "nutrient-disease" relationship for fluoride had *strengthened* [107]. This is surprising considering that in 2001 the NAS had released a report claiming fluoride was

"… generally not regarded as an essential dietary component."[29] [84]

This was in regard to cattle. In this comparison fluoride is non-essential, but there is a disease associated with less…

I need to point out that I compared both groups of authors of the 2001 and 2002 reports (and the reviewers of the 2002 document, there were no reviewers for the 2001), and found none were the same. This example demonstrates that we literally can, knowingly or unknowingly, pick and choose from authoritative sounding bodies to reinforce our opinion.

Consider also the existence of "non-essential nutrients" – which is a category implied in the 2002 document.

I don't know if there's an absolute definition on what constitutes each category of nutrient, essential or non-essential, trace or not. One website that had some definitions and explanations was fitday.com [108]. This is a website that provides an online dietary service. Their definitions made sense to me.

On their webpage an essential nutrient was something the body couldn't make on its own, a non-essential nutrient could be made by the body. Electrolytes were minerals needed in larger amounts – calcium, magnesium, phosphorous, sodium, etc. Trace elements were needed in much smaller amounts, but values and numbers in moles and milligrams per day were not given.

---

[29] They cited **Mineral Tolerance of Domestic Animals**, National Research Council, 1980, in support of the statement quoted.

Using this definition, fluorine would *not* be an essential nutrient, because no signs of deficiency have been found (see Chapter 1, and below). Nor would it be a non-essential nutrient, because it cannot be made by the body. By the definition used here, it would not be a trace element.

The 2014 NZ document [106] claimed the WHO "consider fluorine a micronutrient" – which the WHO did in a 2010 document. There is no citation given in the 2014 document regarding this statement (page 35), though three articles are cited in the paragraph.

Of these, only the 2010 document claimed fluorine a micronutrient, cited in support of the statement, "...actions are needed to provide sufficient fluorine intake..." It is called *Inadequate or Excess Fluoride: A Major Public Health Concern* [109].

The latter title is odd given that the WHO in 1996 said a fluoride deficiency does not exist and there is no "inadequate" amount.

> "No specifically diagnostic clinical or biochemical parameters have been related to fluoride inadequacy. The Expert Consultation was therefore unable to specify a minimum desirable intake." [105]

This was not addressed; the 1996 document is not cited in the 2010 document. Also consider that the only signs of fluoride deficiency that have ever been found in animals have been either outright refuted (as in the case of Messer *et al.* [4, 28, 29, 31], refuted by two experiments [33, 34]) or heavily criticized (as in the case of Schwarz [20, 26, 27] and McClendon [11, 12, 13, 37]) as discussed thoroughly in Chapter 1. The exception to this is the experiment on goats mentioned here.

The 2010 WHO document cited a total of five other documents in the paragraph that claimed fluorine a micronutrient, but the sentence claiming this category for fluorine had no specific citation.

The first of these five was the 2002 document I have already cited above [104]. Here fluorine's necessity was based on prevention of dental caries being of physiological importance. The second was a document called *Air Quality Guidelines for Europe*, 2nd Edition, which had nothing to say about a nutritional role [110].

The third article also cited by Sir Peter Gluckman's team was a 2004 article written by Poul Erik Petersen, who has written much on CWF for the WHO. Petersen's attitude regarding an increase in tooth decay in Africa is:

> "The principal reasons for this increase are growing sugar consumption and inadequate exposure to fluorides." [111]

Petersen cited a document he had written, the *World Oral Health Report 2003* [112]. This is an interesting document, but had nothing to say about whether fluorine was a nutritional essential or not, though it claimed CWF safe and effective.

The same is true for a document regarding salt fluoridation – interesting, but nothing to say about a biological necessity for fluorine [113].

The fifth document was a 2008 WHO document, *Guidelines for drinking-water quality*. This group of experts had written:

"Fluoride may be an essential element for humans; however, essentiality has not been demonstrated unequivocally. Meanwhile, there is evidence of fluoride being a beneficial element with regard to the prevention of dental caries." [114]

A 2006 document cited by Sir Peter Gluckman's team looked at health effects of fluoride but did not take a stand on whether the element was or was not necessary in nutrition (115).

In 1996, the WHO would call fluorine an essential element based on its benefit, in 2008 (and again in 2017) state the above regarding essentiality not being demonstrated unequivocally, and in 2010, call it a micronutrient which as usual, is an undefined term.

I want to make it clear I'm not calling expert *honesty* into question here – with the WHO and the NZ report. But it seems the experts will call fluorine a little less than "whatever suits them"... but the terms are obviously flexible enough, variable enough, and definitions difficult to come by, even searching in WHO documents. This topic gets scant mention; it appears from my search here it can be brushed over. It appears to be considered unimportant when people look at much larger issues of safety, effectiveness, and doing something for the children.

In 2010 the Scientific Committee for Health and Environmental Risks, a European body of scientists, stated that fluorine was not an essential element:

"Fluoride is not an essential element for human growth and development, and for most organisms in the environment." [116]

Their 2011 document contains the same phrase, however both documents claimed CWF safe, beneficial, etc. The 2011 SCHER document [117] was also cited in the NZ Royal Society Report.

If you combine this 2010 SCHER document [116] with the WHO document of the same year [109], you end up calling fluorine a non-essential micronutrient. A cynic may say it all comes down to how you mix your favourite experts together.

In 2005, the European Food Safety Authority (EFSA) wrote:

"There is insufficient evidence for the indispensability of fluoride for human health. Because of the ubiquity of fluoride it is virtually impossible to create an experimental situation free of fluoride.

"Schwarz and Milne (1972) reared several generations of F344 rats in isolators on a fluoride deficient diet (0.002-0.023 mg/kg/day). Rats on this diet showed decreased gain in weight and bleached incisors. Weight gain was improved by fluoride supplementation of the diet (2.5 mg/kg), tooth pigmentation was not. Rats in both the group on the fluoride-deficient and the fluoride-supplemented diet had shaggy fur, loss of hair and seborrhoea, indicative of a probable deficiency of other nutrients in the synthetic diet as well." [118]

In 2013, the European Food Safety Authority (EFSA) wrote:

"No signs of fluoride deficiency have been identified in humans. One cohort study on infants from an area with a low fluoride content of drinking water described a higher rate of length and body weight gain with a fluoride supplement (0.25 mg/day from birth) than without (Bergmann, 1994). The Panel considers that this observation does not provide sufficient evidence to prove a causal relationship between fluoride intake and growth.

> "A lack of fluoride intake during development will not alter tooth development but may result in increased susceptibility of enamel to acid attacks after eruption. However, caries is not a fluoride deficiency disease.
>
> "The Panel concludes that fluoride is not an essential nutrient." [119]

This document was cited in the recent Royal Society of New Zealand report dated August 2014 by Sir Peter Gluckman and Sir David Skegg. I'll point out that this report was not specifically focused on fluorine's status or role in nutrition. The following was written, under the sub-title "Fluoride exposure in specific population groups":

> "A number of public health agencies around the world, including the US Institute of Medicine, Health Canada, the European Food Safety Authority, the Australian National Health and Medical Research Council, and the New Zealand Ministry of Health provide recommendations on adequate intakes (AIs) for nutrients considered necessary for optimal health, as well as safe upper levels of intake (ULs). Fluoride is included among the nutrients assigned AI and UL recommendations." [106]

Recall that the NAS (of which the IOM is sub-group) wrote in 2008 that an AI is used as a placeholder because there is no requirement. Again the term "non-essential nutrient" may apply, if such a term should even exist. This may seem confusing, because "essential nutrient" and "nutrient" mean the same thing (see the list of definitions).

Note the inclusion of the EFSA, who wrote in 2005:

> "The [European Scientific Committee on Foods] SCF did not define adequate or recommended fluoride intakes (SCF, 1993). Other bodies defined adequate fluoride intakes on the basis of the negative relationship between caries prevalence and fluoride intake (FNB, 1997; D-A-CH, 2000).
>
> "There is no convincing evidence that health and development of humans depend on the intake of fluoride, however, due to the ubiquitous presence of fluoride in the environment a zero exposure is not possible under normal circumstances." [118]

What can we conclude from this?

Fluoride is non-essential – meaning we don't *need* any (SCHER, EFSA), but if we don't get enough, we get a disease (IOM). Even though fluoride's not a nutrient (SCHER, EFSA), it *is* a micronutrient (WHO). Fluoride is a "nutrient considered necessary for optimal health"[30] by the EFSA (Sir Gluckman and Sir Skegg's review, page 8), while the EFSA Panel "concludes that fluoride is not an essential nutrient." (EFSA) [119].

These contradictions can happen because as I've demonstrated, the topic of essentiality is one in which criteria change. Another reason is that there's no *need* to look at it – in fact it's probably better for Community Water Fluoridation programs if we *don't* look at it, and if we *don't* have rigorously defined terms with fixed, non-negotiable boundaries. The topic changes depending on our priorities, and what experts have previously written.

---

[30] Consider this statement, and "… lack of fluoride intake during development…" with regard to the information presented in Chapter 4.

Many of these reports have to do with what fluorine *does*, but so few bother looking at what it *is*. I want to be absolutely clear to you that I'm *not* trying to be insulting to *anyone* here, including the experts who work for and within these organizations. The experts *are* very decisive on the safety and effectiveness of CWF and their collective work is often meticulous and detailed.

Sir Peter Gluckman and Sir David Skegg have obviously overseen a lengthy report which outlined their attitudes. They were *not* looking specifically at essentiality of fluorine – something that takes a back seat to more seemingly important issues like safety and effectiveness. Their report had abundant work involved and they could have taken any particular aspect of fluorine that they wanted to a detailed culmination.

The only time the word "deficient" or "deficiency" appears in Sir Peter Gluckman and Sir David Skegg's report is with regard to iodine, *not* fluorine.

In 2017, the WHO repeated what they had claimed in 2008:

> "Fluoride may be an essential element for humans; however, essentiality has not been demonstrated unequivocally. Meanwhile, there is evidence of fluoride being a beneficial element with regard to the prevention of dental caries." [120]

No reason is given for a difference in the EFSA in 2013 or SCHER in 2011 claiming bluntly that fluorine is non-essential, here it 'may' be essential. No new research is shown or discussed.

2.4 Australian Government Literature

Mr. Hamer, the Premier of Australia, said in a Ministerial Statement dated the 9th of September, 1980:

> "Fluoride is a natural dietary component and an essential nutrient for the proper development of bones and teeth." [121]

The statement was given partly as a response to a committee of inquiry that had suggested no changes were needed to the Health (Fluoridation) Act of 1973.

The National (Australian) Health and Medical Research Council (NHMRC) updated fluoride in 2017.

> "Both inadequate and excessive fluoride intakes can affect dental health." [122]

The exception to this was for infants younger than 6 months of age, no AI (adequate intake) had been established. Fluoride had been shown to have no preventive effect on dental decay in these children, according to the NHMRC. This was in line with views put forth by the (American) Institute of Medicine in 1997 [71] and the American Dental Association's Council on Scientific Affairs statement in 2011.

The NHMRC said that 0.05 milligrams fluoride per kilogram of bodyweight per day would suffice for children aged 6 months to 8 years of age, and cited some studies to support 1 milligram fluoride per litre (1.0 ppm) of water as a way to achieve this.

I include this because I have seen at least one expert claiming that fluorine should be used before the teeth erupt [123].

2.5 Textbooks

In Dr. Schwarz's 1972 experiment with David Milne, the gentlemen cited the work of Eric J. Underwood, an Australian author of some very good textbooks on nutrition. One, *Trace Elements in Human and Animal Nutrition*, published in its third edition in 1971, looked at fluorine's essentiality. He wrote that

> "classification … depends upon the criteria employed in determining essentiality."

If survival was used as a criterion, then fluorine was considered non-essential,

> "…for plants, microorganisms, or animals."

> "The results of the experiments [6, 9, 10, 17, 19, 12] … just cited do not permit the conclusion that fluorine is either an essential or a nonessential component of the diet of rats, since different results could conceivably be obtained with diets still lower in fluorine content."

Underwood also claimed that "indisputable evidence" was available which demonstrated that fluorine was

> "required to confer maximal resistance to human dental caries." [25]

Relating this to humans, he quoted Hegsted:

> "If an essential element is defined as one which is ordinarily required for health and well-being, under the usual conditions in which individuals live, then in the light of the above evidence, fluorine must be considered as an essential element in human nutrition." [63]

The 1975 textbook *Mental and Elemental Nutrients* by Carl C. Pfeiffer, Ph.D., M.D, gives us an interesting conundrum:

> "Fluoride has never been proven essential to life, but it is important in human nutrition to help maintain normal bone and tooth structure and resistance of teeth to decay." [124]

It could be argued that if it's not essential, we don't need it – such an argument needs to be considered in light of the information presented in Chapter 4. The question of *how important* is fluoride is a little difficult to address, importance being a subjective question. How important is it relative to elements and compounds that *are* essential? If it's not required for survival, and teeth can grow with extremely low levels of it (0.005 ppm, possibly even lower), it would be less important than iron, less important than calcium, less important than many amino acids, less important than vitamins…

In the introduction to his section on trace elements, Pfeiffer claims that

> "fluorine in tooth enamel is held in a tight complex similar to the mineral apatite. Without fluorine this enamel, and even the bones, become deficient in calcium."

Such a statement is probably based on work discussed in Chapter 6.2 that received a lot of publicity. So fluorine is necessary for proper calcium retention? It is funny that fluorine does not warrant an essential status in his work, if without it we have a calcium deficiency. Pfeiffer mentions the work of Navia, Schroeder, Mertz and Underwood, as claiming water fluoridation beneficial, but he doesn't go into any more details about calcium deficiency caused by lack of fluorine. This perhaps is a little similar to Gautier's idea that fluorine held phosphorous in place, but sixty years after Gautier's theory, Pfeiffer has little more to offer in detail beyond the authors who've mentioned the benefits of CWF.

An Australasian textbook, *Essentials of Human Nutrition*, published in 2002, claims fluoride is "generally regarded" as a "beneficial nutrient" due to the reduction of dental caries when between 1 and 4 mg per day is ingested.

"Most nutritional authorities have not classified fluoride as an essential nutrient." [125]
This textbook cites work from the National Academy of Sciences in the years 1980, 1989, and 1997, pointing out that the 1997 document (cited above) puts fluoride "among the essential nutrients."

These are contradictory statements. They did not go into much detail as to why a contradiction may exist. A few pages after this, they discussed the range between "too little and too much fluorine" being "not wide". If there's a possibility of "too little" this at least implies there is a deficiency state, suggesting essentiality. This is in contrast to the authors' statement about "Most nutritional authorities..." quoted above.

In this investigation I have seen many scientific authorities claim fluorine non-essential, yet often in the same documents, suggest harmful consequences of 'sub-optimal', 'inadequate intake', and 'deficient levels' without explanation and without *detail.* For instance, how do we know a tooth has gone bad because of a problem caused by sub-optimal fluorine, instead of a deficiency or deficiencies of calcium, phosphorous, or anything else? We diagnose and claim this one condition specifically, without differentiating from the rest.

Considering how difficult it has been to create the non-existent deficiencies that we read about in much literature, I have found precious little discussion of it.

2.6 Scientific Articles and Experiments Related to Fluorine and/or Fluoridation

The documents in this section are experiments or journal articles that are not directly related to a necessity for fluorine or fluorides, but have mentioned the topic. Obtaining these you will see they discuss fluorine-deficient water, and compare the element to iodine. There is a lack of depth and discussion on this topic in these documents. The last two examples in this chapter demonstrate that many experts accept very old research.

According to A. P. Black, Head of the Department of Chemistry at the University of Florida, the medical physiologist Sir James Crichton-Browne had claimed fluorine an essential component of tooth enamel as far back as 1892; claiming "while the development of the teeth is proceeding", a fluorine deficiency would result in thinner, weaker enamel[31]. This was mentioned in a February, 1952 edition of the **Journal of the American Dental Association** [126]. Crichton-Browne lamented the loss of fluorine from wheat and flour caused by the

---

[31] *Tooth Culture*, **Lancet:** 2, 1892.

refining process. He critiqued the use of soft, sugary foods. Black quoted a paragraph of Crichton-Browne's work in his article, commenting that this "historic statement" was finally being realised.

The March, 1952 edition of the **Journal of the American Dental Association** contained an article called *Four statements adopted by the Inter-Association Committee on Health*. This body, created in November of 1949, represented six American health and welfare organizations: The American Dental Association, the American Hospital Association, the American Medical Association, the American Nurses' Association, the American Public Health Association and the American Public Welfare Association.

> "The committee serves as a means for the exchange of information so that the participating organizations may cooperate more effectively in improving the health and welfare of the nation." [127]

The statement regarding fluoridation was

> "Too much fluoride in drinking water results in a condition known as dental fluorosis, or mottled enamel; too little is associated with a high dental caries-experience rate. Between these two extremes, however, there is an optimum concentration of fluoride..."

This was very similar to the statement made by Maier in 1950 [91], mentioned previously in the section on the NAS.

The committee

> "... urges the fluoridation of the fluoride-deficient public water supplies of this country as rapidly as plans can be approved by the local medical, dental and health department officials and the state departments of health." [127]

Paragraph 38 of a 1956 American Dental Association publication, *Fluoridation Facts*, repeated this statement[32] [128].

In a 1961 issue, the **Journal of Social Issues** focused completely on fluoridation. The first page of the first article claims without elaboration that

> "Like iodine and other trace elements essential to good health, either an excess or a deficiency of fluorine is undesirable." [129]

Some articles featured in the **Journal of the American Dental Association** have also discussed "fluorine-deficient waters" without addressing whether fluorine deficiencies in people do or don't exist [130-132].

Many chiropractors were initially against fluoridation, however the **American Journal of Public Health** reported on one chiropractor that had words published in a Madison, Wisconsin newspaper:

> "Chiropractors are interested in public health. Fluoridation is an extremely important issue. Chiropractors have a drugless healing profession, but the feeling that fluoridation is medication is absurd. It is an essential nutrient that naturally occurs." [133]

A 1963 article in the **Journal of the Canadian Medical Association** reiterated the observation that

> "... fluorine is evidently not essential for the maintenance of life, some authorities believe that it should be classified as an essential element because of its important role in reducing dental caries." [134]

---

[32] Here the ADA cite *Statement of Inter-Assoc. Com. On Health, Feb. 1, 1952*, quoted in the ADA **Journal** in full [127].

One can see that the reported benefits of CWF have had an effect on influencing those involved in policy-related decisions. Here, if some authorities had their way, the word 'essential' would have its meaning changed to 'important.'

A 1995 article in **The Lancet** called fluoride a trace element [135]. This is relevant because the term 'trace element' is often taken to mean 'micronutrient' or something that is required, but in minute amounts.

A Chinese study published in **Biological Trace Element Research** made the same claim in 2016:

"Iodide and fluoride are essential trace elements." [136]

The following sentence is the first in another experiment from **Biological Trace Element Research**:

"Fluoride, widely distributed in the environment, is an essential trace element for normal tooth and bone development." [137]

No citation was given. This is possibly a consequence of the NAS and other organizations including fluorine in groups of other nutrients as discussed earlier.

In 2017 a paper authored by six scientists, all with very impressive credentials, was published in the **American Journal of Water Resources**. The abstract began with the following sentence:

"fluoride is an essential nutrient for human beings which occur in the surface as well as in groundwater." [138]

This paper cited an article called *The supply of fluoride to man: ingestion from water*, which was contained within the second chapter of the WHO 1970 monograph [102] (p. 18-32), in support of the statement that fluorine was a necessity for proper development of enamel and bone. The six authors probably meant to cite Ericsson's statement as nowhere in Bell and Ludwig's sub-chapter did they claim fluorine to be a nutritional essential, they simply looked at intake from water sources. There is no doubt in my mind that Bell and Ludwig both believed fluorine to be a nutritional essential. The six authors of the 2017 paper did not mention the EFSA or the SCHER [116-119], instead opting for work over forty years old.

A 2015 study looking at fluoride's effect on memory and intelligence published in **Neurotoxicology and Teratology** claimed,

"Fluoride is a trace element that is necessary for the human body." [139]

It went on to state:

"A proper amount of fluoride not only prevents dental caries, but also promotes the use of calcium and phosphorus and the calcium sediment in the bone, stimulates bone growth and maintains bone health (Dean and Elvove, 1936; WHO, 1958)[33]."

While many of the reviews and studies cited in the paper were quite recent, the references cited in support of *this* statement were from 1936 and 1958.

---

[33] H. T. Dean and E. Elvove, *Some epidemiological aspects of chronic endemic dental fluorosis*, **American Journal of Public Health**, Vol. 26, pp. 567-575, 1936; World Health Organization, Technical Report Series (TRS) No. 146.

2.7 Mainstream or Popular Science Books and Websites

This section looks at what books and websites have claimed. The books in this section are not textbooks. They are more likely to have been on bestseller lists, in bookstores, or on a friend's coffee table or bookshelf. I have looked at websites only when they represent the voice of governments, medical bureaucracy or educated intellectuals, because they do have some authority, or they are trusted by the public. The books and websites in this section are not quite in the same category as the media – while they do communicate to the public, they're not a *direct* communicator to the *majority* of the public. These are the books and websites that people who have a greater interest in the topic would read or look at, whereas newspapers are available to everyone.

In the book *The Fight for Fluoridation* by Donald R. McNeil, a typical example of the inaccurate use of the word 'deficient' can be found on page 48:

> "On March 19, 1945, the house of delegates of the state dental society unanimously recommended that deficient water supplies of Wisconsin have their fluorine concentration raised to 1 ppm, providing it was done under strict dental, engineering, and public health control." [140]

In 1970, a book called *Water Fluoridation - The Search and The Victory* was published [47] (and reviewed in the Journal **Science** [141]). It was authored by biochemist Dr. Frank McClure, after a 30-year career with the National Institute of Dental Research (NIDR), a branch of the National Institute of Health (NIH). It was published around the time of his retirement.

There were several discussions in this book relating to fluorine's role in nutrition:

> "Dr. H. H. Mitchell and Marjorie Edman of the University of Illinois in 1953 discussed fluoride as a nutritional factor in the economy of man. They pointed out that although it is invariably present in the diet and is a normal constituent of body tissues, it does not have the dimensions and properties which define an essential body nutrient. Numerous attempts have been made to obtain proof of an indispensable requirement for fluoride but this proof is still lacking."

> "It seems evident, however, that if fluorine is essential for life its daily requirement is extremely small. Laboratory animals have been raised successfully on synthetic diets containing as little as 0.5 ppm fluoride, indicating that the required quantity is more than likely less than 0.5 ppm." [47] (pages 191-193)

(This is the same Mitchell and Edman article [45] mentioned in Chapter 1.2).

This is similar to what Messer *et al.* wrote in 1972:

> "Satisfactory evidence of a deficiency state with respect to fluorine has not been demonstrated despite several investigations with this purpose." [28]

However, there is a contradiction in McClure's book that must be pointed out: on page 193 of his book, two pages after telling us that

> "fluoride… does not have the dimensions and properties which define an essential body nutrient,"

… he tells us,

> "Fluoride has an indisputable beneficial role as a dietary nutrient."

"Nutrient" on its own implies essentiality; this is congruent with medical dictionaries. Yet the word "benefit" is used this time. This *may* be why at least two prominent fluoridation supporters have used the term 'semantics' to describe investigations into a dietary necessity for fluorine (discussed below).

On page 110 of his book, McClure wrote that fluorine was

> "only one of many trace elements unavoidable in human nutrition…"

… without much more detail. On page 273 of his book, he wrote:

> "The problem of religious freedom and fluoridation is related to doctrines of the Christian Science Church. This issue was raised in a Missouri court and the response was a ruling that fluoride is not a medicine but a nutrient found naturally in food and water. It was ruled that in some areas the content of fluoride in water is not sufficient for optimum caries prevention. This ruling is realistic. Fluoride is a nutrient trace element and its status in preventive dentistry is not regarded as medication." [47]

McClure also quoted the 1968 the Food and Nutrition Board of the Nutrition Research Council (NRC), who had called fluoridation "a very important nutritional public health measure…" and mentioned the "nutritional advantages that result from fluoridation of the water supply." He quoted this in his book [142].

This was before the NAS would claim in 1971

> "… the beneficial effects of fluoride on dental health or bone metabolism should be considered as pharmacologic responses, and not as a cure of pre-existing deficiency condition." [69]

(Recall that there were also two experiments concluding fluoride's effect on iron absorption was also pharmacological [33, 34], not correcting a deficiency condition.)

Discussions on this disagreement have been non-existent in the expert literature that I have seen. In a 1970 review of McClure's book in the journal **Science**, James H. Shaw wrote about

> "… the fluoride concentration of a deficient water supply to an optimal level…" [141]

McClure's book has featured in literature dealing with fluoridation. Citing it (without mentioning a page number, maybe these are her words not McClure's), Grace Noda of Portland State University, wrote in her University Honors Thesis:

> "Fluoride was recognized as a trace element found in plants, foods, tissues, and organs of human and animals, and therefore compatible with health and unavoidable in nutrition (McClure, 1970)." [143]

This is an accurate summary of the claims appearing later in McClure's book. There was a point at which McClure said something like this, but he also said the opposite, on pages 191-193. I suppose he said it was a nutrient more often that he said it was not so in a sense Noda is correct, however I believe page 191 is the only page where McClure cites an actual scientific investigation that used McClendon and Rygh's work, and ignored earlier, more detailed work. McClure initially disagreed with Mitchell and Edman's claim, though he agreed with it later in his book. McClure had also authored a section on fluorine in the 1951 American Medical Association Handbook of Nutrition [144]. In this he claimed fluorine was non-essential (based on [6, 9] and [10]).

These examples show us that the words 'deficient', 'inadequate', 'sub-optimal' can be invoked regardless of fluoride's status as a nutrient. You will observe McClure wrote that fluorine does not have the dimensions of an essential body nutrient, but called it a trace element, which is something that *is* (in the dictionaries shown) considered essential, though in technical and less formal literature sometimes it merely indicates presence.

While the NAS publications have given some detail on these terms, at least in the late 1980s, most experts and media didn't really seem to care enough to mention it.

In Chapter 1.1 I mentioned the 1973 review by Nielsen and Sandstead [27] from the United States Department of Agriculture, which had quoted Mark Hegsted:

> "If an essential element were defined as one which has a beneficial effect in health and well-being, under the usual conditions in which individuals live, then in the light of the above evidence, fluorine would be considered an essential element in human nutrition." [63]

In this instance, the word "essential" is expanded to include the word "beneficial".

To be fair, the experts define terms in their scientific literature much more often than in their public statements. I've only seen one media article in which the fact that "necessity" simply means "benefit" has been pointed out.

Now, fluoride becomes essential, even if there is no experiment demonstrating a biological problem or weakness caused by a deficiency state, in an experiment wherein an abundance of necessary nutritional compounds exist.

So in becoming defined as "essential", fluoride only needs to be "beneficial", and stops being "required" or "a necessity". I am yet to see a single expert publicly suggest this may be accidentally misleading. After all, if experts have broadened the term "essential" surely the rest of us should be told?

We deserve an explanation as to *why* this term needs to be broadened. *Broadened* is the only way to look at the pliability of the word. I consider that the word "essential" has been *weakened*, made impotent and compromising – because now something does *not* need to be a requirement (a necessity) in order to be essential.

Put another way, the bar has been lowered for fluoride to get over.

This is important when we see experts in scientific documents and in our newspapers likening fluorine to essential elements and compounds *like* calcium, iodine and vitamins (discussed in detail in Chapter 5). In textbooks on trace elements, death can be caused from lack of potassium, lack of iodine, yet I have never seen a textbook point to death from lack of fluorine.

Consider the following statement:

> "The question of the essentiality of fluoride is really one of semantics. Most researchers consider fluoride essential for proper development of bones and teeth. Whether it is essential for reproduction, growth, and other body functions has been difficult to determine because of the difficulties in developing a totally fluoride-free diet." [145]

For now I'll point out the word 'semantics' though the rest is relevant. The word 'semantics' means 'of meaning'.

The document in which this appeared was written in response to a 1982 pamphlet that claimed Community Water Fluoridation (CWF) to be unsafe; one of its many allegations was that fluorine was not an essential nutrient.

This 1988 document in rebuttal was a

> "special publication of the American Oral Health Institute, Inc., a national, not-for-profit research institute founded in 1984 to promote and protect the oral health of America's citizens." [145]

Of fourteen contributors to this 1988 document, nine worked in, or previously worked in either a department, division, office, or bureau of dental health. All fourteen worked in the United States. They did not elaborate on 'semantics' or definitions.

If you said calcium or iodine was an essential nutrient, and someone said that actually calcium or iodine's essentiality was just a case of semantics, would that be acceptable? I think not. The experts get away with it because few people have really investigated the creation of a fluorine deficiency, or discussed what standards should or should not apply when claims are made regarding a nutritional role.

In October 2013, a similar statement regarding semantics was expressed by New Zealand's Dr. Ken Perrott, in response to one of North American Professor Paul Connett's points in an online debate. This debate appeared on Perrott's website, with each section available for comments from others, one written presentation at a time, every few months, and was eventually made available as a pdf, free to download [146]. The debate began on the 29th of October, 2013 [147]. Here is what Connett wrote (posted 30th October, 2013):

> Page 4: "Fluoride is NOT a nutrient. There is not one single biochemical process in the body that has been shown to require fluoride for normal function..." [148] (His emphasis.)[34]

When addressing this, Perrott wrote

> "This also reduces to semantics – how should 'nutrient' be defined? Paul restricts his definition only to elements involved in 'biochemical processes' – a definition confidently excluding the role of F in bioapatites – bones and teeth. Yet bones and teeth are important to organisms – so the strengthening of bioapatites, and the reduction of their solubility, by incorporation of fluoride is important."
>
> "Perhaps we can agree that F is at least a beneficial element, even if we can't reach agreement on the use of terms like 'nutrient' and 'essential.'" [146] (page 10)

There are quite a few points to be made here [151].

Throughout the debate, Dr. Perrott referred to deficient levels of fluoride:

---

[34] Connett *et al.* in their book [149], (a copy of which Perrott held [150]), used a letter from the presidents of the NAS and the Institute of Medicine that claimed fluoride non-essential. It's unclear in the debate whether Perrott spent any time on this particular citation, if he did he didn't mention it openly, or in detail. The letter quoted the 1989 NAS publication Recommended Dietary Allowances, 10th edition: "These contradictory results do not justify a classification of fluorine as an essential element, according to accepted standards." [81]

(As pointed out earlier in Chapter 2.1, this did not stop the NAS from including it in the category 'Trace Elements' – which could be considered contradictory, because a trace element is usually considered required.)

Page 43: He discusses fluoride deficiencies.

Page 47: He discusses fluoride deficiency right next to selenium and cobalt deficiency, claiming this discovery of fluoride deficiency was not regarded as unusual to him or his peers.

Page 60: He discusses the Li *et al.* study (see below) that looks at a U-shaped "window of benefit" – something seen in essential nutrients, and a demonstration of problems occurring as a result of fluoride levels much less or much greater than about 1 ppm.

Page 85: He discusses natural fluoride levels that are deficient.

Page 204: He refers to fluoride as a trace element, and a micronutrient.

Page 210: He suggests Community Water Fluoridation is not the only method of fixing deficient levels of fluoride in our diet [146].

These statements obviously rest on the assumption that fluorine is a necessity – or, that we can be deficient in things that are of questionable necessity. For him to make such statements, the issue must have some importance.

Dr. Perrott's thinking is abundantly explained on his website. There is an article he had posted in June, 2013, entitled *Is Fluorine an Essential Dietary Mineral?* [152]

Perrott uses 'benefit' as a criterion for essentiality. The WHO has done so off and on since at least 2002, from what I can tell. Hegsted and Muhler were saying the same thing in the 1950s and 1960s. In work regarding 'benefit' as a criterion for necessity I do not see mentioned whether we use this kind of malleable definition for other compounds used in health. The CWF-supporting experts, it seems, never discuss this[35]. Are there any other elements or compounds that use benefit as a criterion for essentiality? If so, then why? If not, then why not? Is it just this one element that gets the special treatment?

I will point out that in Perrott's defence he has made his point plain and clear; he has not been dishonest in his definition with regard to essentiality on this website article [152]. He has simply stretched the word 'essential' to include 'beneficial'. He also discussed a study demonstrating a "window of benefit" that one would typically see with essential nutrients, discussed below.

Please note that Perrott had used the words "... if we can't reach agreement on the use of terms like 'nutrient' and 'essential'" as part of his first response to Connett's statement. It surprises me that neither would go straight for their science dictionaries to find a definition or two. Considering Connett was from North America, and Perrott from New Zealand, this would have been sensible. However, this was a small point in the overall debate.

Dr. Perrott claimed a study funded by the (American) National Institute of Health (NIH), published in the **Journal of Bone and Mineral Research** in 2001, demonstrated a lower number of hip fractures in people in China drinking water fluoridated between 1.0 and 1.06 ppm when compared with lower and higher

---

[35] One exception were the words of Associate Professor Merilyn Manley-Harris in Waikato University's Google Hangout, discussed below.

concentrations, could be used to support his claims regarding fluorine's relationship to nutrition and bioapatites. He discusses this in the debate between the two men mentioned above [146, 153].

How well can Dr. Messer's first criterion be applied to humans? In the NIH study, the authors wrote:

> "In addition, a 3-day dietary survey and analysis for dietary intake of calcium, protein, and fluoride were conducted in a randomly selected 10% of subjects to ensure that all study populations had adequate nutrition and to determine fluoride exposure from diet." [153]

I am unsure if this means one three-day analysis, or one analysis every three days. But it's a good sign, better than nothing. Just consider how difficult it would be to monitor how much of each element/compound a human ate in a day? Or many groups of humans, for many generations. One would have to create a diet that people would have to adhere to for a long, long time. It is no wonder there are only animal experiments to work with. This 2001 study was also mentioned in Sir Peter Gluckman's review for similar reasons, but not in an overt relation to a nutritional role for fluorine.

The Perrott/Connett debate began on the 9th of October, 2013 [147]. On the 15th of September, 2013, barely a month earlier, Perrott had discussed on his website [154, 152] a 2010 document from the SCHER [116].

Dr. Perrott wrote that the document is often discussed in the work of "both sides". The reason he gave was that the document claimed fluoride:

> "... is not an essential element for human growth and development."

However, Dr. Perrott pointed out:

> "Misunderstandings often revolve around precise usage of words like *'essential.'*" [154] (His emphasis.)

I don't know how many meanings the word 'essential' can have, though Dr. Muhler has also expressed thoughts along this line [24].

Barely a few months later, on the 23rd of January, 2014, Dr. Perrott was discussing what this review had said about IQ – he had not mentioned on this page what the review had said about fluorine's non-essentiality for a few months, yet called fluoride a 'micronutrient' [155]. In the previous sentence he discussed 'microelement' deficiencies in selenium, zinc and iron.

Discussing fluorine right next to elements known to be essential is a little misleading, not that I want to imply deliberate dishonesty here, yet this is something I've seen in media again and again (examples are given in Chapter 5). Perrott wrote at the conclusion of his article on a nutritional role that he was not the person to decide if fluorine was essential or not [154]. However what he assumes implies it *is* essential, on this page [155].

'Micronutrient' implies or suggests a necessity, as does discussing fluorine right next to iodine and other elements known to be definitely essential – without needing to use 'benefit' as a criterion for essentiality. Perrott did not elaborate on this, even though the SCHER document was blunt about fluorine being non-essential. SCHER did not use the term micronutrient in this document [116].

However, if you look at the sample of definitions I have at the start of the book, you will see *almost every single definition* of 'micronutrient' or 'trace element' uses a word like 'necessary' or 'required'. Perrott has also commented on his website in a few places regarding Community Water Fluoridation correcting a deficiency just like iodized salt corrects iodine deficiency, and has discussed fluorine in the same paragraphs as other nutrients, which implies that he does consider it a nutrient [158].

He clarifies in the comments section of his page on essentiality (16th June, 2013 [152]), saying that he didn't call fluorine an essential element, although "debatable" because definitions can change. However he had used the terms 'micronutrient' and 'trace element', which at least *imply* essentiality. Presumably these terms do not mean that *here* – one can only presume because they are undefined. 'Semantics' indeed.

The use of the word 'deficiency' means that he is saying we can be deficient in something non-essential.

On a page of his website in 2015, Dr. Perrott discussed fluoride as a drug, claiming it was wrong to label it so. He did not go into any details on the sentence quoted below. He wrote that

"Really, fluoride is in the same class as sodium, potassium, phosphorus, magnesium and selenium." [159]

A couple of years after his debate with Professor Connett, Dr. Perrott wrote the following, in an open letter to Connett (posted on the 14th of July, 2016).

"Your assertion:

'in mammals not one single biochemical process has been shown to need fluoride to function properly'

is simply deceptive – knowingly so." [160][36]

I believe Connett's statement comes from one of his talks. He made a similar statement on page 6 of the debate the two had a few years earlier. This accusation from Perrott is an interesting statement, given that on his own website only a few years beforehand, he had opened an article with a statement addressing the frequently made claim by activists opposed to CWF that fluorine was not a nutritional essential. Of this, he wrote:

"Literally I guess it means that there are no identified biological pathways essential to human life involving F." [152]

He didn't seem to disagree with this earlier statement (June, 2013 [152]) on that particular page [160]. There is a few years' difference here, and he had possibly forgotten.

Dr. Perrott cited a European document that concluded almost exactly the same thing – that fluoride was *not* essential [154]. As well as this, he'd used a quotation he found on Wikipedia saying something similar [152].

As I've mentioned before, Connett *et al.* had cited a letter quoting the 1989 NAS publication, which looked at "contradictory results" from rodent studies that caused the NAS to proclaim fluoride non-essential (though they put it in the 'trace elements' category) [81, 149].

---

36 Perhaps Professor Connett had obtained his statement "… not one single biochemical process…" cited here, from O'Dell and Sunde's introduction: "Fluoride is a structural component of bones and teeth, but there is no evidence that it exerts a specific biochemical function." [89] This textbook (though not this introduction) was cited by Combs in *Essentials of Medical Geology* 5th edition [87], which was in turn cited by the NAS [86].

Perrott claimed so strongly to represent science and think critically, yet in their debate he did not discuss this document, or any of the experiments it was based upon.

Experts have for *decades* been telling the public to trust experts, therefore one would think Perrott would approve when Connett *did* trust a couple of them – namely people from the NAS, big supporters of CWF and not inconsistent about it.

A feature of 'the experts' is that they are so quick to point the finger and accuse many who disagree with them of 'cherry-picking' or 'selectivity' but unable to see when they do it themselves. Dr. Perrott, to my knowledge, has ignored the words of the NAS and the SCHER, even when right in front of him.

His website is called *Open Parachute* because there is a saying that the mind does not work properly unless it is like a parachute – open – yet he did not follow through on finding the NAS document, even though it's online, like Wikipedia.

What is the end result of this lack of investigation? The people reading his website don't see it, don't know about it and don't see the experiments.

At the beginning of 2017, Dr. Perrott's website was getting 4,082 visits per month [161].

Maybe I'm following this a few years too late, but on linking to the Wikipedia article on Dietary Minerals from Dr. Perrott's website [152], I'm seeing fluorine is categorized as

> "Suggested function from deprivation effects or active metabolic handling, but no clearly-identified biochemical function in humans." [162]

The last half of this sentence sounds quite close to what Professor Connett had said, above.

Perrott had quoted this from Wikipedia:

> "However, if one considers the prevention of dental cavities an important criterion in determining essentiality, then fluoride might well be considered an essential trace element." [152]

This statement echoes the words of the WHO in 2002, see above.

Here, 'Preventive' = 'Essential'.

It is interesting that Perrott cites Wikipedia, I can remember being told *not* to use Wikipedia as a source for research when I attended university – at least not for *primary* research, though I can understand it is probably of reasonable accuracy. I'm *not* saying Dr. Perrott has authored a bad article here [152] – on the contrary, it's *good* that he's up front about his terms and definitions.

The article has two headings titled 'benefit' – which demonstrates the overlap between necessity and benefit that we find in expert literature. This is a blurring of boundaries, that we generally *don't* find in the experiments mentioned in Chapter 1. On this note we may want to consider that the experts claim to represent science accurately and objectively, an example can be found in the debate cited previously[37]. Note this lack of precision

---

[37] *The Fluoride Debate*, Dr. Perrott claims his objectivity or claims people who oppose fluoridation lack objectivity on pages 17, 60, 61, 110, 136, 143, 209.

in big city-wide analyses and comparisons used in public health. Sometimes when experts mean "essential" they don't mean "essential" in its traditional sense, they mean it in a sort of lazy Sunday afternoon sense, where it really means beneficial in some circumstances. I'm *glad* Dr. Perrott is open about his definitions at least on this one page, because as I say, I've *almost never* seen this mentioned by the experts in the mainstream media.

In 2012, a paper was published on the website of The Institute of Science in Medicine, discussing statements coming from activists and professionals who did not support CWF. The paper referred to fluoride as a micro-nutrient that was essential for the generation and upkeep of the skeleton and the dentition [163].

No discussion or elaboration on these statements was entered into and no citations to other literature were made.

On the 14th of October, 2013, an "expert panel from the University of Waikato" appeared on a Google Hangout [1]. This was a group discussion filmed with interaction from the public, who could ask questions through social media. The panel contained six experts, four of whom were Senior Lecturers in chemistry, with one in biology and one in psychology. Nobody involved with professional dentistry or public health was present, and no question was asked by the public why this was so. I don't know what the motivation was for the panel to get together, presumably they simply cared about the issue and felt they could help. It is great to see people participating. The discussion lasted for about an hour, with the answer to the question of essentiality lasting about five minutes. Nobody on the panel appeared to know about a single experiment that had tested for fluorine's essentiality, and none of them appeared to know about the recent words of the WHO, SCHER, EFSA or NAS on the matter. This again illustrates a lack of importance of the question of fluorine's essentiality. It looked like the discussion was conducted from the offices of the staff involved, with their own recording equipment. In some places the recording is a little hard to hear, so as with all of the other references used in this book I will suggest the reader visit the source and check for themselves.

The question was asked about twenty minutes in:

> "Considering the natural involvement of fluoride in bioapatites, and the fact that it is ubiquitous in the environment, could the panel clarify the question as to whether fluoride is beneficial or essential? I ask because some reviews describe fluoride as an essential nutrient while others call it an essential micro-element because of the role it plays in bones and teeth."

I have paraphrased the responses to take out unnecessary words, 'ums' and 'ahs', etc. Other than that the responses are here in full.

The question is first given to Dr. Michael Mucalo, Senior Lecturer in physical chemistry.

> "... the benefit of it is that in teeth obviously is the compound that comprises teeth is hydroxyapatite which has got a formula of $Ca_{10}PO_4.6(OH)_2$ and that $(OH)_2$ which is hydroxyl groups is what gets attacked by acid... and the theory is that the fluoride is meant to replace those and produce a compound called fluorapatite which is very insoluble and is more resistant to attack... and I think it has been shown that even if it is ingested it has got a very small improvement for bone strength but, I mean, that's the general view about the benefits of it anyway."

The question was opened to the panel and Dr. Joseph Lane, Senior Lecturer in physical and theoretical chemistry took to the microphone:

"I think whether something is considered to be an essential element or nutrient or whether it's a medication… [problem with microphone]… I think these decisions often get made by courts, and not necessarily by scientists… so, just because a certain decision's been made in a particular country doesn't necessarily mean that's the best description for a word. I think this idea that fluoride is a medication that's commonly used is a position from a high court in Holland, and why are we necessarily considering something to be a medication or not a medication based on the position of one foreign country? I'm not quite sure about. With regard to specifically whether it's an essential element or nutrient, it depends on whether you think having strong teeth is an essential component of a healthy lifestyle… if you think it's not, if you're happy to have your teeth fall out and rot, etcetera, then we'll happily put it in the category of not being essential… but if you want to be able to live a long life that allows you to eat food the whole time, then maybe you'd make the consideration that it is an essential element or nutrient."

Dr. Graham Saunders (inorganic chemistry) also added to the answer:

"I think it would be very hard to prove one way or the other because fluoride is ubiquitous, it's in seawater to 1.2 parts per million, it's hard to avoid it so every creature will have grown up and evolved in an environment containing fluoride. Whether that is actually necessary, one could perhaps think that fluorapatite is less soluble than hydroxyapatite but when bones are first formed, they're seeded on fluorapatite… one could make an argument it's essential if that mechanism applied. So I think it's going to be very hard to prove one way or the other if it's essential or not… it's benefit comes from fluorapatite being much more resistant to acid than hydroxyapatite in terms of the teeth. It also has a perhaps more controversial benefit in terms of bone health in that it slows down loss of calcium in older age, so it can be used and has been used in treatment for osteoporosis but I think that is with much higher doses of fluoride and problems can arise because of that, the patient can develop dental… not dental, skeletal fluorosis as a result of treatment for osteoporosis."

"To conclude I think it's going to be very hard to prove one way or the other whether it's an essential element or not, it quite possibly could be… certainly from a scientific point of view… [hard to hear] a chemical… [hard to hear]… incontrovertible."

The last part of Dr. Saunders' speech suffered from the microphone cutting in and out a little. The conversation returned to Dr. Mucalo:

"Yes, you need to design very careful experiments to specifically exclude fluoride from the diet before you could categorically prove whether it was or was not an essential element, and I think they've done that for things like silicon, where they've tried to prove whether it was essential for the diet but you'd have to do very excrutiatingly careful experiments to do that, so… at this stage I don't know whether anyone's done that yet."

Associate Professor Merilyn Manley-Harris (organic and analytical chemistry) said:

"I think there are many substances which people regard as essential which haven't actually been scientifically proven to be essential."

Now would be a good time to have a look at Appendix 1. The mediator concluded:

"Hopefully we'll give our questioner a reasonably solid answer then."

Stephen Barrett M.D. runs a website called Quackwatch. Indexed on a sub-site, dentalwatch.org, are United States Public Health Service (USPHS) documents regarding CWF [164].

At the top of the USPHS index on his website, Barrett had quoted:

> "The U.S. Public Health Service strongly supports fluoridation of community water supplies. From 1968 through 1979, it issued periodic BULLETINS to help community leaders answer questions and deal with unfounded opposition. Although some are outdated, all were valid at the time they were issued and many refute claims that are still used today."

The following documents look at fluorine's essentiality.

A 1960 document [165], written by a team of nineteen people, most of whom had degrees in dentistry and public health, concluded fluorine essential, "… if teeth are essential to maintain good health of individuals…" The researchers pointed out that no-one had been able to create a diet free of fluorine, meaning that the "minimum fluoride level conducive to optimal general health" was undetermined. This statement was taken from the Food and Nutrition Board of the NAS, in a 1953 document. However, they claimed that "epidemiological and clinical observations" sufficed regarding the level which yielded greatest protection from dental caries, with the lowest amount of dental fluorosis. This team of nineteen were working under two supervisors at the University of Ann Arbor, Michigan. Not a single one of the experiments that I have discussed in Chapter 1 were mentioned addressing fluorine's essentiality in the 1960 document.

One can see the effects that the publicity regarding the work of Schwarz and Messer *et al.* had on the intellectual climate. Note that the earlier, and very good[38] work of Maurer and Day [17], and Doberenz *et al.* [19], were not mentioned in *any* of these USPHS documents. The work of Wuthier and Phillips [18] was ignored by almost everyone; I don't think I have ever even seen it mentioned in activist, anti-fluoride literature either.

A 1970 document quoted the 1968 edition of **Recommended Dietary Allowances**:

> "Fluoride is incorporated in the structure of teeth and is necessary for maximal resistance to dental caries. For these reasons, it is considered to be an essential nutrient." [166]

A document dated January, 1972 from the United States Department of Health, Education and Welfare, Public Health Service, National Institutes of Health, looked at the work of Dr. Schwarz [167] (see Chapter 1). A couple of pages of detail were given regarding the Schwarz and Milne experiment, pointing out that 2.5 ppm in water gave "optimal" results regarding growth rates.

Another one of these "BULLETINS" was a document written about a Nutritionist, Dr. Jean Mayer, from Harvard University, who wrote a column called "Food for thought". The USPHS document claimed his column was distributed to around 100 newspapers in the **Chicago Tribune-New York News** Syndicate. Mayer served as chairman on a couple of White House conferences on aging and nutrition. He blamed dental caries on five things, one of which was "inadequate fluoride in the water"[39] [168]. This was in November, 1972.

None of the other experiments I have mentioned in Chapter 1 were discussed in either of these two 1972 bulletins, even though some had recently been mentioned in the 1970 World Health Organization monograph

---

[38] Recall Dr. Schwarz called it "rather sophisticated" [26].

[39] The others were excessive sugar, poor nutrition, poor dental hygiene and inherited susceptibility.

[102]. This is of interest because the USPHS had *funded* the 1964 experiment by Doberenz *et al.*, which had not found a significant deficiency on rats fed at most 0.005 ppm fluoride. One of Nielsen and Sandstead's criticisms of the Schwarz experiments (see Chapter 1) was that other researchers had healthy mice on *much* less fluoride.

A 1974 document looked at the way in which the 1971 NAS report [69] (mentioned previously in Chapter 2.1) had been "variously referenced by opponents of fluoridation…" and wanted to set the record straight [169]. The document pointed out that the NAS had been long-time supporters of CWF, and quoted Dr. Jaroslav J. Vostal, chairman of the NRC panel on fluorides, who had authored the 1971 report. His statement, dated 7th February, 1974, addressed pages 66 and 67 of the report, a little of which was quoted earlier here. Vostal suggests that

> "A reasonable and correct paraphrase of these statements might be:
>
> Fluoride has without any doubt a beneficial pharmacological effect in preventing tooth decay, but this does not mean that the presence of fluoride in the diet is indispensable for any vital (i.e. important and useful) function, including the integrity of the dental system, in animals or man." [169] (His emphasis.)

This document also pointed to the Schwarz and Milne experiment [20], and the Messer *et al.* experiment on fertility impairment [28], as coming out shortly after the 1971 NAS document [69]. But it did not mention any of the experiments that had concluded fluorine non-essential.

Another 1974 document looked at fluorine's essentiality, "re-emphasized and confirmed in statements by competent authorities" – the Food and Nutrition Board of the NAS, the US Food and Drug Administration (FDA), Dartmouth Medical School, and the laboratories of Dr. Schwarz and Dr. Armstrong [170].

The NAS document was the 1974 edition of **Recommended Dietary Allowances**, pages 98 to 99. It claimed that fluorine's abundance had made a reproducible deficiency in animals "very difficult to produce." According to the USPHS [170], it cited the study by Schwarz and Milne [20], and pointed to the benefits in tooth decay reduction.

Also cited were the words of the US FDA in a Federal Register document – fluorine was listed as an "essential mineral nutrient". There was no elaboration.

This USPHS document quoted excerpts from a letter dated 25th May, 1973, to Senator Hart from Henry A. Schroeder, Professor Emeritus of Physiology from Dartmouth College. These were apparently from pages 201 and 202 the *Safe Drinking Water Act* Hearing before the Ninety-Third Congress, 31st May, 1973 [171]. One is quoted:

> "Standards for the Essential elements, except selenium, which is toxic, are unimportant and can be based on other characteristics (taste, color, staining or enamel) than toxicity." [170]

Schroeder claimed fluorine to be essential and non-toxic here. The work referenced here is from his 1968 experiment [30]. I encourage the reader to consider this work in light of the 1976 experiments cited [33, 34], and the claim that fluorine had a beneficial pharmacological effect upon iron absorption. Schroeder *et al.* claimed that fluorine-fed male mice lived longer:

> "Mice fed [10 ppm] fluoride [in water] and antimony survived as well as their controls."

> "According to measured life spans, male mice fed fluorine lived longer than their controls by 29 to 60 days at 3 intervals, whereas females did not." [30]

In this USPHS document [170], Schroder had been quoted as saying that giving mice 10 ppm fluorine in water was non-toxic. In Schroeder and his team's work [30] fluorine was not detected in the diet[40], nor in soft tissues even after two years (bone was not analysed, though Schroeder acknowledged it accumulates fluorine). No details were given on whether Schroeder and his team felt this lack of detection was usual or not. He began his experiment by including fluorine in the trace element category.

Also cited in the USPHS document were the 1973 paper from the University of Minnesota [4], and the 1972 experiment by David Milne and Klaus Schwarz [20].

A 1977 document discussed a (December, 1976) statement issued by the National Nutrition Consortium,

> "praising the use of fluoridation as a means of providing an essential nutrient to the diets of children susceptible to dental caries." [172]

The use of rodents in these experiments and their applicability to humans was not discussed in any anatomical or dental detail. Nielsen and Sandstead's critique of Schwarz's work was also ignored.

In light of these USPHS documents, it may be worth mentioning the 1974 experiment by Weber and Reid [35] (Reid had worked on the earlier experiment with Doberenz *et al.*, see Chapter 1.1). Weber and Reid's experiment funded by the USPHS was not mentioned here either. It was published in the same 1974 document as the Messer *et al.* summary [31]. This experiment, along with the two 1976 experiments, were not mentioned in any document on this USPHS index, even though the two 1976 experiments that had refuted the Messer *et al.* experiments, were partially funded by the USPHS. I didn't find any of these experiments mentioned or even discussed, not even in the 1977 document. Perhaps this is acceptable because this one came *to* the USPHS, *from* the consortium... but surely the USPHS would have known about the experiments that refuted the claim made by Messer *et al...*? If *they* didn't, surely Stephen Barrett would have? After all, he is an expert. Concerning the bulletins, he did write:

> "Although some are outdated, all were valid at the time they were issued and many refute claims that are still used today." [164]

The examples given by Dr. Barrett of the USPHS demonstrate a bias towards trying to prove a definite need for fluorine in nutrition. Given the date of these documents it is understandable that they would appreciate recent research from 1968 and the early 1970s, yet the USPHS has ignored work that did not suit the conclusion of essentiality. Presumably this is done in order to promote acceptability of Community Water Fluoridation programs. Is it within the realm of honest, objective science for the USPHS to do this? If we're minimizing research that doesn't suit, by accident or purposefully, are we sure we're basing our decisions on firm foundations? The USPHS had no interest *even in studies they had funded*, that concluded fluorine non-essential, at least according to what Dr. Barrett presents. Even the bulletin [169] that looked at the 1971 NAS document

---

[40] Using an Orion Research, Inc. brand fluoride electrode from Cambridge, Massachusetts.

[69] ignored the question of how and why other experiments had found rats perfectly healthy with lower fluoride levels than those Dr. Schwarz used. This was one of three arguments against his conclusion by Nielsen and Sandstead [27]. These examples demonstrate that honesty, as well as deep, thoughtful research, had lost much of their importance, even in the early 1970s.

Consider these examples of USPHS appraisal of evidence with regard to Dr. Rob Beaglehole's recent statement that

"… the evidence is overwhelmingly stacked in our favour." [67]

These bulletins were sent to community leaders in the United States.

Another relevant factor here is the polarization of attitudes to fluoridation. It becomes obvious that if we're on a 'side', showing research that undermines what 'our side' has been saying for a long time, only helps the people on 'the other side'. This is discussed in more detail in Chapter 5, but Chapter 3 will also give some examples of this occurring very early in New Zealand. Here we see an exaggeration of fluorine's necessity, and definitely a refusal to accept the possibility of its dispensability (the word "dispensable" used by Maurer and Day to describe the element [17]).

One of Stephen Barrett's articles addresses Professor Connett. In this article he wrote:

"Connett wants to classify fluoride as a drug (rather than a nutrient or a public health measure) so he can apply drug-related guidelines without considering whether they make sense for fluoride." [173]

Is fluoride a drug? This has not been a focus of this investigation, yet will be mentioned briefly in following chapters where a couple of experts have made relevant comments. Obviously if we can change the definition of what essentiality is, we can probably change the definition of what constitutes a drug.

2.8 Expert Contradictions

The experts consistently present a united front in public. However, in reading their literature, one can find contradictions. The book you are now reading was partly inspired by some of these.

Consider Ericsson's statement,

"For the formation of a caries-resistant enamel, a certain fluoride supply is evidently essential."

He said this after noting that it had been difficult to find a definite answer regarding the need for fluorine.

Compare this with Joseph Muhler's statement in the second chapter of the same document:

"Further study, with the use of diets lower in fluorine content than those reported here, concerning the essentiality of fluorine is needed, especially in regard to the effects on cellular enzyme systems, on normal and pathological calcification processes and on reproduction and initial growth responses." [102]

This is not quite a full contradiction, but does warrant mentioning.

Compare the statement,

"Most researchers consider fluoride essential for proper development of bones and teeth" [145]

… in a 1988 American document, with the statement,

"Most nutritional authorities have not classified fluoride as an essential nutrient" [125]

... in a 2002 Australian textbook.

Neither of these documents presents us with a sample, nor tells us how many 'most' is. Most in the USA/Canada/Mexico? Where else? Most in NZ/Australia? How many is 'most', anyway? Most in the world? Sixty percent of our sample? Three quarters? Seven eighths?

How big is our sample? (What sample?) Most out of a google search? Most out of a pile of textbooks on the shelf of the Professor's office down the hallway? Most out of the people we asked that happened to be in the tea room of the dentistry department on the morning we wrote this chapter?

Nonetheless, one can see why arguments about this element get heated, when a person could seem justified in picking either one of these writings as an authority. I've noticed some reporters are bored and disillusioned with such conflicting information. I decided to stick to one topic for reasons of depth and consistency.

The 1988 document [145] boasted three people from the Ohio Department of Public Health, and one from the USPHS. The authors acknowledged the support and assistance of both departments, as well as the Centers for Disease Control in Atlanta, Georgia, and the USPHS Indian Health Service in Rockville, Maryland.

The 2002 textbook [125] was authored by two people from prominent universities (Otago, NZ, and Sydney, Australia), both using the title Professor of Human Nutrition. The section on fluorine was written by the Australian, along with Marion Robinson (nee Harrison, according to a book review in the **Asia Pacific Journal of Clinical Nutrition** [174], co-author of the paper with Muriel Bell mentioned in the previous chapter), then a retired (now deceased) professor of nutrition from Otago University.

2.9 A Couple of Outliers

Overwhelmingly, those opposed to Community Water Fluoridation (CWF) believed fluorine to be a non-essential element in human nutrition.

On the other hand, the majority of people who supported CWF consistently seemed to claim the opposite in public – that fluorine is, was, and always has been an essential nutrient. In many elaborations it was claimed essential for bones and teeth, and occasionally for growth. Yet in literature supportive of CWF that goes deeper into the topic, we find a greater presence of the belief that fluorine is non-essential.

This section looks at a small handful of outliers – those who oppose CWF but publicly believe fluorine essential, and those who support CWF but publicly believe fluorine non-essential.

I've found only two people to oppose CWF and believe fluorine an essential nutrient. Every other time I have seen the topic of essentiality mentioned by people opposed to CWF they have claimed it non-essential or at minimum leaned toward that end of the spectrum.

One who opposed CWF was Madam Mira Louise James, quoted in the 1957 New Zealand Commission of Inquiry. For want of context, she was criticizing the *addition* of the element, believing that the amount New Zealand's waters was enough.

When asked,

"And you would be fair enough to say that it is an essential thing for human beings to have it?"

She apparently replied,

"Well, if you don't have fluorine you are just unbalanced. It is a very necessary element…" [175]

The second was a person by the name of H. G. Halliwell who wrote a letter published in a New Zealand newspaper.

"In my own work in Palmerston North, before fluoridation was adopted there, we had severe illnesses in dairy stock which scientists traced to excess fluorine in the top-dressing material. This emphasizes the fact that all the "essential" trace elements, in excess, produce toxic effects." [176]

Dr. Frank McClure's book (discussed previously [47]) will suffice as an example of a CWF supporter who expressed at least a slight doubt in fluorine's necessity.

Dr. Mike Berridge works at the Malaghan Institute in Wellington, New Zealand, as a researcher on cancer. In his book *The Edge of Life, Controversies and Challenges in Human Health*, he wrote

"Fluoride – the negatively charged ion of fluorine – was once considered an essential element for human growth and development but contemporary evidence doesn't support that view." [177]

In late 2016, he debated Paul Connett in New Zealand on the TV show *Thinking Green*. He agreed with Professor Connett that fluorine was not an essential nutrient. It was interesting to listen to him say that fluorine is "very similar" to iodine and selenium. Which is bizarre because he said fluorine is not essential… iodine and selenium *are* essential (See Underwood's 4th Edition, pages 280 and 314, or the more recent work of the EFSA).

He said New Zealand soils and waters are deficient in fluoride [178]. This is similar to Dr. Perrott's statements.

We *can* be deficient in something non-essential, according to some of the experts. Like Dr. Perrott in many examples, Dr. Berridge did not give any indication toward evidence of the existence of a deficiency condition in experimental humans or animals.

2.10 Summary

When the NAS cite *more research*, in the form of studies that test for essentiality, they seem to be *more likely* to come to a conclusion of *non*-essentiality [69, 70, 79, 81, 83]. In the literature that claims fluorine essential, the NAS have either used benefit as a criterion for essentiality, assumed essentiality but noted that fluorine's abundance defied the creation of a deficiency, or looked at almost no studies that have to do with essentiality [77, 80, 85, 86].

Publicly, the experts have largely ignored the conclusion of non-essentiality, that animal experiments suggest. Although because no experiment used *absolutely* zero ppm fluorine (except apparently Schroeder's), it can be argued that based on these rodent experiments, fluorine is closer to "*almost* definitely not" an essential nutrient, instead of "definitely not" an essential nutrient. Though this word "almost" is barely significant – if there *is* an amount of fluorine required, it is so small as to be nearly immeasurable in the diet, and on any normal diet one would be guaranteed an abundance of the element due to its consistent presence in nearly all foods. I found no discussion of Schroeder's claim that no fluoride was found in the diet he used.

Applying animal experiments to humans is something infrequently discussed in these writings. Ulf Lindh has suggested that necessity of an element should be demonstrated in "several species" before it is considered essential. Experiments on birds are probably much less relevant than those carried out on rodents, and are rarely discussed in this topic [98]. Nor is the lack of precision (regarding humans obtaining all necessary nutritional factors) available in huge, city-wide CWF experiments.

It appears that the fact that no real fluorine deficiency could be demonstrated in the same way that an iodine deficiency or a deficiency in some other essential element or compound could be demonstrated, was no cause for concern. The experts believe in 'optimal' levels of fluorine, and I believe the experts use the term 'deficiency' interchangeably with the term 'sub-optimal' though I have not seen any literature that discusses this. This is disappointing to me, especially considering the wide age range of some of the literature I'm using, the differing scientific and political natures of the literature, and the fact that I'm going to prestigious and respected sources.

The WHO has called fluorine a micronutrient, suggested it should be classified as essential [109]. This has been done *without* fluorine meeting traditional or conventional requirements of essentiality in trace element research. I have never seen this discussed publicly beyond one small letter to a newspaper editor discussed in Chapter 5.2. This topic is a conversation that must happen if we are to examine the foundation of our understanding of fluorine and the element's relationship to humanity. Recently, the WHO has also claimed fluorine's essentiality "has not been demonstrated unequivocally." [120]

Basing our understanding of a need for fluorine on work done decades ago is imperfect given that in every NAS document cited here, the sample of studies was incomplete. This is probably due to such a massive glut of information on the topic, the obscurity of the subject, time pressures, and perhaps poor cataloging in databases. One cannot expect even the experts to have every nuanced, detailed little aspect of every topic at their fingertips and kept fresh in their minds.

New Zealand experts followed the advice and promotional patterns of American experts (discussed in greater detail in Chapters 3 and 5).

With expertise and prestige comes the power to change the meaning of words: we *can* be deficient in something non-essential. We *can* have 'not enough' of something we almost certainly don't need. The experts *don't need to demonstrate the existence of a deficiency*, in order to claim that a deficiency exists.

In the scientific literature, I have not seen a single expert publicly elaborate on why this is so. Nor have I seen experts criticized by other experts for continuing such behavior for many decades.

The only time the word "deficient" or "deficiency" appears in Sir Peter Gluckman and Sir David Skegg's report is with regard to iodine, *not* fluorine.

It is misleading for experts to discuss fluorine-deficient waters and soils. The reason being that *obviously* if the public believes they are drinking fluorine-deficient water, and eating food grown in fluorine-deficient soil, it follows as *perfect logic* (in the mind of the public) that the public would then become fluorine-deficient. This even though prestigious bodies recommended by experts claim fluorine deficiency in humans has not been demonstrated [103, 105, 116, 117-119].

Afterword

A day before the publication of this book you are now reading (10th June, 2020) I was able to check the 1977 document (footnote 17) cited by Dr. Mertz (footnote 16) in which Dr. Schwarz repeated his claim of fluorine's essentiality. It was based on his work with David Milne [20]. Schwarz (footnote 17) simply cited his work, with no discussion or explanation, and did not address any of the criticisms of his work put forth by two scientists from the US Dept. of Agriculture [27]. (Mertz did not specifically discuss the criticisms of Schwarz's work either.)

3.   What did Experts in New Zealand Say?

Official, less public statements also demonstrate that many public health officials believed fluorine to be an essential nutrient.

It should be obvious that as more research comes to light, as technology improves, as scientific methodologies improve, conclusions in science change. It should also be obvious that one responsibility a conscientious researcher has is that of keeping abreast of new discoveries. In order to fulfil this responsibility, a willingness to actively search for one's own ignorance and change one's pre-existing beliefs is required.

Communications in the 1950s and 1960s largely involved telephone calls, meetings and letters. The speed of communication today allowed by modern technology was impossible.

I will divulge the extent of my research into the New Zealand Health Department archives, so that misunderstandings are minimized. This will indicate to you my "sample size". We live in an age dubbed the 'Information Age' and sometimes a staggering amount of information is available on any one subject. The simple fact that there is so much available means one must select what is relevant often before spending many hours looking for it, or through the file that contains it. This makes it easy to miss a lot, and easy for accusations of favouritism to exist when someone else leaves our favourite document or study out of a sample. I searched all the way through seventeen Health Department files (a little over an inch thick each), and partly through three (wherein I was looking for specific items). These files were archived as part of an Official Information Act, and have been available to the public since 1982. Records from the Health Department archived files are cited with "HD" then the record number. These can be requested through the website https://www.archway.archives.govt.nz/, though permission from the Ministry of Health is required for some files.

3.1 Private Correspondence

In a letter to a Mrs. E. M. Weld of Tauranga, (**Figure 3**) dated 3rd September 1954, the Minister of Health, Mr. Jack Marshall, wrote:

> "... it is quite apparent that a reasonable proportion of fluorine in the diet is essential to good dental health."
> [179]

My Departmental officers would heartily agree with your suggestion that if everybody ate the right food we should have very little dental caries. My Department is continually stressing the importance of good diet but unless we could achieve the absolute prohibition of the sale of white bread, cakes, sweets, ice cream, soft drinks, etc., we are unlikely to achieve our purpose. It is necessary, therefore, to seek other means by which dental health can be improved and it is quite apparent that a reasonable proportion of fluorine in the diet is essential to good dental health. The increase of fluorine intake to the optimum figure will unquestionably bring about a great improvement in dental conditions notwithstanding that people continue to eat unwisely.

Figure 3: Excerpt of a letter from the Minister of Health, 3rd September 1954. HD 125/299 H1 Box 1635.

In a letter to Mr. L. W. Harris, Secretary of the Papatoetoe Anti-Fluoridation Society, dated 24th September 1954, (**Figure 4**) the Minister of Health, Mr. Marshall, wrote,

"It has been accepted by authoritative medical opinion that fluorine is a trace element that is essential for the proper development of teeth and bones..." [179]

I think we must agree to differ as to whether or not "mass medication" is an appropriate term to apply to fluoridation of water supplies. It has been accepted by authoritative medical opinion that fluorine is a trace element that is essential for the proper development of teeth and bones, and it moreover occurs naturally in many foods and in many natural waters. The adjustment of the fluorine content of a water supply to the optimum level cannot therefore be correctly described as "medication".

Figure 4: Excerpt of a letter from the Minister of Health, 24 September, 1954. HD 125/299 H1 Box 1635.

In a letter to the Auckland City Council dated 11th May, 1955, (**Figure 5**) C. S. Hercus, Dean of University of Otago Medical School, wrote:

"There is no question but that fluorine like iodine is an essential component of man's food supply..." [180]

There is no question but that fluorine like iodine is an essential component of man's food supply. In both cases, however, the amount required is extremely minute. Unlike iodine, fluorine is in the main supplied to us in our drinking water. Where the fluoride content of the

Figure 5: Excerpt of the letter from the Dean of University of Otago Medical School attached to the New Zealand Dental Association's submissions to the Commission of Inquiry into Fluoridation of Water Supplies, 22nd November, 1956. HD 125/299/6 H1 Box 1679.

In a letter to the Minister of Health, dated 30th May 1956, (**Figure 6**) the soon-to-be Minister of Health, H. G. R. Mason (at this time he was M.P. for Waitakere), wrote:

"And of course it has long been known that fluorine occurs in the enamel of human teeth, and, I have supposed, has been regarded as an essential constituent." [181]

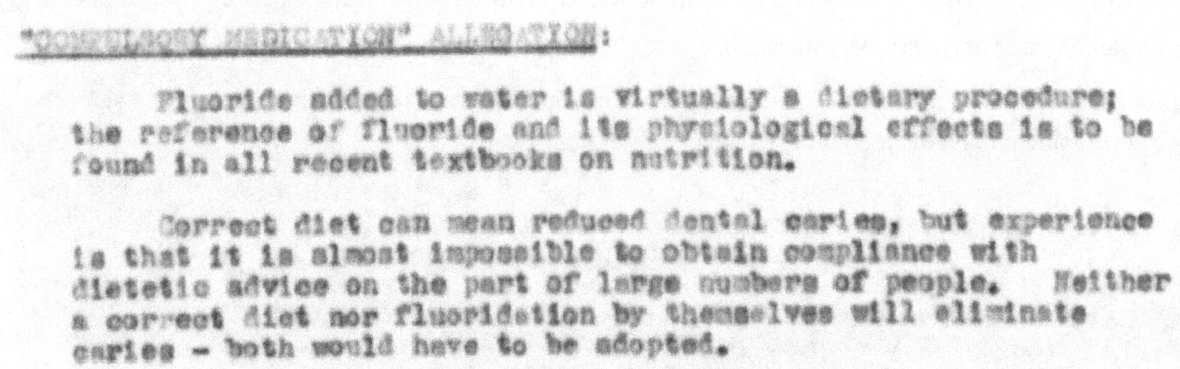

Figure 6: Excerpt of a letter from the Member of Parliament for Waitakere, 30th May 1956. HD 125/299/4 H1 Box 1828.

The document *Fluoridation of Public Water Supplies* (a precis by the Health Department, **Figure 7**) told readers – in response to the "'Compulsory Medication' Allegation" – that

"Fluoride added to water is virtually a dietary procedure…" [182]

Figure 7: Excerpt from Health Department document 'Fluoridation of Public Water Supplies'. HD 125/299 H1 Box 1667.

In the early 1950s the New Zealand experts produced a lot of educational material. Claiming fluoridation a dietary procedure became a convenient defence against the "compulsory/mass medication" argument made by people opposed to fluoridation, but this convincing statement could dissuade someone from looking into the research themselves. Who is going to bother updating themselves with inconvenient research?

When I began studying this topic I wondered "why do experts talk as though fluorine *has* to be a nutrient?" I saw a few statements like the one above, before realizing: if fluorine added to the public water supply is a nutrient, it is not considered a drug, and the experts are justified in their practice of adding it to water. There is no compulsive medication involved, thus the experts have won this battle.

Perhaps the experts think it's not a drug until we're using a huge medically-administered dose, but at these near-1.0 ppm levels the claim made is that fluoride is a nutrient and fluoridation is simply correcting a deficiency.

This statement that fluoridation is "virtually a dietary procedure…" [183] is found repeated on page 2 of the September, 1956 proposal for the 1957 Commission of Inquiry (**Figure 8**).

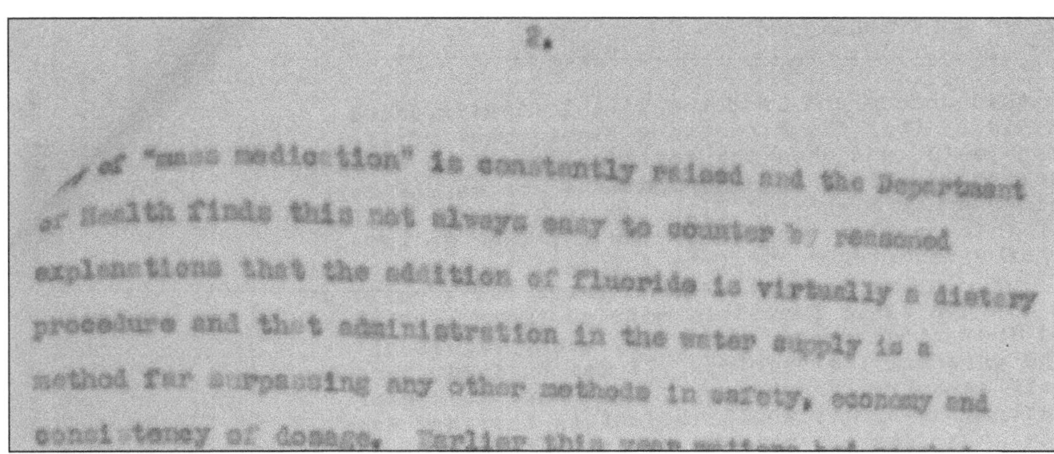

Figure 8: Excerpt of page 2 of the September, 1956 proposal for the 1957 Commission of Inquiry. HD 125/299/6 H1 Box 1674.

The 1957 Commission of Inquiry called fluoridation a process of food fortification. Ironically, this was the year the Maurer and Day experiment (see Chapter 1.1) was published – four generations of rats raised on less than one hundredth of a milligram of fluorine per day, with no teeth problems. The diet was sugar-free, except for what naturally occurred in the food.

In a letter to S. S. Green, Esq., Mayor of Dargaville, dated 3rd April 1958, (**Figure 9**) the Minister of Health, H. G. R. Mason, wrote:

"It has been known for three-quarters of a century that fluorine is essential to the enamel of human teeth ..." [184]

As to your suggestion that the Department should "test every angle", I may say that it would be impossible for one department to cover anything like the work that has already been done by ever so many authorities, persons and bodies in various parts of the world in reference to this problem. There is nothing novel or untried in what the Department is doing. It has been known for three-quarters of a century that fluorine is essential to the enamel of human teeth, and for thirty years or more the problem has been under investigation as to the result of excess or deficiency of fluorine in water supplies. I can remember noticing an article in the Parliamentary Library - it must be twenty years ago - having a bibliography at the end of it showing an immense number of references to investigations of the problem.

When you raise a question and say "This is an aspect which never appears to have been investigated - not even by the Royal Commission", I would point out that the Royal Commission investigated every aspect of the matter that was raised before it

Figure 9: Excerpt of a letter from the Minister of Health, 3rd April, 1958. [REF] HD 125/299 H1 Box 1714.

In a letter dated 26th August, 1958 to a Mrs. Grace Barnes, (**Figure 10**) the Minister of Health wrote:

"Most of our water contains fluoride, but not in sufficient quantity." [184]

He used iodine and goitre as an example.

I have always understood from the time I first studied elementary chemistry that fluorine was a constituent of the enamel of human teeth, and when our teeth are found to be very bad in contrast to the teeth of other nations one cannot help wondering whether a deficiency of fluorine is a cause.   Investigation of this problem, however, does not seem to have arisen from that circumstance but from the fact that the people of a certain State in America - it may be Texas but I would not be quite sure - are notable for their mottled teeth, and investigation showed that this was due to a very great excess of fluoride in the water of the country. It was noticed, however, that their teeth were free from decay. This lead to a most thorough investigation of the whole subject in that and many other countries. The result has been to confirm that fluorides do have this influence in causing enamel to resist decay. Having always had the suspicion that the quantity of fluorine available might be an important influence in the resistance of teeth to decay it would have been impossible for me to express myself as opposed to fluoridation.

"   I quite agree with you as to it being "glaringly obvious "that, the real cause of dental caries lies mainly in faulty "dietary and oral habits - the intake of too much sugar or "starches, also, today, most of our foods are devitalised and "too refined."   The Health Department has been trying to drum this into the people for many a long day, but few people combine the intelligence and will to alter their habits.   It would be a very happy circumstance if those who have done so would help to convert the rest of the country to better habits. Unhappily they seem to think they sufficiently serve if they merely try to prevent people using any other help, and in particular try to prevent them having the help that comes from fluoridating water.

Goitre, for example, is a feature of alpine valleys and of some peoples where the water comes generally from snow or other sources without passing through the earth, and consequently without having in it the necessary traces of dissolved mineral.   As you know, goitre has practically been abolished in New Zealand through iodising our salt and thereby making good the deficiency. We were very fortunate in that this was a local problem and did not have a counterpart in America so far as I know.   Had it been otherwise and the discussion arisen in America we might have had the Americans stirring up the same sort of unfounded argument as they have concerning fluoride, and perhaps we should have had remedies delayed and our people as goitrous as in many districts they used to be.

Most of our water contains fluoride, but not in sufficient quantity. All that fluoridation does is to multiply this quantity several times. It has, of course, no more relationship to vivisection than using table salt in cooking, or sprinkling it on our food.

Figure 10: *Excerpts of a letter from the Minister of Health, 26th August 1958.* HD 125/299 H1 Box 1714.

In a letter dated 18th September, 1958, (**Figure 11**) the Minister of Health wrote a letter to a Mr. Sim, who had forwarded a letter from a citizen to the Minister. The Minister wrote:

"Fluoride in water at one part per million is clearly a nutrient or accessory food factor…" [184]

Fluoride in water at one part per million is clearly a nutrient or accessory food factor and has no harmful effect. It has, in fact, a very beneficial effect in that it substantially reduces dental decay. If fluorides are used as pesticides, wood preservatives or poisons, the quantities needed would be very much larger than the individual would consume from fluoridated water and harm would also result from the use of fluoride as a food preservative in the concentrations needed to inhibit or destroy the growth of food spoilage organisms. There is, therefore, nothing contradictory about the policy pursued by my Department in this respect and

Figure 11: Excerpt of a letter from the Minister of Health, 18th September, 1958. HD 125/299/4 H1 Box 1714.

This was also the conclusion of the 1957 Commission of Inquiry, as mentioned in the previous chapter. The archives show the Health Department had used the Commission's statement – as well as Bell's interpretation of McCollum's 1925 work which will be discussed in the next chapter – and possibly McClendon's experiments, to justify the above statements.

Figures 3 to **11** are not a huge number of documents by any stretch of the imagination, but they do give insight into how the New Zealand leadership were thinking, and what they were communicating to members of the public and the intellectual community. The statements regarding fluorine's essentiality are but one small aspect of a much larger matter. Most of these statements have been made when some angry or interested letter-writer contacted the minister or expert in question.

Statements from the experiments of Messer *et al.*, in 1972, 1973 and 1974 are also relevant. The following statements are taken from the beginnings of their experiments.

In their experiment published September 1972, Messer *et al.* wrote:

"Satisfactory evidence of a deficiency state with respect to fluorine has not been demonstrated despite several investigations with this purpose." [28]

In their experiment published December 1972, they wrote:

"Many attempts to demonstrate the dietary essentiality of fluoride have yielded equivocal results and none of the studies have connected fluoride to a specific metabolic deficiency." [29]

In 1973 they wrote:

"Until recently, attempts to demonstrate whether fluorine is an essential element have yielded equivocal results, despite the use of a variety of diets with a low concentration of the element." [4]

In 1974 they wrote:

"… its remarkably wide distribution throughout nature suggests some biological role for the element. Whether this role is that of an essential trace element, or merely a beneficial effect under specific conditions, has been a contentious point for many years." (p. 425)

"Identification of a specific biochemical function for F remains elusive" (p. 432) [31]

To clarify: all of these papers *eventually* wrote that fluorine was a dietary essential – the four statements shown here are to demonstrate that the authors *did not believe it a necessity* until *after* their work had been carried out.

These excerpts from experiments are the words of scientists, not politicians. Bear in mind one of these scientists was a big supporter of Community Water Fluoridation, so this is *not* the people opposed, this is *not* the voice of activists. The experiments were published in the journals **Science**, **Nature New Biology**, the **Journal of Nutrition**, and in the *Proceedings of the Second International Symposium on Trace Element Metabolism in Animals*, organized by Dr. Suttie, who went on to work for the National Academy of Sciences, a group that has consistently recommended CWF.

The point I want to make is that in reading the letters in the New Zealand Health Department archives, one is given the impression that fluorine was *definitely* a dietary essential – clearly this was not the case. The experts in the New Zealand Health Department were saying "we have evidence of essentiality", without sharing this evidence with the public. I did not find the rodent experiments of the 1930s discussed once, though Dr. Armstrong's refuted 1938 study was popular during the early years of fluoridation.

3.2 New Zealand Experts Following American Experts

With regard to the topic of essentiality, there are some examples of American influence. The following experiment may seem unimportant but is given relevance by its influence on New Zealand views. In 1925, E. V. McCollum and co-workers from the Department of Chemical Hygiene, School of Hygiene and Public Health, at the Johns Hopkins University, Baltimore, and from the College of Dental Surgery at the University of Michigan, Ann Arbor, performed an experiment looking at the impact of diet on rats [55].

This is a *different* experiment to the 1933 experiment discussed at the beginning of Chapter 1.1 [6].

McCollum *et al.* introduced the experiment by claiming that rats used in their experiments had varying degrees of tooth quality. They went on to claim slight confusion regarding the effects of rat diets – the teeth of some animals did not appear to have any problem until later in life, while others had a lot of decay early in life, without the diet appearing defective in any way. The scientists suggested that since many investigators before them had found fluoride in teeth and bones, deficiencies of the element may be a distinct possibility. They believed that because teeth had a high content of fluorine, it may have been one of the structural components of dentine.

This experiment, I believe, will *not* satisfy the most critical of scientific inquiries with regard to any definite conclusion of essentiality, as the amount of fluoride used in the diets were what occurred in the food naturally, then the same but with an added 226 ppm fluorine, a huge amount even for rats. (Rodents have a resilience when it comes to extreme fluoride levels, this is discussed a little in Chapter 6.4). Neither did the scientists tell us how much fluorine was in the base diet, other than the following:

"We have in no instance attempted to control the intake of fluorine in any of our experimental animals…"
They claimed the diets were made of purified foods, meaning,

"… the amount of fluorine ingested in these diets was very small." [55]
Neither this, nor their 1933 experiment is much help in deducing a number to replace "very small" but McCollum and co-workers used a multitude of diets. They reported on only one which produced good teeth, to

which was added 226 ppm fluorine in the form of sodium fluoride. They examined the rats fed the diet which produced good teeth (no *added* fluorine, only what was already in food) and the rats fed the same diet with 226 ppm added fluorine.

Their diet contained mostly wheat, casein, whole milk powder, salt, calcium carbonate and butter fat. The rats on the diet with no added fluoride had fine teeth. They wrote of these rats that mottled areas of teeth were only seen "in a few instances" but that this was also seen on occasion when no fluorine had been added to the diet.

To conclude, I don't believe that this experiment tells us whether fluorine is essential or not. I think it only tells us that *if* fluorine is essential, most foods have the required amount, even after purification (removal of a lot of fluorine).

I discuss this experiment because it has had a large impact on the topic of fluorine's essentiality, and upon fluoridation in New Zealand, though its influence has been indirect. In her work *Nutrition in New Zealand*, Dr. Muriel E. Bell of the Nutrition Research Department (Medical Research Council) of Otago Medical School, wrote a chapter called *Fluoride Deficiency in New Zealand Water Supplies,* in which she claimed New Zealanders had very low levels of fluoride in their teeth:

> "... confirmed the suspicion held by one of the authors (M. E. Bell) ever since she had told her 1926 and 1927 dentistry students of the finding by McCollum *et al*, (**Journal of Biological Chemistry**, Vol. 63, 553-562, 1925) that the teeth of rats were harder when fluoride was added to their diet. It became clear to these authors that fluoride should be tried as a preventive measure for New Zealand children's teeth." [185]

Bell does not tell us how *much* fluoride made the teeth of rats harder. This is true of her book, as well as a recent biography of her life [186]. Consulting the paper by McCollum *et al.*, we find the hypothesis:

> "We tried the inclusion of 226 parts per million of this element in the form of sodium fluoride. We report at this time only the results of feeding a diet which produces good teeth, and of feeding the same diet with fluorine addition." [55]

With regard to results, McCollum and co-workers wrote:

> "The results showed, contrary to our expectations, that the ingestion of fluorine, in amounts but little above those which have been reported to occur in natural foods, markedly disturbs the structure of the teeth."

And:

> "Those rats fed Diet 3619 had excellent teeth."

Diet 3619 had no added fluoride, only what occurred already in the food. McCollum said:

> "... the amount of fluorine ingested in these diets was very small."

Whether it was above or below an average amount of food fluoride is anyone's guess. Putting "very small" into a number or an amount of a particular unit is again, anyone's guess – there are simply no details in this aspect of the experiment. McCollum's statement that

> "... fluorine, in amounts but little above those which have been reported to occur in natural foods, markedly disturbs the structure of the teeth" [55]

... is quite different to Bell's statement that

"the teeth of rats were harder when fluoride was added to their diet." [185]

Once again, it is a question of precision. There is no doubt Bell believed 226 ppm to be harmful, she advocated only 1 ppm be used in New Zealand's water. Bell's book is available through the Alexander Turnbull Library in Wellington. Sometimes works are better defined when contrasted with other work. Kaj Roholm, a Danish scientist cited frequently in literature on fluorine, wrote in 1937 that

> "changes in teeth are among the most easily reproducible and most easily recognizable of all the symptoms of chronic fluorine poisoning... the first description was given in 1925 by McCollum *et al*... very marked changes were observed in the incisors... the quality of the teeth was poor, the lower incisors being very brittle." [187]

The 1925 McCollum experiment doesn't tell us much about using 1 ppm in the water supply. We've gone from 'whatever was in food' – an unknown amount – to 'whatever was in food plus 226 ppm'.

This experiment demonstrates that excesses of fluorine are harmful, it does not tell us much or anything about fluorine deficiencies, whether they do, don't, can or can't exist, due to the fact that there was no attempt to create one. I think it tells us that *if* fluoride *is* essential, there's probably enough in food, or at least the food that was used in *that* experiment. But since we only have one diet shown to us out of a sample of an unknown amount, we'll probably never know, unless someone obtains the raw data used by McCollum *et al*.

The rats fed the diet with 226 ppm fluoride had enormous teeth. (**Figure 12**) They were overgrown and curved back, which the authors attributed to a lack of wear (the upper and lower incisors should grind against each other – this is called 'attrition').

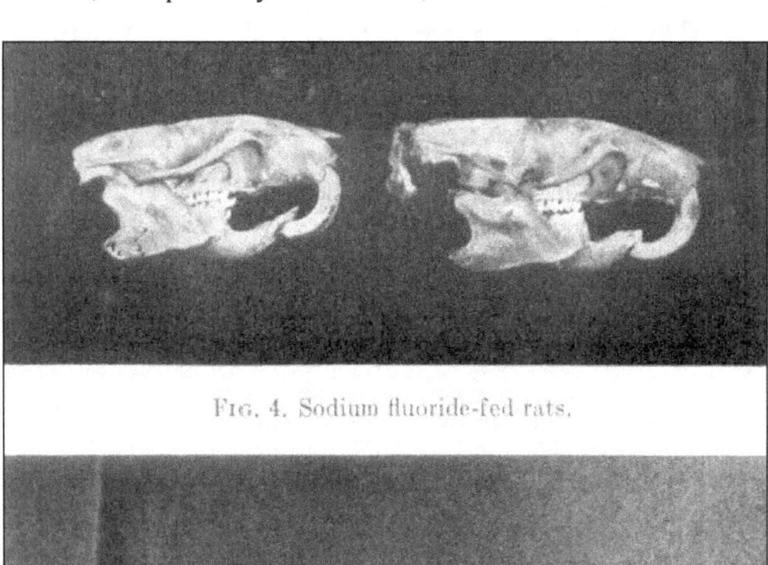

Figure 12. Sodium fluoride-fed rats and normal rats. E. V. McCollum, N. Simmonds, J. E. Becker, and R. W. Bunting, *The Effect of Additions of Fluorine to the Diet of the Rat on the Quality of the Teeth*, **Journal of Biological Chemistry**, Vol. 63, pp. 553-562, 1925 [55]. *Rats in the upper picture were fed 226 ppm fluorine in the form of sodium fluoride added to water. Both sets of rats received an unknown amount of fluorine in food, which McCollum et al. called "very low".*

Wear or attrition is required to stunt growing teeth. Rat teeth grow around 2.5 mm per week. Lack of wear in this instance was caused by the upper and lower incisors not meeting. Other experiments use gently increasing allotments of fluorine. The distortions in incisors occurred not from "stimulation to overactivity"[41], but from lack of attrition. In some instances the upper teeth curved back to the roof of the mouth.

Only the bones of the rats were examined for calcium and phosphorous. The teeth were used for histological examination or fluorine determination. Because of this, we could not learn much about the dental relationship between fluorine and these two elements from this work.

New Zealander Muriel Bell was no doubt a dedicated researcher. Her columns in **The Listener** in 1944 were quite thoughtful. Writing on soil deficiencies, she claimed that extensive rainfall had caused lime and phosphate fertilizers to become depleted, and that these should be scattered liberally over lands. She did not discuss soil deficiency in areas of New Zealand that were unfarmed.

She discussed how lime and phosphate helped increase the calcium content of beans, and how New Zealand was shipping huge quantities of meat overseas, meaning our soils missed out on the minerals in the bones of those animals. She calculated roughly 7,000 cwt[42] phosphate and 35,000 cwt lime going overseas every year because of meat exports [188].

She advocated the use of green manure and crop residue [189], and stressed the importance of magnesium, iron, copper, cobalt, sulfur, iodine, and our dependence on these elements [190].

Her first column on fluorine cautioned against an excess, noting that in the USA

> "... the presence of more than one or two parts of fluorine per million parts of water in the reservoirs serving certain areas was attended by an ugly mottling of the enamel; the teeth became pitted and discoloured, and in severe cases dental decay occurred in these teeth." [191]

Her second article on fluorine mentioned the 1925 work of Professor McCollum (discussed above). She wrote:

> "Some 20 years ago, experiments showed that where rats were fed on diets containing additional small amounts of fluorine they developed teeth that were harder than usual." [192]

She went on to explain, as McCollum did, that rats have incisors that grow continually and must be worn down. In this article she did not mention the amount of fluorine McCollum had given these rats.

She did point out that when she told her dentistry students this in the 1920s, it was of little interest to them. Dentistry was more concerned with *excess* fluorine at the time. This was due to the ability to measure accurate amounts of the element being extremely difficult. She went on to write that those people who had suffered some mottling had been discovered to have less decay. She gave the example of two cities in Illinois with 1.8 ppm fluorine having between a third and a half the decay rates of two (unnamed) cities with concentrations of 0.1 and 0.2 ppm [192].

She opened her third column on fluorine by claiming that in New Zealand the amount of fillings in teeth, and the number of false teeth were

---

[41] This is quoting the 1925 work. We should be open to the possibility that more recent research says otherwise.

[42] "Cwt" is an abbreviation for "hundred weight" – 112 pounds according to the *Oxford Illustrated Dictionary,* **Oxford University Press**, 1962.

"probably greater than anywhere else in the world." [193]

She wrote of the possibility of "evidence of shortage of fluorine…" and thought work should be done to correct this, if found. She expressed interest in an article (not referenced) published in the **American Journal of Public Health**, desiring to test fluoridation on one population of two cities, both of which drank from the same water supply.

A paper in the 1947 **New Zealand Dental Journal** [36] co-written with Marion Harrison cited work from many American experts, including Drs. McClure, Arnold, and Armstrong. This was the paper that mentioned the 1945 McClendon and Foster experiment in a positive light, but said it was "too early to make pronouncements on studies of this type".

Bell's paper *Medical and Nutritional Aspects of Fluoridation*, compares fluoride with

> "many substances taken into the body that are highly reactive and can accumulate, but are nevertheless needed in small amounts for its proper functioning. People take such substances into their bodies every day, but in the amounts that are customarily eaten, these substances act in a beneficial manner. I should like now to give some parallel illustrations of such reactive substances." [194]

She then mentions iodine, Vitamin A, and Vitamin D. I found this paper in a New Zealand Health Department file dated 1960 (the *file* was dated, the document not, so I can only assume it was written around this time). Fluoridation began in New Zealand in the early 1950s.

I detect no dishonesty in her writings or attitude, just a desire to elucidate and help. It is interesting to read this paper [194]. There is scant discussion of experiments relating directly to fluoride's position or role in nutrition, but there are anecdotes regarding scientists. She mentioned meeting Professor McCollum, who told her that with extra (226 ppm) fluoride the teeth of rats in his 1925 experiment,

> "grew abnormally long and semi-circular in consequence. From that time on I [Bell] told my dentistry students of the effect of fluoride in hardening the teeth of white rats." [194]

That she told this to dental students in 1926 and 1927 is mentioned in her book. One can appreciate that Dr. Bell thought a much smaller amount of fluorine than what was used in these rats would improve the oral health of New Zealanders.

I have often wondered what role American and British attitudes played in our own fluoridation. That our Health Department experts were in close contact with experts from those two countries is evidenced by many letters in the Health Department archives. Activists in New Zealand were in contact with American activists. I believe both groups were quick to apply to New Zealand what had occurred in the USA, and I believe this compromised the integrity and the details of research done by both groups. Regarding a nutritional role for fluorine, what I have shown here is all I have found, though there may be more.

Of the American influence on necessity and deficiency, I have not found anything to suggest that New Zealand experts in the 1950s knew anything of the experiments other than the 1925 McCollum experiment and the 1954 McClendon experiment.

I found a copy of the latter [13] in the Health Department archives, which may explain the belief of the experts, although the experts barely discuss experimentation, much less *criticism* of experimentation, even in their private correspondence. Not a single one of the letters quoted in the previous chapter discussed either of these experiments. That even supporters of water fluoridation like Dr. Joseph Muhler, and the anonymous writer of the article featured in **Nutrition Reviews** [37], had criticised the McClendon experiments seemed to elude the Health Department experts entirely (at least to my knowledge. In fact the only mention of the **Nutrition Reviews** article I have seen appeared in Dr. Joseph Muhler's book with Dr. Hine [49]). I eventually found *one* media article discussing McClendon, but it was about fluorine in tea being of benefit to children as young as one year old. McClendon said it should be sugar-free, and that children should still drink as much milk as ever. It was in a file that spanned the years 1954-1956. This brief, undated article was coupled with another, containing a refutation of its claim from the New Zealand Health Department. Their reasoning was that there were different amounts of fluorine in wet and dry tea [195]. The article featuring McClendon had claimed good results had been obtained on rats, but was unclear whether tea had been the vehicle for fluorine.

I found these after a few months of looking through the archived collections of Health Department files at the National Library, after completing the first draft of this book. This file also contained the abstract of the 1954 experiment. I had originally thought that the absence of discussion around McClendon's work suggested the experts were unaware of experimental evidence of what they *did* believe! That I had only found a couple of articles suggests there is probably some truth to my cynicism.

There were abundant news articles about Hastings (the first city in New Zealand to be fluoridated), about American experts, and about experimental progress in the news of the 1950s and 1960s. Much of these clippings are in the archives. I will remind the reader I accessed only twenty files. The files in the National Library are a separate collection, I did not look in them until I had finished this work.

As mentioned earlier [36], Dr. Bell attended Harvard for a year in the early 1950s, where she interviewed American doctors regarding fluoridation experiments (this word "experiments") used by Te Ara.

Bell believed decisively that fluoride was an essential nutrient. She also believed it was almost harmless in concentrations as high as 14 ppm, excepting fluorosis, which she claimed did not occur at 1 ppm [196]. She wrote this to the Managing Director of Thames Valley Newspapers Ltd., on the 16th June, 1958. Note the earlier quotation from her article in **The Listener** regarding pitting of teeth above 1 or 2 ppm [191].

Captain F. L. Losee, head of the U.S. naval research institute at Bethesda, Maryland, U.S.A., was quoted in **The Evening Post** (Wellington) in 1958:

> "We are satisfied that lack of fluoride causes 60 per cent of all caries. Now we have to find what causes the other 40 per cent." [197]

Regarding Community Water Fluoridation programs, there is a great U.S. influence and presence in New Zealand history with regard to both support and opposition. More evidence of this is given throughout the rest of this investigation.

Dr. Fredrick Stare was Chairman of the Department of Nutrition in Harvard University's School of Public Health. In 1967 **The Evening Post** told New Zealanders he said

> "the mineral nutrient called fluoride not only lessens tooth decay but also lessens the development of a condition of the aged called osteoporosis." [198]

He was to speak in Wellington to 'present a meeting of the Nutrition Society' later that week[43].

A final point I want to make here is that while Dr. Bell mentioned McCollum's 1925 work in her book [185], as far as I can tell she never discussed his 1933 work that concluded fluorine non-essential, or required in immeasurably small amounts, if there *was* a requirement. I never found her or any of the other New Zealand experts mention the other experiments from the 1930s that had concluded fluorine non-essential. This is what I have concluded from reading her columns in the July/August issues of **The Listener**, her book, her paper co-authored with Marion Harrison [36], and her paper *Medical and Nutritional Aspects of Fluoridation*, found in the 1960 Health Department file [194]. A recent biography on her life has provided no reason to change these points of view [186]. If there are other documents in which she *did* discuss McCollum's 1933 experiment, or any of the other experiments pertaining to, or refuting a necessity for fluorine, I am unaware of them.

---

[43] Also of interest: on the 14th March, 1957, Dr. Bell appeared in the Dunedin **Evening Star** with the words of Fredrick Stare M.D. (Harvard) and Dr. Norman Joliffe (New York Health Department), recommending that New Zealand use water fluoridation (copy available in archive [180]). The statements in *this* article had nothing to do with a nutritional role for fluorine, but do demonstrate an American influence on the thinking of New Zealand experts. Diana Brown's book expands on this [186].

4.   How Abundant is Fluoride in Food?

"The World Health Organisation, the World Dental Federation and the International Association for Dental Research have all stated that 'universal access to fluoride for dental health is part of the basic human right to health.'"

- Dr. Jonathan Broadbent, Associate Professor and Head of Discipline of Preventive and Restorative Dentistry at the Division of Health Sciences at Otago University, quoted in **The New Zealand Herald** (Auckland, New Zealand), 7th June, 2013 [199].

"I do not want to appear facetious, but the only way of avoiding fluoride in the diet is not to eat."

- Harold B. Turbott, Deputy Director-General of Health, 19th March,

  1959. MS-Papers-6167-01, Fuller, James Ferris (Brigadier), 1913-2001: Papers, Fluoridation files (Auckland).

When you read the first chapter on the experiments that tested if fluoride was essential, you would have noticed that not a single experiment was performed with a diet containing absolutely zero fluoride, with the exception of Dr. Schroeder's work published in 1968 [30]. This anomaly was never discussed as far as I'm aware. This section will help to explain why this occurs: it is about fluoride's presence in foods.

4.1 Revisiting Experiments that Tested for Essentiality

In referring to some of the experiments from the first chapter, many of the scientists noted the difficulty in making fluoride-free diets. Scientists were able to use distilled water to reduce fluoride intake to what was in food and what was airborne (obviously most thought airborne fluoride was negligent; most studies did not mention it).

In 1933 Sharpless and McCollum introduced their experiment with the following:

"It is widely distributed in soils, rocks, and waters... Fluorine is apparently universally present in plant and animal tissues." [200]

In 1933, Floyd DeEds mentioned the studies done by Gautier and Clausman in 1914 which looked at mineral waters and their fluoride content [7].

Amounts ranged from a fraction of a milligram (Eau d'Evian, between 0.15 and 0.33 milligram at the low end) to more than 6 milligrams per litre (Eau de Vichy, between 6.32 and 14 milligrams. Milligrams per litre equals parts per million). Given that fluoride was abundant in water, it was only sensible to expect it in plants. DeEds pointed out a 1916 study, again by Gautier and Clausmann, that found fluoride in all plants analysed, with the leaves – often the edible part – having the most. He showed about fifty foods, most of which contained less than 1 milligram fluoride per 100 grams. An exception was sorrel (a leafy green) with 13.87 mg.

He referenced a 1907 study by Carles that found fluoride in 88 out of 93 samples of mineral and sea water. The amounts varied between 0.005 to 0.012 grams per litre. These are long before the Willard and Winter method of determination [5].

In 1939, Evans and Phillips cited five studies (from 1888 to 1937) in their introduction that related to "low fluorine diets". Not a single one had 0.00 ppm fluorine [9].

Zoologist Jesse McClendon had responded to fluorine's abundance in nature by inventing his method of growing halogen-free water-culture crops. In their 1953 experiment, McClendon and Gershon-Cohen wanted to use yeast for rat food, but could not find a halogen-free variety [12]. The rain water they used had to be run through an ion exchange resin to remove halogens.

McClendon's experiments are definitely useful when it comes to understanding abundance of fluorine: they demonstrate the lengths to which someone needs to go, in order to create a possible deficiency in the element – not living near industries that emit fluorine, and eating food grown only in purified rainwater. Such conditions are only practical for the scientist. The diet was quite probably deficient in many other factors.

In 1954, Dr. Joseph Muhler discussed his experiment on bone retention. He stated that

"even with exceptionally careful purification the diet still contained traces." [16]

By 'traces' he meant less than 0.1 microgram per gram (0.1 ppm).

In their 1957 experiment, Richard Maurer and Harry Day from the Chemistry Department of Indiana University said:

"Fluorine occurs naturally in virtually all foods and drinking water and it is present in the bodies of all higher animals." [17]

Introducing his 1958 abstract, Joseph Muhler wrote

"Moreover, many nutritionists feel that since fluorides are found, to varying degrees of course, in almost all foods, and due to their wide distribution in the plant and animal kingdom…" [48]

Takao Suzuki in 1969 called a basal diet containing 0.45 ppm fluoride "defluoridated feed." [65]

The 1972 experiment by Klaus Schwarz and David Milne claimed that:

"Food, however, is the main source of Fluorine for animals and man. It occurs in practically all foods and feeds… normal human diets provide fluorine levels which are close to those which we found essential for support of growth in the rat, i.e., 1.5-2.5 ppm of fluorine on the dry weight basis. Figures for human fluorine intake from food vary. An available daily fluorine intake of 4.4 mg, including fluoride from fluoridated drinking water, was found for adult men in careful balance studies." [20, 201]

In 1972, Armstrong *et al.*, in discussing other related works, wrote,

"…these studies have been hampered by the ubiquitous occurrence of fluoride in natural foods and waters with the result that it has been very difficult to prepare a diet devoid of fluoride…" [29]

The 1974 experiment authored by Klaus Schwarz said that:

"the element occurs in practically all foods and feeds and food is the main source for animals and man, aside from drinking water." [26]

In 1974, Armstrong, Messer and Singer wrote of fluoride,

"... its remarkably wide distribution throughout nature suggests some biological role..." [31]

The 1974 review of literature by Nielsen and Sandstead on fluorine's role in nutrition told us:

"Foods containing high amounts of Fluorine are seafood and tea, with grains and cow's milk containing much less." [27]

The fact that outliers exist regarding fluoride concentrations in food makes looking at total intake difficult.

4.2 Other Research into Fluoride Levels in Foods

Wilson, writing in 1846, said

"it was impossible to doubt, after the facts I had observed in the laboratory, that fluorine must be no infrequent constituent of well and river as well as of sea water." [75]

In 1949, biochemist Frank J. McClure from the United States National Institute of Health authored a study published in the official journal of the United States Public Health Service and the office of the Surgeon General, **Public Health Reports** [202].

I recommend it to anyone interested in a particularly detailed study, at least for its time. It is available on the *National Center for Biotechnology Information* (NCBI) website. McClure looked at the fluoride content of animal tissues, meat, fish, hen's eggs, cow's milk, seafood, tea, citrus and non-citrus fruits, cereals, vegetables and tubers, wine and other foods like nuts. His numbers stop at two decimal places, so while there are foods with recorded 0.00 ppm fluoride, this may not be perfectly accurate, something with 0.001 ppm will be rounded down to zero. There *may* be *foods* with no fluoride at all, but at least to my knowledge, there is no *diet* with no fluoride at all.

In McClure's investigation his research is out of date, but abundant. It *is* of historical significance because we can use this to determine (roughly) if fluoride content in food is increasing, decreasing, or staying the same. The majority of the reports McClure cites are American, but some European studies are also included. In this study there is almost no food without fluoride (as mentioned above, but he did record some foods with 0.00 ppm). This was in 1949. McClure suggested that without measuring fluoridated water intake, scientists concluded a daily intake of between 0.25 and 0.32 mg per day in one study, 0.45 mg per day in another [203].

In 1953, a review by H. H. Mitchell and Marjorie Edman, from the Division of Animal Nutrition at the University of Illinois, Urbana, was published in the January issue of the **Journal of the American Dietetic Association** [45]. The authors lauded the benefits of CWF, and reiterated statements others had made about the abundance of fluorine in seafood and tea, saying in New Zealand tea may contribute between 0.45 and 0.93 mg per day. They said 50 gm of sardines may provide 0.8 mg per day.

The reader may find the words from CWF advocate Dr. Norman Joliffe's 1956 New York City Health Department document slightly amusing:

> "... minute traces of fluorides are to be found in practically all foods. It has been said that the only way to avoid fluoride in food is a diet of cabbage, beets and cauliflower, cooked in distilled water." [97]

n 1959, Joseph Muhler wrote on claims for and against a necessity for fluorine. He authored one chapter on the necessity of fluorine. He wrote,

> "... since fluorides are found, to varying degrees of course, in almost all foods, and since they are widely distributed in the plant and animal kingdom..." [24]

While fluoridation advocates often speak of deficiencies and sub-optimal levels, sometimes they'll say the opposite in public. For example **The Lincoln Star**, a Nebraskan newspaper in 1961, told Americans that:

> "Members of the [International Association for Dental Health] panel, in a news conference, said fluoride is a nutritional substance naturally found in a wide range of foods. The range is so wide, they commented, that it was almost impossible to work out a diet free of fluoride for experimental animals." [204]

A study from the **Journal of Public Health Dentistry** in 1995 told us that

> "Wide variations in fluoride intake among children make estimating fluoride intake difficult." [205]

A document from the U.S. Department of Health and Human Services, published in 2003 states that,

> "Conflicting results have been obtained from animal experiments addressing whether fluorine is an essential element. Much of this conflict appears to result from the great difficulty in preparing an animal diet that has negligible amounts of fluoride, but otherwise allows normal animal growth and development." [99]

4.3 National Academy of Sciences Research into Food Fluoride Levels

I don't believe an entirety of research is necessary to illustrate the point that fluoride is abundant in natural and city water and therefore, food. Here I will discuss only a few publications from the American National Academy of Sciences (NAS) regarding fluoride's abundance, from 1952 to more recent times. These levels are at the conservative end of the spectrum.

In the 1952 publication **A Survey of the Literature on Dental Caries** the NAS mentioned diets fed to rats that contained between 1.28 ppm (basal diet) and dried mackerel at 84.47 ppm [5] (page 337). The latter value is from McClure's report mentioned earlier [202]. They claimed that about twenty percent of the fluoride from canned salmon (19.34 ppm) and mackerel was stored. However, some deboned fish contained none at all.

In 1971, the NAS pointed out that scientists found it difficult to create deficiencies of fluorine, in order to test if it was essential or not. Citing Joseph Muhler's PhD thesis from the University of Indiana, they wrote:

> "Attempts of early nutritionists to develop a diet that was sufficiently low in fluoride to determine whether fluorine was an essential element were hampered by the widespread occurrence of fluorides in their dietary ingredients. Most of the early studies were carried out with diets that contained at least 0.1 ppm of fluoride, and perhaps even more." [69]

In 1974, the NAS reiterated their statement that creating diets low in fluoride was difficult:

"Recently developed sensitive procedures for fluoride determination have made it possible to detect at least traces of fluoride in practically every natural water supply and foodstuff analysed." [70]

In 1977, the NAS publication **Drinking Water and Health Volume 1**, stated that:

"Recent studies indicate that the total intake of fluoride is as high as 3 mg/day rather than the earlier figure of 1.5 mg/day, primarily because of increases in the estimated levels of fluoride in foods[44]."

To quote them on fluoride levels in food:

"Among the foodstuffs notably high in fluoride are fish, particularly those, such as sardines, that are eaten with the bones. Fish-meal flour, which is produced from the whole fish, is also high in fluoride. Tea is unusually rich in fluoride. Milk and most fruits are generally low in fluoride. Vegetables vary greatly in fluoride content." [206]

In 1989, the NAS publication **Diet and Health Implications for Reducing Chronic Disease Risk** said that the fluoride content of food processed with fluoridated water was three times higher than food processed with non-fluoridated water [207]. They said baby foods contain "high" levels of fluoride, and that the highest consumption reported was for children under five, 0.3 mg. In support of this, they cited a study done in 1974. The most recent study they used in support of their research in food fluoride levels in this section was ten years old, 1979.

In 1993 the NAS told us in **Health Effects of Ingested Fluorides** that fluoride content of food depended on fluoride content of water and soil (and the solubility of fluoride compounds in soil), something obvious, but easy to overlook [208].

In this 1993 document the NAS suggest that quite low amounts exist for daily fluoride intake. They discuss a study from 1980 regarding infant (six-month-old) intake from four areas of the United States, which found between 0.21 and 0.54 mg per day. They said intake from two-year-olds was "directly related" to the concentration in the water supply, and that estimates put adult intake at about 1.2, 1.8 and 2.2 mg per day in areas fluoridated at 1.0 mg per day. I find 1.2 mg per day unrealistic, it suggests that adults would barely drink a litre of water or beverage made from fluoridated water each day, and would take little fluoride in through their foods.

In 2006, the NAS claimed near one hundred percent absorption (bioavailability) from soluble compounds such as sodium fluoride in water. According to this document, absorption lowers by 10 – 25 percent when fluoride is ingested with foods,

"particularly those with high concentrations of calcium or certain divalent or trivalent ions that form insoluble compounds…" [85]

---

[44] The NAS cite Spencer, H., I. Lewin, E. Wistrowski, and J. Samachson, *Fluoride metabolism in man*, **American Journal of Medicine**, Vol. 49, No. 6, pp. 807-813, 1970.

4.4 World Health Organization Research into Food Fluoride Levels

Dr. Joseph Muhler wrote in the 1970 monograph:

> "Since fluorine is so universally distributed in the plant and animal kingdoms, the preparation of a diet totally free from fluorine is a real challenge." [102]

This document was used in the promotion of CWF in New Zealand in the early 1970s [209]. In 1994 the WHO published a document [210] that would be cited in 2016 as

> "the existing authoritative WHO publication offering advice and technical support to countries."

This statement was made by Poul Erik Petersen and Hiroshi Ogawa, in an editorial for the June issue of **Community Dental Health**, 2016 [211].

This 1994 document claimed that unprocessed foods contain between 0.1 and 2.5 ppm fluoride. It contained one of the highest measurements in food I've ever seen, 21-761 ppm range for fish protein concentrate, apparently due to fish bones. The authors give a few examples of food with little over 4 ppm. They claim tea contains between 3 and 400 ppm, while infusions may contain "up to 8.6" ppm, although as noted before, this is dependent on infusion procedure, time, tea variety, etc.

This WHO document pointed to desalination as a way to decrease fluoride content of water [212]. Intake of fluoride from bottled water is also difficult to measure due to differing amounts in sources of water.

The 2016 document mentioned above, stated that:

> "It is important that fluoride exposure be known and health administrators be made aware of exposure before the introduction of any fluoridation or supplementation programmes for prevention and dental caries." [213]

In support of this statement, they cite a 2014 WHO document prepared by Dr R. J. Baez, (University of Texas, Health Science Center, San Antonio Dental School), Dr Petersen, and Dr T.M. Marthaler, (from the University of Zurich, Switzerland), which elaborates on this:

> "However, when fluoride is ingested by young children, very mild dental enamel fluorosis may occur. Because of the numerous sources of fluoride available today, the risk of enamel fluorosis must always be borne in mind. Thus, public health administrators should assess the total fluoride exposure of the population before introducing any additional fluoridation or supplementation programmes for caries prevention." [214]

In reading so many papers and articles regarding parts per million in water, in food, it is refreshing to consider "total fluoride exposure" as the authors of this WHO document recommend.

4.5 Discussion

In this section I have kept strictly to what experts such as the United States National Academy of Sciences (NAS) and World Health Organization (WHO) claim. In this book I'm not covering European and Asian journals, as well as some news clippings, that have suggested greater levels in food than what the NAS or WHO claim.

The purpose of this chapter has been to demonstrate that levels of fluorine in food differ throughout the food chain. Thus the large city-wide experiments involving the counting of holes in teeth and the addition of fluorine compounds to water supplies are less than perfectly practical for the purpose of testing if fluorine should have a nutritional role as there is no real precision regarding daily intakes of fluoride through food, drugs and other vehicles. Were an experiment to be performed on humans in order to attempt to demonstrate a fluorine deficiency, the use of a more precisely controlled level of fluorine in food must be used. Yet here we inevitably run into the problems of creating deficiencies in other elements while removing fluorine. With regard to the statement at the start of this chapter, that

"... universal access to fluoride for dental health is part of the basic human right to health." [199]

We already have "universal access to fluoride" – to the point where scientists cannot make a reproducible deficiency of the element. This has not stopped New Zealand experts using the word "deficiency" – even when they state it's non-essential [158, 178]. Dr. Broadbent's statement here [199] can be held next to an article he co-authored which described fluoride as "ubiquitous in the environment" [215].

Regarding concern over fluorine deficiency, allow me to say that even if all of the activists alive *wanted* to take our fluoride away, and could be bothered doing so, it would not and could not happen simply because of the abundance of the element. The human race would have to go and live on another planet to avoid fluorine.

Those critical of the experts should understand there was seemingly little to explain the poor quality of modern dentition, that appeared sensible in academic literature. Removal of sugar was historically considered a good thing, but the responsibility of the public, not politicians or food manufacturers. The "well-balanced diet" was considered sufficient in every other way, so it was only logical that fluorine was the factor considered missing, leading to poor teeth. This was the picture presented not only to the public but to academics. One example comes from Colonel J. Fuller, writing in the January, 1956 issue of the **New Zealand Dental Journal**:

"The severity of dental fluorosis is accentuated if nutritional status is abnormally low[45], a factor of no relevance in New Zealand." [216]

I include this not to focus on dental fluorosis, but on the fact that Fuller's statement is indicative of a belief that the "well-balanced diet" was abundant enough to render concern about dental fluorosis unnecessary.

Statements like this help to explain the insistence of the experts that a fluorine deficiency does exist, without a precise demonstration of a fluorine deficiency. This is a dissonant feature of the experts' usual claim to abundant evidence in support of their points of view.

Both supporters and opponents of CWF considered the addition of excess refined sugar a harmful thing in the civilized diet. While the experts have considered the junk food industry a threat to public health for a long time,

---

[45] Fuller cites Massler and Schour, *Relation of endemic dental fluorosis to malnutrition*, **Journal of the American Dental Association**, Vol. 44, No. 2, pp. 156-165, February 1952. Fuller went on to claim that mottling was found all over NZ, related to soil types, not drinking water (here he cites Hewat and Eastcott, *Dental Caries in New Zealand*, Medical Research Council of NZ. When Fuller wrote this, Hewat and Eastcott's article was awaiting publication).

it has certainly taken a while for them to even start discussing the regulation of this industry... with its huge multi-million-dollar advertising campaigns, often targeted at the same children the experts wanted healthier.

The food industry defended their campaigns, an example can be found in Sharon Beder's book *This Little Kiddy Went to Market: The Corporate Capture of Childhood*.

> "The food industry also argues that achieving a balanced diet is a parental responsibility and that government regulation of junk-food advertising represents the intrusion of a 'nanny state' into private lives." [217]

I've never seen it discussed, but does this mean on the other hand, that *freedom* of junk food companies to advertise represents the intrusion of a 'business state' into private lives? Consider how the quote given here is worded: protecting me from seeing an advertisement for junk food is regarded by the food industry as an intrusion. *The advertisement itself is not considered an intrusion.* Government *protection* from advertising is an intrusion. It's presupposed that *I want* to see the ad[46]. It's presupposed that consumers seeing advertisements for junk food are not only good for businesses, but good for consumers.

This gets more interesting when one considers that many of those opposed to fluoridation had championed the avoidance of junk foods, and the use of natural foods, going back many decades [218]. I am certain that here we find a point of agreement in what has often been an unpleasant debate, on the occasions that it has been debated (one example is given in the Berridge/Connett debate where both scientists agreed junk food was a problem [178]).

Policies regarding the subsidization of healthier foods, with the taxation of junk food, are (at the time of writing) on the outer ends of the political spectrum in New Zealand [219].

The fact that no evidence of a conclusive fluorine deficiency has ever been demonstrated in humans, has been ignored in mainstream New Zealand media and most academic literature since the beginning of CWF. Even nowadays, the experts still talk of deficiency [146, 158, 178], need [220], and liken fluoridation of water to iodisation of salt and the importance of other vital nutrients [221]. One wonders if access to such a thing *need* be established as a human right by prestigious organizations, especially considering in the instances given here it can be seen these organizations seldom believe in the existence of fluorine deficiencies (see Chapter 2).

In the August 2014 review from the Royal Society of New Zealand and the Office of the Prime Minister's Chief Science Advisor, the word "deficiency" was only used with regard to iodine, not fluorine [106].

In this document the authors reference the WHO as claiming fluorine a micronutrient (see Chapter 2.3):

> "The WHO considers fluoride a micronutrient with a beneficial effect on oral health." [106].

I know of only one criticism of the WHO for this [222]. I have not seen any public discussion regarding a reason why the WHO considered[47] fluorine essential based on benefit, and the SCHER and EFSA consider fluorine non-essential, based on their lack of findings with regard to deficiencies in humans.

---

[46] I don't.

[47] "Considered" – past tense used because the 2017 report from WHO, *Guidelines for Drinking Water*, 4th edition, claimed "Fluoride may be an essential element for humans; however, essentiality has not been demonstrated unequivocally." (page 372)

It is fascinating to note that the WHO, in their own writings, discuss the sugar industry's attempts at disrupting WHO's sugar recommendations [223]. This was because the WHO recommended less sugar than the sugar industry had in mind. Dame Helen Clark wrote in a facebook post that the sugar industry were using the same techniques as the tobacco industry as far as distorting the scientific evidence around the substance [224].

Consider this in light of Poul Erik Petersen, writing for the WHO regarding an increase in tooth decay in Africa:

> "The principal reasons for this increase are growing sugar consumption and inadequate exposure to fluorides."
> [111]

It *is* a good thing he can mention excessive sugar. But as for fluoride – he does not consider exposures to essential elements like calcium possibly inadequate, it is taken for granted that their exposure is adequate. I personally feel that this is an assumption that could sometimes lead to problems. If children are not getting enough calcium, enough iodine or protein (see Chapters 6 through 6.5) and their teeth decay, it could be taken as evidence of "inadequate exposure to fluorides". I have found very little written on such a possibility.

5.   What Do the Experts Say in Newspapers and the Media?

"'We are satisfied that lack of fluoride causes 60 per cent of all caries. Now we have to find what causes the other 40 per cent,' said Captain F. L. Losee, head of the U.S. naval research institute at Bethesda, Maryland, in Dunedin yesterday."

- U.S. Researcher Here To Solve Caries Mystery, **The Evening Post** (Wellington, New Zealand), 23rd May, 1958 [197].

"Although fluoride should probably be regarded as essential, there is no evidence so far from human studies that overt clinical signs of fluoride deficiency exist. No specifically diagnostic clinical or biochemical parameters have been related to fluoride inadequacy.

- **World Health Organization**, 1996, *Trace Elements in Human Nutrition and Health*, p. 187-193 [105].

This chapter will "zoom out" toward a more societal overview of not only what experts say in media regarding a nutritional role for fluorine, but of influences that may effect what experts say. It has been difficult finding information on fluorine's essentiality in scientific literature, but I can say bluntly that finding *detailed* information in public literature is even *more* difficult.

Nevertheless, on occasion when it does appear, the experts claim essentiality with little discussion of research. This is true for Australasian media. American media gave publicity to some of the experiments discussed in Chapter 1.1, though *only* experiments that concluded fluorine essential. From the sample of newspapers I have looked at, refutations, criticisms and contradictions relevant to these were not publicized by supporters of fluoridation.

For the past six or so decades, experimental evidence has demonstrated to us that fluorine is either definitely or almost definitely non-essential in nutrition, this at least true for rodents (see Chapter 1). Rodent experiments and their conclusions have in the past been considered acceptable for use in documents discussing fluorine's role in humans. I have found no recent arguments against their relevance.

In their commissions, reports, and official literature, the experts have in some instances represented these rodent experiments well. In some cases they have changed criteria of what constitutes an essential nutrient.

Eight of the papers in Chapter 1.1 concluded fluorine essential, nine experiments concluded it non-essential. Don't confuse 'number of experiments' with 'number of papers published from these results' – Schwarz performed one set of experiments and published two papers, and Messer *et al.* performed two experiments and had four papers published.

Therefore in our newspapers we should see, through the years, about a half-and-half claim of essentiality and non-essentiality from the experts who support Community Water Fluoridation, assuming that the experts represent research accurately – this is based on a simplified view of a "number of conclusions" without examining methods and real conclusive strength. So this view would *not* take into account scientists who may have exaggerated or understated the importance of their work.

This gets more complicated when we realize that all of the experiments that concluded fluorine essential were either criticized or outright refuted; for example McClendon and Gershon-Cohen, and the work of Messer *et al.* Schwarz's work received three criticisms I'm aware of – all of which were in the Nielsen and Sandstead paper, though the 1989 NAS document [81] pointed at the Weber and Reid experiment in contrast.

The experiments concluding fluorine non-essential were seldom criticized, to my knowledge. There is a reason for this beyond the fact that these experiments may have provided better nutrition or healthier surroundings for the rodents. The experiments at that end of the spectrum were not discussed as frequently, thus they avoided criticism simply by being less well-known. Consider the example given regarding Dr. Stephen Barrett's website and the United States Public Health Service (USPHS) (Chapter 2.7). The scientists writing the USPHS documents wrote nothing about the experiments that had concluded fluorine non-essential[48], so experts learning only from those documents would also not know about them. More examples are shown throughout Chapters 5.1 and 5.2.

Working with a hypothesis that experts tell the truth, and do their best to represent the scientific evidence accurately, *and* have access to and awareness of the entirety of experiments (though this last point is doubtful in many cases) one should see the great majority of experts claiming that fluorine is *non*-essential in nutrition, with only a small number of experts advancing the argument that it *is* essential, this of course using the standard requirements of biochemistry – and of course around the early 1970s we'd see an upsurge in the number of experts claiming fluorine is essential… but we'd also see a bit more scepticism regarding the work of Dr. Schwarz, and we'd see the experts responding to the 1976 experiments that invalidated the work of Messer *et al.*

Yet what we see is the exact opposite: on the rare occasion when the subject comes up, *all* of the experts tell us publicly that fluorine *is* an essential nutrient, *almost every time it is discussed…* with only four deviations that I have found, only one of which was in a newspaper. Another two can be found online, to a total of six (these two are not "full deviations" either – they do not acknowledge their disagreement with other experts in public).

---

[48] Even the experiments the USPHS funded!

Three of these deviations are discussed in Chapters 2.7 and 2.9 – they are Dr. Ken Perrott, who claimed an ambiguity ('semantics'[49]) about the issue, but went on to discuss fluorine deficiencies; Dr. Frank McClure, who told us fluorine was non-essential on page 191 of his book, then "a nutrient trace element" on page 273 of his book; and Dr. Mike Berridge, who told us fluorine was non-essential in his book. He also told us this on TV, then discussed fluorine deficiencies of the soil – so these deviations are not *full* deviations by any means.

The fourth *did* appear in an American newspaper, it is discussed in Chapter 5.2. It is also not a full deviation – it claimed fluorine essential, but pointed out this was based on benefit, not necessity.

Bear in mind that fluorine being non-essential does *not*, and should not, instantly make Community Water Fluoridation (CWF) poisonous, useless, unsafe or ineffective.

Some experiments *did* claim to have created a deficiency in rodents [13, 20, 28, 29], but even a small sample of the experiments that refuted or challenged these conclusions [17, 18, 19, 33, 34, 35] are not well discussed. In media, the experts have been consistently silent on this point. At first glance this is understandable given the obscurity of the topic, yet I believe reader judgements will be subjective here. It's difficult to know what the experts think about these latter experiments because the experts don't appear to *know* about them, unless we dig around in National Academy of Sciences (NAS) and World Health Organization (WHO) literature with specific, pedantic diligence.

The experts who claim the existence of deficiency in public mostly[50] don't seem to notice that the experiments regarding deficiency say the exact opposite – that fluoride is so *abundant* the creation of a deficiency was impossible without going to bizarre lengths – McClendon's water tanks, and Schwarz's trace element isolators – or poor diets, as in the case of the Messer *et al.* experiments. In 2013, we still don't have evidence of a deficiency in humans [103, 105, 116-119], but we *do* have about sixty years' worth of newspaper and other articles claiming or implying we *are* at risk of fluoride deficiency. Newspaper articles are listed in Appendix 1.

Why does this happen?

One obvious reason was given at the end of the previous chapter: the experts believed that the 'well-balanced' diet was sufficient, except for fluorine. Tooth decay had been very prevalent from the 1920s to the 1940s, therefore it made sense to many experts that the diet was deficient in fluorine. The benefits of CWF were also used as a criterion for fluorine's necessity.

Another reason can be seen in some of the statements from experts in support of CWF. People opposed to fluoridation claimed it "mass medication" – but if fluorine was a nutrient everyone was deficient in, and CWF corrected this deficiency, then this claim of mass medication could be regarded as less relevant, maybe even totally irrelevant. The experts' claim that *water* is deficient is a way of getting around the inconvenient fact that no real deficiency in humans exists.

---

[49] The 1988 document *Abuse of the Scientific Literature in an Antifluoridation Pamphlet* [145] also argued that fluorine's essentiality was 'semantics'.
[50] **The Lincoln Star** (Nebraska) article mentioned in Chapter 4.2 is one exception [204].

Following chapters go deeper into reasons why the experts' public claims are sometimes opposite to statements found in the publications of prestigious bodies the experts recommend reading.

I have not investigated social media, for these reasons:

- It's often extremely poor intellectually.
- It's very time-consuming.
- Comments often have a wasteful, imprecise nature and are quickly forgotten.
- Comments can be deleted or edited, meaning extra work must be done to access or view these.

I consider an historical analysis to be long overdue. What we believe now has been influenced by the research of previous years, and the way in which it has or has not been publicized. This is obviously true for social media and online articles as well as formal research. It's a generalization, but modern experts rely on, and have been influenced by the work of experts years before.

Therefore a mistake, a misinterpretation, or a lie (I think it is probably easier to see a lie than a mistake), can potentially have a huge effect.

I have summarized the information yielded from the New Zealand and Australian media. American media was bigger and more exhaustive, so I have simply used some interesting examples discussed in detail afterwards. I saw the same trend in American media with no substantial exceptions. The experts consistently ignored any experiment concluding fluorine non-essential. They claimed fluorine a nutritional essential with minimal discussion until the early 1970s. This was about the only general difference between USA and Australasian media: the NZ and Australian media did not seem to discuss the Messer *et al.* or the Schwarz experiments in the early 1970s. When I use the term "experts" I mean those public intellectuals to whom the media give a platform, and who promote Community Water Fluoridation.

I studied the experiments that you read in the first chapter, comparing the respective expert comment in media with the NAS publications I could find.

I wondered why, when I looked into WHO and NAS literature, I saw so little discussion on the topic of how relatable animal experiments on deficiency and essentiality were to humans, and how sparse the molecular research into the formation of teeth, and what nutritional components were required, was mentioned in the topic.

What amazed me was how quickly the experts had publicly concluded fluorine deficiency was a problem, and why there were no real questions on why the experts said teeth were poor due to fluoride deficiency, and not calcium, phosphorous, or some other deficiency? This was discussed *a little* in the 1974 Trace Element Symposium in Wisconsin (see Chapter 1.1 regarding the Messer *et al.* experiments), but I have found such complications go unmentioned in media. The same is mostly true for the changing of definitions.

In the summary of Chapter 2, I wrote that the experts *don't need to demonstrate the existence of a deficiency*, in order to claim that a deficiency exists. To this we may add that the public don't need to know about this justification in expert thinking.

5.1 Numbers and the New Zealand Media

"I used to argue, hopelessly I'm sure, that every reporter should carry a history book in their back-pocket."

- Robert Fisk, Middle East War Correspondent. Speaking in Sydney. Quoted in *Robert Fisk explains Iraq, history and journalism:* Address to Sydney audience, 12th October, 2005 [225].

I estimate I have sampled at least five thousand newspaper articles and letters dealing with Community Water Fluoridation (CWF). Some of these have dealt specifically with the topic of fluorine's essentiality, usually mentioned as a minor issue, though there have been a few articles in the American media that have given the issue centre stage (discussed in the next chapter).

I searched through one and a half thousand documents available on the National Library of New Zealand's database in Wellington. This yielded items from the late 1990s to around 2015 in New Zealand and Australian news media, with some items from the Pacific nations.

I searched through another one and a half thousand Australian newspaper articles using the database *Trove*, available online at http://trove.nla.gov.au/. This database was recommended to me by a librarian at the National Library of New Zealand.

For Australian and New Zealand newspaper articles and letters used in this investigation, see Appendix 1. For detail on search terms and inclusion criteria, see Appendix 2.

I did *not* specifically search for experts likening fluorine to nutrients known to be essential, nor did I search for the words "deficiency" and "mass medication", yet I found these claims, and have included them.

None of the *recent* NZ media articles that I found used a claim of essentiality to refute the "mass medication" argument. This may suggest that the experts have been less than totally organized in their refutations, or that at least some experts have stopped believing fluorine to have a nutritional status. If this was the case, they did not say so publicly. Many activists and people opposed to Community Water Fluoridation (CWF) still claim it to be mass medication (994 of the 1,557 submissions to the Hamilton City Council in 2013 were listed as making the "violation of human rights/mass medication" argument [226]).

My search included many newspaper clippings from the New Zealand Health Department archives, available in Wellington. There are a few files specifically full of news clippings. The years I looked through were 1951-1967. I have also used the database Newspapers.com for American newspapers, as well as kept my eye on local papers.

The experts have never presented their research regarding fluorine's essentiality publicly, with any real depth in the Australian or New Zealand media that I have ever found beyond a very occasional textbook citation. This has helped keep the discussion around this issue shallow.

The analysis in this chapter looks at the number of times fluorine's status or role as an essential nutrient was mentioned by the experts in New Zealand and Australian media. I've also included the number of times the element was compared with nutrients like iodine, the number of times the experts claimed fluorine deficiency existed, and the number of times a claim of essentiality was used to refute an allegation of mass medication.

Out of this sample of Australasian media articles and letters, only a little over a hundred mentioned fluorine's role in nutrition. This is a good indication of how poorly monitored this topic has been.

All of the media articles that *did* mention the topic, and claimed fluorine an essential nutrient, were in support of Community Water Fluoridation (other than the deviations mentioned previously and Dr. Lindsey mentioned in the next chapter[51]).

There was not a single letter or article I found that supported CWF *and* claimed fluorine non-essential in nutrition, though there were many that claimed CWF beneficial but did not mention the topic of a nutritional role for fluorine at all.

Many times the NAS and the WHO have been invoked by supporters, yet their insistences on fluorine's essentiality have been sporadic and contradictory. This is contrary to the impression one gets reading the newspapers, and none of the experts seem to notice. If they do, they don't seem to speak up about it. Publicly, the experts are united. When these bodies of scientists/experts (NAS, WHO, etc) go into detail, they usually conclude fluorine non-essential. It is often with minimal detail, or using benefit as a criterion for essentiality that they conclude fluorine essential, yet the experts who communicate their work to the public don't comment on this.

Thus, only one half of the "spectrum of conclusions" is represented by experts who are supposedly objective. Experts ridicule people opposed to fluoridation for selectivity and bias, and this may be correct in some instances, yet in this topic it can be observed that the experts have been doing exactly what they have always accused those they disagree with of doing for many decades.

For now, I will discuss this analysis. It is not perfect by any means – for a number of reasons.

Firstly, people phrase statements differently, and a small amount of the time meanings are unclear – but I would estimate only about ten percent of the time at the most.

Another reason has to do with size and precision. Media studies I've seen confine the data to a certain time period or a certain number of newspapers, and while I have made a few restrictions on my work (see Appendix 2) the search has been very broad – I simply used every media article from New Zealand and Australia I could

---

[51] I've focussed mainly on print media like newspapers, and a few experts may have been left out of the sample. There are a huge number of websites on CWF; I've avoided most of them.

lay my hands on that discussed the topic. This is partly due to the sparsity of mention on the topic – I have only a little over a hundred articles!

A reason for this is that not all newspapers have been digitized.

I contacted Fairfax Media about obtaining digitized records of my local newspaper, **The Dominion Post**. I thought it would be great to have *everything* experts had said about fluorine's nutritional role, in one newspaper, complete.

In order to see the entire timeline of the newspaper from the 1930s to now, I had to look at clippings donated to Wellington Public Library, use two databases at the National Library, and go to the Fairfax offices in Wellington where the Librarian of the Fairfax Information and Research Services Team "made an exception for me" which allowed me to see records between 1978 and 1994. Articles on public health and dentistry had been clipped out, but letters to the editor had not. In order to find letters between these years, I would have had to search individual newspapers in microfiche, the letters had not been highlighted or catalogued in any way. Thus it would have been incredibly time-consuming to obtain a complete archive or file of this paper, unless I wanted to read through sixteen years of letters (also about five of the microfiche articles were scratched and unreadable).

This would have been manageable – experts often conduct an educational campaign before fluoridation is discussed in a City Council meeting, so assuming one knew when towns near Wellington were fluoridated, one could look through papers about six months previous to, and immediately after towns had voted or had meetings on the subject. I do not think I found enough New Zealand letters prior to 1995 to include in this study.

Letters to editors are important because they represent (at least on the surface) what the public, and sometimes the odd expert, thinks. While it's important to look at what *experts* say, I believe it is also important to examine what the *public* says. This is relevant because it tells us how *believed* the experts are. If the experts are accurate, the public's belief will be accurate. If the experts are mistaken, the public will be mistaken. Both of these statements are based on the belief that the public trusts the experts.

I have used letters to editors of magazines and newspapers in this regard, while someone writing an article has been given the title of expert – simply because they are the one the media has put forward to speak, they have warranted a position of authority. However this is a slippery slope to base a conclusion upon, because letters to editors are not truly reflective of public understanding as they are sometimes written by marketing, communications, or public relations companies with a vested interest in the topic[52]. This is discussed later.

Newspaper editors may receive hundreds of letters on a controversial subject. Often they will print a reasonably sensible selection of a topic, although editors can and have influenced campaigns to fluoridate community water

---

[52] Activists also write a lot of letters. In many instances experts, newspaper editors and councillors feel overwhelmed by the response they get. For example, in Hamilton recently (June of 2013), 1,385 letters were sent opposing fluoridation, and 170 were sent in supporting it [226]. Of this total, at least 25% were from people outside Hamilton.

supplies[53]. Many, but not all of the articles, are written by or feature an expert with a scientific, medical or dental title. Obviously, in letters to editors, the people are *not* considered experts, but if they have a title their letter will carry more influence, so I have mentioned this in Appendix 2.

Table 10 summarises the data I've found looking only at what experts have said – all the articles and letters that were included claimed fluorine or fluoride was an essential nutrient.

The claim often made by experts that only the experts seem to understand, and therefore represent science with any accuracy is reason enough to study the experts.

From the totals in the left-most column the rest of the statements are taken. For instance, from a total of 56 Australian media articles claiming fluorine an essential nutrient, 13 of these 56 (*not* an *added* 13) likened it to nutrients known to be essential, 6 of these 56 claimed a fluorine deficiency. Some articles may have more than one claim.

Essentiality is either claimed or implied in these articles, in both instances this has warranted inclusion.

Regarding repetition of articles: no article was used twice, though this becomes difficult to police when different people quote from the same fact sheets [227] (though I suspect this example may be a case of pure public relations). Also consider trends and popularity in science. Over the last sixty or so years, experiments regarding the topic of essentiality are not discussed in Australasian media (at least that I'm aware).

The seasoned media hound will inquire about syndication. I've never worked in media so this was something I did not consider until late in the investigation. It did not strike me as important until I began trawling through American media. An example has been given in Chapter 2.7 regarding the nutritionist Dr. Jean Mayer. It appears to be something potentially complicated by national and local news. I believe minor newspapers are more likely to have local stories that have less to do with issues like business and politics. The Research Librarian at Fairfax Media told me that "historic syndication records aren't centralized, or shared." I remember seeing some overlap in New Zealand media in some of the Health Department files, but it was nowhere as extensive as American media, which should come as no surprise.

The Australian letter [228] that mentioned two textbooks contained seven paragraphs, five of which claimed that fluorine was an essential nutrient. It was compared with iodine in the second paragraph. The two textbooks mentioned in the letter were *Quantitative Trace Analysis of Biological Materials* by McKenzie and Smythe [229], published by Elsevier in 1988, and *Fluoride in Waters* [230], published by Her Majesty's Stationary Office, London, 1982.

The first textbook was co-authored by the writer of the letter, Hugh. A. McKenzie from the Protein Chemistry Group at the John Curtin School of Medical Research at the Australian National University in Canberra. Lloyd E. Smythe was from the Department of Analytical Chemistry at the University of New South Wales in Australia. This is a large book, with 700 pages. It contains some excellent points in the introduction, which was written by

---

[53] This is a separate subject, and very interesting. I am not investigating it beyond a cursory nod in this book.

editors McKenzie and Smythe. Some of these are very relevant, including lab variability, specificity of deficiency (deficiency of a given element can only be fixed by that element) and Bertrand's rule, which is summarized in a 2005 paper authored by three researchers:

> "… at low levels the benefits increase with intake towards an optimal plateau, beyond which there are increasing costs as the regulatory mechanisms are overwhelmed and excesses become toxic." [231]

In McKenzie and Smythe's textbook, death is claimed to be an effect caused by extreme deficiency. In this investigation I have seen precious little claims of someone dying from lack of fluorine, nor did McKenzie point to this in his letter.

ARTICLES MENTIONING FLUORINE'S/FLUORIDE'S ROLE IN NUTRITION IN AUSTRALIAN AND NEW ZEALAND NEWSPAPERS

From a total of about 4,000 articles relating to fluoridation[1], all written by or quoting experts who support CWF	Total number of articles[2] claiming fluorine/fluoride an essential nutrient	Number of times fluorine likened to other nutrients, e.g. iodine	Number of times fluorine deficiency claimed	Number of times Mass Medication claim countered with essentiality	Details
AUS Media articles	56	13	6	2	One NAS document cited[3]
AUS Letters to Newspaper Editors	15	4	2	0	One NAS document cited[4] in one letter, and two textbooks cited[5] in another letter
NZ Media articles 1993-2017	14	0	2	0	
NZ Media articles 1955-1992	26	3	11	5	
NZ Letters to Editors 1995-2016	22	11[See 6]	3	2	

Table 10*: Data summary of articles and letters in NZ and Australian newspapers where essentiality is claimed or implied.*

1) I estimate 4,000. Firstly, searches were performed at the National Library of New Zealand in Wellington. This was 1,500 items, mostly from New Zealand, but some from Australia. Beyond this a search of twenty files at the Health Department archives, and the archives of Wellington's **Evening Post** at Wellington Public Library and the Fairfax building. I'm unsure exactly how many more this added, but I will estimate around another thousand, of mostly New Zealand articles. Another 1,500 Australian articles were found through the database *Trove*, this was suggested to me by a librarian at Wellington's Alexander Turnbull Library. All articles in the table presented here were relevant to Community Water Fluoridation.

As pointed out, from 4,000 articles not every article or letter that appeared in response to search terms was even related to CWF, though the majority were. Sometimes the word "essential" was used but not in any way related to nutrition.

2) This also includes advertisements, 3 in Australian media.

3) Presumably **Dietary Reference Intakes for Calcium, Phosphorous, Vitamin D and Fluoride**, National Academy of Sciences, 1997; the article was from 1998.

4) **Earth Materials and Health: Research Priorities for Earth Science and Public Health**, Committee on Research Priorities for Earth Science and Public Health, National Research Council, p. 37, 2007. This was discussed in Chapter 2.1.

5) These are discussed below.

6) Four of these articles did not use the term 'essential nutrient' but still compared the element to nutrients definitely essential.

The chapter in McKenzie and Smythe's textbook on fluorine was authored by John W. Shortland of the State Pollution Control Commission of New South Wales, Australia. His investigation of fluorine's essentiality is brief yet faulty:

> "The question of fluorine as an essential element has been addressed by Ericsson (1970), National Academy of Sciences, NAS (1971a) and Underwood (1977). Underwood refers to evidence of the essentiality of fluorine for growth and reproduction of rats and mice and Ericsson comments that for the formation of a decay resistant tooth enamel, a certain fluoride supply is evidently essential." [229]

Then Shortland began his second sub-chapter, *Occurrence and forms of fluorine*. Shortland's discussion on essentiality ends after quoting Ericsson. I have looked at all three of these documents in this investigation. They are (as referenced by Shortland):

The 1970 WHO Monograph *Fluorides and Human Health*, pages 13-16. This included Ericsson's introduction to the document. The last sentence of Ericsson's statement is quoted accurately here by Shortland:

> "The question 'is fluorine an essential element?' has naturally been raised. It has not been possible to find a definite answer owing to the difficulty of producing a diet for animal experimentation that is fluorine-free but adequate in every other resepct. However, there are indications that traces of fluorine are necessary for normal mineralization, and possibly also for normal reproduction. For the formation of a caries-resistant enamel, a certain fluoride supply is evidently essential." [102]

Only the end of Ericsson's statement is cited, and not Muhler's or Venkateswarlu's more thorough presentations that were ambivalent, calling for more research.

The 1971 NAS document (pages 66-68), *Is Fluorine an Essential Element?* in **Fluorides, Biological Properties of Atmospheric Pollutants**. I quoted from this document in Chapter 2.1:

> "It cannot definitely be concluded from these experiments that fluoride is nonessential for the nutrition of these species."

> "if fluoride is a dietary essential for the species studied, its requirement must be extraordinarily low. Indications that fluoride might be essential for any other species are also lacking, and the beneficial effects of

fluoride on dental health or bone metabolism should be considered as pharmacologic responses, and not as a cure of pre-existing deficiency condition." [69]

Underwood's 1977 textbook is the fourth edition of *Trace Elements in Human and Animal Nutrition.* The first sentence of this work by Underwood is:

"Several attempts[54] in the past to demonstrate an essential function for fluorine in rats fed diets reported to contain as little as 0.005 ppm F were unsuccessful."

It's true that Underwood "refers to" evidence regarding growth, yet he also "refers to" the 1974 Weber and Reid experiment [35] that demonstrated no difference between two groups of rats. He also pointed out that Messer *et al.* said nothing about why they needed such high amounts (50 ppm) of fluoride to obtain fertility in their mice.

Yet Shortland is basically correct, Underwood knew nothing of, or did not include the two experiments from 1976 [33, 34] that refuted the work of Messer *et al.* Underwood wrote:

"On the basis of these findings fluorine must be regarded as an essential element, despite the absence of a specific biochemical lesion or a satisfactory explanation of the cause of either the anemia or the infertility. The situation is complicated further by the findings of Weber and Reid..." [232]

It is forgiveable that Underwood did not know of the 1976 experiments considering his work was published in 1977, and he was possibly in pre-publication when the experiments came out. These experiments were not mentioned in the National Academy of Sciences writings until 1983 (again in 1989), unless I am mistaken[55]. I never saw them in newspapers, nor in the USPHS bulletins so it is very probable they were completely beyond the experts' awareness. It was probably difficult to keep on top of the most recent research decades ago. Shortland did not mention the 1976 experiments in 1988. It potentially indicates that none or few experts knew about them (further exemplified in the next chapter.) In comparison, Dr. Schwarz's first set of experiments that concluded fluorine essential for growth was in a Californian newspaper the day after he presented them (before their publication). Reading McKenzie's letter, so authoritative and definite on the matter, one considers that maybe Shortland's work would not have been published had he been overly thorough.

In Chapter 20 of the fourth edition of his book, Underwood wrote of anemia:

"Trace element x can be vital at one point in this [metabolic] chain, and trace element y at another. A simple or conditioned deficiency of either element would therefore lead to the same end result in the animal, although the cause would obviously be different. For instance, anemia can be a manifestation of iron, copper, nickel or cobalt deficiency, or of selenium, zinc or molybdenum toxicity." [233]

Underwood obviously did not consider that there could be anything wrong with the diet Messer *et al.* used. He probably assumed they would have followed a standard procedure. Perhaps this tells us something about scientists – that they expect other scientists to state if their work is not up to a decent standard. This example demonstrates the problem in simply going along on trust. He had read and cited the 1974 document [31] and

---

[54] Underwood cites Doberenz *et al.* [19], Maurer and Day [17], and Sharpless and McCollum [6].
[55] They were discussed in 1977's **Drinking Water and Health** (p.390) not in relation to essentiality. Suttie's name was spelled "Suttee".

seen Messer's claim of marginal iron and copper levels, though perhaps did not consider their claim of anemia with scepticism.

Of the 1971 NAS document, Shortland had nothing more to say than that it "addressed" the issue. That the document almost flatly disagreed with his conclusion didn't matter to him. Perhaps this makes sense given that Underwood's work was more recent. Shortland's appraisal does give the impression of more uniformity among experts, something promoters of CWF have always claimed, and used to their advantage.

McKenzie and Smythe gave their own opinion of Bertrand's rule, which they called

> "the schematic representation of the dependence of a biological function on the concentration of a nutrient."
> [229]

At the upper limits the organism goes into three phases as intake of the nutrient increases: marginal, toxicity, death. Rising from the lowest concentration there are three stages: death, deficiency, and marginal, before optimal levels are reached. Not even "marginal" has been demonstrated conclusively for fluorine, and as shown here, Shortland's explanation did not give evidence of deficiency, though it claimed to. I am not critical of what he included but of what he did not include. McKenzie and Smythe are exaggerating when they include this element in the category of "Selected 'essential' trace elements" as their contents page indicates.

The second book recommended by McKenzie, *Fluoride in waters, effluents, sludges, plants and soils 1982: methods for the examination of waters and associated materials*, had nothing on essentiality in the contents. The word 'nutrient' did not appear in the book at all. This is a book describing biochemical analytical techniques, however it said fluoride, in the right amount, is beneficial.

The Australian letter written regarding the 2007 National Academy of Sciences publication stated:

> "The NRC [sic] has considered the health effects of fluoride in drinking water in 1951, 1977, 1993, 2006 and 2007. The last report concluded fluoride was an essential element for human life based on its role in cellular functions involving metabolic and biochemical processes." [234][56]

The NAS *did* conclude something similar to this (see Chapter 2.1). The NAS cited the 2005 textbook *Essentials of Medical Geology* [87], which cited the study from Chow [88] and the *Handbook of Nutritionally Essential Mineral Elements* [89]. (It also cited the improvement in decay reduction in Grand Rapids as evidence of deficiency, discussed in a 1950 study [91].) The *Handbook* claimed there was:

> "… no evidence that it [fluorine] exerts a specific biochemical function." [89]

This is a little different from the letter. The letter ignored all the times the NAS had claimed fluorine non-essential (exactly as American experts did in American media).

A newspaper clipping dated 21st July 1964 in the **Taupo Times** (New Zealand) put forth a question and answer styled article from a resident of Taupo who was against fluoridation of Taupo's water. The second Q & A was:

---

[56] In 2008 the WHO claimed fluorine *may* be essential but didn't elaborate beyond saying research was equivocal [114]. This may be irrelevant because in 2002 they called it essential based on the physiological importance of resistance to dental caries [104], and in 2010 they called it a micronutrient [109], citing their 2002 work. See Ch. 2.1 for more on the NAS, and Ch. 2.3 for the WHO.

"Q: Will fluoridation of water supplies ensure an accurate dose?

A: No. It depends on how much water is consumed. If twice as much water is taken, you get twice as much fluorine." [235][57]

The matters raised in this contributed article are not necessarily the opinions of this newspaper, but are published in accordance with the principle of allowing both parties in any controversy free access to the correspondence columns.—The Editor.

The word 'dose' appeared three times in the article. You can see a disclaimer (pictured, **Figure 13**) that was placed in the middle of the anti-fluoride question that addressed safety.

On the 23rd July 1964 the **Taupo Times** featured Dr. Bruce Rice, described as a "one-time chief dental officer for the World Health Organisation" who wrote to the editor to "re-answer" some of the questions properly.

To quote the question of concern here:

"Q: Will fluoridation of water supplies ensure an accurate dose?

A: To apply the word "dose" to fluoridation is completely erroneous as fluoride is not a medicine but an essential nutrient. We do not speak of "dosing" when we put salt in our vegetables or supply our families with milk for its calcium content." [236]

Dr. Rice ignored the 1957 and 1959 work that had concluded fluorine non-essential [17, 18]. He was possibly using the 1958 NAS document that Dr. Fredrick Stare had cited (see Chapter 5.2).

I'm not familiar with WHO work before the 1970 monograph [102], but their Technical Report Series No. 146 (1958), *Expert Committee on Water Fluoridation: First Report*, did not discuss a role of fluorine as a nutrient.

It should come as no surprise that the newspaper put no disclaimer in Dr. Rice's article. The World Health Organization has obvious prestige; their words do not need to be interrupted with disclaimers or rejoinders. This demonstrates two things. One being that the media are more accommodating when it comes to expressing the view of the powerful and prestigious, and the second being that even if the people opposed to fluoridation have some accuracy in their statements, this is irrelevant because the experts are assumed to know better.

Another point demonstrated not so much by the disclaimer but by the statements of Dr. Rice is that fluorine must not be seen as a medicine, it *must* be a nutrient.

A resident lacks the prestige of experts. We all know who the WHO is, or at least we can go and find their publications. From this perspective it makes perfect sense that the newspaper is justified in including a disclaimer with the resident's letter and not in Dr. Rice's.

The letter against fluoridation dated 21st July may have been in response to the **Taupo Times** printing on July 14th of the same year, the words of "a Government publication" (unnamed):

"Q: Are there other trace element deficiencies in New Zealand?

A: Yes. Iodine deficiency is common. Many soils are deficient in copper, molybdenum, and cobalt. Fluoridation of water supplies is really the correction of a trace deficiency." [237]

---

[57] This letter from the resident opposed to fluoridation made a similar claim to the Maier study (cited by the British Geological Survey, Chapter 12 of *Essentials of Medical Geology* 5th edition [87], see Chapter 2.1):
"The quantities of fluoride ingested are generally dependent on the amounts of water consumed." [91] (page 1122)

In these Q&A formats, it is often not stated who chooses the questions.

These examples are no different.

In a 2013 interview on New Zealand's TV One News, presenter Susan Wood asked Dr. Jonathan Broadbent[58] (supporting CWF) and Dr. Lawrie Brett[59] (opposing CWF) how they could have such differing opinions on the same research, but in the investigation I have done, we can see the people in the fluoridation debate are *not* always looking at the same research.

And it can be easily demonstrated why people may argue over research: it says completely different things depending on whether we look deeply or stay on the surface. It will cause many to shut their ears and refuse my voice, but I have demonstrated that on this issue of whether we really *need* this element, the experts who support fluoridation do *not* all agree… until they're in the media.

My research here has demonstrated that experts advocating CWF have a bias towards exaggerating a necessity for fluoride. The word exaggeration is an understatement. Consider that this bias is almost *total* – the only public deviations still manage to make fluoride appear necessary in some way, or that we're missing out on it [158, 178]. Much evidence demonstrates that this is possibly quite unrealistic, so if the experts were really interested in being accurate, we'd *at least* see some deviation and disagreement, instead of this public uniformity.

5.2 American Experts in American Media

"Though long ago settled in many communities with little conversation, how a candidate felt about fluoride could make or break a political career."

- Stephanie Desmon, W.Md. *anti-fluoride lawsuit dismissed by federal judge*, **The Baltimore Sun**, p. B1, 6th September, 2003.

A consistent claim since the 1950s has been the likening of fluorine to nutrients, notably but not only iodine. This was possibly a result of McClendon's work, though I found his name only once mentioned in American media [238]. Another was the claim of deficiency, which appeared very consistently.

Regarding the claims of trace element status, many dictionary definitions of 'trace element' or 'micronutrient' seem to have a word like 'requirement', 'needed', and/or 'necessity' in them, it seems presumptuous to call fluorine a 'trace element' without having ever identified a specific deficiency in humans [103, 105, 116, 117-119], but this obviously depends on our definition of 'trace element', so we're back in semantics. All definitions I found demand a requirement for the element, but there may be some definitions that don't. On this note, perhaps it is the dictionaries that should relax in their strictness; Underwood's fourth edition pointed to

---

[58] BDS, PhD, PGDipComDent, Associate Professor and Head of Discipline of Preventive and Restorative Dentistry in the Department of Oral Rehabilitation at Otago University's Division of Health Sciences.
[59] Practicing Dentist for over 30 years in Kamo, Whangarei. Graduated in 1974 from Otago Dental School having also studied chemistry.

difficulties in "drawing a line of demarcation" around these elements given their natures. Some experiments *did* claim to have created a deficiency [13, 20, 28, 29], but even a small sample of the experiments or reviews that refuted or challenged these conclusions [17, 18, 19, 33, 34, 35] are not discussed in media. The experts are strangely silent on this point. It's difficult to know what the experts think about these latter experiments because the experts don't appear to *know* about them. Examples have been given previously; more follow.

In scientific literature sometimes the experts who support Community Water Fluoridation disagree on whether fluorine should be considered essential or non-essential.

Nomenclature here: macronutrients generally refer to fats, proteins, and carbohydrates. Minerals can be further divided into two categories: major minerals, and trace elements (the term 'element' here is relaxed sometimes to include compounds containing more than one element). I'm not sure if CWF-supporting experts concern themselves with these categories or not, because they generally don't relate fluorine to other elements beyond simply claiming it's like them. The books focusing on "trace elements" that I've seen don't include calcium, phosphorous and the elements required in larger amounts in this category. Some experts suspend a boundary between the two categories; Dr. Fredrick Stare is one example mentioned in this chapter. New Zealanders will be aware of Dr. Perrott's *Responding to Tracey Brown on fluoridation* article online (13th October, 2015) in which he classes fluoride with selenium, sodium, phosphorous, potassium and magnesium. Of these, only selenium is considered a "trace" element according to Underwood's fourth edition, yet one is reminded of Underwood's difficulty in creating boundaries. The public sees little to no disagreement between experts if they stay within traditional media.

Consider the sample of information in Chapter 2, compared to the newspaper articles discussed here. Obtain more information, enlarge the sample if you like, see if my conclusions hold – that regarding fluorine's essentiality, the more public the information, the more one-sided it becomes in the experts' hands. Remember that the experts are mostly presented as objective, knowledgeable and neutral, or claim these characteristics.

It's normal that in less public research, more detail is sometimes given, and in more public research, less detail is given. It makes sense that this should occur for convenience's sake – we don't need all the fiddly experimental details in our newspaper, but in *this* instance, the message from experimental evidence, and the message from experts in our media, are very different. When the experts talk in media, they are quick to cite the National Academy of Sciences (NAS) as claiming fluorine a dietary essential. A quick glance at the WHO and the NAS reveal claims with much less consistency. What these organizations have claimed regarding fluorine's essentiality has changed over the years, yet is presented to the public by experts as *always* stating fluorine is essential. When the NAS and the WHO have said fluorine non-essential, this has consistently been ignored by experts.

In private committees and groups, when experts look at evidence in detail often they do *not* believe fluorine to be essential – or they are at least interested in providing *some* of an entire spectrum of conclusions and research. This is honest of them, and the reason I believe few, if any, are deliberately lying.

But when experts speak in our mainstream media on the topic of fluorine's essentiality, only one end of a spectrum of conclusions is presented. The conclusions and statements of other research, it seems, is too 'far out' to say, for unknown reasons.

Ironically, this presented end is the end of the spectrum consisting of research that scientists have criticised more heavily – and when I say "scientists" I *don't* mean "activists opposing CWF". Consider that the following two papers criticized or refuted the work done in the early 1970s that had concluded fluorine essential. Nielsen and Sandstead began the section on fluorine with the words:

"A beneficial function of fluorine has been known since the late 1930's when..." [27]

They went on to criticize the conclusions of Dr. Schwarz. Another example is the 1976 experiment that demonstrated the conclusions of the work of Armstrong *et al.* as incorrect. Tao and Suttie began their experiment with the words:

"Although the value of an optimal dietary intake of fluoride in reducing the incidence of dental caries in the human population has been recognized for some time[60], data which would support the inclusion of fluoride in the list of those elements essential in animal nutrition have been lacking." [33]

So this is strictly *not* the dissident, antifluoride activist literature. Yet this review and this experiment go undiscussed in media, even though they are scientists not activists, and have said Community Water Fluoridation *is* beneficial, but fluorine non-essential.

American media gave publicity to the research of Dr. Schwarz, and the experiments of Dr. Armstrong *et al.* in the early 1970s. As far as I can tell, Australasian media left this out. This is an interesting time period to study. Examples here will help to demonstrate points made previously.

In Chapter 2.1 I showed that the NAS reflected the spectrum of conclusions with a reasonable commitment to accuracy, although they cited less and less experimentation on this topic as time went on. This is understandable when we consider that almost no work was forthcoming after the 1970s. Yet in considering this, it is also interesting to see examples wherein very old research is used in very recent documents[61].

In 1939, Evans and Phillips claimed that less than 50 microgram per kilogram of body weight was required daily in rats, if there was a requirement. In 1957, Maurer and Day called fluorine "dispensable" in a very good experiment[62], that was, from what I can tell, almost never mentioned in media, except by people opposing CWF.

I have wondered if the experts are not aware that such research exists, not even that such research *could exist* that may call their conclusions into question (a researcher studying internal documents or reading more of the trace element symposiums may have more success in supporting or refuting this). We can see there are lengthy

---

[60] Work by F. Brudevold is cited here by Drs Tao and Suttie, *The role of fluorides in tooth chemistry and in the prevention of dental caries*. In: **Handbook of Pharmacology**, vol. XX/1, pp. 173-230 (Smith, F. A., ed.), Springer-Verlag, New York, 1966. This is a different section of the book than that which Dr. Schwarz cited (see Chapter 1.1). Page 180: "The fluoridation of a water supply is a duplication of nature's way of providing necessary fluoride."

[61] For instance see the example given in Chapter 2.1 regarding the twelfth chapter of the textbook *Essentials of Medical Geology* 8th Edition (2005), and at the end of Chapter 2.6 regarding the study published in **Neurotoxicology and Teratology**.

[62] Recall from Chapter 1.1 that Dr. Schwarz called it "rather sophisticated" [26].

discussions on this topic, but by the time it gets to media, the complications are omitted and the experts are calling fluorine an essential nutrient without reservation.

Also relevant, is that current technology used by media allows *one* message to be transmitted to many people. I'm not saying this is inherently right or wrong, good or bad, in fact it's very useful when it comes to things like emergency broadcasts and crisis situations that demand a prompt, unified response. Yet in lengthy, scientific discussions taking place over many years, the integrity of information can be compromised as details are omitted for the sake of convenience. While everybody may get the same helpful message in some instances, we may also get the same mistake in others.

Finding statements in American newspapers relative to fluorine's role in nutrition before about 1955 was difficult. In the 1930s three experiments looked at a requirement for fluorine in the rat, and concluded there was none, or almost none.

In 1944, 1953 and 1954, Jesse Francis McClendon's experiments were published. He fed poor quality hydroponically grown food to rats drinking fluorine-free water, and to rats with fluorine added to water, though *this* group of rats were also fed normal, soil-grown food in an unknown ratio. His first two experiments were criticized for their "departure from standard experimental procedure" and for showing no details on fluorine content of rats before and after the experiment. He claimed fluorine prevented cavities in the rat molars and pronounced it essential. It is unclear to me if his work influenced any of the public claims shown here.

In February 1955, Washington's **Daily Chronicle** wrote that

> "Chehalis Dentist Edgar Johnson told the Chehalis Chamber of Commerce members … fluoridation is not mass medication. Dr. Johnson… quoted the National Dairy Council which lists fluorides as nutrients essential to the formation of the teeth and bones."

According to the article, Dr. Johnson

> "… said fluorides cannot be both a nutrient and a medicine at the same time." [239]

In March of the next year, a headline (**Figure 14**) in a New York newspaper carried a similar message. This was the headline of a letter three columns wide. It was written by W. W. Westerfeld, Professor of Biochemistry at the State University of New York, at the Medical College in Syracuse.

The Professor wrote (partially pictured below):

> "It is completely erroneous to consider the fluoridation of water as medication."
>
> "The amount of fluoride needed in the diet is extremely small, but its need is none the less real."
>
> "No one knows what would happen if we consumed a diet completely free of fluoride; therefore we do not know if fluoride is absolutely required in the diet." "By this criterion, dental caries is a deficiency disease due to an inadequate intake of fluoride, in the same way that rickets is a deficiency disease due to an inadequate intake of vitamin D: the only difference..." [240].

(It's no wonder people get offended, exasperated and confused over fluoridation – compare this statement above regarding 'deficiency disease' with a 1960 statement from Mrs. David Abrams, Chairman of the Fluoridation Committee of the Intermediate Department of the Woman's Club of Beckley:

"Fluoridation is not a medication – it does not constitute a remedy or treat an existing disease, the chairman said…"[63] [241]

She went on to say it was a nutrient. Also consider the 2013 words of the European Food Safety Authority [118] discussed in Chapter 2.3.)

In the 1956 article, under the sub-heading **Fluoride Not Drug**, the Professor wrote:

Water Fluoridation Supplements Diet; Medication Claim Disputed

"Thus a dietary essential which is required in small amounts to prevent disease…"

Figure 14. Water Fluoridation Supplements Diet. **The Post-Standard** (Syracuse, New York), p. 39, 18th March, 1956.

ican public. The amount of fluoride needed in the diet is extremely small, but its need is none the less real.

No one knows what would happen if we consumed a diet completely free of fluoride; therefore we do not know if fluoride is absolutely required in the diet. But we can say that with an optimal concentration of fluoride in the diet the tooth structure is a good deal more resistant to decay and therefore a more healthy tooth.

Deficiency Disease

By this criterion, dental caries (decay) is a deficiency disease due to an inadequate intake of fluoride in the same way that rickets is a deficiency disease due to an inadequate intake of vitamin D; the only difference is that fluoride provides something less than complete protection against caries because other factors are also involved in tooth decay.

He claimed that fluoride

"… could not be classified as a drug, even in this nebulous way [of giving large amounts]." [240]

He did not mention McClendon's work but there is a possibility it helped him come to these conclusions.

In April of 1956, Dr. Carl Weatherbee, Head of the Millikin University Chemistry Department, spoke to the Decatur, Illinois City Council in support of fluoridation. His main points were listed in **The Decatur Daily Review**.

Perhaps he had also seen McClendon's work, because his fifth point was

"… [fluoride] is necessary as a food nutrient." [242]

In January of 1957, the **Honolulu Advertiser** carried a letter written by Marjorie Abel, Chief Bureau of Nutrition of the Board of Health, which discussed how

"Dr. Harry Arnold, Jr., called fluoridation the addition of a nutrient. Fluorine is one of 50 chemical substances known to be essential to human health. I cannot see that the addition of fluoride to the water supply is any different from the addition of minerals and vitamins to bread, milk, butter and margarine and to the cereals." [243]

---

[63] This statement may have been lifted from the 23-page pamphlet *Fluoridation Facts: Answers to Criticisms Against Fluoridation*, published by the American Dental Association, April, 1956. Pages 10-11: "Fluoridation does not constitute a remedy; it does not treat an existing disease." This of course was in response to the "mass medication" charge. "Adding sodium fluoride to the water supply is no more a medication than adding table salt…"

In August, 1957, Indiana University's Richard Maurer and Harry Day had their study *The Non-Essentiality of Fluorine in Nutrition* published in the **Journal of Nutrition** [17].

From what I have seen in American newspapers, it was ignored by the supporters of Community Water Fluoridation, except when pointed out in a debate between Dr. Robert Roy Kintner (against CWF) and Dr. N. E. Wessman (for) [238]. The response to Kintner from Wessman was that it was irrelevant because Maurer and Day still claimed fluorine beneficial for prevention of decay.

Maurer and Day were also ignored in a letter apparently authored by 'Food and Drug Research' that claimed fluorine an essential nutrient, appearing in a 1958 issue of **The Evening Times**, a Pennsylvania newspaper. "Fluorine in this ["vital trace"] quantity is a food element, not a medication and not a poison." [244]

That this experiment was largely ignored is surprising given its quality. Indiana University was well known for work on toothpaste [245], evidenced by many news articles discussed in Chapter 5.6.

In April 1959, the year-long experiment by Wuthier and Phillips of the University of Wisconsin was published in the **Journal of Nutrition**, in which the scientists claimed that:

"No significant protective effect against dental caries was observed from any of these fluoride levels studied."
[18]

This also was ignored by the experts, with Dr. Ellis Sox, the San Francisco Health Officer, discussing the necessity of fluorine in the formation of teeth in San Rafael's **Daily Independent Journal**, a few months later [123].

I have found seven articles published in the year 1960 authored by Dr. Fredrick Stare of Harvard University's Food and Nutrition Department. In all seven he claimed fluoride was an essential nutrient - in none of them did he mention the experiments of the late 1950s even once [246, 247].

Something should not *need* to be an essential nutrient in order to simply do good. Dr. Stare frequently cited a 1958 document, a revision of the National Research Council's **Recommended Dietary Allowances**. He wrote:

"... did you know... fluorine is listed as a nutrient we need – just as we need vitamin C, calcium, or protein?"
[246]

Consulting the document, we find this is true. Fluorine *is* listed with manganese, copper, phosphorous, and others, just before the 'trace elements' section. Quoting the NAS:

"... [fluoridation] is a means of supplying a nutrient important for the formation of caries-resistant enamel."
[248]

The document *does* cite the 1957 Maurer and Day study, along with others (perhaps this qualifies as an *indirect* citation to the Maurer and Day study, but note Stare does not mention *that* particular experiment). The references are listed here:

Francis A. Arnold, **American Journal of Public Health**, Vol. 47, p. 539, 1957.

T. J. Hill, H. T. Dean and P. C. Kitchin, *Dental Caries and Fluorine*, Washington: American Association for the Advancement of Science, 1946.

National Academy of Sciences – National Research Council. Publication 294. Washington, 1953.

T. F. Dixon and H. R. Perkins, *The Chemistry of Calcification*. In: *Biochemistry and Physiology of Bone*, edited by G. E. Bourne. New York: Academic Press, 1956.

Richard L. Maurer and Harry G. Day, *The Non-Essentiality of Fluorine in Nutrition*, **Journal of Nutrition**, Vol. 62, pp. 561-573, 1957.

The first (Arnold, 1957) is a study looking at the eleventh year of CWF in the town of Grand Rapids, Michigan. Dr. Joseph Muhler among others has suggested that because CWF is beneficial, fluorine should be classed as an essential nutrient, even though in experiments on humans it is difficult to perform accurate measurements of nutrient intake, and one cannot control for every single variable.

The second (Hill, Dean and Kitchin, 1946) is a book compiled from the work of many authors of the time – Dean, Ockerse, Arnold, Armstrong, and others. I have not found anything indicating that there is a study on fluorine's nutritional role carried out in the same way the studies I have cited in Chapter 1.1 have been carried out, but it appears there is some information that may be relevant to the investigator – namely one of Armstrong's initial studies on teeth resistant to caries, and a study on African people, fluorine and dental caries by Ockerse.

One can see benefit as a criterion for essentiality, long before Mark Hegsted ever suggested it. To paraphrase: "We added fluoride to water, our statistics showed less holes in teeth afterwards, therefore they were deficient in fluoride." In some ways it appears to make sense. However, in doing this we've side-stepped the more inconvenient, annoying question about other deficiencies being masked by fluorine, and seemingly demonstrating the existence of fluorine deficiency beyond the shadow of a doubt. The experts are so definite in public, yet this aspect of their foundation is imprecise.

The third reference is a NAS document called *The Problem of Providing Optimal Fluoride Intake for the prevention of Dental Caries*. I have been unable to obtain a copy of this document. The fourth, Dickson and Perkins' 1956 work, appears to be *very* specialized (this is the impression I get from a review of the book published in the **Archives of Disease in Childhood** [249]).

You can find the Maurer and Day study discussed in Chapter 1.1. Neither Stare nor the NRC mention the blatant contradiction in using the study:

> "Thus it is justifiable to conclude that under some conditions fluorine may not have any value in nutrition or even in the maintenance of dental health."

> "The investigation has demonstrated that under the rigorous experimental conditions employed, fluorine is not a dietary essential."

> "… its value in the body is apparently limited to the promotion of resistance to dental caries." [17]

Note that the work carried out in the 1930s was not included in this NAS document. Nor was McClendon's work, yet perhaps this was because it had been heavily criticized in **Nutrition Reviews**[64] only a few years earlier (see Chapter 1.2).

---

[64] The journal was published by Harvard where Stare worked.

However, a 1962 article featuring Dr. Stare could possibly have addressed this: it quoted him as saying

"Fertilization of the soil has very little to do – practically nothing to do – with the nutritive quality of the crop grown in the soil."

This was in response to "misinformation" that was coming out in fashionable books of the time claiming naturally grown foods were superior to store-bought foods, which Dr. Stare dismissed as

"… just a bunch of charlatanism and nonsense." [250]

Sometimes newspaper staff have a wonderful sense of humour. Perhaps the title of the article is a dig at Dr. Stare - *Books, Articles not Doing Food Industry any Good.*

Dr. Stare continued the assertion that fluorine was definitely an essential nutrient throughout the 1960s. His work made an impression; in 1963 Dr. Robert Broad, Commissioner of Health for Tompkins County, New York State, quoted him in a letter printed in **The Ithaca Journal** [251].

In 1964, the National Academy of Science published the sixth revised edition of **Recommended Dietary Allowances**. They wrote:

"Fluoride is incorporated in the structure of teeth and confers maximal resistance to dental caries. In this sense, fluorine is necessary for optimal health."

They mentioned that CWF was

"a very important nutritional public health measure in areas where there is a deficiency." [252]

They used four references to support this statement. One was the 1953 NAS document [253], one was a report from the British Ministry of Health [254], and the other referred to two articles published in the ADA's journal in 1962. One began by saying there had been opposition to all manner of medical processes but fluoridation was here to stay, and the other was about safety [255]. The article about safety pointed to McClendon's 1953 experiment regarding the claim for a need for fluorine in reproduction, but said the work was "unsubstantiated". As of the time of writing I've not obtained the NAS or the British documents; perhaps these will open up new avenues of research.

The word 'deficiency' is inappropriate based on the research I have seen, however I have few to no problems with people discussing benefit. It's possible beneficial effects attributable to fluoride occur because it is sometimes masking a deficiency of some other compound or problem in another area, similar to the way a person with poor adrenal glands will be stimulated by daily caffeine. I haven't yet seen this discussed in the literature at all, beyond the two 1976 experiments.

Two other references in the NAS 1964 document dealt with mottling, three addressed safety. This document basically agreed with Dr. Stare's claim. The NAS ignored the experiments of Maurer and Day, and Wuthier and Phillips. Is this fair enough? After all, these experiments had used rats. In 1963, an abstract of the Doberenz *et al.* experiment was published, in December of 1964 it was published in full [19].

Dr. Stare had consistently been accused of taking 'bribes' – for want of a better term – to produce and publicize research that suited the food industry. He responded to one accusation in a letter printed in **The Cincinnati**

Enquirer in 1960, claiming that General Foods Corporation along with other industrial, private individuals and foundations, and even branches of government, had provided funds to support research at his department at Harvard [247].

He said money was only taken when it was given with no strings attached, though looking at some articles on research funding at Harvard, it appears that this statement is idealistic. A 1935 article said, "the university ordinarily follows a donor's suggestions in such matters…" [256]

A 1949 article in the **Portland Press Herald** (Maine), discussed a gift of $50,000 to Harvard. The gift was from Mallinckrodt Chemical Works of St. Louis,

"available for advanced studies in chemistry without restriction as to use… Provost Paul H. Buck hailed the gift as a sign that 'enlightened management now realizes it can best serve the cause of private education as a free enterprise if it provides free funds without attaching limiting restrictions.'"

"Harvard noted that a large proportion of the funds available to universities and colleges are 'earmarked for specific purposes…'" [257]

Another 1949 article (**Figure 15**) was very expressive about the millions given to Harvard. A 1960 article discussed a "momentous" gift of a little over a million over a ten-year period from General Foods Corp.,

"for expansion of the nutritional laboratories of the Harvard School of Public Health."

This was the largest gift from "any business corporation for the capital purposes of Harvard University." [258]

SOUTHERN ILLINOISAN.

SECOND THOUGHTS
————By David V. Felts

ANNOUNCEMENTS of further bequests to Harvard, which now has an endowment of $182,824,335 according to the World Almanac, are read with a measure of irritation by alumni of colleges which would really be set up in business with a mere million, or half that amount.

They can imagine a stenographer in the office of the Harvard treasurer opening the mail and announcing: "Here's another million dollars. What shall I do with it?" Under such circumstances the treasurer might say, "Oh, set it over in a corner for the moment; maybe we'll find a place for it later."

A couple of weeks ago headlines reported "Harvard receives Gift of $8,626,506." Gifts of less than a million to Harvard are not news, except in the community in which the donor lives, or has lived.

That eight million dollar "gift," really was not new; it was just another installment paid out of earnings of an endowment trust established 40 years ago.

When Gordon McKay, Pittsfield, Mass., shoe machinery designer, died in 1903 he established an endowment trust, leaving life incomes from the estate to various individuals. Income from the estate beyond the sums necessary to pay the annuities was accumulated by the trustees for Harvard university. When these savings amounted to one million dollars in 1909, the Gordon McKay Endowment was created and as various individual beneficiaries died, additional amounts were added.

Thus far the McKay endowment had paid more than $15,000,000 to Harvard.

It should be mentioned, in passing, that in addition to the McKay payment, which had been anticipated, Harvard received between July 1 and September 30, gifts amounting to $1,342,296—miscellaneous.

Figure 15. *Second Thoughts.* **Southern Illinoisian**, p. 4, 23rd November 1949.

A 1979 article looked at a $100 million donation to Emory University, in the form of three million shares of Coca-Cola,

> "of such magnitude 'that every time Coca-Cola [stock] goes up $1, the endowment increases by $3 million or thereabouts'" [259]

said Henry L. Bowden, chairman of Emory's board of trustees at a news conference.

There is a building named for Mr. Woodruff, the 90-year-old donator, on what is sometimes called "Coca-Cola U." Note this is *Emory* University, *not* Harvard, where Fredrick Stare worked. A 1994 article discussed how the founder of ABC (American Broadcasting Company) and his wife donated $60 million to Harvard Medical School; this was originally reported in **The New York Times**. The Goldensons, (the givers), were graduates of Harvard Law School, and had a neuroscience building named after them [260].

A 2005 book looks at conflicts of interest in universities in detail [261]. Journalist and author Jennifer Washburn discusses hearings ordered by the American Congress after President Bush appointed John D. Graham, the longtime director of the Harvard Center for Risk Analysis (HCRA), as the government's "regulatory czar" at the Office of Information and Regulatory Affairs. The HCRA educated about 500 people a year. According to Washburn, the hearings showed that the HCRA solicited money from tobacco firms, and downplayed the risks associated with second-hand smoke.

Harvey Fineberg, a dean at the Harvard School of Public Health, demanded a $25,000 cheque from the tobacco company Phillip Morris be returned. John Graham wrote to Phillip Morris to ask if the money could instead be sent through a subsidiary, Kraft Foods.

This raises questions regarding the funding of experiments. I'm using the following as a hypothetical example. If we read the conclusion of an experiment to find that second-hand cigarette smoke had no effect, then see the study was funded by the tobacco industry, we can see an obvious conflict of interest, and we're sceptical, less likely to be convinced by the study's conclusion. But if the money for the experiment instead came through Kraft Foods, we'd possibly be more likely to believe the study's conclusion because we wouldn't think it so suspiscious, unless we knew that Kraft Foods was a subsidiary of Phillip Morris.

When we're looking at who funded experiments we have to look a lot deeper than simply asking "who funded this study?" We nowadays need to ask, "who funded this study, and of whom is this company a subsidiary?"

Of accusations regarding money influencing experimental results, Stare wrote,

> "a 'changed tune' because of money to me is beneath my dignity even to comment on." [247]

He called Coca-Cola "a healthy between-meals snack" and "extolled the virtues of sugar in coffee", according to one obituary [262]. Stare died in 2002, leaving a legacy **The Economist** called in their obituary, 'at times, contradictory' [263]. Stare was famous for recommending Americans drink a cup of corn oil a day, something the food industry would probably have loved him for.

Author Kevin Myron writes that Stare was mocked for claiming fluoride an essential nutrient, but I never saw evidence of this from anyone who supported fluoridation [263, 264]. There may be some. He was criticized for other things; Mark Hegsted apparently said after complimenting Stare for getting good people together for research, "If he'd just get off this sugar and additive kick." (See the piece by John Hess below.)

Myron suggests that by 2002, two thirds of America's water was fluoridated,

"adding extra resistance to the country's already perfect teeth."

I am surprised at this statement. I believe it is given in humour. In 2012, according to the NAS, $11 million was spent on children's dental caries treatment under sedation in Philadelphia alone [265].

Myron laments of Stare:

"But his reasonable voice was that of the lonely prophet crying on a mountain of burgers, buns and fries, washed by rivers of sticky drink." [263]

Stare was a bit of an outlier. Nonetheless, I don't see any criticism of him regarding his claims of fluorine's essentiality from other CWF supporters.

According to John L. Hess of the **New York Times**, writing in **Saturday Review**:

"That same year [1941], the food industry set up an educational arm called Nutrition Foundation, which engaged [Stare] to publish, at Harvard, a scholarly digest called **Nutrition Reviews**, which he was to edit for the next 25 years."

Hess also quoted a statement from one of Stare's books: "eat your additives, they're good for you." Elizabeth M. Whelan, one of Stare's co-authors, had said

"... availability of soft drinks to children does not pose any known health hazard that would harm them." [266]

She believed 'junk food' should be called 'fun food' – and promoted for this, not safety. Presumably, this means to just gloss over the issue of safety altogether. According to Hess's article, in a public argument with Mark Hegsted, Dr. Stare asked if Mark knew that cola drinks were a good source of phosphorous.

In November 2017, I saw Dr. Rob Beaglehole of the New Zealand Dental Association mentioned in the news: he was asking the government *again* to consider sugar tax[65], junk food advertising bans, etc. Coca-Cola seems to have anticipated, or reacted to this very quickly – they must have a very conscientious advertising department[66]. Currently Wellington, where I live, is awash with ads for new, sugar-free Coke. It would be ironic if Coca-Cola had developed something *worse* than sugar to put in it [267]. Banning junk food *advertising* is a step in a sensible direction if we care about tooth decay or health in general. Recently, New Zealand health professionals seem to be taking a stronger stance publicly against sugar and the effects of its consumption on the young, but this may well be just lip service, a pretense as little seems to occur in terms of policy, advertising and production. This needs to be part of a larger discussion about the rights of corporations.

---

[65] The World Health Organization has been recommending a sugar tax since at least 2016, see *WHO urges global action to curtail consumption and health impacts of sugary drinks*, 11th October 2016. This is the recommendation of Dr Douglas Bettcher, Director of WHO's Department for the Prevention of Non-Communicable Diseases. "... people living on low incomes, young people and those who frequently consume unhealthy foods and beverages, are most responsive to changes in prices of drinks and foods and, therefore, gain the highest health benefits."

[66] What springs to mind is Ben Bagdikian's 1983 book on corporate media, *The Media Monopoly*. Bagdikian lists pages of corporations that have interactions with media. I think a modern, New Zealand equivalent investigation is appropriate.

I recommend the article by Hess without reservation. He claimed in 1978 the food industry was spending $3 billion a year on advertising.

In 1962, one of Stare's articles on fluoridation, *It's Not A Drug At All*, appeared in the **Honolulu Advertiser**. Dr. Stare wrote:

> "Some good people oppose fluoridation on the basis that the fluoride added is a medicine or a drug. This is misinformation because fluoride is not a medicine or drug. It is a mineral nutrient, as are calcium, iron, phophorous, and many other minerals." [268]

In 1966, the Port Huron **Times Herald** (Michigan) wrote about a court case (*Dowell vs Tulsa* – they gave no more information than that) that concluded water fluoridation is:

> "No more practicing medicine or dentistry, or manufacturing, preparing, compounding, or selling a drug, than a mother would be who furnishes her children a well-balanced diet, including foods containing vitamin D and calcium to harden bones and prevent rickets, or lean meat and milk to prevent pellagra." [269]

In 1970, Dr. McClure's book *Water Fluoridation: The Search and The Victory* was published [47]. It contained slightly contradictory information regarding a nutritional role for fluorine, but did state the element had not been proven indispensable (see Chapter 2.7).

The 1970 World Health Organization monograph was reviewed by ninety-three people, all with impressive qualifications, including Dr. Fredrick Stare of Harvard and Sir John Walsh of Otago University, New Zealand [102].

In this document Dr. Muhler had said more research was needed, not necessarily that fluorine was or was not essential in nutrition [270]. He did not take a firm position in his conclusion (though he did not mention the 1934, 1939 and 1959 experiments, and the 1954 editorial from **Nutrition Reviews**).

The public statements of the experts like Fredrick Stare in newspapers suggested they did not agree that further research was needed – fluorine was a dietary necessity, and that was that.

I've mentioned that in 1971, the NAS produced a report, **Fluorides: Biological Properties of Atmospheric Pollutants**, which looked at a handful of experiments and claimed fluorine non-essential, however they were open to change, should new evidence come to light.

The title of this document does not suggest a nutritional role, yet the authors were quite thorough in the appraisal of essentiality – an entire two pages. The main focus of the document was fluoride pollution, not nutrition. Some of the NAS' other work on nutrition had less opinion and information on fluorine's essentiality than what was presented in this document. The United States Public Health Service (USPHS) didn't like the way this document was discussed so openly by people opposed to CWF [169].

I should point out that all three of these publications were authored by advocates of CWF, supported CWF as a safe and effective way to promote resistance to dental caries, and expressed reservations about fluorine's essentiality.

How did the American media react to the influx of this new information? I searched American newspapers in the database newspapers.com for the phrase "fluoride essential" in the year 1971.

I arranged the hits newest first – this would put those closest to the end of the year 1971 first. The purpose of selecting this arrangement would give dentists and experts who spoke in the media the longest time to read these documents, as they *surely would* because these three authorities were cited frequently. These were not just anyone, they were prestigious experts. Muhler and McClure had been working with fluoridation for over twenty years. McClure's 1949 work was cited in the section of the 1970 WHO document Muhler had written, and the NAS had been recommending fluoridation for many years. I was assuming the dentists and experts would be keen to know what these authorities were saying, and because the dentists and experts care about us, they would obviously be honest with us, and keep at least the American people abreast of advances.

I read through the first forty hits. I should remind that not all newspapers and media have been digitized [271], and I looked only at newspapers, not other media in this particular search.

Here is one of the bigger headlines I found in the American media [272]:

FLUORINE HELD ESSENTIAL

It was the second headline of a two-part article featuring Dr. Schwarz (see Chapter 1.1) who was discussing his research on rats with trace element isolators.

A picture showing Dr. Schwarz holding one of his rats was captioned with the claim that fluorine was essential for humans (**Figure 16**). The fact that this goes unquestioned tells us that the use of rat experiments is acceptable, according to the experts (though Dr. Armstrong suggested the application of his own experiments on mice to humans as 'problematic', discussed below).

Dr. Schwarz presented his findings on the 28th of December, 1971. This article was published the next day. I'll point to the caption, which claims fluorine essential for humans. Note that he's not holding a *human* in his hands. In his experiment, Schwarz left the details to textbooks:

> "The metabolism of fluorine in mammals presents several features which support the concept that it is essential." [20]

The article was written by the paper's Medical Science Editor, Ben Zinser, who did not point out or ask why previous research had found rats perfectly healthy on lower amounts of fluorine than Dr. Schwarz had used [17, 18, 19]. Presumably he did not know.

This question regarding other research with diets less in fluoride than Dr. Schwarz used was critical, or at least very important in validating or invalidating his work. It was probably the most important question Zinser could have asked. Schwarz mentioned the 1957 and 1964 experiments in his 1974 paper, but in the paper *this* article was discussing he had not mentioned them; only the Phillips, Hart and Bohstedt experiment from 1934 [8].

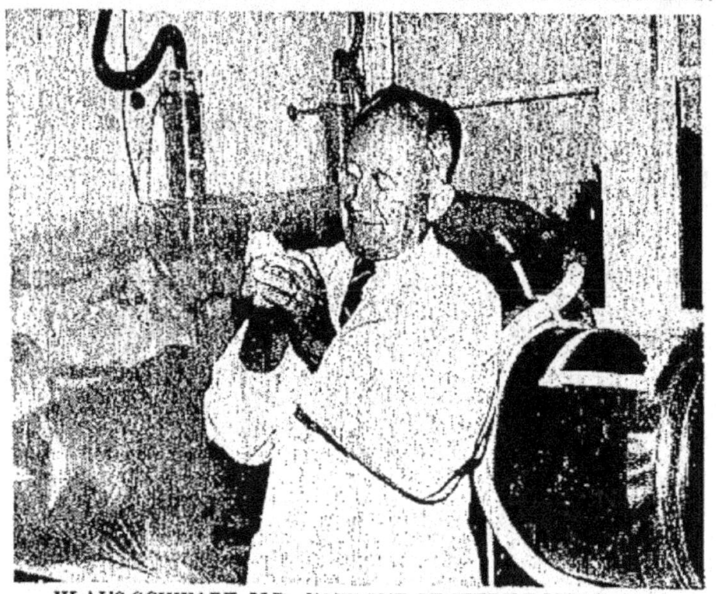

Figure 16. Fluorine Held Vital for Survival, Growth. **Independent** *(Long Beach, California), p. 25 (and 28), 29th December 1971.*

He mentioned this with regard to the fluorine levels of milk, not with regard to a need for fluorine. He must have known about the other experiments because he cited page 183 of the 1970 WHO monograph which featured Venkateswarlu's discussion – and this *did* look at many of the experiments that had used less fluorine than Schwarz's. If Schwarz told Zinser about any of these earlier experiments, it wasn't printed.

Zinser had promoted CWF openly in at least one article [67] prior to this article featuring Schwarz. Within the larger context of what experts say in media it fits in with the flow of claiming a nutritional role for fluorine with little criticism of such a claim.

If Zinser did not think of asking the question about previous research, then ideally Schwarz should have told him, but perhaps this is wishful thinking; Zinser's previous article (see footnote) had pointed to 8,500 "scientific reports on fluoridation" and claimed the question of safety nonexistent. Schwarz's relaxed attitude became apparent at the 1974 symposium [31] (see the quote at the beginning of Chapter 1.2).

Schwarz claimed in this article that "more than half of the fluoride compounds in the body are derived from food."

The paper quoted Schwarz:

---

[67] *Scientific Foes of Fluorides Dwindle*, **Independent Press-Telegram** (Long Beach, California), p. 22 and 23, 14th September, 1969. He did not claim the element a nutritional essential in this article, but did point to Dr. Stare as an expert without discussing corporate ties. His claims were criticized by Gladys Caldwell, *Critic Answers Fluoride Article*, same paper, p. 22, 28th September, 1969.

"It is fair to assume that with the increasing refinement of our staple foods, attention should be paid to the fluorine intake of growing animals and children to guarantee that the large amounts of fluorine needed during growth are adequately supplied."

"Rats were maintained on highly purified amino acid diets which contained all the known dietary agents in sufficient amounts." [272]

It is true that Dr. Schwarz concluded fluorine essential for human nutrition, the newspaper is *not* lying. But it is important that Zinser did not know or mention experiments that had produced perfectly healthy rats on diets considerably lower in fluorine than Schwarz and Milne used. At least six had done so. The health problems typical of Schwarz's rats were not discussed (see Chapter 1.1). The USPHS bulletins discussed in Chapter 2.7 mentioned Schwarz and Milne's work [169, 170].

The point I want to make here is that three authorities (the WHO, the NAS and Dr. Frank McClure of the National Institute of Dental Research) – for years treated with respect – are left out of the media, their investigations and conclusions of fluorine's lack of essentiality, their doubts, are not relevant enough to warrant mention… in spite of the fact that the experts had been claiming fluorine's essentiality a way to obviate the "mass medication" argument.

Yet Dr. Schwarz's work was in the papers the day after its presentation.

There are a few other things relevant here. The NAS report was mentioned in the **Indianapolis News**, p. 49, 16th December, 1971. It looked at air pollution – 120,000 tons of fluoride into the atmosphere every year, but "…no direct hazard to man…" Fluorine's nutritional aspect was not mentioned.

An Ontario newspaper, **The Ottawa Journal**, (p. 91, 14th September, 1971) published an article called *Scientists concerned on Side Effects*, that mentioned a 1969 WHO report that claimed the overwhelming mass of evidence regarding fluorides was that they were safe, and that they may even be necessary. Assuming there was only one 1969 report (there may have been more), it was published in July, and devoted less than a page to CWF, simply pointing out that all other respected authorities were claiming no side effects except for a reduction in tooth decay [273]. The Ontario newspaper also quoted Canadian researcher John Marier as saying "'nobody is counting' to watch exactly how much fluoride is being consumed" – monitoring fluoride intake levels being something the WHO recommends nowadays (mentioned in Chapter 4.4). Note this in contrast to the constant claims of deficiency in media when the subject is touched (see examples given here, in Chapter 5.1, and in Appendix 1). I have not investigated whether the New Zealand government monitors fluorine levels in food. Perhaps citizens of Canada and the USA were offended by the amount of pollution industries were creating around the beautiful lakes of the Ontario/USA border in the early 1970s [274].

I also searched for "fluoride not essential World Health Organization" in the years 1970-1971 and took the first forty. Nothing relevant in US newspapers. These searches were done through the database Newspapers.com.

A search for "Nielsen Sandstead fluoride essential" in the years 1972-1977 yielded no hits. These were the two scientists who disagreed with Dr. Schwarz's claim of essentiality; one reason given was that others had found perfectly healthy rats on diets even lower in fluorine [27] (see Chapter 1.1). This is not mentioned in any article discussing the work of Dr. Schwarz. This demonstrates the ignorance, either with or without purpose, of the experts and media.

There was scant mention of the McClendon experiments either, from what I have seen. It is difficult obtaining older newspapers, but these could have been the go-to experiments for experts throughout the 1960s, yet were barely mentioned.

A search for "Tao Suttie fluoride" in the years 1976-1980 also yielded no hits [275]. These were the two scientists who refuted the Messer *et al.* conclusions of essentiality. Searching for the names of scientists does not guarantee a result if one exists, partly due to incomplete digitization, but also because sometimes the result is mentioned, but the scientists' names are not. Spelling errors in an article may lessen the number of results. But it is important that these names were not found.

Writing in a 1973 issue of **The Morning News**, Dr. Fredrick Stare mentioned Dr. Messer's work on mice:

> "Addition of fluoride to the intake of female mice with demonstrated impaired fertility restored their reproductive capacity." [276]

When Joseph Muhler said fluorides and fluoridation were wonderful for decay prevention, this news was welcomed by the media, and there are articles quoting him as expert [14, 15]. When he writes in a World Health Organization document [102], that contrary to what the experts have been saying for at least fifteen years [239] – that more research was needed before fluorine could be called an essential nutrient, this didn't get a public mention. If I'm wrong on this, and it *has* been mentioned in an article I missed, it didn't appear to change what at least the majority of experts were saying.

Muhler's 1970 writing *possibly* inspired the work in the early 1970s[68]. Though this work was criticised and refuted (see Chapter 1.1), the experts went on claiming fluorine's essentiality as if nothing had happened.

On behalf of proponents and advocates of fluoridation I see constant reference to fluorine as essential nutrient with little discussion on rat vs human experiments – when the National Academy of Sciences or someone else important-sounding uses rat experiments to conclude that fluorine *is* an essential nutrient, this can be shown to the American public with headline after headline. When such an important-sounding group uses rat experiments to conclude that fluorine is *not*... the experts ignore this, and continue quoting the conclusion that suits them. Perhaps this is not considered 'biased' or 'selective' or 'cherry-picking' because the fluoridation programs that no doubt ensue from this information are all done with a desire for greater public health. But it is biased if one regards purity and completion of information, as well as neutrality of science and objectivity (concepts which the experts claim to be committed to).

---

[68] Please consider the amount of power a man in Fredrick Stare's position would carry. He reviewed the 1970 WHO Monograph *Fluorides and Human Health* so was probably aware of Muhler's and Venkateswarlu's thinking (unless there was a lot of ghost-writing in the 1970s, and Stare's name was used without him supplying any real feedback). I've contacted the WHO on this and they have not replied. Also consider that the other expert reviewers failed to raise this issue. It brings into question their potential influence on the direction of research.

Dr. Fredrick Stare couldn't *stop* quoting the 1958 National Research Council conclusion in newspapers when they then referred to fluorine as essential. Maurer and Day, Wuthier and Phillips, the 1970 WHO monograph that *he*, Stare, apparently reviewed, Doberenz *et al.*, and Joseph Muhler's change of criterion after ten years, weren't mentioned in any articles of his that I've seen. Interestingly though, the NRC did mention a few of these, and Stare frequently discussed the NRC in public, provided they agreed with him.

Dr. Stare and others had been claiming fluoride an essential nutrient throughout the 1960s, all the while claiming the science on fluoridation was settled. Clearly, it was not.

I wondered why there was such an amount of research in the early 1970s. Why not just leave our understanding with the Doberenz *et al.* experiment? (Maybe Mark Hegsted's words in 1967 can answer this, see Chapter 1.2.)

All experts in the USA, like our New Zealand Ministry of Health, were claiming fluorine essential without reservation from at least the mid-1950s onward. Armstrong and Messer didn't even need to do these experiments because all of the experts already believed fluorine was essential in nutrition. Shortly after 1970, with three scientific publications released, all claiming doubt around the necessity for fluorine in nutrition, we have a flurry of studies concluding fluorine essential.

The years 1971-1973 saw Dr. Schwarz's work come to light.

Two other experiments were carried out at the University of Minneapolis in 1972, a paper summarizing these published in 1973 with a final write-up appearing in **Trace Element Metabolism in Animals-2** in 1974.

Fredrick Stare mentioned the experiment by Messer and Armstrong on reproduction in mice in a 1973 newspaper [276]. "… attempts to demonstrate whether fluorine is an essential element have yielded equivocal results…" The word "equivocal" means "open to more than one interpretation".

So if conclusions were open to more than one interpretation, why did the experts *publicly* present *only* one interpretation for a couple of decades? And why did *all* the experts do this? And why wasn't this pointed out by the people writing the science columns? One wouldn't expect journalists to notice much occurring in obscure experiments, but the people who write the science columns would be expected to be more knowledgeable, or at least a little *varied* in their opinions, given the sheer amount of knowledge and information available. Why did the experts *not mention in public* when *other experts* in committees such as the National Academy of Sciences and the World Health Organization considered these other interpretations?

How can the public make up their minds without seeing a full complement of research? What about city councillors, who are much more likely to be making the decision?

The topic of fluorine's essentiality is such a niche that this information is so easily dismissed and ignored, but it does come down to whether we actually *need* the element – and what the element *is* in relation to us, not just whether it is of some added benefit or not.

It is less acceptable when experts are selective, "cherry-picking" research that suits them[69], due to the massive amount of resources, networks, and knowledge, in comparison to that which average members of the public have. Experts not only claim objectivity, they are consistently presented as objective, rational, and capable of critical thinking by the media, who seldom seem to question expert objectivity beyond giving room in their newspapers to people opposing fluoridation. While activists may be selective in their approach to science, they're usually not getting paid for their work. Some even take time off work to investigate or present [277]. They usually don't have the huge resources that funded universities and laboratories do. Obviously *all* presentations of science involve some selectivity – the only way someone can *not* be selective is to go into great detail on *all* aspects of every experiment, *all* aspects of every document, which is very difficult – but more difficult for non-experts.

To my knowledge Dr. Stare did not publicly mention any of the experiments cited by Drs. Muhler and Venkateswarlu in the 1970 WHO monograph, nor did he mention the monograph itself, that he, Dr. Stare, apparently reviewed [102].

The 1973 article contained a question and answer format. In response to the question

"Why do you so frequently refer to fluoride as an essential mineral nutrient when few other nutritionists do?"

Drs. Stare and Kerr had replied:

"I don't know who you have in mind when you write of 'few other nutritionists' not referring to fluoride as an essential mineral nutrient. All the nutritionists I know consider fluoride a mineral nutrient and have done so for at least the last 10 years..." [276]

They went on to mention the NRC and the 1973 Messer *et al.* experiment, and *not* the recent writings of Dr. McClure [47], the WHO [102] and the NAS [69] that had come out in 1970 and 1971.

The conclusions of Messer *et al.* were based on a fallacious assumption – that low fluorine levels had caused fertility impairment and low haematocrit in the blood of mice – when the reality was that these problems had been caused by low iron and copper levels.

In 1976, two experiments addressed this; in 1974, Dr. Messer had mentioned that there were low copper and iron levels in these experiments. The experiments were repeated twice with abundant iron and copper, published in **The Journal of Nutrition** and in **Proceedings of the Society for Experimental Biology and Medicine**. They also claimed fluoride's benefit was pharmacological, not nutritional, nor a necessary part of any metabolic process.

When the Messer *et al.* experiments came out, they were mentioned in American newspapers [278], some articles of which were Dr. Stare's [279, 280]. Sometimes Dr. Schwarz's work was discussed with them [281]. It is worth mentioning that in larger media, one article may be repeated many times in many newspapers, thus a small number of articles or newspapers cited does not necessarily mean a small outreach. One example is the advertising for Crest toothpaste [14], another is the USPHS document discussing the Dr. Jean Mayer column that

---

[69] See the USPHS/Stephen Barrett M.D. example given at the end of chapter 2.7.

was syndicated to about 100 newspapers [164]. I may cite one article, yet this *may* indicate hundreds. Without details into newspaper syndication, such a thing is hard to know [271].

In Chapter 2, I presented evidence that when the NAS looked at more research regarding essentiality, they were more likely to come to a conclusion of non-essentiality.

I'm reminded of this in reading the words of Dr. Armstrong as presented in the media:

> "Whether the findings in mice can be applied to man is problematical, Armstrong said. The average human diet has been calculated to contain 0.3 to 0.5 parts per million. Although this level is approximately that of the low-fluoride diet given the mice no deficiency state has been found in humans."

> "Fluoride is a naturally occurring element that can be found in soil, air and water and in virtually all foods."
> [278]

See the three paragraphs (**Figure 17**). Here the words "important bit of evidence" are used. I'll remind that "tentative inclusion" were the words used in 1974 [31]. The words of Armstrong *et al.* are of little relevance given that their work was refuted [33, 34]. The article appeared a few times with minor variations [278, 279, 280]. Though Dr. Armstrong expressed an incomplete certainty, other experts did not, including Dr. Jean Mayer mentioned already [282]. To my knowledge, the words "without convincing evidence" went ignored.

The experiments of 1976 [33, 34] were ignored, as the experts continued their claim that fluorine was a dietary essential from 1976 to the early 1980s [283].

I found only one newspaper article that mentioned the 1974 trace element symposium in Wisconsin [275]. This was where Dr. Schwarz made the statement that

> "... essentiality, like beauty, is in the eye of the beholder." [31]

It was also where Dr. Messer admitted that the diet used in the experiments earlier that decade at the university of Minneapolis, discussed in media so much, were carried out with a diet low in iron and copper. This may have meant little to an aspiring science writer.

Recall that Nielsen and Sandstead, and Tao and Suttie, both expressed the belief that Community Water Fluoridation was beneficial in terms of tooth decay, and also expressed the belief that fluorine should *not* be considered an essential nutrient.

Even *this* was too difficult for the experts writing in media. *Here* a limit was placed on debate. That word didn't get out in the media illustrates that in this instance, the question of essentiality of fluorine *is* important.

The experts would have lost some element of prestige, had they or the medical column writers in the media reminded the public of the experiments that had occurred in the early 1970s, that by 1976, were not looking so accurate. Reminding the American public could have led to confusion – "so do we need it or not?"

Both media *and* experts would have lost a part of their infallibility. Yet acknowledging the 1976 experiments would have had a *third* effect: it would have made the people opposed to fluoridation look correct. After all, they had been saying for a long time that fluorine was *non*-essential, quoting the 1971 NAS document, as confirmed by the USPHS writing on Dr. Stephen Barrett's website [169].

> Their finding, reported in the current issue of Science, is one of the first to contend that adequate levels of fluoride are necessary to a balanced diet, at least in mice.
>
> In the past such a theory has been advanced by some authorities in connection with human beings, but largely without convincing evidence.
>
> A l t h o u g h the Minnesota findings suggest that fluoride may also be an essential nutrient in the human diet, there is, as yet, no direct evidence that this is true. The mouse study, however, is an important bit of evidence in support of the theory.

Figure 17. Three-paragraph excerpt. Source: *Fluoride Called Vital for the Diets of Mice*, **Arizona Republic** (Phoenix, Arizona), p. 38, 7th October, 1972.

At least half a decade of media claims would have been called into question by the publicizing of the 1976 experiments. This would have worked in favour of the people opposing fluoridation. Another reason *why* the experiments were not discussed would no doubt be that few people knew about them.

In January of 1976, Dr. Stare told readers of **The Hartford Courant** that fluorine was one of the

"micronutrients, or trace elements, essential for humans..." [284]

along with zinc, selenium, manganese, copper and more. Dr. Stare didn't acknowledge these experiments in public. Both were funded, at least in part, by the USPHS. Recall that Stare had known about the Schwarz experiment, also funded by the USPHS, a little ahead of time.

In 1977, an article in a July issue of **The Gettysburg Times** (Pennsylvania) claimed that,

"The American Medical Association's Drug Evaluations manual refers to fluoride as an 'essential nutrient.'" [285]

Dr. Stare, along with Elizabeth Whelan, told readers of the **Tampa Bay Tribune** much the same in May of 1978 [286]. In 1979, Neil Solomon M.D. wrote an article in the **News Herald** (Ohio), telling readers that the Food and Nutrition Board of the NAS classified fluorine as an essential nutrient, though he didn't say which document this was mentioned in, and he didn't talk about any of their documents that said the opposite [287].

Maybe he was talking about a document called **Nutrient Requirements of Swine** in which the NAS wrote that fluorine was "required by one or more species, probably are also required by the pig but at such low levels that their dietary essentiality has not been demonstrated." [77]

In 1974 [70] and 1971 [69] the NAS had looked at the question in depth, and come to the conclusion that fluorine was non-essential. This seems to be a recurring theme, when the experts put some effort into the question, they either conclude 'non-essential' or 'it's a question of semantics' along with 'no signs of deficiency found in humans' [118]; this of course helps the issue come off the media conveyer belt as 'essential nutrient' with so many of us being deficient, and the experts presenting a unified, certain front.

Another relevant piece of information from the World Health Organization (WHO) was presented in the 1970 monograph. The following statements are credited to I. Zipkin[70].

---

[70] Professor of Biochemistry, Division of Periodontology, School of Dentistry, University of San Francisco, California, USA.

"Fluoride is a unique ion that it continues to deposit in the calcified structures after the other constituents of bone have already reached a steady state. Thus, the major constituents – calcium, phosphorus, magnesium, carbonate and citrate – reach their maximum concentration early in life and remain essentially unchanged, even after administration of large amounts…"

Zipkin goes on to say that fluoride showed

"… a tenfold increase in bone following ingestion of each of four drinking waters with fluoride contents of <1.0, 1.0, 2.6 and 4.0 ppm, respectively." [288]

In this way, fluoride behaves differently to the "major constituents" of bone. I did not find this pointed out in any of the newspaper articles in the 1970s.

It is also worth considering *which experts* the media go to – or which experts go to the media. The Messer *et al.* experiments were discussed so openly in the media, but Dr. Suttie's statement was not quoted:

"There certainly has been a number of people who have produced diets which are probably somewhere between 0.1 and 0.3 ppm fluoride and have not obtained any response from additional fluoride. Because of this, I think it is premature to call fluoride essential at this time." [31]

In Chapter 1.2, I discussed how Dr. Armstrong's research in 1938 led him to the conclusion that teeth with less dental caries had more fluorine in their enamel [56]. I also discussed how his 1963 research invalidated (his word, not mine) the conclusion of this 1938 study, once he had taken age into account [57]. Age was not appreciated as a factor in fluorine levels in the 1938 study. In 1964 Dr. Armstrong featured in an article in the **Minneapolis Tribune**. After discussing Dr. Armstrong's 1964 testimony in the Irish High Court, and his work on analytical methods, the author of the piece wrote

"He [Dr. Armstrong] also showed that sound teeth contain more fluoride than decayed teeth." [289]

Even Armstrong's *own research from the year earlier* did not get into the newspaper article. This 1964 article stated the conclusion from the 1938 experiment, instead of the invalidation of this arising from the more recent 1963 experiment. Whether this is due to Armstrong's influence, or the article author's, or some other factor or person, is unknown to me. This example of Armstrong ignoring the more stable conclusion of his own studies is found on page 21 of George Waldbott's 1965 work, *A Struggle with Titans*.

In 1981, Fredrick Stare authored an article published in **The Tampa Tribune** with one of my favourite headlines: *Nutritionists Consider Antifluoridation Actions Criminal* [290]. The text body does not say *how many nutritionists* consider these actions criminal, this is left for the reader to deduce. Stare told the American public that they should obtain a book called *The Tooth Robbers* by Stephen J. Barrett, M.D. and Sheldon Rovin, D.D.S., M.S [291].

Presumably it was the authors of this handbook, along with Dr. Stare and Virginia Aronson, R.D. (also of Harvard's Department of Nutrition) who were the nutritionists doing the considering here. Stare and Aronson explain their point of view: "… the existence of unnecessary tooth decay is practically a felony!" They pointed to an area where they considered the anti-fluoridationists were wrong:

"The health food fanatics fear that fluoride is an unnatural 'poison,' despite the fact that fluoride is an essential nutrient…" [290]

The Tooth Robbers also made a similar claim:

"Like iron, zinc, and several other minerals, fluorine (in the form of fluoride) is classified by the National Academy of Sciences as an essential trace element in human nutrition." [292]

If only the Consumers Union, who authored this section, had said which NAS document they had picked (by the 1980s there were a few) and why they *did not* pick some of the others, it would have been helpful for researchers[71]. Eighty pages later, we come upon a section written solely by Stephen Barrett, M.D., who discusses the claims of the anti-fluoride people, who were according to him, robbing the public of their teeth:

"Instead of telling you that fluoride is a nutrient essential to life, they call it a 'poison.'" [293]

On pages 119 to 125 of *The Tooth Robbers* we find advertisments that the authors tell us are "primarily for educational purposes." "Designed for newspaper insertion", "community mailings", "handouts", "PTA meetings", "city council meetings" and so on. Six of the seven ads contain the following sub-heading and text:

"Fluoride Is A Nutrient, Like Calcium" (Their emphasis.)

"Fluoride is not, strictly speaking, a drug. It's a nutrient like calcium, thiamine, niacin, riboflavin, Vitamin D – and all the other nutrients we need for good health." [294]

I could go on [295].

I have no issue with Dr. Barrett and his co-authors in 1980 disagreeing with the World Health Organization's 1970 claim regarding the differences in regulation of calcium and fluorine in bone, yet it would certainly help if they pointed out *why* they disagreed – or the ways in which people who may have been still quoting the WHO were behind the times. In 1986, the WHO reiterated the words of Zipkin (quoted previously) [288], that fluorine "accumulates in the skeleton throughout life and the fluoride content of the bones represents a reliable guide to an individual's lifetime exposure to fluoride" [296].

We ought to be asking if there is any criticism from the WHO about this kind of disagreement. This is not such an unreasonable request given the prestigious reports and groups of experts discussed in Chapter 2.

It might be due to something observed in the 1960s. John E. Mueller Ph.D., at the time Assistant Professor of Political Science at the University of Rochester in New York, wrote an article in the journal **Western Political Quarterly** about seven cities in California. Regarding campaigns to fluoridate these cities, Mueller wrote:

"Newspapers performed several important functions. Endorsement of fluoridation is virtually an essential ingredient (though certainly not a sufficient one) for pro success in a controversial campaign since a noncommittal attitude implies doubt as to the value of the measure." [297]

I can partially appreciate why *journalists* may be hesitant to discuss this, but surely some of the *scientists* who were championing the WHO 1970 monograph publicly should have commented somewhere?

---

[71] But maybe not helpful for CWF programs.

We are left believing that something is far more important than it really is, that it always works in all conditions and that something "ubiquitous" is incredibly rare; all the while we can pat ourselves on the back at how "objective" and "critically thinking" and "rational" we are. In this topic the only experiments that were publicized were those that affirmed what experts already believed[72]. I have scratched my head on why this occurs for some years now. It has been a very difficult subject to research because it is never discussed. Some reasons for this are suggested in the following chapters.

5.3 Semantics?

In 1989, the NAS looked at experiments attempting to create deficiencies in lab rats, and concluded "these contradictory results do not justify a classification of fluorine as an essential element, according to accepted standards." [81] However I'll point out that they included fluoride in the category 'trace elements'.

Is a trace element something necessary? Required? Needed? If it is, then the NAS has been somewhat ironic in saying 'contradictory results do not justify...'. (We mustn't forget the need for the inevitable "both sides": *also* in 1989, in another document, the NAS called fluoride "an integral part of the food chain" but did not define this in greater detail [80].)

Does fluorine *have to* be essential to be good?

If it's a question of semantics, as the people who claim to have debunked the infamous John Yiamouyiannis' work on fluoride claim it is [145], then surely we would expect more than the occasional expert to be publicly saying it's *not* an essential nutrient...? And *not* comparing it to calcium, iodine and the like, or talking about deficiency... that it took me eight years to find one[73], in a 2005 letter, is quite amazing. This exception was a dentist, Dr. Lindsey, from Colorado who pointed out that while fluoride is not necessary for sustaining life, the Institute of Medicine and other organizations,

"... consider fluoride a nutrient in a category of nutrients vital for preventing chronic disease or illness." [298]
This appeared in 2005. That something like this took so long to appear, and is the opinion of just one intellectually diligent dentist, is quite incredible.

Also pointed out was that a previous claim of non-essentiality based on stricter standards of biochemistry made in the newspaper was "erroneous". Fluorine was considered a nutritional essential because:

"Expecting dentists to keep up with and control the amount of dental decay that typically occurs without the help and benefit of fluoridation is like expecting firefighters to keep up with and control a house fire without the help and benefit of hoses and water." [298]
Without fluoridation, there would be "much needless pain and suffering."

---

[72] In his 2005 response to Paul Connett's "*Fifty Reasons to Oppose Fluoridation*" (page 16) Dr. Cutress did the same thing that the American experts did in media – cited Messer's 1972 work without mentioning the 1976 experiments. That Cutress' work was peer reviewed did not stop this. Available from <u>dentalwatch.org</u>.

[73] Remember the other 'deviations' – McClure, Perrott, Berridge – are not *full* deviations, because they have used terms like 'micronutrient' and 'deficiency' as one would for an essential nutrient.

This dentist did not discuss the abundance of fluorine in nature and in food; this is a reasonably consistent feature of expert behavior in media. The same can be said regarding the relationships of other elements and compounds known to be essential to tooth decay, as well as the regulation of junk food advertising. Neither of the letter authors mentioned any of the experiments in Chapter 1.

This dentist had probably not seen the decades of likening fluorine to iodine and other elements known to be essential, nor the claims of deficiency. If we were to use normal standards – those derived from protein biochemistry, discussed in this work in the first two chapters – then of course claims of similarity to calcium and iodine, and the claims of deficiency would be erroneous.

We've literally had decades of experts telling us the element *is* necessary for building halfway decent teeth and bones, and sometimes we've been told it was necessary for growth. Neither this dentist, nor the newspaper staff, considered these decades of exaggeration prudent to mention.

This is the only aberration in expert opinion that I have found in newspapers.

Why get nearly 100% uniformity in expert opinion? Surely given the vast volume of research *alone* we should have nuanced, individualized, detailed discussions. This is partly due to the nature of media – the ability to provide one single message to millions of people. It has overridden some of the contradictions and complications within the scientific literature.

Is it correct or sensible to use standards of categorization derived from protein biochemistry for fluorine, or for any other element? Most trace elements are components of hormones, vital amino acids/vitamins, or required for enzyme activation. Fluorine is not required for any of these.

If an exception should be made it should at least be acknowledged that this is not the way things are done normally. The words of Merilyn Manley-Harris of Waikato University could be the first step to some more detail (quoted in Chapter 2.7).

Yet the experts will probably claim that fluorine should be considered essential based on importance. So how important is it? Is it as important as calcium? It can't be, because calcium is *definitely* essential. Is it as important as magnesium, as phosphorous, as iron? Again, it can't be, because those things are *definitely* essential...

People who work with their hands and with physical things, *must* call things what they are, in order to interact precisely and purposefully with the world. When a builder asks their apprentice for the hammer, they don't mean the screwdriver. But bureaucrats and policy-oriented intellectuals deal with abstractions – word meanings – which are easily malleable. Laws and policies change, and in order to adapt, they probably should. I would argue changing word meanings is necessary much of the time in legal and bureaucratic endeavors. But to be useful, change must clarify the current system, not cloud it further. This is how our laws stay abreast of technology and other dynamic influences. Upon hearing this change of word meaning, a person who professionally must refer to things accurately, may believe this behaviour to be dishonest.

Many of those opposing fluoridation were aware of at least *some* of the research regarding fluorine's essentiality. A little history is required. In the mid-1960s Dr. George L. Waldbott's book *A Struggle with Titans* was published. He claimed fluorine non-essential, citing the 1957 work from Maurer and Day. He suggested that Dr. Fredrick Stare was claiming fluorine a nutrient because he was funded by industries involved in sales of fluorides and fluoride pollution, implying Stare was dishonest or biased[74]. He discussed the September, 1961 issue of **Nutrition Reviews** which he claimed was sponsored or funded by companies profiting from fluoride promotion, namely Swift, Procter and Gamble, and Reynolds Metals. I don't have this issue, but accusations like this probably would have "insulated" Waldbott's more loyal readers against a belief in fluorine's necessity when the work in the early 1970s appeared that concluded fluorine essential. Also, if people were aware of experiments concluding fluorine non-essential, a study concluding it essential *could* be dismissed as contradiction, or treated with scepticism and uncertainty. Precisely *not* what experts wanted. Also recall from Chapter 2.7 that the United States Public Health Service (USPHS) claimed people opposed to Community Water Fluoridation (CWF) were citing the 1971 NAS document [69] that claimed fluorine non-essential.

I don't believe *anyone* cited the 1954 article in **Nutrition Reviews** [37] that had pointed out the obvious flaws in McClendon's 1953 work except for Dr. Joseph Muhler [24]. But this appears only semi-relevant as I hardly ever saw the work of McClendon mentioned in media. Obviously a hydroponic diet largely absent of animal products was only semi-applicable at best to humans of the time.

When people opposed to fluoridation give evidence of fluorine being non-essential, the experts respond with the charge of 'semantics' because semantics are what many intellectuals engage in. Semantics, changing word meanings, is what many experts *do* in a bureaucracy when they're writing reports and changing policies, so when the people opposed to fluoridation state it's non-essential, the experts change the terms to suit themselves. They change the criteria.

This has the added effect of letting experts "off the hook" when it comes to looking at evidence that fits the normal criteria of creating a definite deficiency.

You'll note a complaint of the 1988 document that rebuked the work of John Yiamouyiannis pointed out that Yiamouyiannis cited three experiments that concluded fluorine essential. No details were given. These were probably the papers from Messer *et al.* and Schwarz. In his 1986 and 1993 work, Yiamouyiannis pointed out Messer's own admission of low iron and copper in the diet, Tao and Suttie's work, and Nielsen and Sandstead's critiques of Schwarz's work (see Chapter 1.1). In the eyes of his readers, Yiamouyiannis would have appeared less biased than the experts, at least on this issue. He was looking at (at least parts of) "both sides".

I've only found the charge of 'semantics' levelled twice – when someone opposed to fluoridation claims fluorine non-essential in nutrition. However, I assume it may have appeared more frequently. I have not looked at much British or Canadian literature, and only on the surface of Australian work.

Concluding fluorine non-essential is arrived at via a normal method of investigation – the same criteria used for calcium, iodine and other compounds and elements. The same criteria that came from protein biochemistry:

---

[74] See Waldbott, page 272. On page 137 he claimed Stare was syndicated in 40 newspapers.

- It is present at a relatively constant concentration.
- If the element is removed from the diet, the animal should show symptoms of deficiency (this may take generations).
- If the element is returned, the symptoms should eventually disappear.
- We should be able to replicate this in many species.

This is a simplified list from the discussion in Chapter 1.

It is this conclusion that many people opposed to fluoridation have adhered to since the beginning of their opposition when they looked into available experimental evidence. My investigation has primarily focused on supporters of CWF and not on the people opposed, and you can easily see why – I couldn't quite figure out what the experts were doing at first. The number of experiments claiming CWF as a preventor of tooth decay is discussed in Chapter 6.

The experts may claim fluorine's essentiality to be semantic in nature, yet this claim is only made when people opposed to CWF point out to the experts that experts have been misrepresenting research on the topic for many decades.

That their research was criticized even by their own peers, and people who believed fluoridation a good thing, was interesting to me. That these criticisms almost never reached the public was even more interesting.

This situation should not exist, if the experts really *do* represent a totality of quality experimentation accurately. The experts should *not* misrepresent scientific literature for many reasons. Most reasonable people would not expect perfection, we're only human and all make mistakes. It's difficult keeping abreast of all the knowledge [299], but the experts *insist* that they are the only ones really qualified to discuss the matter. The experts have the most expensive and thorough educations, the most long-winded, hard-earned titles, affiliations and post-nominal letters, the most experience performing studies, the most experience reading technical literature. Sometimes to even cite a name and a place of work requires a small paragraph. Experts have advantages that are fraternal and in terms of experience, such as the knowledge of which are the best databases to find answers to complex questions, wherein less educated people would have to seek assistance to know where to look. Experts have communication networks in the form of peers, closer contact with journal editors, closer contact with groups such as the World Health Organization and the National Academy of Sciences, and the possibility that they fraternize with people from these organizations is very real. Perhaps they are more likely to get replies to their letters from these organizations than non-experts. The possibility that their careers have included, or will include, working for and within these, and other organizations is also very real. They have more resources that are easier to deploy than the rest of us, in the form of influencing experimental investigations, arguing for and against where university or research grants are and are not allocated, in many times they are given work and added job security by corporate funding, as in the cases of Dr. Fredrick Stare and his team at Harvard, Dr. Jesse McClendon and Dr. Joseph C. Muhler and the team at Indiana University.

Thus, given their resources the experts should have *no trouble* at least mentioning to the public the entire spectrum of research. In an investigation such as this, where there is certainly cause for argument, the argument for and against each end of the spectrum of experimental conclusions should be presented. Both ends of this spectrum should ideally be presented by the experts, in the expert literature *and* in public media, given that the experts claim to *not* "cherry-pick" the studies that suit them, they look at *all* the evidence, as they can tell us [67, 300].

Yet the experts are wanting when it comes to full disclosure on this topic. This is demonstrated by comparing scientific literature with media, and is discussed in the following chapters in more detail. This is *not* so apparent in academic reports that experts will read, and the public will probably *not* read. The NAS serves as a great example: some of their investigations have been as deep as could be expected (although some may say still wanting) on this niche topic in some publications.

It appears that it is in public the restriction comes into being. It has to do with not disrupting the fluoridation programs.

Consider one of Matt Jacob's points, paraphrased in a 2013 National Academy of Sciences document:

"Sodium fluoride is a chemical, but there is no need to refer to it as such." [301]

The reason given is understandable: middle-class mums don't like the idea of their children imbibing artificially made chemicals - the environmental movement and other such influences have had an effect on their thinking.

Jacob is the Director of Communications and Outreach at the Pew Foundation's Children's Dental Health Project (CDHP) in Washington D.C. According to his LinkedIn profile, "his media outreach has helped secure coverage in the **New York Times**, CNN, **Philadelphia Inquirer**, NPR's 'Morning Edition' and the **Huffington Post**." "CDHP received one gold and two silver awards from the National Public Health Information Coalition for three newspaper op-ed columns that Matt wrote and placed." Mr. Jacob's specialties are: "Framing issues ... Developing media/communication campaigns ... Managing crisis communications ... Translating research into clear, compelling messages."

While this document is from 2013, "clear, compelling messages" are not something new.

It's staggering that it has taken a very small number of the experts six or so decades to accept that fluorine is non-essential, but I see little evidence that the experts, or any journalists interested in fluoridation acknowledge the initial exaggeration[75]. Most people will probably have some empathy for the argument "it doesn't *matter* if fluorine is essential for human nutrition, it matters whether amounts added to drinking water are effective in reducing tooth decay, and safe." I have some respect for this argument. I do think reducing tooth decay is more important than haggling over whether some experiment sixty years ago used the right number of rats or an acceptable level of copper, or kept the rats on the diet long enough. But I'm brought back to the fact that the experts *have* been playing favourites with the research on something *fundamental*. Namely, whether there is an actual *need* for this element. While they've been doing this, they've been claiming that they're neutral and objective in their appraisal of research.

---

[75] Kevin Myron claimed Dr. Stare was mocked for his claims of fluorine's essentiality, yet provided no evidence [263].

One reason why the research demonstrating no need for fluorine was ignored is that so much focus was taken up by benefit and safety. Experts had spent so much time and effort instilling in the public the importance and the benefits of CWF as a way in which to reduce dental decay, the expert that held fast to a claim of non-essentiality while still proclaiming safety and benefit would have looked like a quirky stick-in-the-mud.

Since the beginning of CWF, the program had been associated with common sense, reason, and progress. If scientists said it was a step forward, people who disagreed were considered opponents of progress. The only people publicly claiming fluorine non-essential in human nutrition were called "antifluoridationists" – a term unappealing in its length and fanatic implication. The "-ist" suffix implied a religiosity, the "anti-" prefix implied a negativity in outlook. These people had been ridiculed since the beginning of the public health measure. Associated in prestigious intellectual documents with luddites, flat-earthers, and people who opposed pasteurization, the wheel and vaccines, they were not taken seriously by supporters of CWF [255].

Their communication was often – not always – of a very different nature to that of the politicians and councillors they attempted to influence. It could be argued easily that the lack of familiarity many of them had with formal academic argument worked against them. Examples can be found in letters to ministers and councillors found in New Zealand Health Department archives, and in letters to newspaper editors, as well as pamphlets produced by groups. Such writings were penned often with an urgency and an intensity in stark contrast to the patient, long-winded and more cerebral intellectualism of the more educated that *appeared* much less biased because of its professional appearance. An in-depth look at weaknesses and biases in more formal as well as activist literature opposed to fluoridation is beyond the scope of this book.

It is much easier to explore *what* people are doing than it is to explore *why* they do it. Chapters 5.4 to 5.8 touch on *why* we see what we see in public.

5.4 Essentiality within the Context of Opposing Sides

"I would argue that the abandonment of an interconnected view of the community is deeper and more dangerous than ever before. Its cause is not due to a natural inevitability but is held in place, almost artificially, by the bitter divisions of our world. This predilection for division, a division which maintains a binary morality of 'them' and 'us', finds its traditional expression in the terms 'communist' and 'anti-communist'. I would suggest that this division has become a kind of global disease that scars and corrupts the best and most humane aspects of our liberal Western traditions."

- Alex Carey, *Taking the Risk out of Democracy*, The Orwell Diversion, p. 133, 1995 [302].

"You decide at the outset... they're wrong, and you're right... and once you've made that decision you don't have to think any more. Once the decision was made that we were the good guys we could do anything we wanted."

- Historian Howard Zinn, interviewed on C-Span. *In-Depth: Howard Zinn*, BookTV [303].

Details within the smaller topic of fluorine's essentiality are sacrificed due to the polarization of the fluoridation debate. In an issue where we do or don't do something, we end up with a polarized issue with some saying do, and others saying don't. The fact that we only have two options with regard to action should not necessarily mean that investigations ought to suffer, yet inevitably this happens.

This chapter looks more at points of view than action. A document on the media's approach to polarization in science is *Science and the Media: The Good, the Bad and the Ugly*, by Anna Salleh [304][76]. Salleh discusses the work of Sandman, a corporate risk consultant, who says journalists do not *create* outrage, but they do "nurture, focus, organize, amplify" and "stick a microphone in front of it".

Sandman points out that scientists value communication that is abstract, impersonal and neutral, more tentative than certain (see Dr. Armstrong mentioned in Chapter 5.2 describing the relating of his experiments to humans as 'problematic' [sic] as one example [278]). Yet journalists,

> "favour alarm over reassurance, extremes over the middle, opinions over data and outrage over hazard."

> "Journalists prefer to frame stories as conflicts between two extreme opposing viewpoints. For this reason, controversial science is very newsworthy." [304]

When I began investigating this topic, I thought I'd found the elusive middle ground. How wrong I was.

> "Balancing different views is considered a method to ensure fair reporting... a way of finding *truth* which is seen to lie somewhere in between two extreme views[77]" [304] (Salleh's emphasis.)

Yet the issue here, on fluorine/fluoride's essentiality/non-essentiality is that the public is given only one segment of an entire picture of research... *with absolute certainty that it's the only end*... not even *the only relevant end* (of a spectrum of research). Just *the only research that exists.*

---

[76] Ph.D. in Science Technology and Society at the University of Wollongong. She has a BSc and a Masters in Journalism.
[77] The work of Rosen, *What are journalists for?* New Haven: Yale University Press, 1999, p 120-121 is cited here by Salleh.

Simplifying a complicated issue is not conducive to scientific accuracy. Once it becomes about winning, instead of about truth, each side has a definite incentive to employ a bias to refute whatever the opposition presents, and such biases are often not discussed or admitted to, due to the competitive framework. (This on top of all of the other biases we may have, and the biases of the researchers we cite, of which we're unaware.)

Once the adrenalin gets pumping, if we're on one of these sides, we may get more rigid and stubborn in our beliefs, and see an attitude of never backing down as a good thing, as "sticking up for what's right". This gives us little motivation to consider points of view not our own, even if they're accurate and logical and backed up with common sense and evidence.

It would be *very bizarre* for one person or one group of people to be right about *everything* or wrong about everything, yet we imply that we think this is what is going on if we are so stubborn that we refuse to budge on anything and shut our ears and eyes to anything beyond our comfort zone.

The implication that truth lies 'somewhere in the middle' is imprecise and unhelpful, especially when both parties are not pressed with citing or declaring where their information comes from, the methodological differences used in attaining it, or the inherent biases within it.

The journalist holds the microphone in front of the expert, then in front of the activist. While this kind of reporting may be great for expressing different points of view, it does lead to very passive journalism. The journalist does minimal investigation to find out how much of what people say is or is not true. Why would they? They don't have to, given that they've got their 'fair' report. They've "balanced" the "different views" which implies truth is somewhere in the middle. They've done a good days' reporting.

Journalists are not scientists, so it is understandable that they have reluctance to give scientific opinions. While commitment to reporting that is fair to many points of view is commendable, I think truth takes a back seat in the absence of thorough investigation.

Consider journalistic objectivity: in a sense, the journalist *is* telling the truth. After all it's true that the person representing one side said what they said, and the person representing the other side said what they said.

One might point out that the experts are representing one end of the spectrum, and the people opposed to CWF are representing the other. Regarding fluorine's essentiality, this is true in media, but it should *not* be, if we have a hypothesis that experts present scientific information accurately and objectively. Experts should be presenting research that claims fluorine non-essential if this hypothesis is true. 'Objectivity' implies one does not mind if one's previous position is shown to be true or false. Reports from bodies like the NAS were in many instances expressing a different point of view than experts in media. This was not discussed. Evidence presented here (comparing media with reports and experiments) suggests that experts *do* select data and conclusions that fit their hypothesis to a rather extreme degree. Media imply that experts are impartial by referring to them as experts, and not looking overly at reports that contradict what experts claim.

We learn something of the scientific community when we realize that if we simply want to *see* a different end of the spectrum of research – *not* to worship it, *not* to conclude it's perfectly true, but just to *see* it – we need to turn away from what scientists are saying in *public* and look a little deeper.

The end of the spectrum of research presented by Dr. Fredrick Stare and most of the other experts exists, and it *should* be looked at... but so does another end. Yet this end is ignored. Even *scientists* had little to say about it. So if we are to criticize media, this is only the surface of the issue.

I believe framing the issue in two extreme areas in total opposition with each other encourages other scientists to trust experts more, purely because to challenge that idea even a little makes one immediately out of step with scientific expertise, in the eyes of the media and their audience (which is almost everyone). Readers of scientific literature will be hard-pressed to find molecular biologists, anthropologists, nutritionists, biochemists and the like who are of varying degrees of scepticism about the nutritional status of fluorine *in public* – yet in scientific documents, a less than complete unity of agreement can be seen.

In some ways, the case for or against fluorine's essentiality is a grain of sand – it's irrelevant, because what really matters is the safety and effectiveness of Community Water Fluoridation, not the 'semantics' of categorizing an element as essential or not.

However, the case for or against fluorine's essentiality is a foundation upon which so much of CWF rests – after all, the experts often avoid the "mass medication" argument by claiming that fluorine is an essential nutrient, not a drug, and that fluoridation of water is a process of food fortification [183] (see Chapters 3.1 and 6.5).

The fact that no such thing as a real fluorine deficiency could be demonstrated in the same way that a calcium deficiency or a deficiency in some other essential nutrient or compound could be demonstrated, was no cause for concern. The experts believe in 'optimal' levels of fluorine, and probably use the term 'deficiency' interchangeably with the term 'sub-optimal' though they don't appear to know this. They seem to believe, based on the number of times the element is likened to vitamins and iodine, that it really is essential.

I have not seen much elaboration on why this is so, but I will suggest that associating fluorine with calcium or iodine (for example), will help sway community leaders and the public into accepting fluoridation programs.

That public belief in the part of the spectrum visible to the public happens to benefit the employment prospects of the experts, is a very possible indicator of bias, and an incentive to not look deeply into the issue.

One can see why there would be aversions to publicizing the research discussed in this investigation in media. One reason is that public may lose trust in media. Just because we read something one day, a few years later it might not be considered true. The public may become more sceptical toward fluoridation programs.

This research is also ignored because simple trust may be lost in experts who sounded confident and certain of themselves. Perhaps the necessity for speed in modern media, combined with trust, has had impacts on fact-checking. Logic alone suggests this is important.

Also, the only people who were claiming fluorine to be non-essential *publicly* before about 2005 were those opposed to CWF – the antifluoridationists. There were obvious reasons why nobody would want to be associated with them: they had been consistently ridiculed in media. A public acknowledgement of fluorine's non-essentiality would only serve to help their cause, a cause which many experts had long considered a threat to public health.

Previous chapters provided some reasons relating to scientific literature why the argument of essentiality was used so definitely. The following examples will help explain why this occurred in media- and government-related contexts.

Dr. Frank Bull, a dentist and Director of Dental Health from the State Board of Health in Madison, Wisconsin, gives us an insight here that may explain the certainty of the experts. The following quotes are taken from a 1951 conference featuring many professionals from the USPHS and State Dental Directors, including Dr. Leonard Scheele, Surgeon General.

> "First you need a positive policy by your state dental society and your state board of health. Now, I mean a really positive policy. Don't put any ifs, ands, buts, or maybes in the thing, because the minute you do you kill it. You simply give ammunition to the fellow who is against it."

> "I could read you some policies that could furnish plenty of ammunition to the opponents of fluoridation. Let's not do that. You have got to get a policy that says 'Do it.' That is what the public wants, you know." [305]

This meeting was mentioned in a 1952 issue of the **Journal of the American Dental Association**.

> "If we want to argue about it, let's get up a debate before our dental organizations and talk the thing out. But when we are inviting the public in and the press in, don't have anybody on the program who is going to go ahead and oppose us because he wants to study it some more." [306]

A year later, Dr. Bull discussed the responsibility of the dental profession in the **Journal of the American Dental Association**:

> "Using terms such as 'medication' or 'artificial fluoridation' helps to defeat the program. The minute doubt is created in the minds of the public, any public health program is doomed to failure." [307]

Complex information – actual *detail* – was probably perceived as being too long-winded to be appropriate for easy public acceptance. It would only be tiring for experts to not only keep themselves abreast of research, but to repeat all the gritty details to the public every time the issue was raised.

Also of interest in Bull's latter statement is that the public is put in a passive position – the public are not creating their own doubt from their own free thought and their own logic and reasoning, selecting their own facts and sources. The doubt is created as if by someone or something else from outside the public mind. The public are *not* a self-governing body even with regard to their opinion, their beliefs are given to them from outside. Dr. Bull does not give the public credit for their capability of original thought and self-guidance.

This is also demonstrated in one of the "many ideal features" of fluoridation that are listed in Dr. Bull's article:

> "It requires no special effort or participation on the part of the individuals of a community." (p. 150)

"The present standards of public health were achieved by telling the public definitely and emphatically what they should do... this is exactly what must be done with the present fluoridation program if the public is to adopt it." [307]

In the same issue of the **Journal of the American Dental Association**, February 1952, Dr. Milton E. Nicholson[78] remarked that

"Fluoridation is extremely important from a public relations viewpoint..."

"... it is not sufficient for a practicing dentist to 'damn with faint praise' when a patient wishes to discuss the process. He should not pass on to the patient his personal opinions or hastily formed impressions but should use the facts which are readily available to him. ... he will be able to take the lead in preventing misunderstanding and confusion and also be instrumental in bringing to his community one of the best..."

Regarding contradictory information appearing in the press, Dr. Nicholson had written:

"The confusion must be eliminated and the scepticism of the public must be removed if progress is to be made in fluoridation." [308]

Another mention of public relations came from the **Journal of the North Carolina Dental Assocation** in 1955:

"During this year the Public Relations Committee has stood by, ready to furnish speakers to defend or propose Fluoridation. This has proven a very valuable support and should be continued." [309]

With regard to water fluoridation the experts have been quite adamant that fluoridation is a matter for experts to discuss, and the public should not be involved in the discussion.

For example, Dr. Carl Weatherbee, quoted in a newspaper from Illinois, said in 1956:

"There should be no referendum – laymen should not decide about health." [310]

Sir Leonard Wright, Mayor of Dunedin, New Zealand, said in a 1958 newspaper article called *Dental Association's Attitude Criticised*,

"Fluoridation is a subject the public does not know much about. It is a subject for experts."

The association was criticized by the mayor for waiting until the public wanted fluoridation before initiating it, an attitude he called 'wishy-washy'. The same article also demonstrated the willingness of the city council to trust the experts, even with minimal knowledge:

"Councillor H. Brown said that if fluoridation would bring about improvement to public health – 'and I believe it will, although I have no facts about it' – we should make some decision soon.'" [311]

Consider a 1963 statement from the Mayor of Kaitaia, New Zealand:

"It is quite true that I have been subject to pressure from the Health Department to avoid a referendum, the reasons given to me being that the ordinary public are not capable of making a decision, and that the councillors were better able to decide on such an important matter." [312]

Such attitudes demonstrate and have helped cement belief in expert infallibility. This may explain the fact that when claims are made likening fluorine to calcium, phosphorous and vitamins, other scientists completely

---

[78] Associate Professor of Public Health Dentistry, School of Dentistry, University of Pittsburgh and clinical dentist at the Bureau of Maternal and Preschool Service at Pittsburgh's Department of Health.

uninvolved in the fluoridation debate (for instance biochemists and nutritionists) often don't give any feedback. The experts know what they're doing, and the rest of us should keep quiet.

Dr. Frederick Stare made a similar point in a Q&A column called *Finding Out About Fluoridation* in response to a question regarding the safety of sodium fluoride:

> "For a lay person to start evaluating scientific data on most any subject is fraught with difficulties. Nowhere is this more evident than on the subject of fluoridation. Most lay people will not even know the difference between fluorine and fluoride, and they are as different as night is to day... it makes no difference whether it comes from the sodium or calcium salt – or other fluoride salts. Why not accept the word of your dentist, physician or health department that fluoridation is safe? Any of them can refer you to 'scientific data,' but can you interpret it properly?" Dr. Stare suggests NRC publication No. 294, and **Journal of the American Dental Association**, Vol. 65, No. 5, November 1962 – "ask your dentist to let you borrow his copy of this issue, devoted entirely to fluoridation." [313] (NRC publication No. 294 is from 1953 [253].)

This exclusion of the public from decision-making may seem undemocratic to many. In reality it is a key feature of democracies and not unusual. Professor Noam Chomsky[79] quoted historian Joyce Appleby[80]:

> "[The Federalists expected] that the new American political institutions would continue to function within the old assumptions about a politically active elite and a deferential, compliant electorate..."

> "George Washington had hoped that his enormous prestige would bring that great, sober, commonsensical citizenry politicians are always addressing to see the dangers of selfcreated societies." [314]

In the wake of 1960s activism, Samuel Huntington, Professor of the Science of Government at Harvard, discussed democracy in a 1974 publication written for the Trilateral Commission. The youth of America were challenging the systems of power, leading to what Huntington and his co-authors[81] called a "crisis in democracy" – the publication's title. Huntington claimed that

> "... some of the problems of governance in the United States today stem from an excess of democracy... Needed, instead, is a greater degree of moderation in democracy."

> "The arenas where democratic procedures are appropriate are, in short, limited." [315]

Huntington likened the management of a society to a battlefield, which would result in disaster if soldiers instead of generals were put in charge.

In looking at newspaper articles on fluoridation, one finds the word "propaganda" used to describe opposing viewpoints.

It is important to point out that *publicly*, the word 'propaganda' is *always* used in reference to an *opposing* viewpoint or information, (almost) never one's own. To generalize, a person who opposed fluoridation may claim government or business propagandizes, and a person who supports fluoridation may claim activists propagandize.

---

[79] Institute Professor Emeritus, Department of Linguistics and Philosophy, Massachusetts Institute of Technology.
[80] Professor Emeritus for the History Department in the University of California.
[81] Michael Crozier, founder and Director of the Centre de Sociologie des Organisations in Paris; and Joji Watanuki, Professor of Sociology at Sophia University, Tokyo.

This is because the word *propaganda* nowadays has a negative connotation: it implies deception. Due to negative connotations in the word after its association with the enemies of Britain and the United States after the Second World War, one does not typically claim the information presented by oneself to be propaganda. However, exceptions can be found, and it is interesting that they are not found in public writings such as newspapers. In the writing of the more educated, one finds the word used to describe information presented *by* the more educated.

The New Zealand Health Department archives contain some examples of this. I have found no example of them defining the term 'propaganda' in any way, though they used the term to describe material produced by people opposed to fluoridation frequently. That they use the term to describe their own material is interesting, and unusual when contrasted with public statements.

In a letter to Dr. F. S. Maclean, the Director-General of Health, dated 6th April 1954, Dr. C. N. D. Taylor, New Zealand's Medical Officer of Health, wrote of a talk he was to give to the Junior Chamber of Commerce in Hastings. He mentioned (**Figure 18**) that there was

> "… every possibility that the Junior Chamber of Commerce will throw their weight behind our fluoridation propaganda." [316]

In another letter to Maclean dated 5th May 1954 (**Figure 19**), Taylor wrote of how he had

> "… advised the Jaycees in Hastings who have undertaken to forward a detailed statement on how the money is spent. It is probable that most of it will be spent on advertising propaganda…" [317]

The letter also lamented that the local newspaper was no longer going to give publicity to his views, meaning that

> "Propaganda in future will therefore have to be paid for to a large extent."

The letter also used the term 'propaganda' to describe material given to the people opposed to fluoridation by another group, the New Zealand Voters Association.

Compare these two statements with a newspaper clipping from the **Hawke's Bay Herald Tribune** dated the day before, the 4th of May 1954. It discussed a motion carried on the evening of the 3rd of May, that

> "… all units of the New Zealand Junior Chambers of Commerce, by educating the public in the true facts of the fluoridation of municipal water supplies…" [318]

The word 'propaganda' was not used publicly (unless describing work opposing CWF), only in private. In public, the words 'true facts' were used.

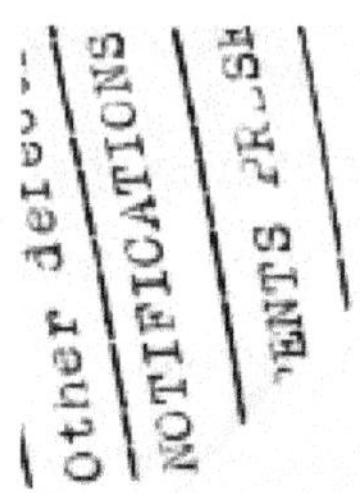
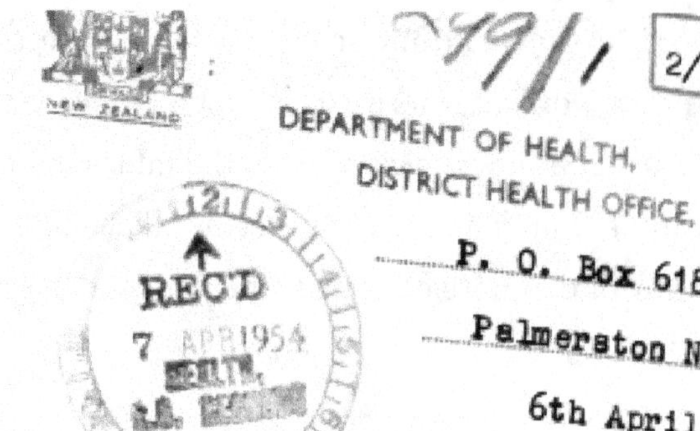

DEPARTMENT OF HEALTH,
DISTRICT HEALTH OFFICE,

P. O. Box 618,

Palmerston North,

6th April, 1954.

The Director-General of Health,
WELLINGTON.

FOR ATTENTION: DR F.S. MACLEAN

FLUORIDATION OF WATER

Thank you for your memorandum of the 2nd April, re the above.

For reasons which I will be able to better explain when I see you later this week, I do not think a public meeting to debate fluoridation would serve any useful purpose in Hastings. However, as I advised you by 'phone I have been invited to speak to the Junior Chamber of Commerce in Hastings next Monday evening and there is a possibility that a speaker will also be invited from the Anti-Fluoridation Society.

As reporters are bound to be present this should serve a useful purpose, particularly as there is every possibility that the Junior Chamber of Commerce will throw their weight behind our fluoridation propaganda.

I will know more about this by the time I see you on Friday.

(C.N. Derek Taylor)
Medical Officer of Health.

Figure 18: *Fluoridation of Water. Letter, Taylor to Maclean.* HD 125/299/1 H1 Box 1634, 6th April 1954.

5th May, 1954.

The Director-General of Health,
WELLINGTON.

ATTENTION DR F. S. MACLEAN

FLUORIDATION - HASTINGS WATER SUPPLY.

Your memorandum of 3rd May, reference 125/299/1.

1.   I thank you for arranging a £50 grant towards the campaign
funds for the support of fluoridation. I have advised the Jaycees in
Hastings who have undertaken to forward a detailed statement on how
the money is spent.   It is probable that most of it will be spent on
advertising propaganda and it will be particularly useful for this as
from the end of this week the local Paper has declared that it is not
prepared to publish any more correspondence on the matter.   Propaganda
in future will therefore have to be paid for to a large extent.

2.   The Jaycees in Hastings suspect that the "New Zealand Voters
Policy Association" are feeding the anti fluoridationists with
propaganda material.   They are anxious to find out as much as possible
about this Association and I would appreciate it if you could arrange
for somebody to see if they are able to pick up any details about the
Association and its policy.   I received a rude letter from them in
March.   The letter-head read - "New Zealand Voters Policy Association,
P. O. Box 1672, Auckland.   Hon. Secretary, E. C. Browne."

Figure 19: *Excerpt of letter to Maclean.* HD 125/299/1 H1 Box 1634, 5th May 1954.

In another letter to Maclean, dated 3rd February 1956, (**Figure 20**) Taylor wrote of the "Society for Fluoridation"
and how he would help the society:

> "I have sent the Society some sixty odd references, which I have collected in anticipation of their formation,
> and these can be used as a basis for their propaganda." [319]

4.   The inaugural statement of the "Society for Fluoridation",
announcing its aims and objects, was given good publicity in the Herald-
Tribune on 1 February.   The statement announced the Society's intention
to "use every means at our disposal to inform the public on all matters
relating to fluoridation if a referendum is decided upon".   It went on
to state further that "............any misleading or incorrect statements
such as had been published in the past would be publicly corrected".
I have sent the Society some sixty odd references, which I have collected
in anticipation of their formation, and these can be used as a basis for
their propaganda.   I have also sent them suggestions for articles,
letters and replies to letters already written by the opponents and will
continue to do this from time to time although to be really effective
they will soon have to learn to stand on their own feet.

Figure 20: *Excerpt of letter to Maclean from Taylor.* HD 125/299 H1 Box 1667, 3rd February 1956.

A letter from W. I. Paterson, Medical Officer of Health, to H. B. Turbott, then Director of Dental Hygiene, dated 31st August 1959, (**Figure 21**) discussed the possibility of above-average fluoride levels in waters of the Nelson District, based on a comment from a dental nurse who had inspected children's teeth in the area. The letter contained the phrase

"This lead might be worth following up for propaganda purposes." [320]

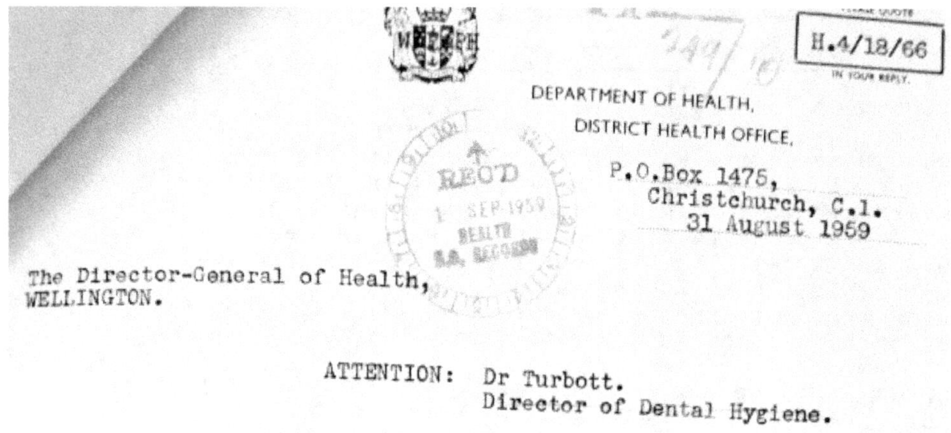

DEPARTMENT OF HEALTH,
DISTRICT HEALTH OFFICE,

H.4/18/66

P.O.Box 1475,
Christchurch, C.1.
31 August 1959

The Director-General of Health,
WELLINGTON.

ATTENTION: Dr Turbott.
Director of Dental Hygiene.

FLUORIDATION

Last week I was told of an interesting possibility in connection with natural fluoride in New Zealand waters.

A personal friend of mine, Mr T.J. McKee, a geologist and head of a mining company, has been interested in opening up some extensive deposits of baryta which occur in the waterbeds of the Baton and Wangapeka Rivers, Nelson District. He has found that the baryta and other rocks in the area are extensively fluorinated. If the project is proceeded with, the fluorine will have to be removed and will be recovered as a bye-product Ca F$_2$.

He was sufficiently interested to go to a farmhouse in the Baton Valley and inquire about their teeth. He was informed that they had exceptionally good teeth. During the conversation he tried to see if any mottling was present, but there did not appear to be any evidence of it on this casual examination. The farmer volunteered the information that the dental nurse had remarked on the hardness of the teeth of one of the children when she had to do some drilling, and he told Mr McKee that other families in the valley were the same.

This lead might be worth following up for propaganda purposes. If the waters of these streams do in fact contain more fluoride than is usual in New Zealand, a dental survey of the people living in the valley might be able to correlate with it an improvement in dental health. I understand that only eleven families live in the Baton Valley, but from memory there would be many more in the Wangapeka. A good many of these might use rain-water for drinking and cooking, but nevertheless it would be interesting to know whether there is anything in this story.

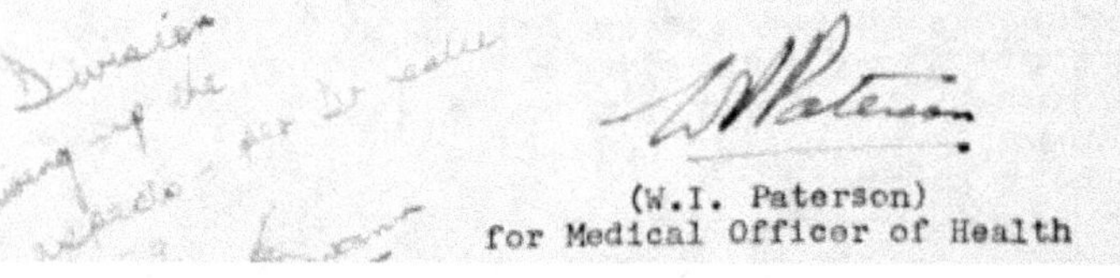

(W.I. Paterson)
for Medical Officer of Health

Figure 21. *Letter to Paterson from Turbott.* HD 125/299/10 H1 Box 1734, 31st August 1959.

A document dated November 1959, (**Figure 22**) authored by S. Hickling, the Deputy Medical Officer of Health, discussed the referendum in the town of Masterton and contained the phrase

> "Long before any education or propaganda on behalf of fluoridation in the town was dreamt of, this opposition group had been working steadily and insidiously against it." [321]

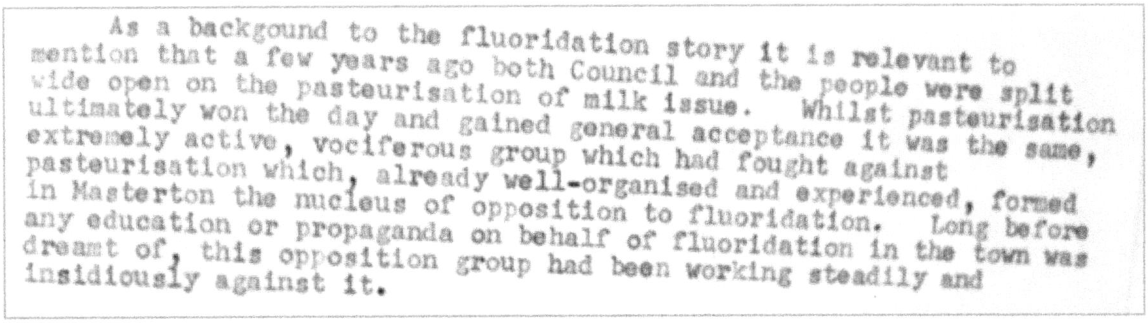

As a backgound to the fluoridation story it is relevant to mention that a few years ago both Council and the people were split wide open on the pasteurisation of milk issue. Whilst pasteurisation ultimately won the day and gained general acceptance it was the same, extremely active, vociferous group which had fought against pasteurisation which, already well-organised and experienced, formed in Masterton the nucleus of opposition to fluoridation. Long before any education or propaganda on behalf of fluoridation in the town was dreamt of, this opposition group had been working steadily and insidiously against it.

Figure 22: *Fluoridation Referendum – Masterton – November 1959, p. 1.* HD 125/299/10 H1 Box 1734.

The implication is that if people don't like being propagandized, they are insidious.

A letter from L. F. Jepson, Medical Officer of Health, to the Director-General of Health dated 4th February 1960, (**Figure 23**) used the word to describe the information presented by opponents of fluoridation, *as well as* the activities of the medical and dental professions.

> "The local doctors and dentists will continue their active chairside propaganda..." [322] (The second sentence after point 2.)

The Ministry sometimes believed it was sensible to have professionals communicate the benefits of fluoridation programs to small groups, often allowing them to take the issue outside the media. This got around the media's presentation of "both sides". A study of this in itself is a large undertaking.

There are many more examples of the Health Department staff claiming people *opposed* to fluoridation propagandize [323], yet I believe these examples demonstrate that the experts knew there was a strategic nature to their own public communications.

It is extremely serious to accuse others of less than honourable intention here, especially when many of the people involved have since died and are no longer here to defend themselves against such an accusation. As well as this, many of these people cared about child health, and their desires to help improve it should not be scoffed at. In selecting individual letters only one moment of an entire story is shown.

I would like to share more from the 1959 document cited earlier (**Figure 24**) regarding Masterton's referendum. The document outlined reasons for the loss, and what could be done in future to make the citizens vote for fluoridation. It was written by S. Hickling, the Deputy Medical Officer of Health.

It also it looked at the "education of a community to the acceptance of fluoridation".

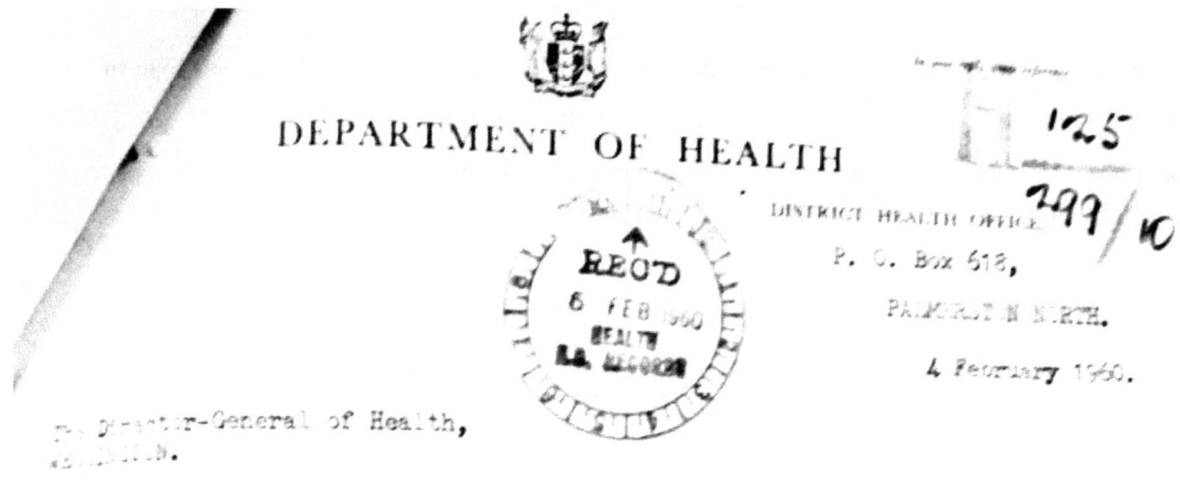

DEPARTMENT OF HEALTH

125
299/10

DISTRICT HEALTH OFFICE

P. O. Box 618,

PALMERSTON NORTH.

4 February 1960.

RECD
6 FEB 1960
HEALTH
H.O. RECORDS

The Director-General of Health,
WELLINGTON.

FLUORIDATION

1.   At a meeting of the Marton Borough Council held last week the Council voted by a majority of 5 to 2 against the proposal to fluoridate the Marton Borough water supply and I understand from Mr Meads, the Mayor, that it is not intended that any further consideration will be given to fluoridation by the present Council.   The local Citizens' Committee at Marton is continuing in office. Meetings of the Committee will now be held irregularly and on an informal basis as in the past.   However, the members have undertaken to continue to contribute short articles to the Press, to answer local propaganda by Anti-fluoridationists and to continue as before with their active underground campaign, particularly amongst Plunket mothers, schools, dental nurse and the doctors.

2.   Similarly in Levin the local Committee have agreed to continue their efforts.   The local doctors and dentists will continue their active chairside propaganda and it is proposed when the holiday season is over to arrange for speakers by invitation to address the small groups and again any correspondence that eventuates in the Press will be answered by members of the local committee.

L. F. JEPSON
Medical Officer of Health

Figure 23: *Fluoridation letter from Jepson, 4*[th] *February 1960.* HD 125/299/10 H1 Box 1734. *There were 2,488 votes against with 1,583 for, from a total population of 9,114 people. Most did not vote.*

```
3.    Specific suggestions for improvement along these lines are :-

      (a)   At present the School Dental Service is so smoothly
            organised that most parents do not fully realise how
            much dental treatment their children do need.    Could a
            small card be prepared for children to take home to their
            parents at the end of each course of treatment or at the
            end of each year, recording the treatment which has had
            to be given during this period, possibly also with a
            running total?

      (b)   Could articles be prepared for publication dealing with
            some of the more serious complications which have
            followed dental caries, preferably by someone actively
            dealing with these problems in hospital for example?

      (c)   A regular page in the Health Bulletin should be devoted
            to a 'Fluoridation News Letter' with jottings and short
            articles of interest from New Zealand and overseas.

      (d)   Although we all consider it most unlikely that fluoride
            tablets could give the same benefits as fluoridated water,
            it is essential for the persuasion of the layman that we
            try to obtain some figures to demonstrate this.

      (e)   As presumably one of the first material benefits of
            fluoridation would be a reduced spending on the School
            Dental Service, every effort should be made to obtain
            a state subsidy for local authorities deciding to proceed
            with fluoridation schemes.

      (f)   That a close affiliation be promoted amongst Fluoridation
            Committees, both with other district committees and with
            the national committee.    The attendance of two district
            committee members - one departmental and one non-departmental
            - at each national committee meeting might be worthy of
            consideration.
```

Figure 24: Excerpt from Fluoridation Referendum – Masterton – November 1959, p. 5. HD 125/299/10 H1 Box 1734.

Hickling wrote (**Figure 25**) that

"… the education of a community to the acceptance of fluoridation must be a matter of years rather than months."

```
      In retrospect, I feel that what was done could scarcely be
faulted - it was merely that not enough was done.    Acceptance
of fluoridation is not a natural instinct, particularly when the
status quo is fed and bolstered by the fears and doubts of
antifluoridation propaganda - it is something which requires
education and persuasion.    Practically every vote for fluoridation
means that someone has had to be converted and I am sure that the
two omissions in the campaign which resulted in insufficient
conversions were :-

1.    Most important of all, the period of real effort was altogether
      too short - the education of a community to the acceptance of
      fluoridation must be a matter of years rather than months.
      In this regard, the unfortunate delay whilst hopes were high
      that the Council would rescind its decision to hold a
      referendum has been mentioned already - one important result
      was that the original Interim Committee was not expanded into
      the wider Association until two months before the referendum.
```

Figure 25: Excerpt from Fluoridation Referendum – Masterton – November 1959, p. 6. HD 125/299/10 H1 Box 1734.

I will remind the reader that these archives have been open to the New Zealand public since 1982. The only time I've ever seen them come close to being mentioned in media was in a 1990 article in the **Dominion Sunday Times**. This is discussed a little more in Chapter 5.8 and Appendix 3.

The majority of Masterton's citizens voted *against* this measure, yet **The Evening Post** (Wellington) ran an article in 1957 with the headline *Fluoridation Wanted by Masterton*. Reading the article we find that the City Council and the Mayor approved of the process.

"The first move should come from the public." [324]

This was the Mayor's opinion. At the writing of the article there had been no move from the public – interesting considering the headline. Yet in the referendum the majority of citizens voted *against* fluoridation. We can see a subtext here regarding who *is* the town of Masterton, at least according to the newspaper: it is not the people of the town. It is only the Councillors and Mayor, only the leadership.

The belief that dentists should propagandize has been expressed at least once (see Appendix 7) in academic literature. Dr. John Knutson wrote an article entitled *Water fluoridation after 25 years* that was published in the April 1970 issue of the **Journal of the American Dental Association**. At the time he was Professor of Preventive Dentistry and Public Health at the University of California Medical Center in Los Angeles. The introductory statement of Dr. Knutson's article is repeated here in full:

"Dentists will make an outstanding contribution to fluoridation programs when they see their responsibility not only to educate but also to propagandize. Complete knowledge of the detailed scientific literature is not a prerequisite for this important community role. Many competent commissions have reviewed the voluminous data on the practical effectiveness and safety of fluoridation programs." [325]

Knutson discussed what he considered potentially the "greatest deterrent to meaningful political engagement of dentists in the promotion of water fluoridation" – the belief that in order to participate, dentists needed to "have full and complete knowledge of the detailed and voluminous scientific literature" pertaining to fluoridation's impact on dental and general health. Knutson wrote that "They need not." "Committees or commissions competent..." had already done the detailed work.

A survey funded by a Public Health Service fellowship for the National (American) Institute of Dental Research was discussed in a 1968 issue of the **American Journal of Public Health**. The article was authored by John E. Mueller.

This is a reply by Dr. Mueller to favourable commentary on his previous article:

"For one thing, the very admission that there is disagreement on the issue, that 'doctors disagree,' is enough to cause many to join the antifluoridation camp. The public seems to demand unanimity of professional opinion on this issue, but on a school bond issue, for example, the mere existence of debate is not so likely to have such an important effect. Additionally, water fluoridation has not proved to be subject to compromise." [326]

In 1981, Robert Isman, D.D.S., M.P.H., wrote in the **American Journal of Public Health**:

"The American Dental Association, as part of its nationwide Public Education Program, has contracted with a public relations firm to conduct speaker training sessions involving role playing and videotaping speakers. While this training is not aimed specifically at fluoridation, but rather at creating well-rounded spokespersons for dentistry, it can be focused somewhat on fluoridation." [327]

Mueller's "unanimity of professional opinion" (above [326]) can perhaps yield a reason why we see such a stark difference when we compare complexities of experimental evidence and textbook explanations with what the experts say in public and in the simplified, promotional literature from official bodies.

The experts must unite to achieve their goal. Another reason for this unanimity is given in Mueller's 1968 article. This was part of his conclusion:

"... when the average voter is confronted with arguments for and against fluoridation, in an objective format without conspiratorial overtones and in a noncampaign situation, he is likely to find opposing arguments to the measure more persuasive than those in its favor." [328]

The times may have changed, and more modern surveys may yield different results. I have not investigated this[82]. While experts of the 1950s complained about the scepticism of the working class, more modern experts criticize the easy access and freedom the internet gives.

New Zealand's Dr. John Colquhoun[83] gives us another suggestion about experts:

"The commitment to be maintained by a strong sense of professional solidarity, and a shared concept of themselves as professionals with scientific status, which distinguishes them from outsiders and insulates against doubts and uncertainties." [329]

Australian social scientist Brian Martin once wrote:

"Especially when a contentious public issue is at stake, experts band together. They are reluctant to publicly expose each other's mistakes, since it might hurt their cause." [330]

Isman noted that

"emotionalism surrounding the issue has made it difficult to generate public support outside of the health professions." [331]

We must consider that most experts have probably just been going with the flow. Consider the USPHS documents from the early 1970s, now available on the website quackwatch.org (discussed at the end of Chapter 2.7). These were "...bulletins to community leaders..." which would have helped give our experts (doctors, dentists, nutritionist media personalities, etc) a one-sided perspective – a perspective that would suit fluoridation programs. Obviously if community leaders had seen a good 50/50 or so discussion on the question of fluorine's essentiality, this may have led to confusion and less commitment on their part. This is relevant in light of Dr. Frank Bull's statement:

---

[82] The Health Department archives contained information suggesting that in the 1950s and 1960s younger, more educated citizens were more favourable towards fluoridation.

[83] Principal Dental Officer for Ministry of Health in Auckland until 1984.

"First you need a positive policy by your state dental society and your state board of health. Now, I mean a really positive policy. Don't put any ifs, ands, buts, or maybes in the thing, because the minute you do you kill it. You simply give ammunition to the fellow who is against it." [305]

Does this mean that telling the truth would obstruct public health?

The experts needed a way to address the "mass medication" argument, and the most logical way to do this was to invoke a necessity for fluorine. The more conventional methods of nutritional categorization had to be slackened somewhat in order to obtain this. Consider Drs. Berridge and Perrott saying it's not necessarily an essential nutrient, yet NZ's soils and water supplies are deficient in it [146, 158, 178].

On this question of telling the truth, elaboration is required. The examples given here demonstrate the relationship that the experts believe they have with the public, and the responsibility they have to the public. Experts believe the public don't know what's uplifting for them, and the experts need to intervene or the public is just going to harm themselves. The important thing here is that experts (and community leaders) *don't want* to deliberately mislead people. They *don't want* to lie, they want to *improve public health*.

However, the belief of a *need* for fluorine is near-totally flawed in its fundamentals, and the experts have gone along with it hook, line and sinker, in a very trusting manner with no real scepticism. This happens even when reports from professional bodies that experts cite as authorities express disagreement with them on this issue. The fact that disagreements are not mentioned publicly help them appear minimal. This is not how a scientific investigation is performed, and it is certainly very far from "objective".

Consider the recent review by Sir Peter Gluckman that pointed out that the WHO claimed fluorine a micronutrient, without pointing out that this was due to benefit and prevention, not due to necessity or a real, proven essentiality. While this review cited the words of the SCHER and EFSA, it did not show they disagreed with calling fluorine a micronutrient.

I believe fluorine's status as nutrient has been entrenched and insisted upon by educated intellectuals partly because of their own sense of CWF being the moral thing to do, but also to serve their own reputations and prestige. This also allowed for a lack of concern and scrutiny toward the food industry which employed some of the experts involved here. The words of Dr. Frank Bull I consider evidence that promotion of fluoridation programs were more important to some than a diligent commitment to objectivity. In that approach a "positive program" that says "do it" is not really helped by nitpicking, haggling and disagreement.

There are some things that have escaped the eyes of promoters of CWF, even when right in front of them.

Dr. Frank Bull was from Wisconsin. This was the first American state to achieve fifty cities fluoridated [332]. No doubt his techniques of promotion worked in helping cities adopt the programs he recommended.

Compare what you've seen in this investigation regarding claims of fluorine's essentiality from dentists, and the words of Dr. Knutson mentioned earlier [325] with the more recent (2013) words of Associate Professor Jason Armfield, of Adelaide Dental School, Australia:

"Dentists are a valuable source of accurate public health information regarding water fluoridation because they already are an important source of preventive dental information for the general public[84]." [333]

For a long time I scratched my head on why I saw such a cluster of insightful thought, and such a variety of experimental methods and conclusions in scientific literature, yet saw lockstep conformity and convenient catchphrases from experts in the public eye and media.

This may sound like an insult to journalists, but it's not: consider that in many instances, the journalist is simply holding the microphone in front of the expert. Public health is an important topic, and most journalists probably feel out of depth claiming they knew the latest research, when it would only be sensible to refer to a person who studies such things professionally.

Yet one can see the experts do not present research with complete objectivity. Many experts support fluoridation out of altruistic motives, with the exaggeration of a necessary nutritional role that is part and parcel of much official and some scientific literature.

There were a few things that slowly came to light that helped explain why I saw such a divergence between what was said in experiments and official reports, compared with "objective" experts in media. One was the Health Department documents from the 1950s that opened my eyes to the constant claims of awful teeth around the second world war, and to the letters quoted in this chapter regarding propaganda. While there were some dishonesties about the way the Health Department behaved in the 1950s, I did not see any desire to hurt or harm anyone. One explanation for the divergence was the way the "mass medication" claim was dismissed with the claim of a nutritional role for fluorine.

Another was the propaganda model of the mass media put forward by Professors Herman and Chomsky in their 1989 work *Manufacturing Consent*. They believed:

"… among their other functions, the media serve, and propagandize on behalf of, the powerful societal interests that control and finance them." [334]

According to Herman and Chomsky, the claim that media and intellectuals perform functions in the service of powerful interests makes sense in light of a free market system in a business-run society where there are groups sometimes in concert, sometimes in competition, working towards various goals. This is far more realistic and reasonable than any 'conspiracy theory' idea, although I have found so little on the financial or profit-related aspects of CWF it is difficult to judge this aspect of the propaganda model's relation. Regarding expert statements in media, I *don't* think (at least the majority of) experts knowingly lie. The literature is replete with claims of a nutritional role, and while evidence and research that disputes this is sometimes readily and easily available, it is not discussed. This lack of discussion may *appear* to be dishonest. I am confident that in the case of the majority of experts it is *not* dishonest, most experts are simply repeating what other experts have said,

---

[84] A study is cited by Armfield here: Roberts-Thomson KF, Spencer AJ. *Public knowledge of the prevention of dental decay and gum diseases.* **Aust Dent J**. 1999; 44(4):253–258. [PubMed: 10687234]

without scratching the subject too deeply. Yet what about the experts that *do* read about the experiments that refute a nutritional role? It is difficult to generalise in answering this question.

I believe it is the use of the word *propaganda* in describing the government's own information in private, while not using the word in public, that justifies at least a partial consideration of a propaganda model of the mass media, though this should of course be extended to include, and I think in this instance primarily focus upon, the intellectual class that promotes CWF.

Applying such a thing to only media would be narrow because fluoridation is not a subject limited to the media; in fact one can see they are often last in a chain of communication that reaches the public. This topic of a potential nutritional role for fluorine is a little different in that while the issue is occasionally mentioned *in* media, it is not an issue in which the media claims to have much expertise – it is the *experts* – the politicians, the ministers, the educated professors, that largely do the talking, and it's a little more complex than simply being on a side.

By going to nodes of power, the interests of the people who already have power are expressed, and discussions can be framed in the terminology and presuppositions of those people. The experts' claim of an essential role for fluorine may be considered a presupposition of CWF promotion.

A point made by Herman and Chomsky is that intellectuals believe much of what they hear from those with prestige above them. They need to, in order to promote it well; if they didn't believe it, they would find it much harder to promote. I believe intellectuals in turn project this expectation of subservient complicity onto the public. For example, one of the articles in **The Dominion Post** recently referred to people in rural District Health Boards as "hillbillies" if they didn't go along with the government's plan to fluoridate all of New Zealand [220]. The propaganda model has three orders of prediction. It was not until some time after I completed the first draft of this book that I could give an example of the third (see Appendix 8). Even if intellectuals *don't* believe what they say, there are filtering mechanisms in the system that limit debate and expression, for instance the "both sides" competitive mentality, as well as abuse, and the need to not alarm or shock the public.

In *Reshaping the Truth*, Australian sociologist Alex Carey claimed:

> "There is a remarkable correspondence in attitude to truth between pragmatists and propagandists. Both justify the promotion of false beliefs wherever it is supposed that false beliefs have socially useful consequences." [335]

Something becomes true if it has socially useful consequences. Fluorine becomes an essential nutrient because this will ensure the public are less likely to oppose the addition of the element to water supplies.

One of Colonel Fuller's points on how to promote fluoridation was:

> "Do not let yourself be placed on the defensive. On no account approach the subject [of CWF] as if you have need to defend it." [216]

When we read scientific experiments we often read uncertainties, people putting their experiment in the bigger picture. Recall McClendon suggesting that maybe not all nutritional requirements were known to scientists, as one example. Another might be the experts at the Waikato University Google Hangout, unsure if experiments had tested extremely low amounts of fluorine. Dr. Armstrong said that applying work carried out on mice to humans was problematic.

Perhaps this is why so many people feel such scepticism about fluoridation – it *requires* the simplification of something technical and elusive into catchphrases and clichés designed for public approval.

All of the public relations and the insistence that what experts believe and say is scientific, has interrupted a slow, patient, scientific appraisal of this matter (the question of essentiality). While scientists may consider fluoridation to be about the whole body, dentists may consider it about the teeth, people opposed to fluoridation will have their own multitude of concerns, one of which may be the way in which the programs themselves are reflective of the entire political culture of the society. We all draw boundary lines in different places. For this reason the experts may feel justified in completely ignoring what they ignore, and the activist may feel justified in being frustrated when they see this, report after report, decade after decade.

Writing in the book *The Tooth Robbers*, (this was recommended by Harvard's Dr. Fredrick Stare to the American public in 1981 [290]) Stephen Barrett M.D. and Sheldon Rovin, D.D.S., M.S., discuss writing letters to editors in a section called *Fighting for Teeth: Fluoridation Campaign Tips.* They write that the fluoridation supporter is met with a difficult situation when people opposed write letters to their local newspaper editor – responding "tit-for-tat" allows the audience to feel that there is some controversy about the matter, which is bad for the fluoridation publicity campaign. Yet leaving letters unanswered gives "the antis" free reign.

> "If you blitz the newspaper with 'pro' letters, you may get more space for your ideas; but if the antis respond in kind, they too will get more exposure." (page 73)

The authors are wary of the delicate situation, that it may easily get out of hand. They suggest meeting with the newspaper editor early in the campaign.

> "Your approach should make it clear that many members of the community will admire a firm stand on the part of the newspaper."

> "A meeting with an editor should be attended by several of the most prominent members of your organization, including the citizens' committee chairman, the steering committee chairman and the editor's dentist and personal physician. A small amount of written material which has key points high-lighted for easy reading should be sent a few days beforehand." (page 73)

> "Key people at local radio and television stations should be approached and educated in the same manner before any controversy becomes heated." (page 74)

The reader is advised to start the meeting by asking for the editor's help – asking first of all whether he doubts the safety and effectiveness of fluoridation (this document or the authors are so old there is no consideration of female leadership). Oh, and does the editor have any suggestions for your campaign? Would the editor like to *join* your campaign? Barrett and Rovin point out that the editor will probably decline joining on grounds of journalistic objectivity, but "no harm in asking". The reader is then advised to "point out the nature of antifluoridation propaganda" and request that the editor follow such articles and letters with corrections "explaining their fallacies."

Recall from Chapter 5.2 that one of the final sections of their book contained many advertisements claiming a nutritional role for fluorine, most of which likened it to calcium [294].

The actions endorsed in *The Tooth Robbers* and the use of the public relations industry are highlighted in one of dentist Dr Michael Easley's statements:

> "The last technique effectively used by antifluoride extremists is <u>Subversion of the Media</u>." [336] (His emphasis.)

Another example of experts speaking to community leaders to prevent them from believing the words of the people who voted for them can be found in the July, 2015 report of the Childrens' Dental Health Project (CDHP), managed by Pew Charitable Trust. A lesson from San Jose was

> "Inform public officials and key stakeholders of the typical arguments that critics use so they are 'inoculated' and are far less susceptible to the myths that they will hear as the public dialogue intensifies." [337]

The implication here is that the experts believe that public officials will simply believe the experts. Why don't the *public* simply believe the experts?

The propaganda model suggests that the public read less official information, and are therefore exposed to less propaganda. The public are more likely than experts to read activist, or unofficial information. The experts really believe the truth of what they write. It's easy for them to believe it, after all they've written it, and it couldn't be wrong when all the other experts can insist that it's true as well. It's in well-known, admired journals, and everyone has an important and long-winded title, so a lot of prestige and respect is involved. Following from this is the logical conclusion that the information from experts and leaders must be true.

The experts are more willing to believe what they read if it comes from other experts. They're more sceptical of public, or 'non-expert' information. This is partly because the information experts receive has been through the reviewing process, so experts trust it. The public, on the other hand, can see the world going to hell in a handbasket right in front of their eyes, so it's much harder for them to believe all is fine and fair in terms of the consequences of expert influence. As you can see, the experts' self-criticism is quite a painless process.

We see in the 2015 CDHP document the belief that the public cannot tell the truth. The public do not represent any group with political power, they have *their own – and the society in general's* best interest at heart. This makes them incapable of telling the truth, thinking rationally, according to the CDHP.

Incidentally, the words "sugar", "junk", "food" and "industry" don't appear once in the CDHP/Pew document.

A 1980 article in the **Journal of Public Health Dentistry** looked at fluoridation campaigns throughout the year. The authors noted that

> "... need for public education is important, but to win fluoridation campaigns, a political approach must be strictly followed in the later stages of the campaign." [338]

They wrote

"The following tactics have proved useful in towns that were successful in adopting fluoridation -"
and followed this with seven tactics for the willing expert.

"Obtain strong endorsements by the mayor, city council, and other community opinion leaders."
In small towns where community leaders are more independent and proud of it,

"... committees should be open and vocal about their support for the measure and seek as many local public endorsements as possible."

"The 'freedom of choice' issue is exploited thoroughly in a small town and must be dealt with before the campaign starts. Strategies must encourage an objective comparison of the value of fluoridation, against the value or supposed abridgement of free choice."

"... the real key to success in small towns is to identify the 'power source' of the community. Influential citizens are not always obvious – they may be in any occupation and not necessarily in city government. They may be the owner of a florist shop or water plant operator. If the campaign leaders can find the 'power source' and convince them of the merits of fluoridation, the election will be won."

There is no suggestion of ensuring the 'power source' has access to the most up-to-date research. Reading this article, one cannot help but wonder about the disparity in terms of resources and money available to the 'two sides'.

"The hiring of a seasoned political person to help coordinate campaign activities is a definite plus to any campaign – large or small."

The article noted the importance of professional medical people in supporting the campaigns. An added bonus to this was that if these people worked at a local health or science centre, "students and teachers can be a source of manpower to work the telephone banks, provide door-to-door canvassing..."

"Professional organizations have also been a source of campaign funds."

"All ethnic and religious groups in the community should be reached, if possible."

"Good media support will help overcome the distorted messages and 'scare tactics' of the antifluoridationists. Conversely, those opposed to fluoridation will use the media as much as they can." [338]

The latter sentence is interesting in light of what Dr. Robert Isman (one of the co-authors of this 1980 article) wrote in his 1981 article on public relations, quoted previously [327]. The paragraph on media continued:

"... many of the successful campaigns in 1980 attempted to limit the access of the antifluoridationists to the media by minimizing *all* contact with the media (such as debates)... it is important to note that editorial endorsements by newspapers can be very influential and should be sought." [338]

The experts want "good media support" and "editorial endorsements" yet "the 'anti's' have become especially skillful at using radio and TV." No examples or citations of radio and TV use were given. The experts also recommend a "seasoned political person" to help with the campaign, and have funds available from professional organizations. Such one-sided behavior is more easily condoned if there is a very fundamental belief that whatever experts say is correct (this also obviates the need to double-check and keep up to date with research).

On the 31st July, 2016, two thirty-second advertisements made by New Zealand-based activist group Fluoride Free NZ screened on four prime time television ad spaces [339]. There were six complaints about the ad or ads, none were upheld. The ads were timed to coincide with some talks Professor Paul Connett was giving in New Zealand. The media responded. Radio New Zealand interviewed Peter Griffin from the Science Media Centre [340].

Griffin said he attended Professor Paul Connett's talk in Petone, Wellington. He told interviewer Jesse Mulligan that there were no scientists present, however in this comment it is obvious that he was discussing the *audience*. In this interview (11th August, 2016) *and* in an interview two months later (12th October, 2016) RNZ *did* state that Paul Connett was a retired chemistry professor. Quoting Mr. Griffin:

"There was just Paul, there were no scientists there." [340]

We do not hear *how* Griffin knew that nobody in the audience was a scientist, nor are any of Connett's other audiences around the world discussed. Surely one would have to ask everyone there, just a quick show of hands may have sufficed, but there was no explanation as to how Griffin knew this. The significance is difficult to judge.

Mr. Griffin was introduced by Radio New Zealand's Jesse Mulligan as being "among many in the science community..." Griffin has a Bachelor of Communication Studies in journalism, and a Master of Arts in Creative Writing [341]. This is not mentioned in the interview. He's among many in the science community, but not a scientist, nor does he have a scientific qualification. I do *not* have a problem with him expressing his ideas, research and opinion in the media, but it says a lot about how to become an expert. I am opposed to the "experts only" views that occur as a result of our system. Neither Peter Griffin nor Jesse Mulligan think it relevant to the audience that Griffin does not *have* a scientific qualification, after he has pointed to a lack of scientific training in an audience.

Acknowledging such a double standard would make both media and experts look hypocritical, so there is no incentive to include such information. This may also demonstrate to us the lack of a knowledge of history – for many decades non-experts like the Jaycees have participated in support of CWF. You'll note in the 1980 document cited previously [338], there was no cause for concern if an endorsement came from a florist or a water plant operator. Mr. Griffin's words are treated with the same respect as any professor of dentistry's words would be.

Griffin concluded no-one in the audience was educated enough to appraise the evidence. How is *he* then able to appraise the evidence, given that *he* is not a scientist?

We learn something about journalism if we watch for long enough: Jesse Mulligan is *not* supposed to investigate this issue on his own and tell us what *he* has found out, digging where no-one else has dug. That such a thing is not suggested, implies that all media need do is go to an expert. Implied in this is the claim that there is literally no relevant information beyond that of which experts speak.

I believe most experts don't know that the PR industry has been involved in fluoridation's promotion.

Public relations violates an important aspect of the traditional left wing: the ability to elect leaders from within one's own ranks. In PR, a celebrity might be used as in advertising, but overall, the communications have their origin in the unknown. The public are supposed to trust the person they do *not* know over those they *do* know.

In PR, the experts are chosen for their ability to present a point of view conducive to the maintaining of power and wealth. The poor base their decisions on what is in the interests of business leadership, believing it beneficial for themselves, and this naturally leads to the poor undermining themselves [342]. Avenues of activity that uplift and help the poor gain wealth and power are not presented so overtly to the poor.

The belief that media antagonism is a check on power is a self-serving belief, because it allows journalists to believe they're "fighting the power". If we're already antagonistic to power, we don't need to be *more* antagonistic to power. Being *more* antagonistic to power would not make sense. A certain amount of antagonism to power is *necessary* for the media to believe in their commitment to what they believe their role to be.

Therefore the media *can* present the odd activist who says fluorine is non-essential, the odd activist who might discuss potential profits made by an industry, and the experts don't like this and will quite possibly criticize the media for presenting such antagonistic views.

The media in some instances are quite open about the sycophantic relationship they have with industry. For example, in their 2004 book on the public relations industry, Sheldon Rampton and John Stauber quote the Press Association's (PA) website:

> "The Press Association's unique position at the centre of the media industry in the UK enables us to provide support for many PR and marketing campaigns." [343]

I did not find this quote, but I did visit the PA's website. The PA can tell us they put industry first; the following is from the 'industry monitoring' section of their website:

> "Whether you are looking to maximise your organisation's positive coverage, or are in the midst of a publicity crisis, Mediapoint gives you the means to respond quickly to news regarding your company, industry or market, straight to our captive audience of media clients.
>
> **Commenting first to protect your brand**
> "Mediapoint allows you the opportunity to offer your comments to journalists before the story hits the headlines, significantly increasing the likelihood of your analysis being picked up by the UK's national and regional media.
>
> **Agenda setting and Informing PR strategy**
> "Access PA's news diaries so you know what the UK's media will be covering ahead of time, allowing you to plan PR activities in advance." [344]

You can see here the fundamental nature of the media/business relationship: the media gives business opportunity to say what business wants. Business is not in a defensive position as it would be in investigative journalism that is antagonistic to power. Governments have also used the PR industry in the past. The American Center for Disease Control is one government agency that has used the industry recently. The website PR Week deals with news relevant to the PR industry. In 2012, they reported:

> "... the Centers for Disease Control and Prevention awarded communications contracts worth more than $12 million combined."

> "Washington-based [PR firm] Hager Sharp won two multi-year contracts worth about $6.2 million in total. The first contract requires it to conduct initiatives for the Heart Disease and Stroke Prevention Division and the Division of Oral Health."

> "The CDC also awarded Hager Sharp a two-year contract to support communication and education efforts for oral health issues, including community water fluoridation." [345]

A glance at the Hager Sharp website confirms the CDC as a client, but does not go into specifics. The CDC is not a business, yet they are not completely immune to corporate and political involvement [346].

Again, a different picture emerges if we read the intellectual fodder provided for public consumption. Bob Brockie, author of the science column in Wellington's local paper **The Dominion Post**, wrote on the 7th of October, 2013:

> "A big problem is that the anti fluoride lobbyists have the propaganda field to themselves. No noisy organization promotes fluorine or challenges the antifluoridationists." [347]

To me this echoed the way in which businessmen play the victim. In the week following, articles would appear in the NZ media discussing how much was actually spent on advertising to influence the referendum: "a few thousand" from the people against (their own money), and $47,000 by the District Health Board (taxpayer money) to promote fluoridation [348].

Who comprises Bob Brockie's audience? He authored the weekly science column, so his audience are the critical thinkers; sceptics, intelligent, scientifically oriented people. His claim simply demonstrates how little is known on this topic. His claim reaches the public with no criticism or accompanying note from his editor, and no correction a week later once other newspapers have shown it to be unreasonable. Then again, propaganda is something the *other* people do, almost never the one doing the pointing. At this time, I believe **The Dominion Post** had a daily readership of about 275,000 people in Wellington, New Zealand's capital city.

5.5 Abuse

"Probably the best tactic for the pros (if the arguments can't be successfully ignored) is direct, harsh, and sarcastic personal attack on the authorities and the people quoting them. The pros point to the absurdity of some of the more extreme arguments sometimes made by anti-fluoridationists (even if they have not been made in the campaign) and seek to imply that all the arguments are of this sort. This tactic can backfire, however, and takes considerable political finesse."

- John E. Mueller (Political Scientist, University of Rochester, New York), *The Politics of Fluoridation in Seven California Cities*, **Western Political Quarterly** [349]. The word "pros" refers to supporters of fluoridation, the word "authorities" refers to the more medically inclined and qualified opponents of fluoridation.

"The effects of fluoride are multiple and complex. In order for a consensus to emerge on these the debate needs to focus on the evidence rather than on the character of those producing the evidence."

- Dr. Bruce Spittle, *Killing the Messenger*, **Fluoride** (Journal of the International Society for Fluoride Research), Vol. 28, No. 4, pp. 178-179, 1995.

"... I can promise the nutters they won't take the fluoride out of my water without a fight."

- Sean Plunket, quoted in **The Dominion Post**, 8th June, 2013 [350].

"... no credible people support the fluorophobics' view."

"Like parasites, opponents steal undeserved credibility just by sharing the stage with respected scientists who are there to defend fluoridation."

- Michael Easley D.D.S., M.P.H., *Community Water Fluoridation in America: The Unprincipled Opposition*, p. 9, 1999 [351].

"'They come with their own group of professionals, eminently qualified and respected people in their area and it places local politicians in a very difficult position,' [Hutt City Councillor Ken] *Laban said.*

Laban said the District Health Board's response in the past had been to dismiss the arguments of fluoride opponents rather than address them.

'The argument was to say that they were bad, they were idiots and we'd be crazy to listen to them.'"

- Hutt City Councillor Ken Laban, quoted by Blake Crayton-Brown, *Hutt DHB: anti-fluoridation lobby has upped its game considerably*, 11th September, 2015, http://www.stuff.co.nz/national/health/71348455/hutt-dhb-antifluoridation-lobby-has-upped-its-game-considerably.

It is ironic that some of us who want to increase public health often want to do it with hurtful, intimidating words.

Perhaps this is simply part of being human. It relates to the statement Howard Zinn has made, quoted at the beginning of the previous chapter. If we're the good guys it's OK for us to control and dominate other people. Being the bad guys, whatever those others want to do must be wrong.

Appraising the effects of abuse is very difficult as these effects differ person to person, culture to culture. Yet I believe abuse has had an inhibiting effect on debate, discussion and information. Some people are thick-skinned, some are thin-skinned. Some people care more than others about their careers, promotions, and prestige. Some people are very proud, some are willing to concede points if they don't know. Some always want to get the last word in. Some are stubborn, some are polite.

It is arguable that the media do not help by printing abusive comments. This is an easy argument to make as I don't enjoy reading insults. Yet I think making the media inoffensive would probably do more harm than good. Painting our anger, our offence, rosy-coloured would be very misleading, making it even harder to see how our personalities shape our "objective opinion". I don't share the comments and examples in this chapter to start a fight; I share them so we can be honest about our biases, our lack of self-control. Five minutes on a social media fluoride page will probably yield a lot more insults than you'll read here, but what I include here relates to print media, continues in an historical vein, and may help to partially explain attitudes and behavior of not only each side, but also of journalists and newspaper editors.

One example of abuse is from Wellington's **Dominion Sunday Times** dated 1st April, 1990. The title of the article is *Fluoride Gets a Kick in the Teeth.* This is a misleading title given some of the statements in the article:

"The position of the pro fluoride groups seemed unassailable, the antis dismissed as loonies."

"Once every reporter's joke, the anti-fluoride campaign looks set to demand fresh attention." [352]

I have never found a single comment on this last statement. Not in academic literature, media or *anywhere* – have I seen it mentioned that if a group were "every reporter's joke" that this may have detrimentally influenced media coverage of issues or information. This is a particularly important point when we consider that fluoridation is often settled by referendum.

John Mueller wrote:

"Newspapers performed several important functions. Endorsement of fluoridation is virtually an essential ingredient (though certainly not a sufficient one) for pro success in a controversial campaign since a noncommittal attitude implies doubt as to the value of the measure." [297]

The 1990 article contained more:

"Papakura dentist John Bell laments what he sees as a blow to primary health care. He likened 'fluorophobes' to child molesters."

Dr. Bell explained:

"'I know that sounds emotive but I say it because they are assaulting people with diseases and illness. The punter out there is going to have to get angry and do something about it, because they are the ones who are going to suffer.'" [352]

Again, I have never found a single comment regarding the likening of these people to child molesters. A sub-headline of this article reads "It's always been a dirty fight". *This* book was written with the hope that it may become a cleaner one. It is relevant to this topic of essentiality because it seems Dr. Bell believes people will suffer without fluoride, something very abundant (see Chapter 4) even before additions to water are made, and something we have no reproducible evidence of deficiencies in [105, 116-118] (and see Chapters 1 and 2).

The fact that abuse is consistent over the years has almost definitely had some effects on restricting discussion. Would the head of a prestigious university department be just as willing to hire someone labelled 'as bad as a child molester' in public? This article had to do with Principal Dental Officer of Auckland, John Colquhoun, who had changed his mind about Community Water Fluoridation (CWF) being safe, effective and beneficial. The insult was not directed specifically at Dr. Colquhoun, but at all opponents of CWF.

These examples of abuse demonstrate what the conclusion of non-essentiality is really up against. When we take a microscope to the matter, close to 100% of the experts who've mentioned the subject agree in print media fluorine is a nutritional essential. And while the media allows people with differing views free expression, gives them a fair half and sometimes *more* of the opinion column to express this, abuse has a curbing effect on their credibility, and possibly a silencing effect on other members of the public and journalists.

In 2013, a four-day tribunal occurred in New Zealand's city of Hamilton to decide if the city should stop or continue CWF. This was an event in which people on both sides of the fluoridation debate could share their attitudes, beliefs and research.

Shortly after the decision was made to cease the addition of fluoride to Hamilton's water supply, the Science Media Centre (SMCNZ) published an article called *Hamilton's fluoride furore makes splash* on their website on the 7th of June 2013 [353]. The article was barely a couple of sentences but had links to thirty-two other articles in the media from sites like Radio New Zealand, Radio Rhema, TVNZ News, **New Zealand Herald**, **Waikato Times**, and other mainstream media.

The list contained only the media outlet, then the story headline. Twelve of these headlines are openly abusive or disrespectful to the councillors who voted to cease fluoridation, or people opposed to fluoridation.

The action to cease fluoridation, or the people who wanted it gone, were called in headlines "absolutely gutless", "disappointing", "defying all logic", "nutters", "anti-fluoridation will harm children", "regret", "decision baffles". Some of the other headlines were "health experts slam decision", "a blow for Hamilton Maori", "Expert disappointed" "decision slammed by doctors", "Health advocates rue city's decision…"

I've yet to find an answer to the question "why didn't the media *attend* the four-day tribunal in Hamilton?", given that they appeared to care so much about the issue. Also, had it been broadcast on mainstream TV, it would have been an opportunity *for the entire country* to hear (supposedly) the *best* arguments, and hopefully the most up-to-date research on both sides, which *obviously* would save *so much time* for future council meetings all over the country. It would have been a good way of showing the entire country a selection of arguments from people on either side of the debate.

The tribunal was in June. The Hamilton City Council believed that a tribunal was an acceptable forum for deliberation and appraisal of points of view. These are a couple of points from their *Extraordinary Council Open Agenda*.

> "A tribunal style hearing was held. In addition to the substantive presentations, 141 individuals or representative organisations presented."
>
> "Staff are satisfied that the Council is undertaking a robust decision-making process that complies with the Council's obligations under the Local Government Act 2002. The Fluoridation consultation process has been appropriate for identifying and understanding the views and preferences of all interested and affected persons so as to satisfy the Council's obligations under section 78 of the Act and the options identified and the level of analysis set out in this report and the Submissions Analysis Report (Attachment 1) are appropriate to satisfy the Council's obligations under section 77." [354]

There was a lot of abuse when the council decided to cease the fluoridation program. A referendum occurred months after, in which the majority of Hamilton residents voted to restart CWF. One potential reason for the media not showing, and the public's lack of interest in seeing the four-day tribunal is given in the **Waikato Times** in October 2013:

> "Waikato DHB Medical Officer of Health Dr Felicity Dumble said ultimately, the referendum result was 'an example as to why it's not a good idea to use tribunals, which grossly over-represent the position of small interest groups, when it comes to making public health decisions for the whole city.'" [355]

Dr. Dumble's statement here is odd given that the experts who supported fluoridation also presented their case at the tribunal. Mayor of Hamilton, Julie Hardaker said:

> "My council and I have sat through four days of what I would regard as a very, very good process, listening to and receiving info, evidence, data, statistics, expert advice from both sides of this debate." [355]

Two exceptionally qualified, intelligent people, Mayor Hardaker and Dr. Dumble [356], think differently on the best way to simply look at evidence!

This can be explained a little. It is obvious that Dr. Dumble agreed with the DHB point of view before the tribunal, yet Mayor Hardaker's point of view before the tribunal is more difficult to ascertain. Being trained in law, she probably thought it fair to hear "both sides". Yet Dumble is a doctor, and a DHB member, and probably feels justified in not listening to the other side. Remember Dr. Frank Bull's advice:

> "Don't put any ifs, ands, buts, or maybes in the thing, because the minute you do you kill it." [305]

Mayor Hardaker no doubt thought it fair to have an adversarial style of presentation – who can make the better argument? This might seem sensible in any *usual* scientific issue, but this completely violates one of the key principles of support for fluoridation, namely that it should *not* be debated or discussed, unless in a positive light; never doubted. To debate or listen to "the other side" can give the dangerous impression that the other side has something worth saying [357]. Consider many of the statements given in the previous chapter – that fluoridation is a matter for experts, etc, and the words of Doctors Knutson, Bull and Nicholson.

I'm drawn to the fact that these two sides sometimes simply *cannot* seem to discuss the same thing. *Again* I'm offended that we have satellites, cellphones and power pylons all over but we couldn't show the four-day tribunal on mainstream TV.

Councillor Dave McPherson claimed to have initial scepticism toward a tribunal process, but afterwards spoke well of it [358].

The tribunal in Hamilton lasted four days. For readers who believe this not enough time to make a decision or mild investigation on a subject, I will offer some polite, tepid agreement[85]. An article in a Waikato newspaper by DHB member Denise Irvine voiced a similar criticism, upon hearing Mayor Hardaker claim that she'd "learnt a lot over the last few days"[86]:

---

[85] (Depending on the subject of course.) In the introduction I mentioned Charles Darwin's study of barnacles, yet that had more to do with mastery of a subject.

[86] This quote "... learnt a lot..." was apparently on Mayor Hardaker's Twitter account. Assuming Irvine's article is accurate, it would have been between the 5th and 15th of June, 2013.

> "The 'certainly learnt a lot over the last few days' line is actually a bit worrying: it could imply that the mayor thinks that a few days is all it takes to come up to speed on fluoride. (My apologies if I've incorrectly interpreted this.)" [359]

One wonders how much time is acceptable, especially considering some of the expert statements quoted in the previous chapter. Dr. Rob Beaglehole of the New Zealand Dental Association did not spend all that much *more* time than the Hamilton City Council in *his* appraisal or research. According to the **Nelson Mail**:

> "[Dr. Beaglehole] said when he became the Dental Association's spokesperson he spent a week looking at all the evidence on fluoridation to make sure he thoroughly understood the topic and knew all the evidence was correct." [67]

Consider this with regard to the average citizen voting in a referendum. How much time does *the average citizen* spend? Nobody seems to discuss such a thing when citizens vote the way of the experts. I will also point out in 2017 I spent *six months* in the Health Department archives and I still have questions and areas of uncertainty where there is simply no information. When we discuss "all the evidence" how big is our sample size?

Councillor Dave McPherson said of the media:

> "... the media comments, particularly the daily paper in Waikato had been pathetic, not to put too fine a point on it. They weren't at the hearing for a lot of it, they didn't follow the actual arguments that were put at the tribunal, and they came and attacked us for 'not following science' afterwards, well... which science did they want us to follow? And we heard – as I said – scientific arguments from both sides... the media didn't, and they had done an exceptionally poor job of presenting both of the arguments in the tribunal."

> "I have seen the **NZ Herald** coverage, but I'm not certain I'm getting the same **Herald** edition that you're getting up north, so, what I've seen has been much lower key, slightly more even-handed, but not very in-depth for either side. So I suspect that the arguments are not well known at all by Aucklanders, compared with now, by Hamiltonians." [358]

I will also point out that many Junior Chambers of Commerce both in America and New Zealand have publicly supported CWF, without their qualifications or lack of qualifications relevant to science becoming an issue at all, without this aspect of their learning or knowledge even being mentioned, beyond rare occasion [360]. The attitude of media and experts is just that they're happy to have the Jaycees on board and helping with promotion. Such a thing is justified by the words of John Knutson, no doubt applicable here if we simply expand the word 'dentists' to include other intellectuals:

> "Dentists will make an outstanding contribution to fluoridation programs when they see their responsibility not only to educate but also to propagandize. Complete knowledge of the detailed scientific literature is not a prerequisite for this important community role. Many competent commissions have reviewed the voluminous data on the practical effectiveness and safety of fluoridation programs." [325].

Abuse lets people know where boundaries of acceptable opinion, statement and behaviour lie. Some of the claims of the people opposed to CWF in letters to politicians and newspaper editors were expressed heatedly, emotionally or without precision, and sometimes they too were abusive. It was in public where the experts really shone in their abuse. In private letters to individuals, it can be seen that politicians were polite and respectful. City councillors were on the receiving end of a lot of abuse.

This consistent ridiculing and attempts at ostracism with abuse, or "flak" has its effect. In discussing a campaign in Palo Alto, California, fluoridation supporter John Mueller reports that

> "The campaign was especially noteworthy for the continual sarcastic attacks made by the pros at the antis and at their authority. This was intended to discredit anything the antis said by discrediting the antis themselves – a technique which appears to be considerably more successful than point-by-point refutation of the anti arguments. In addition, fear of ridicule helped keep 'respectable' members of the community from joining the anti forces." [361]

We can see here one reason *why* people are abusive – it works. Fear of ridicule probably prevents many from participating. Tribal leaders don't want to lose their leadership or be ostracized. Leadership has obvious perks.

Mueller's observation is noteworthy given that experts consistently claim to be scientific and objective. Experts claim it is those people *opposed* to fluoridation who are emotional, not the experts. Yet "fear of ridicule" *is* an emotional thing.

Proud people don't like to admit that they're scared. Just like confidence in expert claims of current science, fear of ridicule is expressed by conforming to the status quo, and therefore is nearly impossible to detect from the outside.

It is sensible to consider one of Dr. Richard Smith's statements here:

> "It may be that some non-financial conflicts of interest may have more powerful effects than financial conflicts, but they are hard to pin down and define." [362]

Smith was editor of the **British Medical Journal** for 25 years. In many instances it is probably easier to monitor financial conflicts of interest, and it makes sense that we should base conflict of interest policies on things we have sound evidence on. Is wanting to be a respectable member of society, the inclination whether blatant or subtle to tow the line, to get that promotion, to not rock the boat, a conflict of interest?

What about the opposite? The desire to stand out, be a bit different, or be seen as more of a fighter, more sceptical than anyone else...?

Including this section on abuse in a book about a nutritional role for fluorine is justified, as abuse functions as "flak" in the sense of demonstrating to experts and the public that certain experiments, conclusions and sometimes by default, the publications that include them, are "off limits" or getting close to being off limits. Given that the majority of work (that I have seen) that opposes CWF concludes fluorine non-essential in nutrition, abuse serves as a boundary for deep investigation into such claims, and therefore communication to the public is compromised.

Experts don't *need* to look into anti-fluoride publications to see the studies and experiments I have discussed in Chapter 1. These papers are discussed in expert literature as well, one just has to be diligent. Experts are quite happy to quote their favourite small portions of this literature it seems, provided it does not disrupt the promotional aspects of CWF.

Activists can be just as abusive as politicians and health professionals. I can remember a couple of examples from the February 2017 submissions here in Wellington. However, the abuse of activists is far less likely to be printed in a peer-reviewed academic journal, or in a newspaper headline.

There are a couple of trends I've noticed in newspapers. Abusive headlines are aimed more frequently towards people opposed to fluoridation. I have seen only a couple towards people who support it.

Both sides will be abusive in the small print, the text, the letters they write.

Abusive headlines give the appearance that the newspaper is abusing those opposed, yet in reading the article we see that it is often a medical expert who is doing the abusing. I have only seen a handful of newspaper *headlines* that are abusive to the supporters of fluoridation. There are some that are titled with a victim role: *Fluoridation of Water a Trampling of our Rights* is one example. This article by Tom O'Connor invokes the Bill of Rights, that suggests we can "... refuse to undergo any medical treatment..." [363] of course, we all know how to argue our way out of that one...

But this headline isn't really abuse – it's not the same as calling someone stupid or crazy. It actually suggests power, something that may be positive, or may engender fear. So in this sense, it may work in the opposite way. There is an attraction to siding with the more powerful in a confrontation or competition, just as there is an attraction to siding with the underdog.

Fluoridation of community water supplies began in America in 1945. An investigation of fluoridation is lacking without a discussion or at least an attempt to seek some knowledge of the political climate of America in that time period.

Both experts and activists from New Zealand were heavily influenced by Americans. This is evidenced by personal letters, letters to editors and articles which are available in New Zealand media and Health Department archives. The fluoridation debate was like our own "mini-America" in this part of the world. This American influence probably altered how New Zealanders would have approached fluoridation if left to their own devices, but this is difficult to tell.

Abuse from people involved with fluoridation in some instances intimidated and threatened councilors. That both sides of the debate were abusive helped to cause standstills, and (in my opinion, though this is hard to tell with precision) make journalists and legislators less likely to speak and write honestly in public on the issue, though some took a brave stand on either side, or for the right to change their mind.

The 1990 article mentioned earlier claimed:

"For years journalists have dodged fluoride issues, partly because they thought it was boring and partly because of the loony mail that was always bound to follow any article." [352]

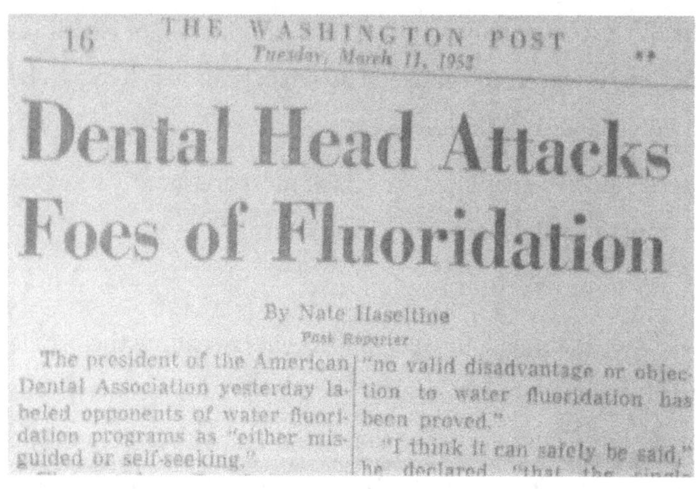

Practical New Zealand journalists probably sniffed the polarizing likeness to McCarthyism, and found themselves under some sort of emotional coercion regardless of who they interviewed. This is my opinion based on the research in this book and the archives used to obtain many of the media articles. I wonder if all of them saw so much of the American research and arguments just played out over here, the same old things in the same old ways.

Figure 26. Dental Head Attacks Foes of Fluoridation. **The Washington Post**, 11th March, 1952.

The following section looks at headlines. I believe they have an impact, or did in the past. First I will show articles with headlines abusive to people opposed (**Figures 26** to **37**). Later I will show articles with headlines abusive to people who support CWF.

Abuse and abusive headlines worked *for* promoters of fluoridation in that they helped minimize opposition to the programs, scaring the more timid or cautious among people opposed, or others – maybe some city officials, some medical professionals, who were uncertain or more sceptical about it, or people who just wanted to wait until they knew more.

Figure 27. Doctors Hit Opposition 'Crackpots'. **Orlando Evening Star** (Florida), p. 1, 19th April, 1955.

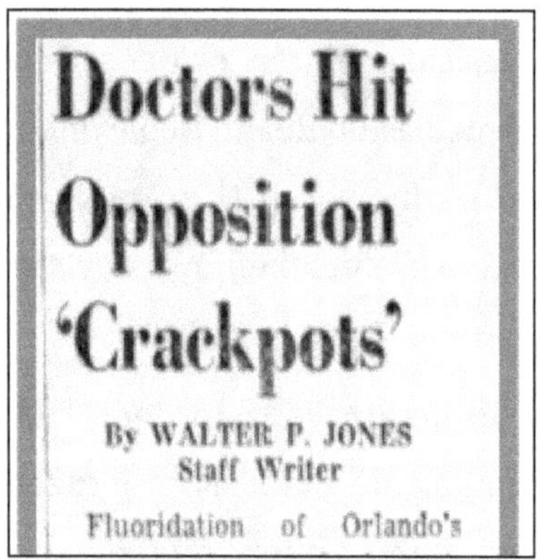

Figure 28. Fluoridation Foes Fear Things They Just Don't Understand, Says Dentist. **Janesville Daily Gazette** (Wisconsin) p. 20, 2nd May, 1957.

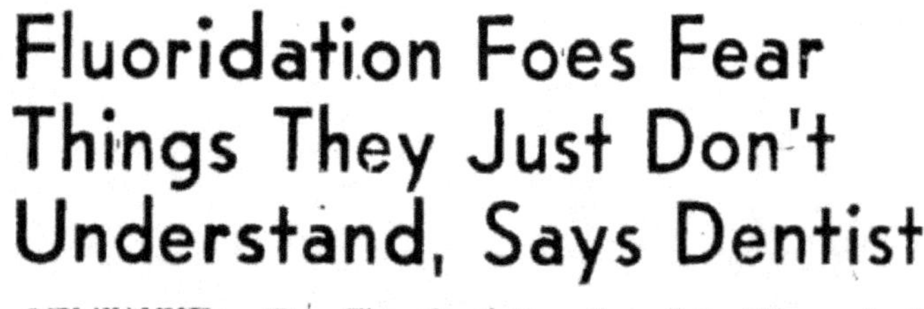

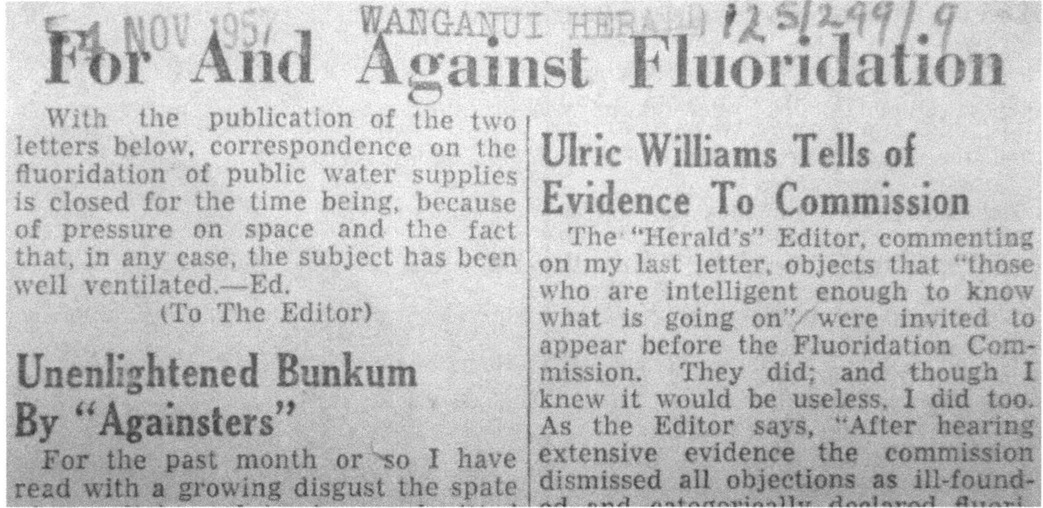

For And Against Fluoridation

With the publication of the two letters below, correspondence on the fluoridation of public water supplies is closed for the time being, because of pressure on space and the fact that, in any case, the subject has been well ventilated.—Ed.

(To The Editor)

Unenlightened Bunkum By "Againsters"

For the past month or so I have read with a growing disgust the spate

Ulric Williams Tells of Evidence To Commission

The "Herald's" Editor, commenting on my last letter, objects that "those who are intelligent enough to know what is going on" were invited to appear before the Fluoridation Commission. They did; and though I knew it would be useless, I did too. As the Editor says, "After hearing extensive evidence the commission dismissed all objections as ill-found-

Figure 29. For and Against Fluoridation. **Wanganui Herald**, 4ᵗʰ November, 1957.

Many of these articles are very old. I argue that headlines like these have affected the approach to CWF in many subtle ways. If you ever wondered why fluoridation was such a political issue [364], **Figure 30** may help. It discussed a resolution that

"urged dentists to use their influence as citizens to replace officials who continue to block fluoridation." [365]

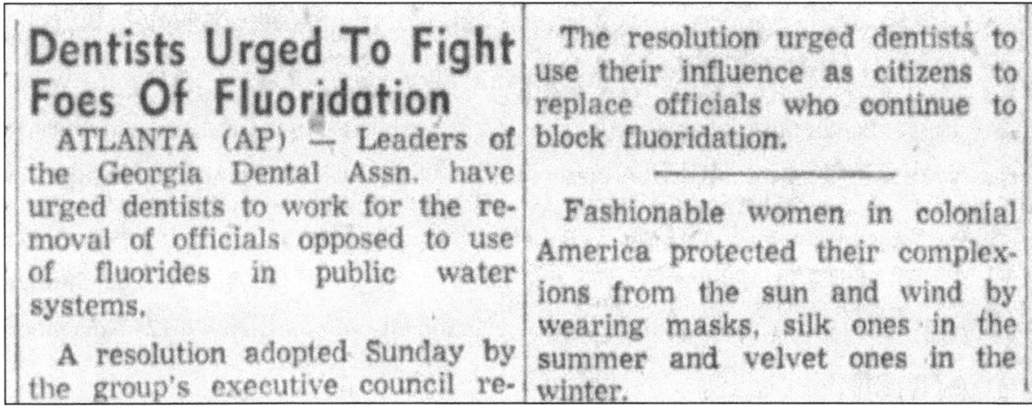

Dentists Urged To Fight Foes Of Fluoridation

ATLANTA (AP) — Leaders of the Georgia Dental Assn. have urged dentists to work for the removal of officials opposed to use of fluorides in public water systems.

A resolution adopted Sunday by the group's executive council re-

The resolution urged dentists to use their influence as citizens to replace officials who continue to block fluoridation.

Fashionable women in colonial America protected their complexions from the sun and wind by wearing masks, silk ones in the summer and velvet ones in the winter.

Figure 30. Dentists Urged to Fight Foes of Fluoridation. **Stevens Point Journal** (Stevens Point, Wisconsin), p. 12, 26ᵗʰ October, 1959 [365].

This may help us to understand the unanimity of public health officials regarding fluoridation programs. Compare this with a recent claim made on one of the Making Sense of Fluoride web pages, that

"No one here is stopping anyone to vote it [fluoridation] out." [366]

One can see that the actions of the Georgia Dental Association (**Figure 30**) were precisely what would stop people from voting it out. This is a less than perfect comparison because of the time gap, yet it is an interesting piece of history.

Three years later in 1962, the **Journal of the American Dental Association** ran an article in the November issue authored by John Chrietzberg, Director of the Branch of Dental Health at the State of Georgia Department of Public Health. Chrietzberg claimed out of 11 referendums for fluoridation in Georgia, all 11 had been won by the supporters. The article focused on policies of Georgia's health department. It claimed:

"No effort is made to denounce publicly individuals who oppose fluoridation." [367]

The resolution for the removal of officials opposed was not discussed.

Dr. Walter C. Kraatz, Professor Emeritus of Biology with 35 years experience wrote the letter, *Fluoridation Foes Ignore Facts* (**Figure 31**). One argument he makes is discussed a little in the next chapter.

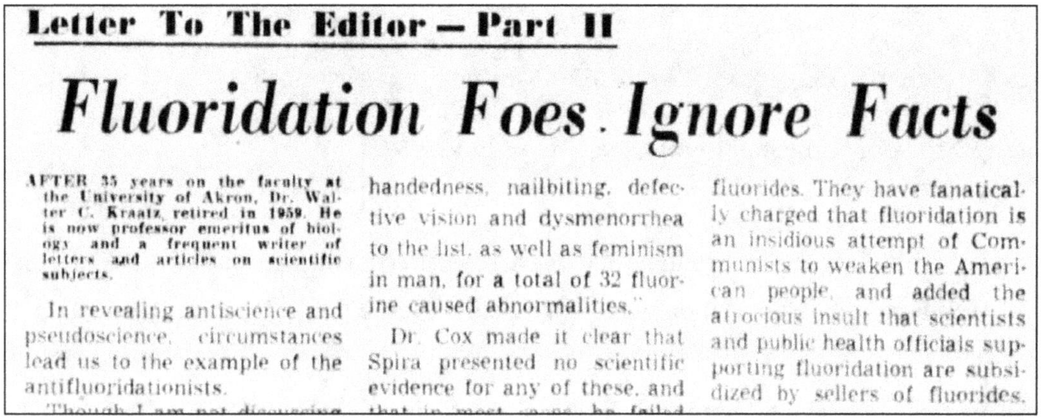

Letter To The Editor — Part II

Fluoridation Foes . Ignore Facts

AFTER 35 years on the faculty at the University of Akron, Dr. Walter C. Kraatz, retired in 1959. He is now professor emeritus of biology and a frequent writer of letters and articles on scientific subjects.

In revealing antiscience and pseudoscience, circumstances lead us to the example of the antifluoridationists.

handedness, nailbiting, defective vision and dysmenorrhea to the list, as well as feminism in man, for a total of 32 fluorine caused abnormalities."

Dr. Cox made it clear that Spira presented no scientific evidence for any of these, and

fluorides. They have fanatically charged that fluoridation is an insidious attempt of Communists to weaken the American people, and added the atrocious insult that scientists and public health officials supporting fluoridation are subsidized by sellers of fluorides.

Figure 31.

Fluoridation Foes Ignore Facts, **The Akron Beacon Journal** (Akron, Ohio), p. 6, 23rd September, 1961 [368].

In the very small article (**Figure 32**) Dr. Fredrick Stare claimed that proponents of CWF "will have to stand up to personal abuses from an odd assortment of food nuts, organic gardeners, John Birchers, pure water enthusiasts and others whose comic chemistry transcends common sense". He claimed that the evidence in favour of CWF was "massive" enough that people who oppose the measure were "misinformed, stupid or dishonest."

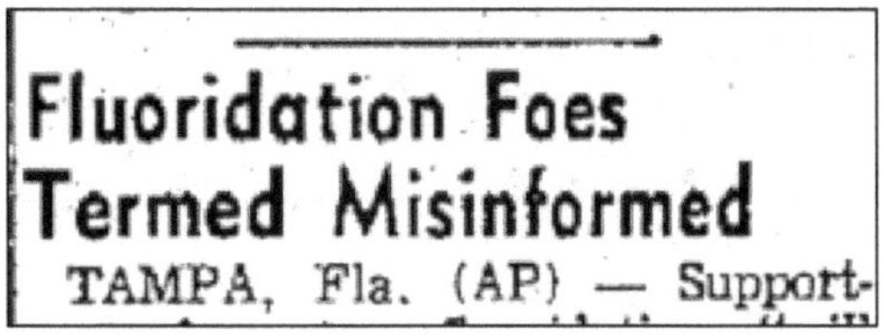

Fluoridation Foes Termed Misinformed

TAMPA, Fla. (AP) — Support-

Figure 32. Fluoridation Foes Termed Misinformed. **The Sunday News and Tribune** (Jefferson City, Missouri), p. 17, 12th November, 1961.

Dr. Fredrick Stare also featured in **Figure 33**. I have cut out the middle.

In This Corner

Why Opposition to Fluoride Is Illogical

(The author of this article has been professor of public health at Harvard University since 1945. This article is reprinted from the March issue of New Medical Materia.)

By FREDRICK J. STARE, Ph.D., M.D.

status.

Our National Academy of Science, recognized as the pinnacle of the nation's scientific community, had this to say about fluoridation in 1958:

"The practice of adding fluoride to water supplies at the rate of 1 part per million is highly desirable as a public health practice in areas where the content of fluoride in natural water

A MINERAL NUTRIENT

Fluoride is a mineral nutrient, not a drug nor a medicine. By fluoridation, one is not treating a disease, but merely adjusting the composition of this nutrient —which, in the food and the waters of many parts of our country, is too low to provide us with even the small amount we need to build and maintain

health societies; and others of similar standing in the field of hea

Figure 33. *Why Opposition to Fluoride is Illogical.* **Argus-Leader** (Sioux Falls, South Dakota), p. 4, 13th March, 1962.

The editor's note in **Figure 34** claimed:

> "This is the first of three special articles about the 18 years of successful experience with the adjustment [sic] of fluoride content of public water supplies in Grand Rapids, Michigan. The author of the series of articles has been a staff writer of the Grand Rapids Press for 37 years."

The article began:

> "Anyone who opposes the fluoridation of public water supplies for the promotion of dental health is considered a 'crackpot' in Grand Rapids."

AFTER 18 YEARS OF SUCCESS:

Opponents of Water Fluoridation Called 'Crackpots' in Michigan

(EDITOR'S NOTE: This is fully discussed by city officials fact, or at least they were suffic- able and willing to dispel misin

Figure 34. *Opponents of Water Fluoridation Called 'Crackpots' in Michigan.* B. G. (Bill) Brown, **The Daily Journal** (Vineland, New Jersey), p. 7, 12th March, 1963.

The "emotional primitives" claim (**Figure 35**) was attributed to Dr. Hillenbrand of the American Dental Association. He was the ADA's journal assistant, then full editor from 1942 to 1945. According to the **Chicago Tribune**,

> "From 1938 to 1951, he was also associate professor of ethics and social relations at the Loyola dental school." [369]

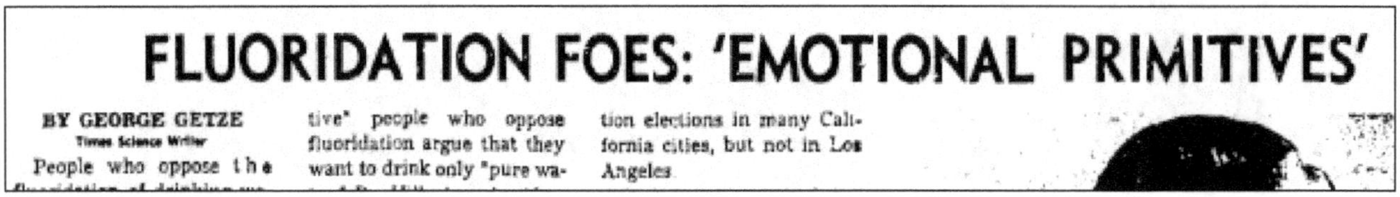

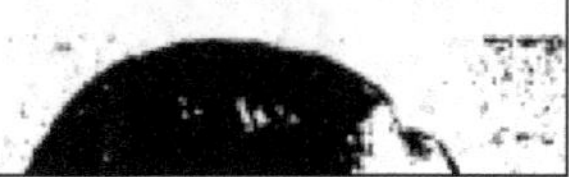

FLUORIDATION FOES: 'EMOTIONAL PRIMITIVES'

BY GEORGE GETZE
Times Science Writer

People who oppose t h e

tive" people who oppose fluoridation argue that they want to drink only "pure wa-

tion elections in many California cities, but not in Los Angeles.

Figure 35. *Fluoridation Foes: 'Emotional Primitives'.* **The Los Angeles Times**, p. 31, 11th May, 1965.

Similar criticism occurred in Wanganui (now Whanganui), New Zealand, where the townspeople were deemed 'backward thinking' by the district medical officer Dr P. M. Allingham for not having CWF (**Figure 36**).

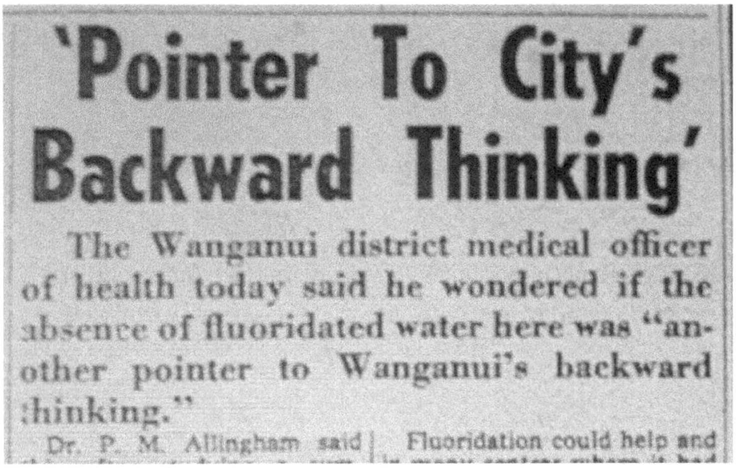

'Pointer To City's Backward Thinking'

The Wanganui district medical officer of health today said he wondered if the absence of fluoridated water here was "another pointer to Wanganui's backward thinking."

Dr. P. M. Allingham said   Fluoridation could help and

Figure 36. *Pointer to City's Backward Thinking.* **The Wanganui Herald**, Vol. 101, No. 30,596, 26th September, 1967.

The article featuring Dr. Fredrick Stare of Harvard was discussed in Chapter 5.2. It recommended reading the book *The Tooth Robbers* by Dr. Stephen Barrett and Dr. Sheldon Rovin. The "criminal" actions were simply to oppose fluoridation (**Figure 37**).

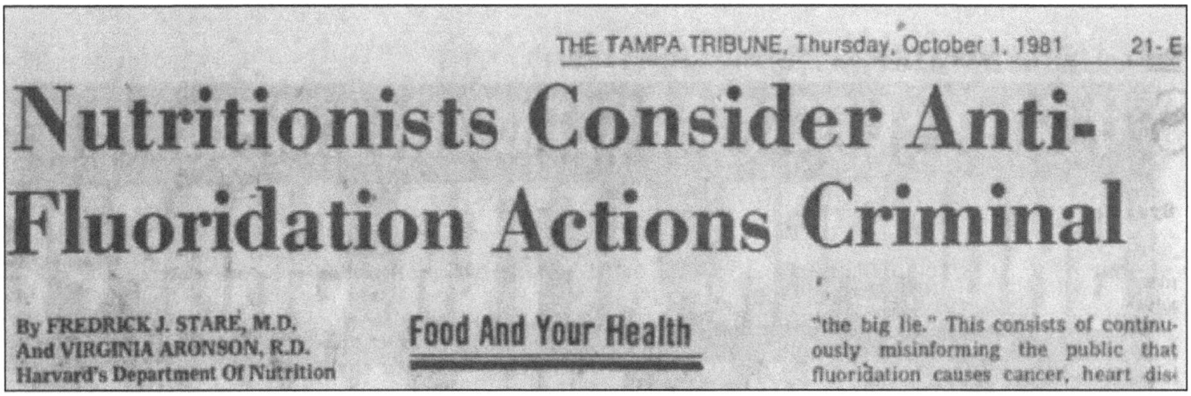

THE TAMPA TRIBUNE, Thursday, October 1, 1981   21-E

Nutritionists Consider Anti-Fluoridation Actions Criminal

By FREDRICK J. STARE, M.D.
And VIRGINIA ARONSON, R.D.
Harvard's Department Of Nutrition

Food And Your Health

"the big lie." This consists of continuously misinforming the public that fluoridation causes cancer, heart dis-

Figure 37. *Nutritionists Consider Anti-Fluoridation Actions Criminal.* **The Tampa Tribune** (Florida), p. 21-E, 1st October, 1981 [290].

The reader may feel that sometimes a debate, or discussion could help. **Figure 38** discusses an occasion where Dr. Kaylan Worley (for CWF) and Dr. John Yiamouyiannis (against) had such a debate. The article helps us to understand why journalists and city councilors have been averse to participating in these debates:

"From the outset the debate was drowned in mudslinging, catcalls, rudeness, slanderous remarks and general disorder. Neither side was able to present a clear-cut argument because on a number of occasions the speakers were hooted down by the crowd."

Worley's approach was taken from a page out of Mueller's book:

"Worley built his argument around the theme: 'Who do you trust?' Then he immediately set out to discredit the speaker for the opponents of fluoridation."

Yiamouyiannis came out no better:

"Although the debaters started out being nasty with each other, later in the debate it became worse. There was so much shouting and howling and yelling that even the speakers at times seemed to forget which side they were on."

"Apparently Guin's recitation of fluoridation supporters touched a nerve among the anti-fluoridationists as Yiamouyiannis rushed to the microphone and tried to stop Guin from completing his statement."

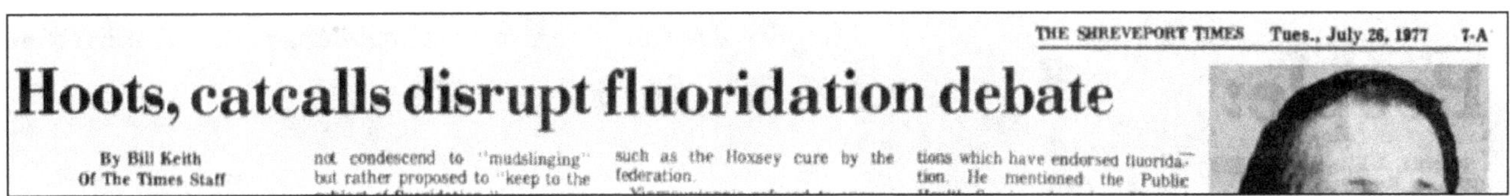

Figure 38. Hoots, catcalls disrupt fluoridation debate. Bill Keith, **The Shreveport Times**, p. 7-A, 26th July, 1977.

Figure 39 and above demonstrate some abusive headlines in the opposite direction. It appears that those opposed to CWF were more likely to threaten violent action against councillors in the earlier days. This behavior has obviously worked against them, helping others justify labelling *all* opponents as crazy, something that worked, according to John Mueller [361]. It also appears that the threats mentioned here were never acted upon.

Figure 39 discussed how four city officials were threatened with business boycotts and violence in "numerous anonymous callers". The number of phone calls was not mentioned in the article. The city was going to go ahead with the plans to fluoridate anyway (with councillors voting four to three), though a petition was to be put up for vote in November of the following year.

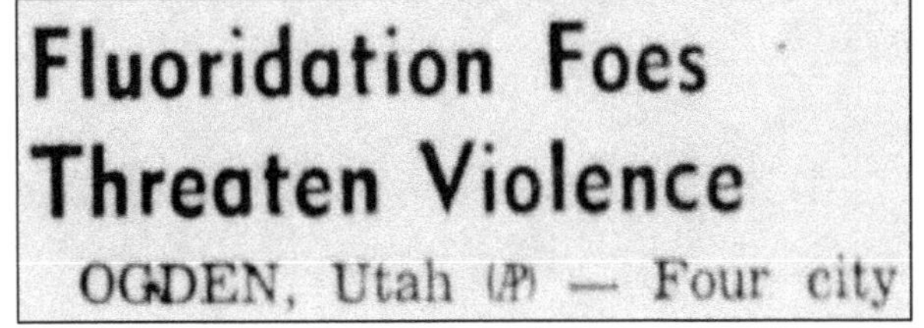

Figure 39. Fluoridation Foes Threaten Violence. **The La Crosse Tribune** (Wisconsin), p. 15, 15th May, 1958.

The "threats" in the letters mentioned in **Figure 40** were simply that people opposed to fluoridation would not vote for the councillors if they did not stop the fluoridation program.

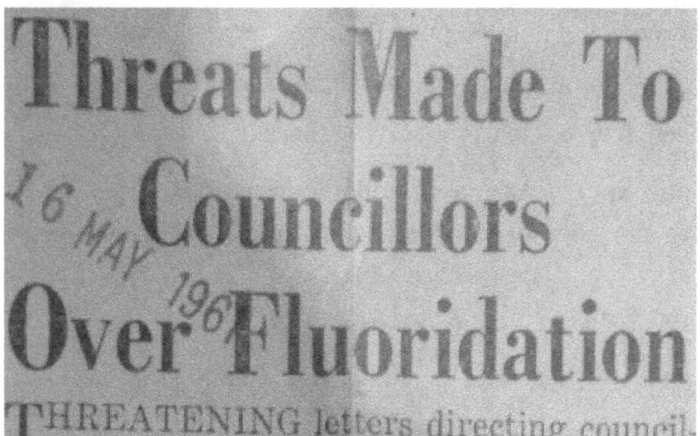

Figure 40 clipping:

Threats Made To Councillors Over Fluoridation

THREATENING letters directing councillors how to vote on the fluoridation issue were produced at last night's meeting of the Lower Hutt City Council.

Nearly every councillor received several letters saying if they did not vote to have fluoride removed from the city water supply they would not be voted for in the next municipal elections.

Far from being swayed by the threats councillors decided by a 10-4 majority to keep fluoride in the city ...

Figure 40. Threats Made to Councillors Over Fluoridation. **The Evening Post** (Wellington), 16th May, 1961.

Three more serious cases can be given.

The threat in **Figure 41** was from a man the councillor knew. He said,

"Remember you are in business... I assure you that if you proceed with this attitude your business will be affected."

The threat was not aimed at harming her person. The article did not state what line of business she was in, or how the caller proposed to affect it.

Figure 41 clipping:

FLUORIDATION ISSUE

Phone Threat To Woman Councillor

TAURANGA, Today (PA).—The business interests of Tauranga's only woman borough councillor have been threatened following her support for fluoridating the borough water supply. She knew he was associat...

Figure 41. Phone Threat To Woman Councillor. **The Evening Post**, 24th December, 1962.

The anonymous threats mentioned in **Figure 41** were on three postcards to separate councillors, all from the same person. The matter was handed to the C.I.B. and the person was warned.

Figure 42 clipping:

Anonymous Threats To Councillors Over Fluoridation

GISBORNE, Today (PA).—Police are investigating anonymous postcards using threats against the Gisborne City Council's plan to fluoridate the city's water supply.

The postcards, warning of the possible "unpleasant consequences" if the decision to ... had obviously originated from the same person and had been posted in Gisborne. "The writer is warned that the consequences could be serious if these postcards ...

Figure 42. Anonymous Threats To Councillors Over Fluoridation. **The Evening Post**, 21st January, 1965.

Letter Threat To Poison Councillors

DUNEDIN, Today (PA).—Three unnamed members of the City Council have been threatened with death by slow poisoning if the council fluoridates the city water supply.

The water and baths committee, which considered a letter on Monday, is not very perturbed about the threat, having noted the contents.

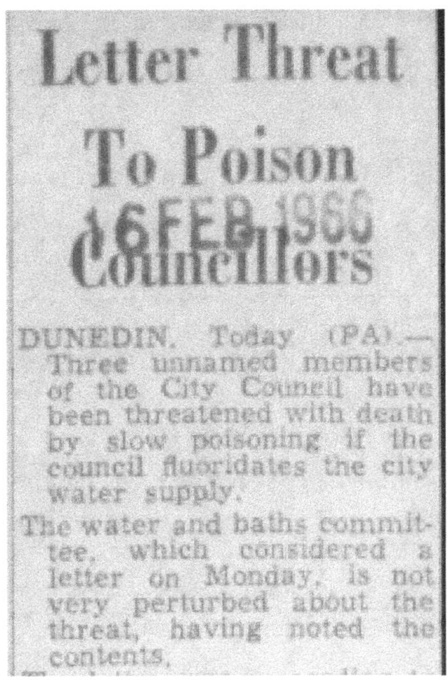

Regarding the threat to poison the Dunedin councillors (**Figure 43**), the police expressed the view that there were a few people who did that sort of thing and they had a decent idea of who it was. Tracking them down was not said to be difficult, as the letter was hand-written. I don't believe there was anything more than a warning from police done about it because it was the only **Evening Post** article I found from 1966.

Figure 43. *Letter Threat To Poison Councillors.* **The Evening Post**, 16th February, 1966.

One other thing was a real arrogance from some of the DHB people and scientists . . . We felt they were treating us as a bunch of morons.

Dave McPherson, Central Hawkes Bay councillor

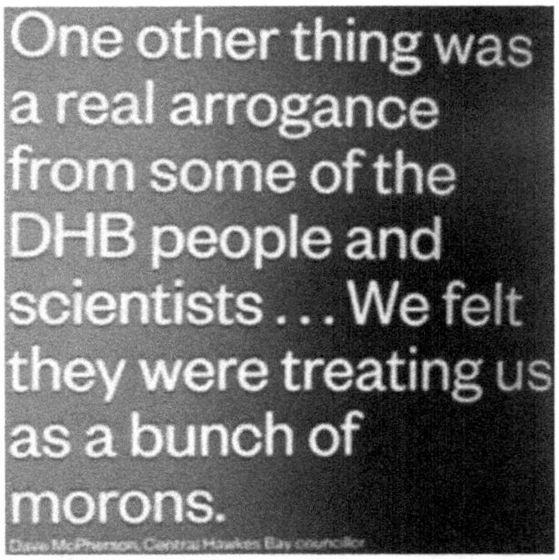

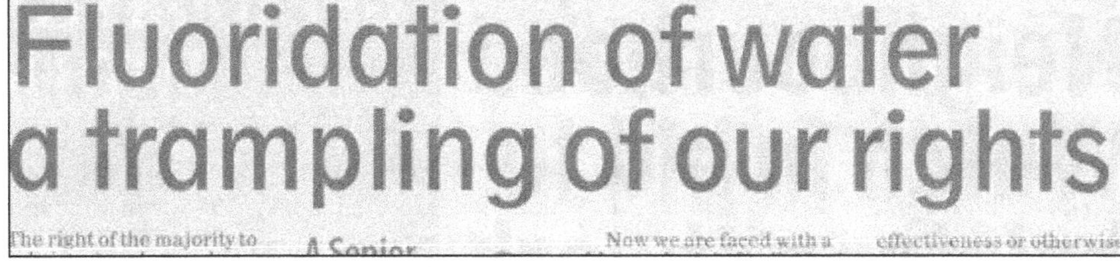

The picture from a recent article in the New Zealand Herald (**Figure 44**) quotes Councillor Dave McPherson, and blows up his comment almost to the size of a headline. The difference in Cr. McPherson's statement is that it is attributed to him, which makes it *his* fact. Normally the media does not attribute the abusive headlines to anyone until we read the small print (one exception is the Whanganui article), which makes it look a little like everyone agrees with it. It appears as a piece of common knowledge, at least at first.

Figure 44. **NZ Herald**, 6th July, 2013.

The headline of Tom O'Connor's article [363] mentioned earlier is shown (**Figure 45**).

Fluoridation of water a trampling of our rights

The right of the majority to ... A Senior ... Now we are faced with a ... effectiveness or otherwise

Figure 45. *Fluoridation of water a trampling of our rights.* **Timaru Courier**, 26th May, 2016.

The topic of abuse is muddied by two things: people opposed to fluoridation consider the very act of CWF a form of abuse, and people who support CWF consider opposition to CWF a form of abuse. When you're on a side, the mere existence of the other side is a form of abuse.

The reader is invited to consider abuse as a 'resource' as expressed in Professor Brian Martin's paper *Analyzing the Fluoridation Controversy: Resources and Structures* [370]. Given that the media are willing to print and even participate in public abuse [350], this may be appropriate.

Abuse from a position of privilege and prestige would obviously have more value as a resource than abuse from no position or little social status.

Nowadays, social and other media have allowed people opposed to fluoridation to voice and vent abuse, just like their counterparts have in the media. The experts can tell us that this is unfair, it's not supposed to happen. For instance, one group of experts has said:

> "Our experience has been that the opponents of fluoridation prefer to indulge in criticisms through the media, pseudojournals, and social media. They also engage in individual attacks in their criticisms of the work. These would be considered libellous in a more litigious society." [371]

The article does not mention the fact that experts have also been very abusive. This demonstrates that there is some ignorance of history here. It may be argued that experts have *encouraged* abuse in some instances[87]; for example if we consider propagandizing people to be abusive, even if it's for their own good (see Chapter 5.4), if we consider the statement of John E. Mueller at the beginning of this chapter, and if we consider dismissing people's arguments abusive, though maybe these are grey areas. It's in some ways a matter of perspective, people opposed to CWF find the experts' reluctance to debate offensive, while experts find opposition, and the desire to debate offensive.

The reader will remember Dr. Michael Easley's comment from the start of this chapter, calling opponents of fluoridation "parasites". Hilariously, the *next* sentence in Dr. Easley's article is:

> "It is impossible to compete against opponents without appearing to discredit them personally." [351]

Experts bemoan the fact that people opposed to fluoridation go online to learn about and discuss the subject, which basically makes it a free-for-all. Experts correctly point out that people are very abusive online, but don't seem to understand that if online is the only place one can speak or write or televise freely for a good few hours, one will go there. In the 1950s the New Zealand Health Department held meetings to get around the media's need to show both sides. It is certainly easier for people to advance goals and ideas in a place without constant criticism and rebuking.

---

[87] An exception to this is Muhler's book with Hine, cited in Chapter 1.2. "One cannot... condemn such honest individuals [anti-CWF], or communities who choose to regard fluoridation as 'crackpot,' for America has remained steadfast as a nation where such individuals can voice objections to personal intervention without retaliation." Fuller's piece in the January, 1956 **New Zealand Dental Journal** cited at the end of Chapter 4 is similar: "Do not question the sincerity of opponents of fluoridation, or call them 'crackpots,' and do not question their right to express their views." Fuller was a Colonel in the NZ Army. Upon his death **The Evening Post** wrote that "Fuller came home dismayed by the state of New Zealand soldiers' teeth – 50% wore dentures..." *Dentist battled to fluoridate water supply*, p. 5, 15th March, 2001. Fuller played a chief role in the New Zealand 1957 Commission of Inquiry.

While the experts are derogatory and openly abusive and sneering towards the opponents of fluoridation, they are *not* abusive towards the junk food industry, and the people who sell sugar-laden products.

In Chapter 5.2 I mentioned that the food industry in America spent about $3 billion on advertising in 1978 alone, and while I don't know how much of that was spent on *junk* food, soft drink or confectionary specifically, we know that the experts get up in arms with the people opposed to fluoridation spending "a few thousand" [372] of their own dollars, on their own advertising.

The experts *criticize* the junk-food industry as a threat to dental health, but I've never seen them be openly abusive to CEOs of junk-food companies, or call their advertising "misleading propaganda" even though it basically is – the message is that an ice cream, a chocolate bar, will be of some wonderful benefit to my life, or a fizzy drink will make me popular. In the thousands of media articles I've read on fluoridation I've never seen any dental expert sneering and name-calling big junk-food businesses. Perhaps such behavior wouldn't work against people with real power, and the anti-fluoride people are an easy target. When push comes to shove, the sugar industry, like the experts, has some real clout [223, 224]. Is the thought of abusing junk-food advertisers ridiculous? Personally I don't think the discussion around fluoridation is helped by abuse. In that sense, yes, it is ridiculous. Yet experts do ridicule relatively powerless individuals and citizens, but *not* mega-corporations.

While minority groups opposed to fluoridation can protest and hire a mail drop or print flyers, in terms of their ability to advertise in mainstream media, they're extremely limited. Yet when they do save up enough money to raise their voice in the public media, it is much less welcomed than junk-food salesmanship. Perhaps simply changing things is one of our fears. Better the devil you know.

I suggest there are too many revolving doors in science, industry and business nowadays for experts to abuse the junk-food industry. It would probably seem very unprofessional as well. After all, it's difficult to call the junk food industry "anti-science". Just consider Coca-Cola has (or had) a Beverage Institute for Health and Wellness ("there's no need to stick to plain water if it bores you") [217]. There has been little protest that they have or had this Institute, considering what they sell and the amount of plastic they sell it in. A recent article in **The Guardian** claimed that by 2050 the plastic crisis would be as bad as climate change [373]. Is that a threat to public health?

A point was made by Dr. Carrie Barber in the 2013 Google Hangout organized by Waikato University [1]. In response to the question about encouraging critical thinking, she said each side could listen to the other, which was difficult, but necessary. It seems fitting that finding truth has something to do with leaving no stone unturned, or no barnacle unturned, using Darwin as example. This does not only involve trekking through old archives and reading studies, or spending hours in the echo chambers of the internet [374], it must also involve listening to others, or reading the work of others… even (or perhaps especially) the work of those with whom we disagree. This is a good point many of us would think… but it's in total violation of one of the key principles of fluoridation, which is that we don't *need* to listen to the arguments given by the people on the other side [357].

There are egos and elitism on both sides. People on each side ought to be careful about becoming exactly what they despise in the others – totally dogmatic and without empathy.

I have read an enormous amount of abuse in this investigation – remember there are snide comments in article bodies, not only headlines. I think the headlines have more of an "instant shock" factor. For a long time I thought the "as bad as child molesters" [352] was the worst accusation I had found, but that's not the worst. Perhaps the threats are the worst, though they're not all of violence. "We won't vote for you" is hardly a threat, coming from people considered to be a minority. The poisoning threat was not really taken seriously; the newspaper had no follow-up article I saw. I'm very happy this, and any other threats never materialized, to my knowledge. But they do demonstrate that the people opposed felt ignored, marginalized, pushed to the edges. Yet herein lies a painful catch-22: when politicians and councillors *do* listen patiently, they end up abused by the *supporters* of fluoridation! Called "anti-science" etc, publicly defamed and shamed, even if they knew nothing about the matter beforehand. Even if they felt it their duty as elected officials, to treat it with the same concern, equanimity and impartiality as they would treat *any* issue.

The most abusive thing I found in my opinion was the public ignoring of the experiments that concluded fluorine non-essential. The work of Armstrong *et al.* and Schwarz got into the papers, it was discussed more in the public eye. McClendon's work was at least discussed in *some* of the scientific literature, if not publicly. The work of others, Maurer and Day, Wuthier and Phillips, Doberenz *et al.*, Weber and Reid, the two 1976 experiments, were almost completely ignored, except for the NAS publications and a few others. But as demonstrated, the experts just picked the publication wherein benefit was the criterion for essentiality, and publicized *that* claim.

This is abusive to science itself, it's abusive to the mums and dads who think their children need fluorine more than they really do, and it's abusive to researchers and readers like you and me. It's unfair on the city councillors and the honest legislators who don't care for upholding a 'pro' or 'anti' position and just want to do the best job they can. If you ask me about the experiments that concluded fluorine essential, I can talk about what so-and-so said in which article, what this or that scientist claimed, which newspapers they were in, yet if you ask me about the experiments that concluded fluorine non-essential, I can't really give as much information and comment from other scientists at the time. I can't talk about them as much because the amount of knowledge available on them is so sparse, other than Schwarz's "rather sophisticated" comment regarding a couple of experiments, and maybe a statement or two from Dr. Muhler. I can tell you what *my* point of view is, but there's no authority or prestige or consensus through popularity and awareness for me to fall back on.

All of us have our collective available knowledge weakened because of this one decisive partiality.

5.6 Are There any Industrial or Financial Motivations for Entrenching Fluorine's Role in Public Health?

"The greater the financial and other interests and prejudices in a scientific field, the less likely the research findings are to be true."

- Professor John P. A. Ioannidis[88], *Why Most Published Researched Findings are False*, (2005). **Public Library of Science Medicine**, 2(8): e124.

"The scientists researching the effectiveness of water fluoridation as well as health officials and dentists do not receive money from sugar, aluminium or any other companies for their research or opinions."

- Professor Jason M. Armfield[89], Debate: When public action undermines public health: a critical examination of antifluoridationist literature, **Australia and New Zealand Health Policy**, 2007, 4: 25, p. 11.

"The Procter and Gamble company of Cincinnati, Ohio, has given more than $200,000 to help finance the Indiana University (IU) fluoride research. The company is now test marketing a new toothpaste, called "Crest," which contains tin fluoride. Under a contract with Procter and Gamble, the IU Foundation is to receive royalties from the sale of the toothpaste."

- Tin Fluoride Best for Tooth Decay, **The Republic** (Columbus, Indiana), p. 7, 19th November, 1955.

"There will be no material on any of our programs which could in any way further the concept of business as cold, ruthless, and lacking all sentiment or spiritual motivation."

- Procter & Gamble, 1965 formal requirement to the Federal Communications Commission, quoted in Ben Bagdikian's *The Media Monopoly*, 1982. A current list of Proctor & Gamble owned companies can be found at https://us.pg.com/our-brands. They include Gilette, Oral B and Crest.

"The twentieth century has been characterized by three developments of great political importance: the growth of democracy, the growth of corporate power, and the growth of corporate propaganda as a means of protecting corporate power against democracy."

"It is arguable that the success of business propaganda in persuading us, for so long, that we are free from propaganda is one of the most significant propaganda achievements of the twentieth century."

- Alex Carey, *Taking the Risk out of Democracy*, Closing the American Mind: The Early Years, p. 18, 1995.

---

[88] Department of Hygiene and Epidemiology, University of Ioannina School of Medicine, Ioannina, Greece, and Institute for Clinical Research and Health Policy Studies, Department of Medicine, Tufts-New England Medical Center, Tufts University School of Medicine, Boston, Massachusetts.
[89] Australian Research Centre for Population Oral Health, School of Dentistry, University of Adelaide, South Australia.

In my opinion the insistence of a nutritional role from the majority of experts has had more to do with refuting the "mass medication" argument and instilling citizen confidence in experts rather than in ensuring any industry achieved their legal or political goals. Yet industries have had legal and political goals, and it would be foolish to deny their influence simply because experts are not focused on this.

Studying this topic has been very difficult. I can say confidently there are *incentives* for industry to influence science in industry's favour, but this of course does not prove or even suggest that someone has done such a thing.

This topic of a nutritional role for fluorine is a topic in which so many experts have espoused views publicly that are almost totally opposite to experimental evidence. We are asked to believe that university training gives people the ability to always pick truth over profit, truth over popularity, truth over any conflict of interest or bias. Yet on this issue of a nutritional role for fluorine, simply by comparing scientific with expert media statements we see scientific statements compromised.

One wonders when honest mistakes, bias and conflicts of interest become acceptable suggestions, even if made gently, tentatively and without grandeur, or without the suggestion that scientists or anyone else involved *wants* to deceive.

This chapter gives examples of some of the ways in which experts disavow any industry bias or conflict of interest. If there are ways in which experts help industry, this is surely one. Another is in making a refusal to look at the topic socially acceptable.

In tracking down more about the entire topic of fluorine's essentiality I was fascinated and a little disappointed by the infrequency of mentions McClendon's work received. I searched for the Aluminum Company of America (Alcoa/ALCOA), the Lever Brothers, Indiana University and some of the other organizations that I thought may have influenced the direction of research. I found a lot of newspaper articles discussing lawsuits directed toward ALCOA and many other aluminium and metal companies as a result of fluoride and sulfur dioxide pollution, with a couple mentioning research grants. In reading an environmental law professor's 1970s work, I found many corporations responsible for fluoride pollution had paid scientists to come to their defence in the courts.

These lawsuits were rarely mentioned in scientific literature.

I suspected that the McClendon experiments were carried out as a result of these lawsuits. I thought this may explain why his work was almost never trumpeted by experts in the 1950s and 1960s as demonstrating fluorine a necessity. I expected to find his work in the newspapers discussing fluoridation in the early years, but I did not – except for the one small article mentioned in Chapter 3.2. (There is the possibility it was mentioned but those papers are not digitized). It did not seem an unreasonable expectation considering I had found a copy of his 1954 experiment in the New Zealand Health Department archives. Neither McClendon, nor anyone else in the scientific literature commented on the lawsuits against ALCOA, from the documents I have gathered here. I've never seen this funding aspect discussed in any of the literature supportive of fluoridation I've looked at in textbooks, pamphlets, government documents and archives, newspaper clippings or reports from prestigious bodies like the World Health Organization. I have also been unable to find anything on the Lever Brothers[90] and their brief interaction with McClendon.

I had a hunch, an expectation that because his work was mentioned so sparsely in scientific literature and media, his experimentation may have been useful in helping ALCOA fight pollution lawsuits, therefore there would be no *need* for it to appear in public. I briefly looked on the Library of Congress website for archived court cases, but found none relevant.

Therefore I apologize to the reader that my investigation stopped at American court cases. These possibly contain information that I believe would be important to resolving the issue of McClendon's small amount of research, and may help to explain why it was not discussed (much, from what I can tell) in media.

It has been difficult for me to find promotional literature from the United States in the late 1940s and early 1950s. Such work could be compared with scientific claims of the time, to see if industries that were selling fluorides had kept their claims to factual information.

However the matter is complicated by the fact that experiments and their conclusions are argued over, sometimes incessantly, and sometimes for many years. Unravelling even the most obvious pieces that make up the strange tapestry of research and claims in the 1970s was not easy.

Assessing motivations is very difficult and I am cautious in casting aspersions upon the integrity of people I have never met, and who may not be alive to critique or disprove what I say. Nevertheless, a few things can be said with certainty.

One is that research over the past hundred years has become more and more corporate-funded. Some have argued this has made it more corporate-friendly [261] (and see Chapter 5.7). Such a thing is hardly a surprise – if funders did not get what they wanted from universities, funding would not continue.

Based on what I have found and seen here I am confident in stating there was at least an industrial or economic *motivation* for the introduction of fluorides to water supplies on top of the obvious desires for reductions in tooth decay. Whether *this* is a factor in the exaggeration of a nutritional role for fluorine is a very elusive thing to ask. Industry's presence is monolithic but subtle.

I requested the help of a retired environmental law professor from California who had written on this topic in the 1970s to help track down more information on McClendon, but no reply was forthcoming. Much journalism on fluoride pollution lawsuits is readily available, some is collected in Appendix 4.

---

[90] It appears they were more successful in Canada than the USA. "In 1914, the average Canadian bought 68 times as much Lever Brothers product as the average American." "In 1929 the average Canadian still bought 272% more Lever Brothers' product than the average American." See Andrew David Allan Smith, *A successful British MNE in the backyard of American big business: Explaining the performance of the American and Canadian subsidiaries of Lever Brothers 1888–1914*, **Business History**, Vol. 56, No. 2, pp. 135-160, 2014.

It appears to me that most American research on CWF has been funded by the United States Public Health Service (USPHS) and the National Institute of Dental (and now craniofacial) Research (NIDR/NIDCR). I have discussed a bias that concerns the USPHS on this topic in Chapter 2.7.

There are at least four industries that have, or have had, something to gain from a favourable image for fluorides: the phosphate and aluminium industries, both of which have in the past sold fluorides used in CWF programs. Both of these industries have had enormous problems with fluoride pollution lawsuits. A third is the toothpaste industry, which has something obvious to gain.

Finally, there is the junk-food industry. Political heat (for example, risk of advertising regulation) is taken off this industry and its products if there is a substance that can reduce tooth decay in the children this industry targets with its advertising.

It is an incredible coincidence that experts seem to provide, unintentionally, the perfect sales pitch for these industries – that fluorine is a nutritional essential. Whether experts knowingly or unknowingly aided these industries by their (experts') public claims for a nutritional role for fluorine is probably impossible to know for the most part.

The junk-food industry is the topic of the next chapter. This chapter will focus a little on the aluminium and toothpaste industries, but more so on experts and the way in which they avoid this topic of an industrial presence. This was the main reason studying this topic was difficult – there is no information on it, in literature authored by experts.

Such a circumstance falls perfectly in line with the hypothesis of the propaganda model: that the majority of expert statements are not unfavourable to those in power (industry), and that such a thing is not discussed.

In mainstream media it has long been presupposed that experts *don't* propagandize for powerful groups and interests, so such a thing need not be investigated. It is very similar to the topic of a nutritional role – presupposed is the claim that experts are objective and represent research accurately, so there is no need to investigate if such a thing is true or not.

In 1982 journalist Ben Bagdikian wrote a book which investigated the corporate ownership of American media. He summarized:

> "Many years ago, a fellowship from the John Simon Guggenheim Foundation permitted me to take a year for study of ownership patterns in the American press. That study made it clear that a transformation was in progress from a traditional family enterprise to corporate ownership." [375]

Bagdikian wrote in *The Media Monopoly* that even though there were three national networks and one thousand TV stations in 1980s America, TV programming was

> "... carefully noncontroversial, light, and non-political in order to create a 'buying mood.'" [376]

In a system where advertisers have increasing influence and control of information, science would cause undue confusion by being overly complicated, or too encouraging of a self-sufficient lifestyle. Bagdikian writes that "diversity of information" suffers as giant firms became bigger.

In 1965, Procter & Gamble[91] gave a formal requirement to the Federal Communications Commission ("as established by the medium's largest advertiser"):

"There will be no material on any of our programs which could in any way further the concept of business as cold, ruthless, and lacking all sentiment or spiritual motivation.

"If a businessman is cast in the role of villain, it must be made clear that he is not typical but is as much despised by his fellow businessmen as he is by other members of society.

"Special attention shall be given to *any* mention, however innocuous, of the grocery and drug business as well as any other group of customers of the company..." [377]

New Zealand and the USA have such a similar message in media regarding a nutritional role for fluorine (and for CWF overall). The same American experts appear in the media of both countries. New Zealanders will be interested in the Americanization of New Zealand media, discussed in Robert McChesney[92] and Edward Herman's[93] 1997 book, *The Global Media*:

"Programs were increasingly adapted to serve sponsor interest: editing cuts to allow advertising time, programs that would coordinate well with advertiser plans..."

"The news itself was gradually 'Americanized,' helped along by the importation of U.S. consultants who specialized in reshaping U.S. news formats to keep audiences watching.[94]" (page 182)

"... global media system has fundamental structural flaws that limit its service to democracy and even stand as a barrier to the development of meaningful self-government. It tends to further centralize media control in a narrow business elite, whose offerings are shaped by advertiser interests; these in turn feature entertainment, the avoidance of controversy, minimal public participation, and the erosion of the public sphere." [378] (page 189)

The authors wrote of a narrowing of choices regarding educational programming with an increase in entertainment. They mention a study by Jeanette Forbes[95] that found between 1982 and 1992 the number of programs of "documentary, news, craft, science, natural history, music" had halved, "and Māori children's programs had virtually disappeared." The only "growth sector" was cartoons, but Herman and McChesney state there was "a huge overall shrinkage of offerings to children."

According to Herman and McChesney, these changes occurred

"... to the delight of the transnational corporation community, International Monetary Fund, and neoliberal governments abroad. Its effect on the public sphere has been strongly negative, as it has replicated and even pushed beyond the model laid out in the United States." (page 183)

---

91 A current list of Proctor & Gamble owned companies can be found at https://us.pg.com/our-brands. They include Gilette, Oral B and Crest.

92 Associate Professsor of Journalism and Mass Communication, University of Wisconsin.

93 Professor of Finance at the Wharton School, Pennsylvania.

94 Herman and McChesney cite political scientist Joe Atkinson, *The "Americanisation" of One Network News*, **The Australasian Journal of American Studies**, July 1994, pp. 1-26.

95 Forbes' unpublished research is discussed in Alan Cocker's paper, *Broadcasting Myths and Political Realities: New Zealand's Experience in Comparative Perspective*, **Political Science**, Vol. 46, No. 2, pp. 234-254, 1st December, 1994.

While one can look back to the 1950s to see the American influence on the fluoridation experts in New Zealand, these occurrences in the 1980s may have helped reinforce the influence of corporations on our thinking over the last thirty or so years.

The American business community has always been conscientious in its approach to education. Corporations do not simply make consumer products and be done with it: they actively promote various values, ethics and ideas [379].

Industry's influence functions in terms of research direction – what is and is not studied. Regarding the changing of laws, such things are obviously done with minimal involvement of scientists, though there has been some excellent journalism that demonstrates industry presence in pollution regulation.

Experts obviously have some conflicts of interest involved here. One can see the amount of pride with which CWF is promoted [371]. When the topic of a nutritional role is considered in more detail than usual, one can observe at least two instances where the "antis" are correct in their claim of a non-nutritional role, and rather than accepting this, the experts deflect with the charge of "semantics". Experts don't like to be wrong.

Media and experts have a symbiotic relationship in that both groups are occasionally useful to each other. It is in the interests of media *and* experts for experts to be trusted in media, therefore it is difficult for media to remain sceptical of experts. I believe media don't like experts to be wrong because this makes experts less trusted, which would make experts less useful to media when they are called on to refute claims made by activists or dissidents. This means media have a conflict of interest in their treatment of experts.

Media have long-term relationships with nodes of power in society; this is convenient and sensible from their point of view. Trusted, or "proven" sources can be treated with less scepticism; this makes sense if there is a long-term relationship, and possible associations beyond the professional relationship. It makes sense that lesser-known sources would be treated with scepticism, as these are not as familiar to journalists or to audiences, and therefore have not demonstrated that they can be trusted. Abuse has helped take the heat off CWF for years, ensuring the journalism around the issue is shallow.

I certainly believe the experts when they claim they've not been bribed – they're not driving flash cars or living in mansions. Yet the propaganda model suggests more subtlety than mere bribes. Propaganda functions better if one is isolated in one's role, one does not need to be aware of roles others play in the dissemination of information or accumulation of research.

Previous chapters discussed the fact that experts have denied much of the science around a nutritional role that does not suit them. Studies that concluded a nutritional role for fluorine were discussed in American media. Studies that concluded fluorine non-essential, and papers and writings that refuted or were critical of experiments that concluded a nutritional role for fluorine, were treated as though they did not exist. If anyone picked up on this, the message they received was simple: conclude in the negative, and work will be largely ignored, at least in public.

Experts don't explore this in any way. In CWF it's unthought-of to suggest that experts and their understanding could be influenced by money, therefore such a thing can be refuted as ridiculous immediately. This is quite consistent throughout expert literature, making a discussion or investigation around such a topic difficult.

I would suggest that if we argue against someone who has been funded by industry, we are not only arguing against their argument, we are arguing against their professional survival. This is particularly true in a society like the USA in which there are highly competitive employment prospects and limited welfare measures.

In the biomedical sciences conflicts of interest and biases have become acknowledged as part of the academic landscape. There are various incentives and organizations that deal with them [380].

Dr. Richard Smith's 2007 book *The Trouble with Medical Journals* pointed to many possible and some real conflicts of interest facing editors of medical journals. One of the most astounding claims of Dr. Smith's is that while editors are often trained professionals in areas of medicine, there has traditionally been no qualification or training that one takes in order to become a medical journal editor, though recently there are groups that seek to rectify the effects of this [381].

Yet in Community Water Fluoridation, one is hard-pressed to find the term "conflict of interest" or "bias" involved at all when one is looking at the work of experts. Such a thing becomes incredibly conspicuous for its absence when compared with normal practices in modern biological sciences.

Such a thing has gone largely ignored for many decades. One reason for this can be the American public's natural aversion to trust big business. As CWF has often been voted on, the trust of the public has always been important. This is partly why experts recognized the importance of public relations in CWF. In 1949, **Fortune** discussed an article in the **Harvard Business Review** which looked at public opinion of big business:

> "A majority of the people… believe that very few businessmen have the good of the nation in mind when they make their important decisions. They think business is too greedy…" [382]

The article mentioned a study by the Opinion Research Corporation at Princeton claiming nearly half the people in the survey believed "business falsifies its financial statements". Obviously dentists and promoters of Community Water Fluoridation (CWF) would not want the programs they were so hopeful about associated with the stereotypical greedy businessmen. One may be able to argue that ignoring any interaction between big business and CWF programs may have been considered a virtuous thing to do, because the programs were believed to be so promising, and any associations with, or motivations of industry, would have put the sceptical American public off the measure, so often decided by referendum.

An American political scientist named Valdimer O. Key wrote in his classic work *Politics, Parties and Pressure Groups* about the complexities regarding the interaction between business and the rest of society.

> "These relationships, complex and chaotic though they may be, add up to a working system in which organized groups, private centers of power, play a basic role. At times their leaders may be animated by the most stubborn and immediate self-interest; at others, they may be animated by more noble motives."

Key wrote not only of the strength and power of businessmen, but of their weaknesses:

"Businessmen are a small minority highly vulnerable to political attack. They labor under serious political handicaps. They lack the strength of numbers. Moreover, their position lacks the moral authority that inheres in the cause of the sturdy agrarian yeomanry or the horny-handed toiler of the factory and foundry." [383]

This latter statement may explain much of the behavior of the business community discussed in this book. Key spent a lot of time discussing the importance of public relations, as a tool the business community can use to help justify its existence. This would be very important for those times when "their leaders may be animated by the most stubborn and immediate self-interest..."

In July of 1951, an article (**Figure 46**) discussing Community Water Fluoridation (CWF) appeared in the trade journal **Chemical Week** [384]. According to this journal's website, the journal is now a leading source of information for the chemical industry worldwide. It was founded in 1914. **Chemical Week** is a trade journal; most of their reporting on Community Water Fluoridation (CWF) in the 1950s was positive in the sense that they did not doubt it worked as intended [385].

The article opened by saying:

"WATER SUPPLY: Addition of fluorides by more and more communities makes a . . . **Water Boom for Fluorides**" (Their emphasis.)

"Only 1% of the nation's water is now treated: thus the market potential has fluoride chemical makers goggle-eyed." (Their emphasis.)

The article discussed how and why they were excited:

"All over the country slide rules are getting warm as waterworks engineers figure the cost of adding fluoride to their municipal supplies. They're riding a trend urged upon them by the U. S. Public Health Service, the American Dental Association, the State Dental Health Directors, various state and local health bodies, and vocal women's clubs from coast to coast."

After noting that some people feared malfunctions in equipment, or mistakes on behalf of personnel leading to overdosing, the article stated that:

"... any apathy or opposition on the part of the public is made up for by the USPHS's zeal in drumming up the program. It is asking for Federal money to develop interest, and there is talk of seeking Federal subsidization of water treatment.

"Beneficiaries: Standing to benefit from the boom are chemical companies and equipment firms." [384]

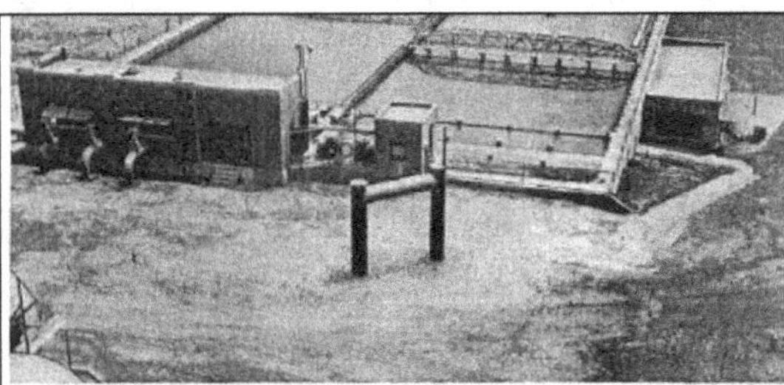

WATER SUPPLY: Addition of fluorides by more and more communities makes a . . .

Water Boom for Fluorides

Fluoridation of municipal water supplies to reduce tooth decay is now practiced or planned by 174 communities.

Backed by the U.S. Public Health Service and various state and local health officials, the treatment is daily becoming more widespread. Smaller cities are leading the parade.

Only 1% of the nation's water is now treated: thus the market potential has fluoride chemical makers goggle-eyed.

All over the country slide rules are getting warm as waterworks engineers figure the cost of adding fluoride to their municipal supplies. They're riding a trend urged upon them by the population) cities have taken the lead in fluoridation, and consequently only about 1% of the national water supply

Still others fear that equipment failures or mistakes on the part of waterworks operators might result in occasional overdoses of fluoride, which would mottle teeth or have even more more serious effects.

But any apathy or opposition on the part of the public is made up for by the USPHS's zeal in drumming up the program. It is asking for Federal money to develop interest, and there is talk of seeking Federal subsidization of water treatment.

Beneficiaries: Standing to benefit from the boom are chemical companies and equipment firms.

Among the chemical suppliers of sodium fluoride, sodium silicofluoride, or hydrofluosilicic acid—all of which may be used—are General Chemical, Harshaw Chemical Co., Blockson Chemical Co., American Agricultural Chemical Co., Aluminum Co. of America, Davison Chemical Corp., and Baugh Chemical Co. Another, Ozark-Mahoning Co., has developed a special formulation of alum and fluoride, called Flural, for this particular application. Most of these firms are now aiming sales campaigns at municipal water authorities.

Feeding must be controlled to 1 part per million within narrow limits.

*Figure 46. Part of the one-page article in the issue of the journal **Chemical Week**, p. 14, 7th July, 1951.*

"Most of these firms are now aiming sales campaigns at municipal water authorities."

"Federal money to develop interest" means the taxpayers pay for the advertising used to develop their opinions on the issue. Taxpayers are not encouraged to seek out sources *they* trust. As quoted in Chapter 5.4, this is seen as a good thing by experts, because "laymen should not decide about health" [for example 310, 311].

Firms "now aiming sales campaigns at municipal water authorities" is blatant. It suggests that people in charge of water would be listening to firms and their salesmen as well as, maybe even instead of, the public.

If we are to test the extent to which industry has been factually accurate in their claims we need to look at campaigns like this.

Most of the advertising I have seen that appeared in **Chemical Week** did not make any real scientific claims, it simply gave the name and details of the firm that was supplying.

I have not found early American promotional material used in these sales campaigns that *targeted* municipal water authorities beyond one Wallace and Tiernan brochure in the New Zealand Health Department archives. There is nothing unexpected about it.

There is something close to an example of "a sales campaign" found in Donald McNeil's book *The Fight for Fluoridation*. This was around early 1946 in Madison, Wisconsin. Two Wisconsin dentists, Dr. Frank Bull and Dr. John Frisch, were desperate for the city to fluoridate the water, but at this time the idea did not have the blessing of the American Dental Association (ADA), which made it hard going. The Madison 'Fluorine Research Committee' spent a few months reading the literature, and called in two experts, one of whom was Dr. Stream.

> "Dr. L. P. Stream, director of research for a New York chemical company, told the committee that rather than foster fluoridation, he advocated use of fluorine-vitamin lozenges, a product his company manufactured under the trade name Enziflur." [386]

This at first glance seems to be a rather small, inconsequential example, but I think it is telling of the economic climate. McNeil's words illustrate there is no elaboration or discussion. In the sentence that followed, he discussed the other expert, who urged caution.

That the experts ignored this **Chemical Week** article is probably due to the unfavourable image of business in America at the time, as illustrated by the **Fortune** article cited earlier.

The fact that people are excited by selling a product is not necessarily evidence that the product is effective or defective, and should not be taken to mean these things.

The experts have discussed the role of industry in CWF. This is one document that claims a real benefit to industry, and yet the experts have never discussed it, to my knowledge. This article is mentioned mostly in American letters to editors in the 1950s and 1960s, I've found twenty-five of these [387-389]. All of these letters were written by people *opposed to* Community Water Fluoridation.

I believe the neglect of this topic by the media had a subtle effect, possibly obvious to some: that *only* the people labelled deluded would discuss this topic of an industrial motivation suggested that there *must* have been something spurious about it, and it could be ignored. Obviously if we're looking at industry and studying industry's influence, we should look at industry's literature, and at reporting on business, given that we live in a society heavily influenced by business.

One letter was critical of the public's trust in the experts, but more interesting was the way the newspaper responded. This was in 1956, in Wilmington, Delaware:

> "I read your editorial of Oct. 29... I must say that I am a little bit amazed that the editors of the **News**, City Council and the public in Wilmington are so complacently accepting [CWF]..."

> "Where there is such a vigorous promotion going on I think we are justified in suspecting an economic motive. The whole fluoridation campaign started when the chemical manufacturers and those who made the equipment saw a golden opportunity. I quote '**Chemical Week**...'"

Excerpts of the article are quoted. The letter is followed by:

> "EDITOR'S NOTE: Readers interested in getting the facts on these and other critical attacks are referred to *Fluoridation Facts: Answers to Criticisms Against Fluoridation*, published by the American Dental Association, April, 1956." [389]

This is one of the few public 'corrections' I have seen. The letter's citation is not perfectly accurate in saying that the "... whole fluoridation campaign started when the chemical manufacturers and those who made the equipment saw a golden opportunity..." as CWF began in January of 1945 and the article quoted is dated in 1951.

In a business-run society, suggesting an "economic motive" is considered a "critical attack", even when some evidence, or a potential gateway to evidence is provided, and to newspapermen, people with the resources and knowhow to track down much of what is available.

I interloaned a copy of the 1956 American Dental Association (ADA) document [390] through my local library. In the contents, discussions on industry are given in paragraphs 8, 10, 12, 33, 36 and 40. The format of this document is given in an easy-to-read, "assertion" then "fact", very similar to Q & A style. You can see from these paragraphs that an economic motive is not addressed.

Paragraph 8 addressed the assertion that because fluorides in industry are hardening agents they would also cause hardening of the arteries. The claim was that these are two totally different types of hardening – one an industrial process, the other a physiological process. There was no citation given for where the assertion (the "Q") came from, but the citation for the response (the "A") was from the Atomic Energy Project [391].

Paragraph 10 addressed the assertion that "fluorides weaken the bones of cattle", something the ADA believed not relevant to CWF. "Dust control measures have been taken to prevent further such occurrences."

Paragraph 12 addressed the assertion that fluorides are by-products of aluminum, which the ADA denied. "The Aluminium Company of America does produce sodium fluoride, but in a special plant, in the same manner as it is produced by others not in the aluminum industry." "... fluoride compounds used for water fluoridation are not a by-product of aluminum plants."

Paragraph 33 dealt with the assertion that CWF will "adversely affect the manufacture of ice", which the ADA claimed had only occurred once, and could be avoided easily.

Paragraph 36 addressed the assertion that the Federal Food and Drug Administration would "take action against processors of foods prepared with fluoridated water." The ADA refuted this by quoting a statement from the FDA.

Paragraph 40 addressed the assertion that CWF would "interfere with food processing which involves yeast fermentation." While the ADA claimed that some food manufacturers expressed caution in the early days of fluoridation, they said there was no problem.

None of these paragraphs dealt with an economic motive for CWF. The editor of **The Morning News** either did not know or discuss why the ADA's pamphlet did not actually address the concerns expressed in the letter.

ALCOA has admitted to selling fluorides used in water supplies until 1961. The company claimed these were not wastes [392].

A 2005 edition of the American Dental Association's *Fluoridation Facts* does tell us something relevant to fluorine's essentiality:

> "Fact. Like many common substances essential to life and good health – salt, iron, vitamins A and D, chlorine, oxygen and even water itself – fluoride can be toxic in excessive quantities... As with other nutrients, fluoride is safe and effective when used and consumed properly." [393]

Regarding industry, the ADA in 2005 addresses the allegation that

> "... fluoridation additives are byproducts of the phosphate fertilizer industry... Byproducts are simply materials produced as a result of producing something else... In the chemical industry, a byproduct is anything other than the economically most important product produced." [394]

The question of a motivation for business to make a profit (and just how much profit is available to be made) is still ignored. It may be easy to conclude that fluoride chemicals are not the economically most important – even without the ADA's 2005 document. There is no elaboration on motivation for business or any aspect of business – employment, jobs, influence, etc.

New Zealand's Director-General of Health, H. B. Turbott once wrote in a document (undated, but I deduce around 1960):

> "The <u>only</u> motive behind fluoridation is a sincere desire to improve the dental health of the population of New Zealand." [395]

I think from *his* point of view, this is justified and absolutely true. Get the document and you'll see there is no mention or detail on the possibility of any benefit to industry. In Turbott's document as well, the issue of economic motivation is ignored. One anti-fluoride pamphlet I found in the New Zealand Health Department archives did include it; this had originated in Ohio (mentioned at the start of reference [387]).

The **Chemical Week** article continued:

> "Drop in the Bucket: Even if all the water in the country were fluoridated, it wouldn't add up to a bonanza for fluoride makers. It has been estimated that 45,000 tons a year of sodium fluoride or 35,000 tons of sodium silicofluoride would do the job, but current output of the silicofluoride is about 40,000 annual tons."

"Nevertheless, it adds up to a nice piece of business on all sides, and many firms are cheering the USPHS and similar groups on as they plump for increasing adoption of fluoridation." [384]

This suggests that the United States Public Health Service may have been subjected to pressure from industry.

Fluoride Relief

Producers of sodium silicofluoride, which is used in water fluoridation, have had their requests for price relief answered in Washington. Last week the Office of Price Stabilization put the chemical under a special ruling designed to eliminate hardships caused by extremely low prices in effect at the time prices were frozen.

Reason for the whole price muddle came about because of the interrelationship between main and by-products. Principal source of the silicofluorides is phosphate rock, a large percentage of which if fluorapatite. During the production of superphosphate for fertilizer, the salts are formed through interaction of hydrofluoric acid, silicon dioxide and water.

In past years these compounds have been definite stepchildren of the fertilizer industry. Silicofluorides have been sold for practically nothing, the costs of production being borne by fertilizer ingredient buyers.

But the snowballing water fluoridation process (*CW, July 7*), coupled with demands for the silicofluorides in other fields such as insecticides, has changed the attitude of fertilizer producers. While the volume of fluorides will never even approach the volume of phosphate sales, they're a nice piece of extra business. Their thoughts: Let the by-products pay their own overhead.

The price now allowed to silicofluoride producers ranges from 7 cents per pound to 8.4 cents, depending on

39

Another company mentioned in the **Chemical Week** article [384] was Wallace and Tiernan, who were selling fluoridation equipment to New Zealand. This was evidenced by a letter found in the Health Department archives, available in Wellington. One was a letter from Robert O. Prael, the Division Representative of a Belleville, New Jersey office, to the New Zealand Consulate General in San Francisco. The letter was sent with advertising material on fluoridation equipment [396].

Another article in **Chemical Week**, September 1951, (**Figure 47**) discussed increasing the price on silicofluorides, from 5 cents per pound to up to 8.4 cents per pound.

"In past years these compounds have been definite stepchildren of the fertilizer industry. Silicofluorides have been sold for practically nothing, the costs of production being borne by fertilizer ingredient buyers."

"But the snowballing water fluoridation process (*CW, July 7*), coupled with demands for the silicofluorides in other fields such as insecticides, has changed the attitude of fertilizer producers. While the volume of fluorides will never even approach the volume of phosphate sales, they're a nice piece of extra business. Their thoughts: Let the by-products pay their own overhead." (Partially pictured) [397]

The second page of the article noted that

"... the 2-cent increase will definitely encourage production."

This second article is something I have seen cited only once, in a letter to a newspaper editor[96] from someone opposed to CWF.

Figure 47. Fluoride Relief, **Chemical Week**, p. 39, September 1951. The article continued on p. 40.

---

[96] *Fluorides Boom to Chemical Firms,* **The Post-Standard** (Syracuse, New York) p. 4, 28th April, 1952.

The McIntosh County Democrat (Checotah, Oklahoma) discussed how an article on flural (a fluorine-aluminium compound, see Appendix 4) in the 1952 **Journal of the American Water Works Association** was written by Jack C. Gillespie, and Dr. Wayne E. White, from the Ozark-Mahoning mining company. Industry could study their own product, write on it and this was not considered biased in any way by the media. They were manufacturing 500 pounds of fluorides per day [398].

The previous **Chemical Week** article [384] pointed out that the chemicals used in Community Water Fluoridation were sodium fluoride, sodium silicofluoride, or hydrofluosilicic acid.

Less than a year after this **Chemical Week** article was published, Dr. Joseph Muhler and three others would publish a report stating only sodium fluoride was acceptable for use in CWF, except for study purposes [399]. This article suggests that tooth decay was not the only factor in the selection of fluoride compounds. Engineering details, such as ease of delivery were important too. Muhler and and his co-authors cautioned that these and other factors such as cost should not supplant thorough testing of these compounds on human populations.

The others were Professor Harry G. Day, one of Muhler's mentors and co-workers, Doctors C. L. Howell, D.D.S.[97] and L. E. Burney, M.D. The study claimed that sodium fluoride would reduce the caries rate by 60-65%.

> "Most of the more recent articles emphasize the fact that sodium fluoride and sodium fluosilicate can be used interchangeably so far as the engineering aspects are concerned, giving no mention of the caries-reducing ability of the different compounds.[98]"

> "Possibly other criteria besides the amount of fluorine available by analysis should be considered when evaluating new fluoride compounds to be used as fluoridating agents of communal water supplies." [399]

The Aluminum Company of America had funded two of the three experiments (that I've discussed) performed by Dr. McClendon [11, 13]. McClendon's experiments (see Chapter 1.1), if one ignores the criticisms (see Chapter 1.2), appear to show at the very least, a temporary dental benefit from fluorine[99].

ALCOA was sued many times in the 1940s for fluorine emissions. Nowhere in McClendon's experiments does he mention his funder has been sued for emissions of the element he's testing for essentiality. This is understandable in his 1944 abstract, but it's not mentioned in *any* of the experiments he did regarding fluorine's essentiality that are cited by the WHO and the NAS. The 7th edition of McClendon's book *Physiological Chemistry* does not discuss it either, though this is understandable given it was published in 1946 [400]. There is also scant mention of the harm ALCOA's emissions had on cattle, crops and produce, even in the small amount of

---

[97] Howell and Burney were from Indiana State Board of Health.

[98] A study is cited here: Bull, F. A., Frisch, J. G., and Hardgrove, T. A. *Methods and Costs of Water Fluoridation.* **J. Am. Dent. A.** 42:29, 1951. This is the same Dr. Bull mentioned in Chapter 5.4. Hardgrove and Frisch were both from Wisconsin, these three men were the ones who really got things going in the early 1950s, at least according to the beginning few chapters of McNeil's book [66].

[99] One may be tempted to claim that "at the most, they demonstrate an essentiality of fluorine" which makes perfect sense, until we see the criticisms of the experiments. I do not see any discussion from McClendon regarding the length of the 1954 experiment. On this I agree with Dr. Armstrong's (*et. al.*) point about experiments not going on long enough.

work that discusses McClendon's[100]. From what I can tell, the first lawsuit against ALCOA was also 1944. I have found only one mention of this lawsuit; it came from an American newspaper [401] with the headline, *Huge Sum Spent To Stop Fumes of Plant*. The headline is not an exaggeration, as the sum was over a million dollars.

However, by McClendon's third paper in 1954 (his second was funded by a South American organization), I find it difficult to believe he was unaware that ALCOA were being sued for fluorine emissions (see the news articles below), and were spending a considerable amount on pollution control, lawsuits, cleaner procedures and equipment development [402].

One suit in Oregon involved a greenhouse. Two people who operated the business filed a $20,000 damage suit against Warren Northwest Inc. (a contracting firm that worked on roads and buildings), alleging that fumes containing fluorine had poisoned plants [403].

Air and water pollution were becoming big issues around this time in the United States. Polluters had a great motivation to create a favourable image for fluorine and fluorides. Nobody that I'm aware of mentions this in the scientific literature on McClendon's experiments, even the few people who were critical of his work. Then again one would not expect environmental politics discussed in experiments.

Nowadays it is not considered strange to inquire about motivations behind experimental funding.

McClendon's work was cited by a couple of the NAS publications until 1974 [70], and the 1970 WHO monograph *Fluorides and Human Health* [102]. It was also cited in the 1953 Mitchell and Edman review [45], which was very decisive in its support of CWF.

In 1948, the **Kingsport News** (Tennessee) reported that ALCOA would spend "millions of dollars" on "engineering and chemical research", "in an effort to diminish damages to nearby cattle and land caused by fluorides from the plant's potrooms" [402].

The emissions increased under intensified wartime productivity, but "extensive damaging effects went unnoticed until eight or nine months ago, officials said." In October of the same year, the **Eugene Guard** (Oregon) reported that ALCOA would spend "more than a million dollars" on its Vancouver plant, to cease emissions [403]. "Numerous farmers have sued Alcoa", the article reads, "contending fluoride deposits injured their cattle and crops." Washing equipment that was installed in response to the first lawsuits in 1944 was "partially effective" in reducing fluoride emissions, the Works Manager, C. S. Thayer, said. (Evidence and information on these original 1944 lawsuits has been very difficult to find.)

Discussing a $900,000 suit brought by 13 farmers, another article from an Oregon newspaper read,

> "The suit contends gases and solids from the ALCOA plant near Vancouver have rendered their Sauvies Island farms unfit for use or sale."

---

[100] A couple of documents that did look at emissions' effects on cattle are *Pharmacology of Fluorides* and *Fluorine Chemistry Vol. IV.*, also cited by Dr. Schwarz in Chapter 1. The 1971 NAS document **Fluorides: Properties of Atmospheric Pollutants** also discussed the subject. I have found it difficult to obtain information regarding the effects of this pollution on people, beyond what is discussed here.

The farmers claimed livestock and crop were killed by gases.

"The federal court clerk said several similar suits against ALCOA are pending." [404]

Environmental law (now Emeritus) Professor William Rodgers authored a book in 1973 which contained two chapters on the aluminum and copper industries of America. Rodgers' work is thick with cynicism and meticulously detailed. It has nothing to say about CWF, yet does show the might and power of the industries, and the consequences of their power. Though their presence is significant, they are elusive.

Rodgers quotes a Manager of a Reynolds Metals aluminum plant, from one courtcase:

"It is cheaper to pay claims than it is to control fluorides." [405]

An interesting statement when held next to the experts' constant concern for "fluoride-deficient water" [158, 165, 389, 390, 406-409, and see Appendix 1]. Appendix 4 discusses fluoride pollution lawsuits.

Donald McNeil *did* mention the journal **Chemical Week** in his 1957 book *The Fight for Fluoridation*, but did not mention any individual article[101]. The purpose of discussing his work is to demonstrate that he did not use the actual journal in the citations he gave.

McNeil wrote:

"Towards the end of 1955, the American Dental Association reprinted **Chemical Week's** optimistic interpretation of the status of fluoridation. The voting population, said **Chemical Week**, had finally become aware that the 'hard core of resistance to fluoridation rests with a relatively small handful of Americans who have caused a stir out of all proportion to the merits of their arguments" [410]

McNeil wrote of the "optimistic interpretation" but did not mention that while the journal agreed on fluoridation's safety and effectiveness, and celebrated the claimed reductions in decay, a large focus of the optimism was regarding profits for industry. In fact, the July 7th article suggested a carelessness regarding accuracy of concentration:

"Still others fear that equipment failures or mistakes on the part of waterworks operators might result in occasional overdoses of fluoride, which would mottle teeth or have even more serious effects. But any apathy or opposition on the part of the public is made up for by the USPHS's zeal in drumming up the program." [384]

He includes the journal in only one paragraph in the text. In the references, the journal **Chemical Week** is not cited at all. I infer he is using second-hand sources for it; these are discussed [411].

On this note it may be worth investigating how many reports and commissions written by experts for community leaders examine an industrial motivation for this public health measure. I have with me also an Australian report for the Honorable J. T. Tonkin, M.L.A., Premier of Western Australia. While fluoride pollution is mentioned a little, the larger subject of industrial motivation, profit, influence and the long-term consequences of such things are completely ignored [412].

---

[101] McNeil's book is interesting and unique partly because he went to a lot of archives in Wisconsin, but I am sure there were omissions – one example is given here, another is given in Chapter 6.4. McNeil barely looked at an industrial motivation at all, though page 139 of his book briefly mentioned ALCOA and Oscar Ewing.

The same is true for a 1953 document written by the Ministry of Health, Department of Health for Scotland and the Ministry of Housing and Local Government of the United Kingdom. This makes perfect sense – this document involved British experts being led and shown by American experts, who did not discuss such things.

A letter titled *Fluoridophobe* from Mrs. O. M. Baxter of California, appeared in the **Chemical Week** issue dated 12th June, 1954. It read:

> "I don't know how much the chemical business stands to make out of selling fluoridation to all the cities and persuading them to poison the people with this expensive chemical. It must be more than people realize, though, to cause them to push such an obvious fraud so hard. I'll never know how they can persuade all these city councils to spend public funds on something that isn't healthy for people and runs against so many people's religions." [413]

She also suggested a Congressional investigation into fluoridation. That issue contained only one full-page advertisement for fluorides, from American Agricultural Chemical Co., featuring a smiling child next to a tap. It read "for healthier teeth". The next issue contained a full-page advertisement on the inside cover featuring an enormous genie wearing a turban trickling a stream of powdered fluorides from his massive hand in the heavens onto a small American factory below.

Of course, there was a response to Mrs. Baxter's letter. Alfred B. Goldbach of New York wrote that his (unnamed) company,

> "... has specialized in fluorine products for over 40 years... neither we nor any other producers has ever made any determined effort to sell this product to various municipalities in the U.S. and Canada... I know of no firm that spent a single penny to intimidate any public or city official..." [414]

Mr. Goldbach did not specify his company name. He knows that neither his, "nor any other" company has engaged in sales campaigns, around the time the journal he was addressing contained frequent advertising for fluorides. Presumably he means advertising that specifically targets water municipalities.

A financial or industrial motivation for CWF was not discussed by Dr. Frank McClure in his 1970 book *Water Fluoridation: The Search and the Victory*; McClure cited George Waldbott's book *A Struggle with Titans*, which contained much discussion on industry's interaction with scientists involved with fluoridation. Surely it would have been easy for Dr. McClure to correct Dr. Waldbott's claims regarding industry, but he left these alone, without giving a reason.

In 2015, the 2014 review commissioned by Sirs Gluckman and Skegg was criticized by dentist Dr. Stan Litras, who claimed the review

> "... limited their literature search solely to evidence that supported their position."

Dr. Rob Beaglehole of the New Zealand Dental Association responded by saying:

> "... Gluckman's review went through 'every single argument that an anti-fluoridationist has ever come up from and picks up the details' and concluded water fluoridation had no proven negative effects." [415]

I don't have much to say here about 'negative effects' but I certainly find it quite narrow of Dr. Beaglehole to suggest that the review by Sirs Peter Gluckman and David Skegg looked at every single argument against, considering the benefits to industry from CWF as a motivation, and the possible tendency of industry to manipulate science in favour of their profits were not even touched on. If industry is funding research, there are pressures for researchers to come up with industry-favourable conclusions.

I must differentiate – Dr. Beaglehole discussed effects, and here I'm looking at motivation of industry to influence the public image of a product.

In Sirs Gluckman and Skegg's review, there was a mention of a book that *did* look at an industrial motivation for CWF, journalist Christopher Bryson's book *The Fluoride Deception* [416]. The 2014 paper quoted only two sentences from the foreword, which was not written by Bryson, and ignored the rest of the book [417]. It was not pointed out (in Sirs Gluckman and Skegg's review) that Bryson did not write the foreword. That Bryson's work involved a lot of interviews and archived material makes fact-checking much of his claims difficult for the layman and the expert alike, yet what surprises me is that there has been no *effort* in even *trying* to increase our collective knowledge by demonstrating the veracity or inveracity of Bryson's work. The archival work and interviews are not acknowledged. Presumably because it claimed a link that experts think is irrelevant or non-existent, it is ignored.

Bryson's work was also mentioned in Australian literature in 2007. Professor Jason M. Armfield of the Australian Research Centre for Population Oral Health at Adelaide University's School of Dentistry wrote a 13-page summary on techniques used by people opposed to fluoridation that he believes undermine public health.

Armfield wrote about "innuendo" – unproven, often derogatory claims made to impugn the integrity, ability and attitudes of others. Citing Bryson's book *The Fluoride Deception*, Armfield attributed the following quote to Bryson, as an example of innuendo:

> "It was an era of thalidomide and plutonium; school segregation and human experimentation; ... atmospheric Hbomb testing and DDT... Fluoridated water was idealized as the ultimate form of 1950's failsafe social engineering". [418]

No page number of Bryson's book was given in Armfield's reference, but I still looked for the quote. I looked in a physical copy of the book, searching the index for 'segregation', 'DDT' 'thalidomide', and other terms. I couldn't find the quote. The book was a first edition published in 2004 [416]. In the index, you can see the word DDT is on pages 234, 235 and 265. The phrase Armfield attributed to Bryson is not on those pages, the words 'segregation' and 'thalidomide' are not in the index.

Frustrated, I thought maybe someone online had quoted the same thing, but cited a page number. This seemed probable, given that Armfield and others claim people opposed to fluoride get so much of their research online. I copied and pasted the quote into Google. One website came up, DoctorYourself.com [419]. The only two responses on the search were from Armfield's article and the DoctorYourself.com website. It seems nobody else had quoted it online.

The quote Armfield uses is made up of the first seven sentences of the DoctorYourself.com website article. The words actually belonged to the author of the website article. It does not come from Bryson's work at all.

Armfield did what many of us could be tempted to do: Googled Bryson's book, selected the first thing found, and attributed it to Bryson. Armfield did *not* do what professors are supposed to do – read the actual book, and see for himself if there is any truth to it. What does he agree with and why, what does he disagree with and why, and what is he uncertain about? He has dismissed years of Bryson's work sifting through archives, reading documents and interviewing people, based on one thing he read on the internet and then attributed to Bryson. This is not warranted.

If you're interested, obtain a copy of Armfield's paper, Bryson's book, and see if you can find the quote. If I've made a mistake here, I'm open to hearing it.

The DoctorYourself.com article also contained an interview with Bryson, a small portion of which I shall reproduce here because it relates to media.

> "DY News: Your book, with its very commendable 110 pages of notes, might be well described as sort of a 'Fahrenheit FL.' What facts, what parts of your book are your critics specifically attacking you over?
>
> Bryson: I don't know that I have any critics. If they exist, they have been profoundly silent, well aware that any attack would be good publicity for the book.
>
> DY News: I think your book is so tightly documented that they haven't a leg to stand on if they try. I noticed that there was an advertisement for your book in the **NY Times**, but am unaware that the **Times** ever reviewed it. Where may we find and read major media reviews of *The Fluoride Deception*?
>
> Bryson: Thus far, there has not been a single mention of the book in the US media, with the exception of **Publisher's Weekly**. I'm certain industry would love to keep it thus."

This interview was from August 2004. The **Publisher's Weekly** review is online [420]. Bryson's book was reviewed in the July 2004 issue of **Environmental Magazine** [421], **Nature** in 2005 [422], but neither mentioned Bryson's claim of looking in archives. One small article in the **Fraser Coast Chronicle** (Queensland) claimed that three copies of the book had been sent in from readers [423].

A **New York Times** article [424] linked to a blog that discussed Bryson's archival work. The author wrote of Baruch's Newman Library that was hosting a collection from the museum of public relations; the author of the blog hurried to see if evidence was included that implicated Edward Bernarys in fluoridation, as Bryson had claimed.

> "Alas, evidence in the Bernays materials at hand was scant. Suspiciously or not, Bernays, seemed to steer clear of fluoridation in his writings. The record, Bryson writes, is to be found in Bernays's letters in the Library of Congress." [425]

I don't want to pick on *all* of Professor Armfield's article, the rest of it may be perfectly accurate for all I know. I discuss it because I see this claim:

> "The scientists researching the effectiveness of water fluoridation as well as health officials and dentists do not receive money from sugar, aluminium or any other companies for their research or opinions." [426]

The fact that experts don't look at the suggestion of industrial influence beyond an instant dismissal, is evidence of an unwillingness to examine the ways in which profit has influenced research treatment and direction. From the articles mentioned here one can see that there *was* a lot of money and influence regarding industry and government in the past. One of the reasons Armfield asserts lack of industry influence is that none of the experts or media have put any effort into examining the professional connections between industry, government and public health, and the possible conflicts of interest that may occur.

What about personal or familial connections? For instance, the Right Honorable Sir Rupert James Hamer was the Premier of Victoria (Australia) from 1972 until 1981. His brother, Alan William Hamer worked for ICI chemicals (now Orica), a firm that sold fluorides. Credit to Australian journalist Wendy Varney for pointing this out; this can also be confirmed with other documents [427]. The 1970s saw a push to increase CWF in Australia.

Recall the statement from Professor Armfield quoted previously [426]. Regarding the funding of studies, surely Professor Armfield should show us a sample of studies and say something like: "I looked at *x* number of studies and none of them were funded by sugar, aluminium industry... etc" or words to that effect? But Professor Armfield does not *need* to show this kind of evidence in this instance, because he is voicing an opinion that all the other experts, and probably much of society, already believe. Whoever peer-reviewed his study certainly believed it; they did not suggest he provide a selection of studies and check their funders.

Even if Armfield *had* supplied a study or investigation like this – taking a few hundred or a few thousand studies and looking at funders and conclusions – the results would be unsatisfactory. The Maurer and Day study [17] was funded by the army. These two worked at Indiana University (IU), where toothpaste companies gave money and probably had a lot of influence. It does not give us a complete view of what occurs if we only look at who funded experiments and ignore the larger societal and economic motives and pressures. Recall the example from Chapter 5.2 of the Phillip Morris tobacco company funding going through Kraft foods, a subsidiary.

Incidentally, the Maurer and Day study which described the two groups of rats (2 ppm sodium fluoride and less than 0.007 ppm fluoride) that "could not be distinguished", led them to call fluorine "dispensable" in nutrition. We could have expected Maurer and Day to say that fluorine *was* essential in nutrition, given that this was a conclusion favourable to the toothpaste companies that were not financing *this* experiment, but did finance much research at IU. Yet at the end of their experiment they wrote that fluorine had an apparent benefit in the prevention of decay, which is not really what their experiment showed, or was even looking for. Perhaps *here* was where the thinking of the times reared its head. CWF was 12 years old by 1957, with Crest toothpaste almost invented and about to participate in the $300 million dentifrice market [14, 15]. Even when fluorine was considered "dispensable in nutrition" it still retained its preventive ability.

Regarding ALCOA funding the McClendon research, Armfield is correct here because technically McClendon's work was not *specifically* about CWF for humans, yet it was cited by Mitchell and Edman as evidence of fluorine's possible essentiality in a report that was very praising of CWF in 1953 [45] (this report was then cited in 1970 by Dr. Frank McClure [47]).

In 1953, the **Rushville Republican** (Indiana) reported that the town of Bloomington was not going to begin CWF until 1955 when Dr. Joseph Muhler would finish his fluoride research.

> "Muhler's project, financed by state, Army and industrial grants, is testing the value of tin and sodium fluorides on teeth of two out of every three children in Monroe County." [428]

Relevant here is that his work is partially financed by unspecified industrial grants. In 1960 full-page ads appeared in American newspapers for Crest toothpaste. Dr. Joseph Muhler was 38 years old, working with stannous fluoride. The advertising commended Muhler on his persistence, even though

> "the conservative ADA continued to decline acceptance of his assertions…"

> "Muhler has assigned his patent to the Indiana University Research Foundation. Procter & Gamble, headed by Neil McElroy, former secretary of Defense, has paid almost $100,000 in royalties to the foundation. Under university regulations, Muhler is not allowed to participate in royalties but a university spokesman said he had been taken care of with a substantial increase in salary that puts him in 'top level ranks'." [14, 15]

In his letter (quoted in Chapter 5.5) *Fluoridation Foes Ignore Facts*, Dr. Walter C. Kraatz mentioned the industry issue in this sole quote:

> "[Antifluoridationists]… have fanatically charged that fluoridation is an insidious attempt of Communists to weaken the American people, and added the atrocious insult that scientists and public health officials supporting fluoridation are subsidized by sellers of fluorides." [368]

There was a lot of money floating around fluorides in 1950s America. An expert can refute a claim simply by suggesting that something is ridiculous. This is the power of prestige. Recall that experts do not correct each other or point out mistakes in each others' work, in public. In this instance, again the expert does not *need* to worry about evidence, because he is voicing an opinion that all the other experts, and probably much of the society, already believes.

In a **Journal and Courier** article in 1970, Leroy Pope reported that

> "The giants of the toothpaste business, Colgate-Palmolive and Proctor and Gamble… aren't quarrelling over any piddling million-dollar gate. They're brawling over a 10 to 20 per cent share of the $350-million-a-year dentifrice market. For weapons they use chinks of advertising and public relations dough running to the millions."

Pope goes on to discuss a report from IU about mechanically brushed teeth with 43 different dentifrices. Cosmetic toothpastes, according to the report, were unsafe. Colgate had started the cosmetic toothpaste movement, and taken a significant share of the market.

> "The IU study was well publicized and many periodicals that printed it pointed out that P&G [Procter & Gamble] was a heavy financial contributor to Dr. Muhler's preventive dentistry at the university. Stung by this, Dr. Muhler denied that P&G knew about his abrasiveness tests until they were completed."

Pope claims Colgate-Palmolive suffered, even though their product Ultra Brite was not mentioned in the IU study.

> "Now Colgate-Palmolive is readying a counter attack, an advertising campaign based on a new toothpaste abrasiveness test by the Council on Dental Therapeutics of the American Dental Association. 'The ADA council had to act because of pressure from association members,' said a Colgate spokesman." [429]

What we see and buy is influenced by what we think, which is in turn influenced by these studies and public relations. One company funds a study that just happens to conclude their competitor's toothpaste is worse…

Big business uses "advertising campaigns" to "[counter] attack" each other, in a war played out among the billboards on our streets, our supermarkets, and the images in our minds. How has toothpaste advertising affected our understanding of fluorides and the necessity claimed for them? Advertising by its nature is shallow, and not focused on long-term consequences. Public relations in many ways is worse because it gives impressions of depth, expertise, concern and neutrality, yet simply wears these as packaging. At its core it is information doing the bidding of people who want to increase and maintain wealth and power [430].

Regarding toothpaste and CWF I want to say I'm *not* attacking anyone's integrity here. Just because someone makes money from their work does not instantly make them greedy. We should *all* be paid well for our work, assuming our work is helpful. The point I want to make here is that it is foolish to completely turn our nose up to the facts that people *are* funded by corporations, and that keeping that money coming does not necessarily make these people bad or conniving, but it is at least a conflict of interest. I'm not interested in impugning anyone's kind-hearted attempts to prevent tooth decay in children, but when we get into corporate boardrooms and competitive economics, a different set of values is prioritized. This is very evident in the following section.

In 2014, the **Journal of Dental Hygiene** published an article which investigated toothpaste advertising aimed at children [431].

This article pointed to the Federal Drug Administration (FDA) guidelines for toothpaste development, which required toothpaste manufacturers to include the following warning on their product:

> "Do not swallow. Use only a pea-sized amount for children under 6. To prevent swallowing, children under 6 years of age should be supervised in the use of toothpaste." [432]

In 1997, the FDA required the following statement to be added:

> "If you accidentally swallow more than used for brushing, seek professional help or contact a poison control center immediately."

The **Journal of the American Dental Association** ran an editorial in the October, 1997 issue dismissing this warning as "unnecessary" and "ludicrous". Editor Lawrence H. Menkin wrote:

> "The Association has always monitored any adverse reactions to fluoride toothpastes through surveys of incident reports in emergency rooms and through contacts with regional and national poison centers.

> "The results of this surveillance leave no room for disagreement: incidents involving fluoride toothpastes do not lead to major adverse outcomes. It appears that other toothpaste ingredients-the humectants and surfactants they contain will induce vomiting long before any toxic effects of fluoride can take place."

> "Those who suggest that the best solution would be the development of a lower-dose fluoride toothpaste for preschoolers must understand that such a venture would be costly, with no guarantee of marketplace success. Since there is no evidence that a lower-dose fluoride dentifrice would have the same caries-reducing effect, expensive clinical investigations would have to precede any FDA clearances." [433]

Note again a stark difference in the fundamentals of perceptions about fluoride. The editor wrote:

> "The antithesis to this much ado about nothing situation recently appeared in media reports warning that children in families that consume bottled water may not be getting enough fluoride."

David Richardson, vice president of regulatory affairs and product safety for the Colgate-Palmolive, expressed a similar opinion:

> "The industry believed that this label was inappropriate for toothpaste and would not be required because it was absolutely diametrically opposed to the public health policy of encouraging the use of fluoride for the reduction of dental cavities." [434]

This statement was quoted in a 1998 **New York Times** article which looked at the issue. The paper quoted a doctor from the FDA, who claimed fluoride was a drug:

> "'There always was a warning,' said Dr. Linda Katz, deputy director for over-the-counter drug products at the F.D.A., 'but I don't think it really hit the message that fluoride is a drug and has been associated with both acute and chronic toxicity.'" [434]

The **Times** claimed that in 1997, only 4,453 cases were made to the Poison Control Center regarding fluoride overexposures, 99% were minor with not one being life-threatening.

The 2014 paper looked at a total of 26 fluoridated toothpastes for children, available from pharmacies in New York City. These were developed by three companies; Colgate-Palmolive, Procter & Gamble and GlaxoSmithKline. All 26 products contained at least one animated or cartoon character from children's shows. Dora the Explorer was the most frequent, appearing on 38.5% of toothpastes. Half the toothpastes had a picture of a food item, mostly fruit (often a photograph), with 24 of 26 toothpastes claiming to be flavoured, usually something sweet – bubblegum, orange, strawberry or the like. Seven toothpastes contained a picture of a full swirl of toothpaste on the tube, in contrast to the warning to only use a pea-sized amount.

> "In 2 of these cases, the swirl of toothpaste was illustrated as an animated character." [435]

While 22 toothpastes contained the warning "use a pea-sized amount", this was *always* listed "on the back of the tube and in a very small font (size 8 font or smaller)." The same was true for the 25 toothpastes that gave a warning that it should only be used by children over 2 years old.

In discussing these results, the authors claimed the small font size for warnings, contrasted with the pictures of food and full swirls of toothpaste created a conflict – if only a pea-sized amount should be used, then only a pea-sized amount should be pictured. If toothpaste should not be swallowed, pictures of food and claims of flavour give the impression that toothpaste should be *treated* like food, and therefore swallowed.

Claiming 21,513 calls were made to the (American) Poison Control Center in 2011 related to "over-consumption of fluoridated toothpaste,"[102] the authors stated "measures need to be taken to deter children from eating toothpaste rather than drawing them to it."

This report referred to an article that looked only at advertisements for fluoridated toothpastes in parenting magazines. Of 117 advertisements featuring in 116 issues of 2 magazines between 2007 and 2011, 30 of 31

---

[102] Bronstein, Spyker, Cantilena, Rumack and Dart, *2011 Annual Report of the American Association of Poison Control Centers' National Poison Data System (NPDS): 29th Annual Report*, **Clinical Toxicol. (Phila)**. 2012; 50.

advertisements that pictured a toothbrush with toothpaste used a full swirl of toothpaste, much more than (the authors suggested at least four times) the recommended, pea-sized amount.

How effectively can the dental industry police this? Colgate currently advertises in the **Journal of the American Dental Association**. Colgate has consistently advertised in the **New Zealand Dental Journal**. In July of 1983, the **Journal** published an editorial by Dr. Harvey Brown, which pointed out that some children swallow "considerable quantities" of toothpaste, which "is not recommended for systemic use."

> "It is therefore with some concern that we note a trend in the advertising of toothpastes to suggest that more is better. Children are depicted loading brushes from end to end with paste or gel in amounts that are too great for small mouths to handle without significant amounts being swallowed." [436]

Dr. Brown wrote very positively of fluoride toothpastes here, yet did state that only about a quarter of a toothbrush's bristles should be covered. He pointed to enamel opacities as a possible problem, urging manufacturers to

> "consider carefully the nature of their advertising and to reduce substantially the size of the orifice of toothpaste tubes." [436]

The Colgate advertising department must have forgotten Dr. Brown's warning, as the April, 1987 issue of the **New Zealand Dental Journal** contains an ad for Colgate toothpaste depicting a full swirl of toothpaste on the bristles. Editors choose to run these ads for financial reasons. The positions of Editor, Scientific Editor and Assistant Editor of this journal had not changed between these years, but the Advertising Manager had changed.

Earlier I quoted Professor Armfield, who claimed researchers were not financially supported by companies, but there is a potential conflict of interest with regard to the toothpaste industry here. Perhaps something can be said for the sheer volume of advertising and communications which must overwhelm the less glamourous and more sober cautions of scientists.

Dr. Leslie Winston of Procter & Gamble Oral Health authored an article that discussed the relationship between universities and businesses. It discussed collaborations between industry and universities taking off in the 1980s, encouraged by government, and organizations such as the Medical Research Council of Canada, and the (US) National Institutes of Health. Dr. Winston's perspective is quoted:

> "University-industry collaborations foster economic growth, improve standards of living and extend humanity's intellectual reach. With these lofty goals a long-term relationship mindset is essential." [437]

An important aspect of industry-university collaboration is the simple fact that the discoveries are made for the purpose of the private interest; they exist for the goal of increasing the ideals of profit, competitiveness and efficiency for corporations. Environmental factors and other externalities like consumer health are not unimportant, but become less important.

Dr. Winston's small article did mention the importance of conflicts of interest, largely regarding whether academia is "unbiased and ethical". On this note, a speech given by Mark Stouse, CEO of marketing analysis firm Proof Analytics, is worth mentioning. The speech was part of a presentation hosted by the Museum of Public Relations in partnership with the Institute for Public Relations. The presentation was from the RAND

Corporation, and was called *Does Truth Still Matter? "Truth Decay" and the Implications for the Practice of Public Relations*. Mr. Stouse said:

> "The bottom line here is that even though [telling] the truth is always the right thing to do… always the right thing to say… if you can't also show how you're going to make telling the truth pay dividends, for business or for a stakeholder, or for an organization, you're gonna have a problem. That is the reality." [438]

The amount of money spent on advertising and PR by toothpaste companies is quite incredible. In 1999, Colgate-Palmolive donated $1 million to the American Public Health Association to "promote health and hygiene worldwide" and to address "looming public health issues" [439].

In 2000, **Advertising Age** reported that Colgate-Palmolive had sales of $2.2 billion. In the early 2000s, the company planned to use Y&R Advertising, a New York firm. They spent a little over $100 million on advertising in the mid-1990s, up to $133 million in 1999. Most of their products enter US markets before going overseas.

This was not much compared to Proctor & Gamble, who spent $1.2 billion on "media outlay" in 1992, $17 million of which was spent advertising Crest toothpaste [440].

In 2015, Procter & Gamble won the prize for Global Campaign of the Year for their *Thank You, Mom* campaign, developed with agency Wieden + Kennedy Portland.

The minute-and-a-half clip featured mothers supporting children who aimed at competing in the 2014 Sochi Olympics. It introduced consumers to P&G's *Raising an Olympian* film series, which followed 28 world-class athletes and their mothers.

> "Securing exclusives with Mashable and The Huffington Post, coverage of the powerful clip set off a chain of media placements for P&G."

> "In Sochi, the company had 17 brands featured in 54 events and moms were treated to 1,200 hours of pampering from brands including Pantene and Olay. Not to feel left out, Gillette, Head & Shoulders, and Braun were on hand to groom dads." [441]

We don't need to go to media critics to see the power advertisers hold over media. Media even admit that they exist to serve advertisers. Michael Jordan, president of Columbia Broadcasting System (CBS-TV; previously Jordan was president of PepsiCo and Westinghouse), told **Advertising Age** in a 1997 interview:

> "We're here to serve advertisers. That's our raison d'etre." [442]

The article is called *Jordan Brings the Heart of the Marketer to CBS-TV*.

Recall Professor Armfield's claim:

> "The scientists researching the effectiveness of water fluoridation as well as health officials and dentists do not receive money from sugar, aluminium or any other companies for their research or opinions." [426]

This was quoted on Dr. Ken Perrott's website[103] [443]. The article also found its way into Dr. Stephen Barrett's website [444], and journalist Sean Plunket's article [350]. These are prominent people who are intelligent and presumably well-respected by their various audiences.

Armfield's paper has been peer-reviewed. Professor Armfield and the reviewer/s ignored work authored by Australian journalist Wendy Varney, whose book *Fluoridation: A Case to Answer* was published in 1986. The reviewer/s of Armfield's paper obviously didn't know or care that Varney included an *entire chapter* on industrial motivations for fluoridation, a "technique" that the academics ignored. If Armfield concentrated *only* on Australian work, he would have had at least some leads to get some potential evidence of an industrial or financial motivation… but he had this in Bryson's book…

In Professor Armfield's defence, his paper was looking primarily at techniques of argument, which lets him off the hook as far as really testing if any arguments are definitely true or false – though falsity is probably presupposed because the people making those arguments are on the other side. His paper dealt with a great many things, but what I've shown here is how one little statement can get out to the public with absolutely no depth of research anywhere along the way[104].

It would be unfair to blame this solely on Armfield. *None* of the experts who discuss CWF show any interest in the possibility of industrial or financial motivation, or any conflict of interest or effect on research such things may have. Don't think I'm disagreeing with everything in his article. On this note, if we find a mistake in someone's work, or something we disagree with, should this be used as an excuse to throw out *all* of that person's work? I wouldn't want *all* of my work thrown out just because I made one mistake, or missed a document that somebody else liked. It's unrealistic to expect that one person or group of people would always get *everything* correct.

People say that the burden of proof is upon the one making the claim. This is fair, yet one can see here that there is a possibility that truth can suffer if we're restricting ourselves from looking at certain things. Our "ask-an-expert" style of journalism is faulted if experts do not explore certain questions.

Overwhelmingly, you can see it is activists who look at this topic of businesses and the profits they may make from a belief in a necessity or benefit for use of fluorine compounds. If they're going to believe such things, surely the burden of proof is upon them. This is perfectly logical. Yet I feel journalists and the experts have a greater responsibility here for honesty and openness. It's difficult for ordinary members of the public to visit libraries, archives, and follow all leads. It must be even harder for someone with barely any resources, and more personal or professional commitments and responsibilities.

---

[103] Of the three hundred comments on this article, not a single commenter discussed the point on industry funding, which demonstrates how poorly investigated this topic is, even among interested parties.

[104] While Professor Armfield responded to both of Professor Connett's comments, he did not respond to Dr. Bruce Spittle's (I checked on the 2nd of April, 2018, https://anzhealthpolicy.biomedcentral.com/articles/10.1186/1743-8462-4-25/comments). Maybe this indicates he didn't know if Dr. Spittle's comments were correct or not.

What do the experts, with all their resources do with the topic of big business involvement and possible or potential conflicts of interest? They deflect the claim, the burden of proof, the following of money, to people who *don't* have anywhere near the amount of resources, putting the burden squarely on the shoulders of people who have a hard enough time looking at, and making sense of things on the surface. The experts allow the activists to fumble around in the academic dark.

I don't think the expert mentality is one resembling that of Charles Darwin's slow and patient appraisal anymore. There is very little impetus to be honest about the possibility of mistakes, and no desire to acknowledge any aspect of history or science that does not suit. This is more like justifying an ideology instead of a search for scientific accuracy.

I don't know if Bryson's claims made from the American archives are accurate or not. The point I want to make here is that ostensibly none of the experts put any effort into finding these archives when the work first came out in 2004. Almost nobody has been interested in verifying Bryson's claims about the archives.

In 2008, Dunedin (New Zealand) City Council and Public Health South "expressed concerns" regarding a program Fluoride Action Network New Zealand (FANNZ) had offered to various TV stations in New Zealand. It was *The Fluoride Deception*, named after the book by Christopher Bryson. The half-hour program was not broadcast because it may have been "alarmist" or "could cause disquiet in the community" [445]. Here we see the experts worried that the public will just believe whatever is put on the television for them to watch.

A televised debate was set up involving three supporters and three opponents of CWF; it was an hour long including ads [446]. Bryson's work was not discussed at all. Dr. John Holmes of the Otago District Health Board and Public Health South claimed fluoride was "essential for life." This was the same year the WHO would write "essentiality has not been demonstrated unequivocally." [114]

The experts may avoid Bryson's work for one key reason: he gave a link between fluoride pollution and CWF, two areas experts have consistently claimed are separate. He claimed many scientists heavily involved in the military and in fluoride pollution authored a booklet called *Our Children's Teeth*[105]. Bryson claims this booklet was used in a fluoride pollution lawsuit when Reynolds Metals were in court. The legal defence for Reynolds argued that because 1 ppm fluoride in the water supply was perfectly safe – healthy, even – there was no way fluoride could have been the harmful element in pollution, therefore Reynolds would not be responsible.

I have not seen this claim discussed in detail. Bryson also linked ALCOA's Francis Frary to Gerald Cox and the National Research Council (NRC) [416] (pages 39, 40 and 259).

Historian V. O. Key points out that not only do businessmen manipulate public opinion; they are in turn manipulated *by* public opinion:

---

[105] A copy exists in Wellington's National Library. The corporate ties were not mentioned in the booklet. It was sponsored by Kellogg's (according to Bryson, p. 323), featured Frank A. Smith, Robert Kehoe and more.

"As industrial power grew and the conscious policy of managing public attitudes to retain that power came to be adopted, big businessmen underwent a curious metamorphosis. They came to act like politicians; or, as they termed it, they became 'industrial statesmen.'" [447]

Businessmen were "sensitive to public criticism" and organized the strategy of their policies "with a sharp eye to the anticipated public reaction". The firms that cultivate public opinion the most seem to be those that have necessity and funds to do so, and are at least semi-monopolistic in nature. Key cautions against believing business is *overly* concerned with public opinion.

The following example of promotion may have influenced experts in Britain. I cannot say for sure what the precise nature of the communications was, but the process is illustrative of a very important point – that those who communicate to us are selling something.

In 1963, the supplement of the **British Dental Journal** contained a small article (**Figure 48**) regarding the promotion of fluoridation [448]. It demonstrates that scientific journals can be influenced by industry.

Fluoridation Campaign

Council have agreed that a publicity campaign should be launched in the name of the Association, on the subject of the fluoridation of water supplies: this has become possible through the generosity of three firms of tooth-paste manufacturers, who will remain anonymous.

24

If the co-operation of the proprietors of certain newspapers can be secured, it is hoped that a campaign may be conducted by means of advertisements in the Press and in magazines. The donations have also made it possible to proceed with the circularisation of letters and pamphlets to all local councillors, and the distribution of posters for display in waiting rooms, clinics, out-patients' departments, factory notice boards, canteens, interviewing rooms in factories, etc. as 'throw-ins' in various journals, including the *British Dental Journal*.

Figure 48. Fluoridation Campaign. Proceedings of the Representative Board, **British Dental Journal Supplement**, 3rd September, p. 24, 1963 [448]. Also cited in *Compulsory Mass Medication* by Clavell P. Blount.

Thus, academic, or science journals may sometimes be considered propagandistic in nature. I hope the reader will consider the 1970 words of Dr. Knutson presented earlier [325] before disregarding this claim.

The "Association" no doubt refers to the British Dental Association. Note that the toothpaste companies involved retain their anonymity, the public and the readers of the **Journal** don't need to know who is communicating to them (or why).

This demonstrates that the toothpaste companies have a direct one-way communication to the public, but more importantly to readers of the **Journal**, namely the experts. We think of experts as more sceptical, yet when it comes to familiar sources they are less likely to apply their skeptism - they don't need to be told who is communicating to them, or who is providing funds. These experts will be advising other community leaders.

That the entire topic of an industrial influence in the science surrounding CWF has consistently been dismissed with minimal investigation appears to me to have obvious effects in terms of what is presented from the experts, to other experts, and to the public. If it's not presented *by* experts, it won't be cheered by the media, and the public probably won't see it, unless they are involved in detailed research.

Mueller's 1966 paper cited earlier discussed a survey by Dr. Arnold Simmel of the New York State Health Department, in which people opposed to fluoridation gave the "aluminum companies are behind it" reason less than six percent of the time [449]. I'd like to point out a lack of detail in the statement that "aluminum companies are behind it". Mueller said this demonstrated the "comparative weakness of conspiratorial and especially of moral arguments."

That the perfectly normal focus of business on profits can be labelled a conspiracy argument is quite interesting [450]. The purpose of business is to make money. No doubt the use of the word "conspiracy" by laymen includes laws believed to be unfair – relaxed punishments for the consequences of pollution, and wealth inequality – *as well as* anything illegal. For the highly educated, "conspiracy" means something illegal, but the less educated see things that are perfectly normal in the standard running of business that they feel unfair – low wages, environmental neglect, laws that appear to favour business over the population – and *their* use of the word "conspiracy" can simply mean the normal operation of business.

I don't believe that even the business community has the ability to deceive absolutely. Yet in this topic it helps to know that many media and journals are mouthpieces of the business community – they are financed by corporations, they print studies funded by corporations, they are full of advertisements for corporate products, and in the case of large media they simply *are* corporations.

Noam Chomsky claimed that a third of all American textbooks in the 1950s were authored or influenced by people working for corporations [451].

Volume one of *Fluorine Chemistry* was authored by fifteen people, among them Willy Lange of Procter and Gamble (P&G); and John Turner Pinkston, Jr. of *The Harshaw Chemical Company*. P&G were big players in the toothpaste industry, and Harshaw advertised fluorides for CWF in **Chemical Week** [452]. Also mentioned was W. H. Pearlson, of the *Minnesota Mining & Manufacturing Company*. I'm unsure if they had anything to do with fluoride sales.

Volume two lists T. J. Brice and D. G. Weiblen of *Minnesota Mining & Manufacturing*.

In volume three, the authors (Hodge, Smith and Chen) thank people who "have permitted us to copy data or who have made available hitherto unpublished data for inclusion": W. D. Bowersox from E. I. duPont deNemours and Co.; DuPont has consistently been a huge polluter in the USA [453].

Even in the beginnings, many thousands of people and organizations were involved in fluorine and fluoridation. While it is very difficult to pinpoint anything specific to the aluminium industry, they must have gained from the widespread acceptance and reputation of CWF.

Their presence and influence is hard to detect if it exists, yet laws, policies and public opinion seem to work in their favour. Ben Bagdikian points out that ALCOA shared directors with Columbia Broadcasting System (CBS) [454].

Environmental Law Professor William Rodgers claimed he was rebuffed when he wrote to J. C. Dale of the Aluminum Association to obtain a study that was "... completed on schedule but not released. Our reason for withholding this is due to the fact that in our view the study was incomplete. We have since provided additional funds to Battelle Memorial Institute..."

Regarding the funding of experiments, Rodgers writes of a "boiler-plate clause" in a contract belonging to Kaiser regarding "Measurement of Particle Size Distribution at Tacoma Works of Kaiser Aluminum":

"plans or data prepared by the researcher or disclosed to him are 'the property of the owner.'" [455]

The researcher is obliged to "limit access" only to Kaiser employees directly involved with the work. Compare this statement with expert claims of seeing "all the evidence" [67, 340, 360].

It is blatantly obvious why the industry-university relationship is normalized: such a relationship works perfectly to suit industry's agenda.

This is by no means evidence of anything deceptive. The way certain information is focused on, and the way certain information is ignored, makes far more sense in light of markets in a competitive society, where corporations are allowed to keep information secret from the public, and the goal of the competition is to make as much money as possible, as quickly as possible.

Is a lawyer a conspirator if they defend their client from a pollution lawsuit? Of course not, they're just a hard-working person functioning according to their professional purpose. Is a businessman a conspirator because he wants to maximise profits? Of course *not*, he's just doing his job, he's *supposed* to maximise profits. It's an economic necessity in a competitive system.

There is, at minimum, a motivation to give fluorine a favourable image. Coupled with so close to 100% of my small sample of experts claiming a nutritional role for fluorine and ignoring anything suggesting otherwise, as well as constant claims of objectivity, there is reason for concern.

When we introduce the public relations industry, and the business community's desire for an increase in profits, we introduce different priorities. One article on public relations discussed how the industry doesn't "spin" any more, they simply "manage the facts" [456]. The interaction of dentistry, government, and public health seem far removed from industry, yet there are relationships here. Bagdikian's work pointed to corporate power and influence on media [457]. Others' work points towards a powerful influence of industry on public health [430, 458] as well as professional media and science.

In 2012, the **New York Times** reported that the New Jersey Utilities Association testified against fluoridation, claiming it would cost water companies anywhere from $400,000 to $64 million [459]. Exactly who this money would go to or how it would be spent was not mentioned in this article.

Recently, the **Tampa Bay Times** ran an editorial which discussed the "conspiracy" (big business) charge. They addressed the implication one activist had put forth that chemical company Mosaic had put pressure on politicians to win the contract to sell fluorides to the town of Pinellas:

"Mosaic spokesman Russell Schweiss said fluoride sales represent about 0.02 percent of the company's estimated \$6.7 billion in annual revenue. The implication there was a conspiracy to win the Pinellas contract is baseless." [460]

I don't think ALCOA will ever be completely free of accusations of foul play with regard to fluoridation.

In 1953, **The Pittsburgh Press** (Pennsylvania), wrote of Dr. Churchill, Chief Chemist for ALCOA, who "first identified fluorides in water – and opened the way for the use of this chemical as a preventive of tooth decay." Apparently this identification was done in 1931 [461]. Grace Noda, mentioned briefly in Chapter 2.7, also pointed out Churchill was Chief Chemist for ALCOA, but did not mention their legal problems over fluoride pollution [143]. Professor Armfield and others deny the aluminium industry's involvement, when ALCOA's Chief Chemist was the first to identify the compound. This was even mentioned in the **Journal of the American Dental Association** [462].

The fact that people nowadays are sceptical about conflicts of interest in research is not proof of any real bias (although the topic is now addressed in the biomedical literature), but taken with the rest of the information presented in this chapter, there is certainly reason to doubt the statement of Harold Bertram Turbott's that:

"The <u>only</u> motive behind fluoridation is a sincere desire to improve the dental health of the population of New Zealand." [395] (His emphasis).

Dental health was certainly one motive, and from *his* perspective it looked like the only motive. But I don't think he looked deep enough to see anything more. The experts say nothing about industrial motivation for CWF, other than it's not relevant.

Even searching legal databases was difficult. The U.S. Library of Congress was one of the few groups that responded helpfully to my emails about tracking down the possible legal applications of McClendon's work. Their database had not only menus for types of law, but types of court. I was out of my depth. I did not find any court cases online that I found mentioned in these newspaper clippings. I found such an abundance of newspaper articles on this topic that I haven't been able to include them all. None of them appear to really scratch below the surface of the topic, though some discuss corporate involvement in government. They still went with an "… activists say…" sort of approach. The claims of activists were often not verified, though journalists have in many instances put quite an effort into reporting the topic.

To look at a bigger picture of corporate influence on media framing, we can see much of the American media has been owned by corporations involved in the production of weaponry. This may go far to explain the pro-war stance of the American media throughout the years. If fluorides used in CWF are by-products of industries that promote war and weapon manufacture (see the end of Chapter 1.1 for a list of funders), then there is at least some pressure on American media to show CWF in a good light. There is probably a great deal of subtlety here, as promoting something that is meant to help children and the poor needs little exaggeration to be considered a good thing.

The pollution suits give at minimum, a motivation to label fluorine a nutritional essential. Without access to internal documents, we are left only with what the corporations give to us in press releases, and work of people diligent enough to keep chipping away at this elusive topic. While Professor Rodgers' work did not look at CWF, it is very interesting regarding the aluminium industry [463].

Rodgers claimed that the Washington State University College of Engineering advisory board were funded largely by trade associations and corporations; Intalco "bought" a seat by funding research on its Bellingham plant impact [464].

The Boyce Thompson Institute received $200,000 in yearly contributions from Harvey Aluminum in 1963. Harvey had paid for a couple of Boyce's people to go to the Dalles area, where Harvey was being sued (see Appendix 4). Boyce's David McLean claimed under cross-examination that the majority of the sponsors for Boyce were the aluminium industry. Others were the National Air Pollution Control Administration of the Public Health Service, and the phosphate industry. No produce growers (suffering the effects of pollution) contributed to Boyce [465].

The history page of the Boyce Thompson Institute (BTI)'s website discusses the noble ideals of its founder, William Boyce Thompson (1869-1930). Research on fluorides is discussed, but there is no mention of the aluminum industry.

> "The BTI group was recognized as perhaps the foremost research group on fluoride effects in the world and developed what are now standard methods for the analysis of fluoride in biological materials and the atmosphere. Studies were carried out in the laboratory and field, and ranged from biochemical and physiological effects to responses on plant yield and quality."

> "As molecular biology became increasingly dominant at the institute, the Environmental Biology Program lost much of its cachet and support and was eliminated." [466]

Rodgers wrote in 1973 that "Boyce Thompson witnesses frequent courtrooms" always on the side of the defence.

> "As 'neutral' experts before state agencies and the courts, as authorities to be quoted, they sell a service, and the service helps the Institute and the aluminum industry. Science strains under twenty years of incest..." [463]

The aluminium industry had written on maximum allowable volumes of fluorides in air pollution in the 1970s. Rodgers' looked at the authorship of the 1971 National Academy of Science publication I have quoted from in Chapter 2.1.

The NAS publication featured Dr. Leonard H. Weinstein and Delbert McCune of the Boyce Thompson Institute, Dr. Frank A. Smith, and Dr. John Suttie. Suttie edited the 1974 symposium in Wisconsin mentioned in Chapter 1, and carried out the 1976 experiment that reproduced the 1972 experiments of Messer, Armstrong and Singer. Suttie was also the author of a document called *Air Quality Criteria to Protect Livestock from Fluoride Toxicity*, written for the Aluminum Association. Delbert McCune, also of Boyce Thompson was the "special consultant".

The 1971 NAS publication claimed:

> "Reviews directed specifically toward fluoride toxicity in livestock as an air-pollution problem have been prepared by Suttie." [467]

Cited here were three studies, the aforementioned Aluminum Association study, as well as two published in the **Journal of the Air Pollution Control Association** [468].

Rodgers has one of the best definitions I have found regarding conflicts of interest:

> "The difficulty is that every nuance, every bias counts in a conflict that turns on parts per billion. The National Academy's, i.e., Suttie's, repudiation of the Columbia River Valley study, for example, could be used to discredit that effort if relied upon in the courtroom. Any scientific judgement about permissible standards, moreover, is fraught with value choices about trade-offs society must make. The hard question is whether it asks too much of a researcher to cash a check from industry, on the one hand, and yet be sufficiently independent to bite the hand that feeds him, on the other, if that prescription is in order."

Rodgers claimed it was not "corruption" that "helped the aluminum industry write the state standards for fluorides."

> "Conscientious administrators, trying to do their best, were simply denied options."

> "The premises of the law succumbed to the planning prowess of the Aluminum Association – the data, the experts, the weight of opinion, the common assumptions came from a single source. Its purpose is to minimize liability for damage caused and prevent disruption of existing technology."

Describing the power of the industry overall, he wrote:

> "Influence is not occasional but routine, not accidental but systematic, not modestly successful but thoroughly so." [463]

In the debate between Dr. Perrott and Professor Connett, Dr. William Hirzy, a scientist formerly of the United States Environmental Protection Agency (US EPA) was quoted:

> "The 'efficient use of natural resources,' viz. FSA (*Hydrofluorosilicic Acid*) in the U.S. is reflected in sale of about 280,000 tons of 23% assay FSA in 2011[106], which at an average price of $2000/ton,[107] resulted in transfer of taxpayers' cash of over $500,000,000 to phosphate producers in 2011 alone." [469]

Hirzy went on to say that most of this FSA went straight down taxpayers' toilets and drains, concluding that the reason FSA was added to water had little or nothing to do with dental health, but was a way for phosphate companies to prevent disposal of FSA in hazardous waste facilities.

Dr. Perrott responded to Dr. Hirzy's claim:

> "His use of the silly conspiracy theory that fluoridation is a way of disposing of industrial waste also raises questions of his credibility." [470]

Surely if Dr. Perrott knew how much or how little money was made or saved by the phosphate industry selling FSA, he would have said. We can only assume that he does not know.

---

[106] USGS Minerals Yearbook 2011. Fluorspar, http://minerals.usgs.gov/minerals/pubs/commodity/fluorspar/myb1-2011-fluor.pdf, accessed 11/01/2013.

[107] http://www.scribd.com/doc/18235930/NYC-Fluoridation-Costs-2008-Feb-2-2009-Letter-Page-1, accessed 11/01/2013.

A quick look at Florida demonstrates it has been influenced hugely in terms of its economy, employment, taxes and infrastructure by the phosphate industry. The Florida Phosphate Political Committee, claims on their website:

"Since November of 1979 the phosphate industry has come together as a group to educate policy leaders and promote the interests of this industry." [471]

Here, industry educates policy leaders because of the benefits business brings to the state.

In California, the **L. A. Times** reported on a lack of public trust in 1969 regarding the influence of polluters on water boards:

"Public hearings on proposals for a new state water pollution control law were highlighted Monday by charges that California's regional water quality control boards are dominated by polluters.

"'Domination of these boards by dischargers of pollutants has created widespread public distrust,' Chief Deputy State Attorney General Charles A. O'Brien told members of the State Water Resources Control Board." [458]

O'Brien did not "question either the motives or integrity of the men who sit on these boards." He said that progress had been made in regulation.

"Yet, the fact remains that spokesmen for the general public and representatives of groups concerned with the effects of pollution on our total environment are in a unique minority on these boards."

"The Chairman of the Board of the Ocean Fish Protective Association, John B. Gaskill, claimed the wolf was guarding the sheep. He thought the state's waters belonged to the people of the state – and that the industries and governmental agencies 'degrading the public's waters have no peremptory[108] right to do so.'"

"The Secretary of the Pico County Water District charged that the Los Angeles Regional Water Quality Control Board was 'dominated six to one by pollution interests.'"

William Rodgers quoted a letter from the Chairman of the Board at Anaconda Aluminum to the Assistant to the President asking for "... any assistance you can offer..." regarding EPA regulations for sulphuric acid pollution [472].

If industry interacts with politicians, its need to perform illegal actions to get what it wants are somewhat lessened.

While it may be difficult finding information on the American aluminium and phosphate industries, it is a little easier finding information on the junk-food industry's interactions with dentistry. One example involves an Australian organization called the Dental Health Education Research Foundation (DHERF).

The organization's Honour Roll of Contributors from the 1979 Annual Report [473] listed seven governors from Colgate-Palmolive [474], Johnson & Johnson [475], Cooper Laboratories [476], Coca Cola Export Corporation, Stafford Miller [477], The Wrigley Co. [478] and the Health Commission of New South Wales.

---

[108] Peremptory is legalese for 'not open to appeal'. I think it's a lawyer's version of 'beyond debate'.

Also included in the DHERF's Members and Associate Members were Arnotts Biscuits, Australian Council of Soft Drink Manufacturers, Cadbury Schweppes, Colonial Sugar Refining, Hardman Chemicals, Kellogg's, and Tubemakers of Australia. One of the Donors was Scanlen Sweets, another was Associated Tin Smelters.

I don't believe the DHERF still operates, but this association may help explain an advertisement on the back cover of the July, 2018 issue of the **Journal of the American Dental Association** for Colgate's Prevident Caramel Sundae Varnish (5% sodium fluoride). There is a picture of a caramel sundae on the box. It appears xylitol is used instead of sugar. "Give kids a new flavor they will love" reads the tagline. "Want your appointments to end on a 'sweet note'?" Colgate asks the ADA's dentists. The picture shows a dentist wearing a lab coat high-fiving a child.

Is it bad that corporations want to promote dental health? I don't think so, but I know that focusing on short-term profits is more important to the corporate world than people's teeth. Are they wanting to repair dental damage caused by their products so they can sell more of the product to the public? These companies are compromised in the extreme.

Of the $202,099 the DHERF spent in 1979, $43,100 was used in promotion of fluoridation. Just under $100,000 was spent on research and educational programmes, publications and films; there is no mention of fluoridation in these two sections. Details are lacking. I do know that IPANA toothpaste were name-dropping the DHERF in their ads, and for their obvious catering to inferiority: phrases like "you're probably brushing your teeth wrong" as a small sub-heading were used, with the phrase "Australians have the worst teeth in the world" was the heading [479]. Were they trying to shame people into buying a product? Caring for teeth is a wonderful thing, but shame as a motivation, perhaps not so much.

It is obvious that the sugar industry would support CWF, as they would believe it reduces the societal impact of their product. I've never seen this DHERF document mentioned in work supportive of CWF, even though it *has* been mentioned in two of Mark Diesendorf's articles (not cited by Armfield, who did cite 3 of Diesendorf's other articles) [480] and in Wendy Varney's book [481].

The DHERF document was published by the University of Sydney. I mention this because the experts and the media always tell us they've looked at both sides.

These claims of looking at "both sides" and "all the evidence" [67, 340, 360] can be reached *with minimal discussion* of the concepts presented here. The experts state something like "these are unworthy of discussion because..." Such a thing does not need to be explained. It is a conclusion borne of implication, borne of the mentality that "we would already know if..."

William Rodgers said it best in 1972:

> "The enduring lesson of the National Industrial Pollution Control Council should provide the touchstone for reform: when members of an industry set out to influence their government, they should be required to do so publicly." [482]

Australian sociologist Alex Carey discussed the corporate values encroaching Australian university staff. He wrote that staff should expect

> "increasing pressure – and temptation – to become more deeply involved in politically motivated research on behalf of corporations." [483]

Another aspect of the power of big businesses Carey briefly mentioned was the funding of chairs at universities in the late 1970s with the express purpose of promoting and defending the free-enterprise system. By 1981 more than forty American university chairs were funded by big business. The first of these in Australia was suggested in 1981, with "'substantial financial support' promised by sympathetic businessmen." [484]

What does the free enterprise system mean for the issue of CWF – or any scientific issue for that matter?

Regarding CWF, this is a topic that I have never seen explored or discussed. Dentistry has consistently approved of a less-regulated market. Note that Dr. Brown suggests that toothpaste manufacturers "consider carefully the nature of their advertising" [436] – a call for industry *self*-regulation, as opposed to suggesting government become involved. When it is believed children are obtaining "less-than-optimal" fluoride levels, experts are quick to suggest government enforce fluoridation schemes. When children are at risk of obtaining excessive fluorides, government intervention is not suggested.

It appears that business should have the right to sell its product and say what it wants about its product. This may appear innocuous and harmless, yet when business can decide not only what research is funded and what is not, and also influences what is publicized and what is not, we are led into a one-sided presentation of information.

An example will help.

British physiologist Professor John Yudkin wrote in 1964 about a conference he attended in France hosted by La Fondation pour le Progrès de l'Alimentation (FIPAL), an organization supported by the French food industry. The object of FIPAL was to "promote the study of food and nutrition and the dissemination of knowledge". Discussing communication from FIPAL's secretary, Yudkin claimed:

> "It's purposes, the letter continued, were entirely scientific and had nothing at all to do with the commercial objectives of the supporting industrial firms." [485]

After making a few enquiries, and seeing a list of other scientists who were to take part, Yudkin believed "this was a body with truly scientific aims." Yudkin responded that he was only too happy to take part.

A few months after this agreement, the secretary contacted Professor Yudkin again, this time with concern that the French press had exaggerated some of Yudkin's claims that had appeared in the prestigious medical journal, **The Lancet**. French newspapers had claimed that Yudkin's work implicated sugar in the etiology of heart disease. The secretary of FIPAL claimed he was in *this* instance writing to Yudkin in his other capacity – that of the head of public relations for the French sugar refining industry.

Yudkin sent the man the articles from **The Lancet** to demonstrate that the newspapers were not exaggerating, apologized for causing FIPAL some embarrassment, and suggested that he withdraw from speaking to avoid further embarrassment.

The secretary responded by saying there was no need to withdraw, FIPAL was an organization that wanted to "obtain and disseminate scientific information without any bias whatever." [485]

Yudkin went to Paris. A year later, Professor Yudkin received another letter from the secretary, who was finalizing the papers for a book to be published. He brought up the topic of Yudkin's paper, which had claimed sugar's palatability was responsible for its high consumption, and outlined the reasons why Yudkin thought sugar could be implicated in the "diseases of affluence" like heart disease.

> "Would I mind, asked FIPAL's secretary, if he omitted the offending passage – it was only one or two sentences – or alternatively could he put in an asterisk at this point, referring to a footnote in which I would say that this was only my own personal view and in fact most other people did not agree with it?" [485]

Yudkin said he "could not reconcile this request" because it was in complete contrast to the secretary's claims that FIPAL was an unbiased, objective organization that was not influenced detrimentally by commercial interests.

> "I did not agree, therefore, to having my article censored. Moreover, as any other author, I took it for granted that what I wrote would be understood as giving my own personal view and no one else's, so that it would be ludicrous to write the sort of footnote he requested."

> "There was a third possibility, and that was that he might wish to omit my article altogether. And this is what happened." [485]

The publication that was a result of the conference included Yudkin's name in the list of contributors yet did not include his study or work.

The story exemplifies the world of the experts: that experts can represent two conflicting sides – on one side, scientific accuracy, and on the other, the prevailing status quo (often corporate profit) – and still retain objectivity. Public relations firms give industry the ability to simply pay experts and media to frame issues in ways that suit industry. A 2010 study from the Australian Centre for Independent Journalism looked at a five-day working week over 10 newspapers, and claimed between 42 and 70% of news had its origin in Public Relations [486].

5.7 The Current State of Affairs Regarding Sugar

"Ideally, the goal of the dental profession is to eliminate itself."

- Dr. Leonard Shackles, President of the Sedalia Dental Society, quoted in *The Fluoride Issue – Conclusion: Children, Adults Can Benefit*, **The Sedalia Democrat** (Sedalia, Missouri), p. 1, 31st March, 1972.

"A great deal will depend on whether or not Australian academics in the social sciences are able to produce a very different track record from their US colleagues. It is already clear, I think, that corporations, with the advantage of relatively abundant funds, will have no difficulty in finding academics who will give the seal of professional credibility to the invariably tendentious[109] policy research conducted from business's viewpoint."

- Alex Carey, *Taking the Risk out of Democracy*, Exporting Free-Enterprise Persuasion, p. 130, 1995.

"When commissioning we had a difficult time finding authors in the developing world who had not already established links with food companies (thus disqualifying them from contributing to the series, per our Magazine competing interests policy), which might be more evidence for concerns about co-opting of international nutrition experts."

- The Public Library of Science Medicine Editors, **PLoS Medicine**, *Series on Big Food: The Food Industry Is Ripe for Scrutiny*, 19th June, 2012 [487].

"Prioritisation of government policies that resulted in short-term economic benefit, over policies related to longer-term health outcomes, was also evident in the literature. This prioritisation was apparent when agricultural policies based on subsidies raised the relative price of healthy foods and lowered the price of unhealthy foods... One effective way issues were framed and reported in the media was that regulation violates freedom of expression and limits personal responsibility."

- Katherine Cullerton, Danielle Gallegos (both from the School of Exercise and Nutrition Sciences, Queensland University of Technology), Timothy Donnet (School of Management, Queensland University of Technology, Brisbane), Amanda Lee (School of Public Health and Social Work, Queensland University of Technology), *Playing the policy game: a review of the barriers to and enablers of nutrition policy change*, **Public Health Nutrition**, Vol. 19, No. 14, pp. 2643-2653, 1st April, 2016 [488].

---

[109] "Tendentious: (Of writing, etc) having an underlying purpose, calculated to advance a cause." *Oxford Illustrated Dictionary*, 1962, Oxford University Press.

"… watering down action on junk food advertising… sends entirely the wrong signal to business, parents, and health professionals."

> - Dr. Mick Armstrong, British Dental Association Chair, quoted in *Clinicians underwhelmed by "watered down" childhood obesity strategy*, by Adrian O'Dowd, **British Medical Journal**, Vol. 354, 22nd August, 2016.

"There is surprisingly pervasive sponsorship of national health and medical organizations by the nation's two largest soda companies. These companies lobbied against public health intervention in 97% of cases, calling into question a sincere commitment to improving the public's health. By accepting funding from these companies, health organizations are inadvertently participating in their marketing plans."

> - Daniel G. Aaron (Boston University School of Medicine) and Michael B. Siegel (Department of Community Health Sciences, Boston University School of Public Health), *Sponsorship of National Health Organizations by Two Major Soda Companies*, **American Journal of Preventive Medicine**, Vol. 52, No. 1, January 2017.

This chapter looks at research on sugar and presents some arguments from the food industry and its detractors. A little history is warranted to understand more recent events. The word "current" in the chapter title is used tentatively, as attitudes are constantly changing. In searching through the early 1950s issues of business journal **Chemical Week**, I came across an article called *Sweeter for Industry*, which discussed an organization founded in 1943:

> "'Sugar' means dessert and candy to most, but to [the] Sugar Research Foundation (SRF) it's a dead-serious business." [489]

This article may help to explain why sugar finds its way into savoury foods. For instance, sausages, savoury sauces and the like sold at my local supermarket contain added sugar.

> "The long-term stability of the market is remarkable. Sugar is the only carbohydrate that has held its own, market-wise, over the past 50 years. It's an industry the economists like to call 'depression-proof.'"

The article then discussed the problem of oversupply, which could have lead to a glut in the market.

> "The simple fact is that almost any conceivable need for sugar could be filled with little strain. Finding new markets for this potential supply is a prime aim of current research."

> "Debunking the once-popular misconception that sugar is the sole culprit of dental decay is an outstanding example of this fence-mending drive. Incidentally, one interesting discovery made by SRF-sponsored researchers is that the sugar in a vegetable is, for all intents, equal in its caries-inducing power to the sugar of candy."

What the article did not point out was something obvious to anyone who has studied biology: a sugar molecule in a vegetable's cell is just one of a huge variety of molecules, a small, sometimes tiny percentage of total molecular composition. A sugar molecule in candy is one molecule repeated over and over, with no minerals or nutritional factors involved. It is not only the overloading of sugar, it is the lack of these other factors that can cause problems.

"The industry feared the long-term implications of government propaganda designed to discourage sugar consumption, promote compliance with rationing regulations. SRF was brought into being to counter this campaign by developing a sound, scientific defense of sugar's place on the dinner table. Within a short time it became apparent that a number of SRF's activities didn't fit the function of a research organization. To spread the word of its work, the industry set up Sugar Information Inc., placed it in the hands of SRF secretary… Neil Kelly… [who] describes his work as 'low-pressure public relations,' [Kelly] emphasizes in no uncertain terms that it's completely non-political, has no lobbying interest."

Note that here, "propaganda" according to industry, is information "designed to discourage sugar consumption".

The Sugar Association was the "fund-gathering" arm of the SRF. This and the Sugar Information Inc., are

"supported by 110 private sugar refiners and processors…" [489]

The article claimed that while there was not much more room in American diets for sugar, the substance could still have many industrial uses. The major portion of sugar sales were in the diet.

In 1953, Dr. Fredrick Stare of Harvard graced the pages of **Chemical Week**, which pointed out that the "30 million-odd obese adults" in America potentially made up a "well-fattened market for the sugarless soda pop".

At this time the synthetic, sugar-free sweeteners took only 0.6% of the American market. This, after American doctors and health professionals were advising the public about health risks of obesity, some apparently believed were caused by sugar.

"Against the mountain of sugar, the total pile of synthetic sweeteners casts an insignificant shadow." [490]

Still, the SRF was

"Directing a $600,000 fund for a big-scale rebuttal to the claims of non-sugar foods."

This is where we step from the science of nutrition into the science of public relations.

"Guiding association member 'educational' advertising, pointing out that sugar – singled out as fattening – is, after all, no more calorie-adding than such publicly approved diet foods as tomatoes or grapefruit."

The SRF directors were reported to have voted to continue the $27,000/year research project at Harvard, under the guidance of Dr. Stare, to

"discover whether or not non-nutritive sweetening agents are of value in reducing diets."

Stare was to direct studies on humans. The article writes of "conclusions, if verified by Stare" were:

"When you're hungry, reach for a sweet (one containing sugar, of course)."

"Sugarless drinks (and foods) serve no dietary purpose; the body still requires the same amount of food because it has not assimilated any sugar."

Of these potential conclusions, the article claimed:

"Quite understandably, the sugar suppliers are interested in establishing proof of Stare's hypothesis; such results (1) would remove the 'fattening' stigma from sugar and (2) could lead to increased sales." [490]

A 1976 article published in the more left-wing journal **The Progressive** notes that the syndicated newspaper columns of both Dr. Jean Mayer and Dr. Fredrick Stare carry the Harvard affiliation, yet "neglect [to mention] the corporate ties."

"Stare has refused to disclose to us the companies which currently employ him." [491]

Two other professors,

"… were reluctant to disclose their current outside affiliations to us. Instead, each referred us to university administrators. Inquiries to the university department heads met with equal evasiveness."

This article was authored by Benjamin Rosenthal, a New York Democratic Representative, and two people from the Center for Science in the Public interest, Michael Jacobson and Marcy Bohm. Their article also reported that the University of Wisconsin's Food Research Institute, while claiming "the scholar himself must be free", had received $635,390 from various "food, packaging and drug companies" in 1975. Donations were from Kellogg ($20,000), McDonald's ($20,000), Nestle ($20,000), Campbell ($20,000), Kraftco ($20,000), General Mills ($10,000), and the Institute of Shortening and Edible Oils ($60,000).

The investigators claimed Dr. E. M. Foster, Director of the Food Research Institute, did not mention "his membership on the board of directors of the Stange Corporation since 1972." Stange manufactured many food ingredients.

These investigators also claimed Dr. Alfred E. Harper, Chairman of the Department of Nutritional Sciences, and head of a National Academy of Sciences committee that worked on recommended dietary allowances of vitamins and other nutrients (for instance on the 9th edition of RDAs in 1980), had said under oath at an FDA hearing that about 20 percent of his income was from consultancy work. He had consulted for G. D. Searle Company (drugs and food additives manufacturing, up to $10,000 per annum), Procter and Gamble, McGaw Laboratories, Abbot Laboratories, General Mills, and Pillsbury. His faculty chair was sponsored by General Foods at M.I.T., and the $50,000 went with him when he moved to Wisconsin.

The article explained why these donations were important:

"Any grant will induce a certain amount of gratitude on the recipient's part and discourage him from being a major critic of the donor – particularly if there is a chance for a second grant." [491]

This is where we need to look – to the *criticism* or *lack of criticism* that comes after these research grants or donations are made. For instance, the 1979 Australian Dental Health Education Research Foundation listed among its members and donors; Cadbury Schweppes, Arnotts Biscuits, Scanlen Sweets and Coca-Cola – researchers need to examine communications from the DHERF in the late 1970s and early 1980s to see if there is any open criticism of these companies and the foods they sell in DHERF communications. If there *was* open criticism of these products from the DHERF, open recommendations to government to regulate junk food advertising, or open recommendations to children and parents to avoid Sugar Sweetened Beverages (SSBs), then this would be evidence of *no or little* bias. Yet if there was *no* criticism of SSBs and the like, no recommendation to restrict junk food advertising to children, and the focus instead on exercise, attitude, an unspecified "well-balanced diet" and (only) parental responsibility, these points of view are identical to those promoted by industry, and this would very possibly demonstrate a biased view. One example is discussed below. Some studies on the topic of advertising to children are discussed in Appendix 6.

I have noticed that there is often an argument when researchers or organizations receive money from corporations – some argue this is an obvious conflict of interest, some argue the opposite. Yet I have found it very difficult finding research on the communications coming not so much from the corporation, but from those who the corporation funded.

In his 2007 book *The Trouble with Medical Journals*, Dr. Richard Smith, editor of the **British Medical Journal** for 25 years, made a very similar claim to that of the authors of this 1976 article: that industry-sponsored studies consistently have conclusions favourable to industry's interests [492].

Again let me say I believe if we argue against someone who has been funded by industry, we are not only arguing against their argument, we are arguing against their professional survival.

Rosenthal, Jacobson and Bohm commented:

> "In sharp contrast to the pervasive and multifarious links between professors and industry, professorial associations with consumer groups are rare." [491]

They give the example that of the 18 professors that responded to a survey they developed, "half of the links" were "token involvement" – for instance, a subscription to the journal **Consumer Reports** or belonging to the organization Common Cause (a watchdog group famous for recommending the cessation of America's attack on Vietnam). They concluded:

> "When interviewing professors about matters that may affect a corporation or industry, reporters should routinely inquire into that professor's industrial ties." [491]

One of the examples given by Rosenthal *et al.* detailed a clinical trial performed by Dr. Robert L. Glass, DMD, DrPH, of the Forsyth Dental Center in Boston, and Sylvia Fleisch, MS, Assistant Director of the Boston University Computing Center. The Forsyth Center is affiliated with the Harvard School of Dental Medicine.

Their trial looked at 1,199 children from 690 families, and their consumption of regular and presweetened cereals. The relationship to the incidence of dental caries was measured over a two-year period.

Funding was not mentioned, but cereals were provided by Kellogg Company. Eight cereals were regular, 6 presweetened. In this study, 979 children's records were used. At the beginning of the study, each child was given an oral prophylaxis[110] and examinations and x-rays of teeth were made. Three examinations were carried out by the same dentist at yearly intervals.

> "Nutritional histories were made for the children through their mothers by trained nutritionists."
>
> "Mothers were asked to encourage their children to eat as much cereal as they liked, and at least one serving daily."
>
> "… the cereal consumption of individual children was estimated from family size and orders of cereal."
>
> "… a considerable range in estimated amounts consumed is evident for both regular and presweetened types." [493]

---

[110] "The removal of calculus, both sub- and supra-gingival, and plaque from the surfaces of the teeth using hand or mechanical instrumentation accompanied by appropriate oral hygiene instruction." *Oxford Dictionary of Dentistry*, Edited by Robert Ireland (Associate Clinical Professor of Postgraduate Dental Education at University of Warwick Medical School), 2010.

Glass and Fleish categorized the children's consumption levels as low, medium or high, because they did not have exact determinations of daily cereal intake. They did show a table of 'number of boxes of cereal consumed per child per year', for regular and presweetened cereal, though the word 'estimate' was not used in the table.

> "Although some of the participating children consumed large amounts of cereals containing up to 45% sucrose, the results of the several analyses carried out demonstrate no association between dental caries and cereal consumption."

They showed a graph comparing the children in their study with standard Massachusetts children; at 7 years old the DMF (Decayed, missing or filled teeth) was just over 2 in both groups, at age 10 it was close to 5, and at age 13 the DMF was 10. There was only one very small point in which the children they studied had a higher DMF than the standard Massachusetts children.

They went on to discuss the fact that most studies regarding sugar intake had been carried out on animals, and that they believed in extrapolating these to humans care must be taken regarding differences in eating habits. They discussed the famous Vipeholm study, mentioning that "sucrose taken at mealtimes and in other than a sticky vehicle failed to produce increased caries activity." The study was published in the April issue of the **Journal of the American Dental Association** in 1974. In July of that year, letters from two dentists who each criticized the study were published.

Herschel Horowitz, D.D.S.[111], of Bethesda, Maryland, wrote claiming that the appraisal of measuring intake was faulty because *family* intake was measured, and *individual* intake was simply estimated by dividing the number of people in a family by the total amount of cereal.

> "To merely add up boxes of cereal and divide by people is merely a meaningless arithmetical exercise." [494]

Dr. Horowitz believed a more precise measurement of individual intake could have been achieved.

Dr. Howard J. Greene, DDS, of Colorado Springs, claimed that he found the study

> "... unacceptable on any reasonable scientific or epidemiological grounds."

The first reason was that Glass and Fleisch did not consider other nutritional factors; Dr. Greene pointed out that children could have eaten

> "... candy all day and failed to practice proper oral hygiene... (a reasonable assumption in our culture), what difference would a breakfast cereal make?"

That the children had rates of 2.5 DMFs in the first year of the study, and around 4 in the second year, he inquired whether this "... reflects an unacceptable rate of pathosis..." which he thought should have indicated to the researchers that some cariogenic factor was operable in the children's lives. He claimed that

> "... the few remaining cultures in this world where our type of diet is unknown have practically negligible DMF rates during a comparable period."

---

[111] National Institute of Dental and Craniofacial Research. One obituary in the **Journal of Public Health Dentistry** (Vol. 64, Special Issue 1, 2004) claimed "He loved a good argument in the strict sense of that word (i.e., a reasoned exchange of views) ... Hersh knew that truth only advances when suppositions are held up to the light and given a good shake. He was one of the best at shaking suppositions." This is credited to Brian A. Burt.

He wondered if the children put sugar on the unsweetened cereals, as this was not mentioned.

His "… training in epidemiology and simple common sense caused me to recoil."

He pointed to the "sophisticated razzledazzle with regression analyses, correlation coefficients, analyses of variance, and F ratios" which lead to a "statistically significant irrelevancy—a phenomenon I find all too common in so-called scientific literature today." [494]

Dr. Fredrick Stare also contributed to the discussion. His letter was published in the September issue of the **Journal of the American Dental Association** [495]. Dr. Stare pointed to several phrases in the Glass and Fleisch study;

> "Nutritional histories were made for the children through their mothers by trained nutritionists."
>
> "These figures (estimate of cereal consumption) were verified on an individual basis through the dietary histories taken by nutritionists."

Dr. Stare pointed to Dr. Horowitz's statement that "it is impossible to determine with accuracy the exact amount of food ingested…" Stare wrote:

> "I agree with this statement, but then this all hinges on what degree of accuracy is desired. In summary, diet histories were taken by well-trained nutritionists at varying times during this study. However, we did not think the results were sufficiently accurate to clutter up this paper with the results; but they did provide a verification on an individual basis of the estimate of cereal consumption." [495]

According to Rosenthal *et al.*, the study was praised later in 1974 by the Cereal Institute (a trade group), in a press release titled *Scientific Studies Prove Cereals Don't Cause Cavities, are Vital in Nation's Diet*. The Institute was responding to consumer groups that had petitioned the FDA to remove high-sugar cereals from the market. Rosenthal *et al.* claim that the Cereal Institute left out the fact that Kellogg Company had contributed to the study. [491]

Regarding the timeline of events here – the Kellog study was published in April and the letters critiquing it were published in July, but as for the dates of the petition and press release, I am uncertain. The 1974 Glass and Fleisch study was also cited in the National Academy of Sciences 1989 publication **Diet and Health: Implications for Reducing Chronic Disease Risk** (pages 279 and 638), without comment on its quality.

In 1980, the National Academy of Sciences published a document called **Public Policy Options for Better Dental Health**. One of the claims it made was that total reduction of sugar resulted in 90% less dental caries [496]. This was based on the infamous Vipeholm study, now regarded as a classic, which concluded that the risk from sugar was largely from eating in between meals [497]. It also claimed that only 25% of sugar was added to foods by consumers, implying 75% was added by food manufacturers. Media ought to consider this when they lay blame at the feet of parents for children's high-sugar diets.

In 2000, **Advertising Age** reported that Coca-Cola had an estimated $200 million deal with Time Warner's Turner Broadcasting System that allowed the company to advertise on TBS Superstation, TNT, CNN/SI and the Cartoon Network [498]. Because of the company's proprietary status, Coca-Cola was allowed a first look at

Turner's developing sponsorship avenues, for instance virtual product placement. The **Age** reported that Coca-Cola spent a little over $350 million yearly at this time advertising in the USA.

In 2001, Coca-Cola reportedly gave $150 million (US) to Warner for rights to use Harry Potter in junk food advertising to children [499] (UK's **Telegraph** reported £95 million [500]). This was protested globally by over 40 organizations. Coca-Cola made a 3-year, $18 million donation to Reading is Fundamental, a group established in 1966 to address illiteracy in America. This was one of the conditions of using the franchise, another was that there was to be no product placement in any of the movies. The latter was probably quite an easy condition for the company to bear. I have found no research on the amount of profit made by Coca-Cola from the deal.

In 2003, the **Journal of Public Health Dentistry** featured a guest editorial from Dr. Jonathan D. Shenkin[112], which criticized the American Academy of Pediatric Dentistry Foundation (AAPDF) for receiving nearly $1 million from Coca-Cola, to support research, and promote "'personal responsibility' for oral health, nutrition, and diet." The academy represents 5,600 pediatric dental specialists. Dr. David Curtis, President of the AAPDF claims the organization "is certainly not clear on exactly the role that soft drinks play in terms of children's oral disease." [501]

Shenkin's editorial also called out the US National Soft Drink Association (NSDA) for consistently denying any link between excess caloric or soft drink intake as a cause of health problems, including "displacement of calcium in children's diets".

> "We can be assured that the NSDA and Coca-Cola would likely focus any pediatric dental public information campaign on the lack of toothbrushing and professional dental prophylaxis and not on the frequency or volume of soft drink consumption as the cause of tooth decay." [502]

The Center for Science in the Public Interest suggested the AAPDF leadership should resign [503]. Not all soft drinks contain sugar; some are sweetened with other ingredients. [267]

According to an article in American journal **Mothering**, the Minnesota Dental Association "vigorously supported" a bill that would ban SSBs from schools, only to have it die at the last minute

> "as the result of successful maneuvering by professional lobbyists from Coke and Pepsi." [504]

The authors of this article claim to have spoken to many dentists who were "appalled", yet did not want to publicly challenge AAPDF over this "because they feared retaliation." The article claims that Dr. John Rutkausaks, AAPDF's Executive Director, stated that the relationship between SSBs and dental caries was "certainly not clear". Dr. Joel Berg, President of the AAPDF, has been quoted as claiming that

> "… all foods can cause decay. To blame a product for the problem is somewhat inappropriate, given that it's how the product is used that can cause the problem." [504]

What Coca-Cola receives for their donation is obvious from one article published on **PR Newswire** in 2006 entitled *Nation's Dentists Get Behind Fluoride Awareness Campaign for Kids*. The article discusses not only AAPDF but another initiative with an organization named Spring! by Dannon that would help raise awareness

---

[112] DDS, MPH, Clinical Associate Professor of Health Policy, Health Services Research and Pediatric Dentistry at Boston University.

about the importance of drinking fluoridated water. The article is 1,700 words long, and the word "sugar" does not appear. Nor do the words "soft drink". The Senior Brand Manager of Spring! by Dannon, claimed:

> "Parents who prefer bottled spring water to keep their kids healthy and hydrated now can choose the convenience of bottled water, confident that they are also providing essential fluoride…" [505]

The last part of the article did state

> "Do not put your child to bed with a bottle containing anything but water…"

The latter article may have been an ad for Dannon; ten years earlier they were spending $10 million yearly on advertising [506].

One statement from the **Mothering** article:

> "It was painful for us to watch the turmoil that the Coke deal had set off within AAPD [Foundation], an organization that typically is on the side of children. It was also difficult to witness the convoluted rationalizations and self-serving excuses that AAPD leaders put forward to justify their position, when basically they just wanted the money. We have seen the same process at work when cash-strapped school administrators and teachers deny the harm of selling soda in schools… administrators are not bad people… we believe, they are well-intentioned individuals trying to support organizations that are strapped for funds."
> [504]

In studying this issue of funding from the soft drink companies and the food industry, one thing I have very rarely seen discussed is the amount of taxes corporations pay, compared to the amount of profits they make for owners and shareholders. Surely if they can afford to spend so much on research and advertising, they can afford a substantial increase in their taxes. Perhaps our science would not only be better in quality, it would be more democratic if laws prohibited corporate funding of science, and with research funded by governments, ratified by public vote.

While there is much evidence to suggest junk food advertising works, not everyone involved in the healing profession thinks advertisements for junk food and Sugar Sweetened Beverages (SSBs) should be minimized. There *is* a belief that advertisements don't work at all so there is no need to ban or restrict them – this was expressed by a spokesperson for Tony Abott, the Australian Minister of Health in 2007 [507].

The Australian Government's healthy eating ads were being drowned out – advertising from junk food companies were outweighing them fifteen-fold.

> "As Mr Abbott has previously said it's not junk food advertising that is causing obesity, it's an unhealthy lifestyle."

Here is a good example of the propaganda model: one of the top authorities in Australia, expressing an opinion that *perfectly* suits – and is identical to – that of big business interests, *not* people. An "unhealthy lifestyle" was not defined, with an obvious consequence: nobody has to take responsibility, has to change their behaviour, except the consumer. No laws or regulations need to change.

When we go to the scientific literature, it's very easy to find articles claiming junk food advertising *does* function according to its intended purpose (see Appendix 6).

Obviously in studying a nutritional role for fluorine, many are quick to discuss the myriad effects of not only various other foods, but *advertising* of foods. Experts and intellectuals in media claim that parents need to take responsibility for what their children eat, that parents need to "just say no" [508].

Compare this demand for parental or self-control with the information presented in Appendix 6. In looking at research, it can be seen that marketers consistently do their best to undermine parental authority. Marketers deliberately exploit the "cool" factor of rebelling, so when parents "just say no" their efforts are less effective.

In 2011 the South Australian Health Minister, John Hill, claimed almost the exact opposite of his predecessor (Abott): the "key problem" is "voluntary self-regulation". Hill claimed most parents wanted government regulation, according to phone surveys.

It has been pointed out that the industry uses "personal responsibility" as a way to encourage consumption:

> "It should be noted that the ideology of personal responsibility is an entity in its own right albeit strongly influenced by industry as a strategy to increase consumption." [488]

An article comparing "Big Food" with "Big Tobacco" suggested that while there were certainly differences, one key similarity (of many) is to:

> "Focus on personal responsibility as the cause of the nation's unhealthy diet." [509]

In 2011 Coca-Cola gave over $70 million to various organizations, including the American Diabetes Association (*Diabetes Education & Outreach in Latino Community, Live Empowered*, $125,000), American Dietetic Association Foundation, (*Kids Eat Right*, $100,000), Big Sur International Marathon, (*Just Run*, $50,000), CAN DO Houston (*Let's Move in Magnolia Park*, $25,000), Children's Medical Center Foundation (*Center for Obesity*, $25,000), Good Sports, (*Youth Sports & Fitness Programs*, $200,000), Illinois African American Coalition for Prevention, (*Mind, Exercise, Nutrition, Do It! (MEND)*, $100,000), National Black Nurses Association, (*Preventive Health Action Team "PHAT"*, $100,000), Portland After School Tennis & Education, Inc., (*Eat Wise & Exercise*, $25,000), University of Alabama at Birmingham, (*Exercise Study*, $300,000), University of South Carolina Educational Foundation (*School-Based Childhood Obesity Prevention Program*, $200,000), Vive en Forma, (*Vive en Forma*, $100,000), YMCA of Greater New York (*Food & Fun/Move to Improve*, $50,000), and $5,000 to the Women's Health Symposium of the National (US) Dental Association.

> "With an enduring commitment to building sustainable communities, our Company is focused on initiatives that reduce our environmental footprint, support active, healthy living, create a safe, inclusive work environment for our associates, and enhance the economic development of the communities where we operate." [510]

In 2013, they donated $10,000 to the National Dental Association Centennial Anniversary Convention. In 2014, they donated $100,000 to the NDA-HEALTH NOW (Health Equity, Access, Literacy, Technology & Hope) program of the National Dental Association [511].

A paper published in March of 2015 on the **Public Library of Science Medicine** website received attention from many involved in the issue of sugar research [512]. The paper investigated the National Caries Program (NCP) of the National Instititute of Dental Research (NIDR) in the 1970s. All three authors were affiliated with the Philip R. Lee Institute for Health Policy Studies and the Department of Medicine at the University of California in San Francisco and other educational organizations.

The **New York Times** reported on this issue. One article by reporter Anahad O'Connor summarized the work of Kearns, Schmidt and Glantz quite well [513].

Kearns *et al.* wrote:

> "Reflecting the research priorities of the sugar industry, the 1971 NCP research priorities ignored strategies to limit sugar consumption and focused instead on fluoride delivery, reducing the virulence of oral bacteria, and modifying food products with additives to counter sugar's harmful effects[113]. Ultimately, the NCP, which drove the US dental caries research agenda for more than a decade, failed to significantly reduce the burden of dental caries..."

> "The documents show that the sugar industry knew that sugar caused dental caries as early as 1950 and did not attempt to deny... Instead, through trade associations, the sugar industry adopted a strategy to deflect attention to public health interventions that would reduce the harm of sugar consumption, rather than restricting intake." [512] (page 12)

The authors claimed a 1950 Sugar Research Foundation document demonstrated the desire to "deflect attention" from the belief that sugar was the primary factor in cariogenesis [514]. They state there was no obvious reason why the NIDR took the position that sugar reduction was unachievable, possibly due to "limited access to industry documents" – something much journalism and research has suffered from. If policy makers want to help researchers, journalists and the public, they should create and enforce laws that prohibit corporate secrecy.

Deflecting attention away from a problem is a good strategy for industry because it is difficult for its critics to call it dishonest. Industry is not so much guilty of manipulating data which is obviously dishonest, but simply deciding on entire directions of research.

Another article by Kearns with Gary Taubes looked at the influence the sugar industry had on people like Dr. Fredrick Stare, who along with his department, "had a long history of ties to Big Sugar." The article began by discussing two Sugar Association executives winning the 1976 Silver Anvil award from the Public Relations Society of America for "the forging of public opinion" (words of Kearns) and "establish [ing] the safety of sugar as a food" [515].

The University of Colorado, South Carolina, and West Virginia, have lent their support for Coca-Cola's "Energy Balance" Network in 2015. This was discussed by the CSPI [516] and the **New York Times** [517].

The Network claims that weight-conscious Americans are too concerned with calories and sugar, and need to focus more on exercise.

> "'Most of the focus in the popular media and in the scientific press is, 'Oh they're eating too much, eating too much, eating too much' — blaming fast food, blaming sugary drinks and so on,' the group's vice president,

---

[113] Here the authors cite National Institute of Dental Research (1971) Opportunities for participation in the National Caries Program. http://catalog.hathitrust.org/Record/003436264. Accessed 16 May 2014.

Steven N. Blair, an exercise scientist, says in a recent video announcing the new organization. 'And there's really virtually no compelling evidence that that, in fact, is the cause.'" [517]

Scientists involved, one with 25 years experience researching in food science, another a university dean, claimed they were not biased because of the money. The article's author wrote:

"It is unclear how much of the money, if any, ended up as personal income for the professors." [517]

Stanton Glantz, Professor of Medicine in the Division of Cardiology at the University of California, claimed that industry had deflected concern from sugar for about five decades [513].

Regarding sugar and children, there is much that can be said. Some research has been collected in Appendix 6. Many people want Sugar Sweetened Beverages (SSBs) regulated, taxed, banned from advertising, and removed from schools.

The article published in **Mothering** claimed:

"... Coke is continually hunting for opportunities to sink its financial talons into any organization that might even indirectly influence its ability to sell soda at schools." [504]

This article claimed Coca-Cola had funded educational organizations like the American Association of School Administrators, the National Association of State Boards of Education, the National Association of Secondary School Principals, the National Alliance of Black School Educators, and the Boys and Girls Clubs of America (BGCA), which the authors claim "curious" due to BGCA's "Cavity-Free Zone" program of oral health.

In 2017, the (US) Centre for Science in the Public Interest (CSPI) and The Public Health Advocacy Institute initiated a lawsuit, "on behalf of themselves and the general public" against Coca-Cola and the American Beverage Association (ABA). Their brief contains 186 points in which they claim Coca-Cola and the ABA corporation misled the American public. These range from simple things like always using slim models in advertising, to complicated scientific aspects of sugar metabolism that the plaintiffs claim had been distorted and misrepresented in public [518]. Coca-Cola disagreed with these claims [519].

The CSPI document cites research pointing to Mexico, where SSB consumption made up 9.8% of total energy intake, compared with what they claimed the American Heart Association recommends – a 3% maximum [520]. In 2009, Mexicans drank about 665 Coca-Cola drinks per year, the highest in the world [521]. They also drank the most bottled water in the world, per capita [522]. In America, Mexican immigrants continued this because they were uncertain if American tap water was safe, after the issues at Flint, Michigan.

A **New York Times** article discussed an educator who gave small seminars on dental health to people; the **Times** quoted her as saying; "We've been told: If you don't drink Coca-Cola, you're poor..." [523]. The article did not say where this attitude came from. Diabetes was the leading cause of death in Mexico in 2012, killing 87,600 people according to WHO data [524].

In the USA the beverage industry interacts with schools; this has become a small yet occasionally significant source of revenue for the schools. It's not an immediate money-maker for the SSB companies, but it does give them exclusive market rights to particular schools and long-term brand loyalty in children who will be future customers. A 2006 study of 120 school beverage contracts in 16 states performed by the CSPI found only 12 to 58% of the revenue from selling non-nutritious drinks went to the school; the rest going to the beverage corporation (with an average of 33% for the school and 67% for the corporation). There was still an incentive for schools to have these contracts, as they were a source of revenue. On occasion, schools were given cash advances for taking contracts.

> "Sometimes a cash advance is tied to subsequent commissions on beverage sales. When a cash advance is tied to commissions on sales, it serves as a pressure on a school/district to ensure that a sufficient volume of beverages is sold to cover the cash advance." [525]

Though not all of companies' revenue is profit, they also found long-term benefits: many times the contracts were exclusive, meaning not only sales, but marketing and advertising were exclusive.

Value of non-cash benefits for schools, such as computers, programs, uniforms (complete with drink brand logo) and scoreboards were difficult for researchers to ascertain. The highest value items were scoreboards ($2,500-10,000), cash bonuses for teachers, and college scholarships. The CSPI quote Peter Healey, former marketing director of Coca-Cola:

> "With soft drink consumption, early preferences translate into later life preferences. It's a lot easier than getting consumers to switch their brand preferences later on." [525]

The CSPI cite a 1998 study that claimed that children between 4 and 12 purchased and directly influenced annual sales of $24 billion. Children as a demographic were thought to influence about $500 billion in family and others' spending [526].

Provisions in contracts allow companies very strict control over soft drink sales in schools. The study concluded by claiming that many schools were getting a raw deal. Most of the money was going to corporations, not to schools.

A Canadian study discusses how schools have been "... forced to view their students as customers..." [527].

The Center for Science in the Public Interest has investigated the issue of SSBs in schools in the USA:

> "Sales in schools account for less than one percent of overall beverage sales in the U.S., according to CSPI's analysis. CSPI found schools earn an average of $3.72 per student per year from beverages sold through vending and other venues outside of the school meal programs."

> "Much progress has been made improving the beverage mix in schools—90 percent fewer beverage calories were shipped to schools between 2004 and the 2009-2010 school year, according to an audit by the beverage industry. Still, 88 percent of high school students and 63 percent of middle school students have access to sugar drinks at school, largely in the form of sports drinks." [528]

There is a popular movement among parents, teachers and activists to remove SSBs from schools, both in the USA and in New Zealand.

Juliet Schor discussed the influence of corporate-developed educational material in her 2003 book *Born to Buy*:

> "… a Kellogg's breakfast curriculum presents fat content as the only thing to worry about when choosing breakfast food. There is no mention of the sugar and salt in Kellogg's cereals. A first-grade reading curriculum has the kids start out by recognizing logos from K-Mart, Pizza Hut, M&M's, Jell-O, and Target."

> "For corporations, one of the appealing aspects of Sponsored Education Materials (SEMs) is that they can market covertly, and thereby more effectively." [529]

One reason for the willingness of teachers in the USA to include these materials has to do with money: Schor writes that around 2003, teachers were estimated to be spending about $500 each year of their own salaries on reading material. Corporate materials are often given free of charge. The information is slanted to suit the provider. Incineration of plastic was called "recycling" in one waste curriculum. Procter & Gamble distributed a curriculum called Decision Earth, which told students clear-cut logging was good for the environment. Distribution ceased when attorneys general in 11 states investigated its claims. All but one "expert" in a video claiming plastics were not a threat to the environment, worked for the plastic industry.

> "Businesses are willing to spend millions of dollars on crummy classroom materials, but have proven unwilling to pay taxes to support high-quality, serious curricula for the nation's children. There's a national discourse paying homage to equality of opportunity, but schools in low-income districts have far fewer resources and are more likely to turn to insidious products…" [529]

In her 2009 book *This Little Kiddy went to Market*, Sharon Beder discussed the influence of businessmen on schools:

> "[Business leaders] argue that, because teaching methods affect business, they have a right to influence them. The irony is that the failure of corporations to pay their fair share of taxes has been a major factor in depriving schools of the necessary resources to provide a high-quality education." [530]

The **New Zealand Dental Journal** in 1960 wrote of the interaction between the biscuit business and schools in England, described as an "educational vested interest":

> "There is a growing practice amongst the representatives of Biscuit Manufacturers of approaching head teachers of schools with the suggestion that they should buy biscuits at a special concession price and sell them to the children at normal retail prices, keeping the difference for school funds. This is happening in a country where the School Dental Service is the responsibility of the Minister of Education." [531]

This may help explain why the British have had a reputation for poor quality dentition.

In 1991, **The Evening Post** reported that the German high court had ruled that Milupa, a company making baby food, had to pay damages to children,

> "… whose teeth were harmed by its sugared teas. Medical studies estimate 100,000 German children suffered damage to their teeth from the teas. Many had to have their baby teeth extracted." [532]

In 1995, one panel of experts from the American Academy of Pediatrics recommended that "A variety of resources should be developed to help parents teach children that commercials are designed to sell products." [533] A 2010 American article claimed young people would see 21 food advertisements daily, most for foods "loaded with sugar and fat" [534].

A 2012 American article that looked at compromises between the First Amendment rights of corporations, and the rights of children to be protected from the consequences of advertisements for unsafe food, claimed American children saw on average, thirteen junk food adverts daily on TV, this comprising about 30% of all paid TV advertising to children [535].

Radio New Zealand's (RNZ) news program Checkpoint with John Campbell recently reported on an experiment from the Wellington branch of Otago University that New Zealand children are exposed to an average of twenty-seven junk food ads every day [536].

Louise Signal, Associate Professor of the Department of Public Health, put cameras on 168 children over four days (Thursday – Sunday), and monitored the advertising they were exposed to. Reporter John Campbell asked Dr. Signal:

> "How important is it do you think that we control the messages that children are getting, and do you think that's possible in a democracy?"

He was suggesting that parents may not be able to have a say in what messages corporations send to children. Corporations need to have the same freedom of speech rights as people, in order to maximise profit. It is argued that advertising is part of these rights. Yet freedom of speech rights for someone like you or me does not give us the ability to advertise on television or on billboards unless we're extremely wealthy. While some of us may do this occasionally, only the extremely rich can do it consistently.

I believe a discussion on the behaviour and regulation of the food industry *must* involve the question of subordination of the legal rights of corporations. They must *not* have the same rights as people, because they have so much more money, power, (in the form of close ties with government), knowledge (in the form of research), ability to shape and control knowledge (in the form of research funding and financing), and outreach in the form of advertising and public relations, than any person or group of people can at present.

It is a shame that the tobacco fiasco was not part of a wider discussion on the rights of corporations. We're wasting time if we're having these tiny talks about how should Coca-Cola, Nestle, GE etc, advertise and communicate without putting it into a larger context of the regulation of corporate rights, and the fact that the most destructive of these companies never really expire, they are often simply engulfed by a larger body. One of Bob McChesney's arguments from a 2003 documentary was that "freedom of the press" should not only be the right of the press to express their points of view, but of the public to hear multiple points of view, not only information acceptable to advertisers [537].

Dr. Eric Crampton, an economist with The New Zealand Initiative, recently wrote an opinion piece arguing against sugar taxes, in which he claimed that:

> "They presume poor people are too dumb to make the 'right' choices and must be guided by their betters."
> [538]

Yet this "guiding by their betters" is what advertising and public relations do all the time. In fact it is one of the basic conceptions of life in the modern world – that experts know what is true and the rest of us should trust them, above our own judgement. Coca-Cola, also opposed to a sugar tax, is one of the funders of The New Zealand Initiative, but Dr. Crampton assured RNZ that this was his own point of view, which was not influenced by the funding.

It is also interesting to see Dr. Crampton describe sugar taxes as "classist" – especially when we see the following: a 2012 Reuters article looked at the behavior of soft drink companies and the food industry. It claimed that despite mounting scientific evidence that their products are harmful, they have never lost a battle of any significance in the US. Reuters analyzed lobbying records of industry from 2009. All 24 states that considered taxing SSBs saw the matter dropped.

> "The groups have spent more than $175 million lobbying since President Barack Obama took office in 2009 — more than double the $83 million spent in the previous three years, during the Bush Administration.
>
> The totals do not include broader lobbying efforts by the Chamber of Commerce, the National Association of Manufacturers, and media and advertising interests that also opposed the federal plan."

Dr. Crampton's article did not mention the behaviours of the SSB or food industry when profits are potentially threatened. This Reuters article also discussed how the two major soft drink companies behaved when Congress was considering sugar taxes:

> "In a stark example of lobbying muscle, PepsiCo Inc, Coca-Cola Co, bottlers and the American Beverage Association spent more than $40 million lobbying in 2009 when Congress was considering a soda tax. That was more than eight times the $4.8 million they had spent the previous year, the analysis showed. After the proposal died, the groups cut spending to $24 million in 2010 and $10 million in 2011." [539]

Perhaps some would consider such incredible wealth concentration *classist*. Some would also consider refusing to subsidize healthier foods classist, when it is more convenient for the poor to purchase cheaper food. I do not think a sugar tax will solve anything without making healthy foods cheaper. Perhaps taxes on unhealthy food *are* classist – then the poor wouldn't be able to eat *anything*! Lowering the cost of healthy food so that poor people can afford them would be a far more egalitarian and sensible approach.

In 2006, schools in New Zealand began banning food high in sugar. This was part of a $70 million campaign against obesity, coinciding with a week-long World Health Organization Asia/Pacific meeting [540].

In 2017, the website stuff.co.nz reported that $2 lunch packs full of poor quality food were being sold in dairies in Auckland, mainly to children [541]. Pictured here (**Figure 49**), is close to what a person could buy for $2.

The work of Alex Carey [302] and others [261, 334] help to show us why nowadays universities produce intellectuals whose opinions perfectly echo the ideas and suit the goals of industry, of the business leaders' desire for power and profit. Studies conforming to industry's point of view are abundant like junk food advertising, and vastly outnumber the patient, precise work scientists are ideally thought to do. This may lead to studies that are not funded by industry, studies not favourable to industry in terms of conclusion, being outliers in their results. Outliers can be treated as mistakes and dismissed.

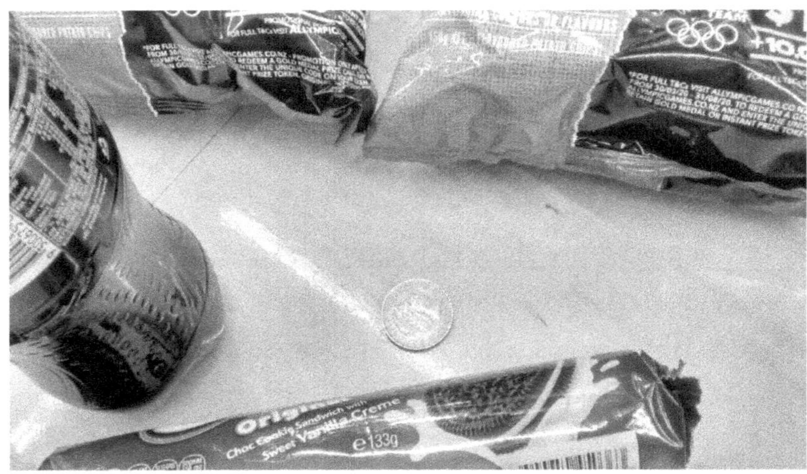

Figure 49. This is a recreation of a 2017 photo demonstrating the buying power of $2. Source: Eleanor Black, Unhealthy 'lunch packs' costing $2 marketed to children, stuff.co.nz, 29th September, 2017, [541]. Note the potato chip companies are involved with the Olympic Games.

In discussing junk food advertising, notice how healthy the people in junk food ads appear – do they have healthy-looking, white teeth? Are there any visible fillings or crowns, or ugly staining in their teeth or malocclusions? Are these people slim or obese? Are they balding, with bad eyesight? Are they lethargic and suffering the effects of malnourishment, something probably very common in junk food users? If junk food is always advertised using healthy-looking people, this gives a misleading impression of these foods.

The WHO of course, have written on their guidelines for sugar intake in 2015:

"Although previous attempts to influence WHO did not lead to a change in sugar recommendations, there have been concerns that vested interests would seek to influence the process of updating dietary guidelines." [223]

In 2003, Kaare Norum, Professor Emeritus of the Department of Nutrition from Oslo University's Medical Faculty was to chair a reference group to help the World Health Organization (WHO) develop a document outlining a "Global Strategy on Diet, Physical Activity and Health" (GS), aimed at prevention of Non-Communicable Diseases (NCDs). A paper Norum wrote on the influences from industry and trade groups that were lobbying the WHO directly and indirectly through member states appeared in a 2005 issue of the **Scandinavian Journal of Nutrition** [542].

Norum's article discussed the extensive, two-year process behind the setting up of the GS. The GS was based on the scientific work of an expert committee of 30 people from around the world, chaired by Richardo Uauy, a professor in paediatrics and nutrition from Chile[114]. Over 100 scientists were involved. This process resulted in a Technical Report Series document, number 916 (TRS 916) [543], "Diet, nutrition and the prevention of chronic diseases". Norum writes that the creation of this document was "open, translucent and peer reviewed". It was a heavily scientific document, which gave nutrient intake goals, like a previous, 1990 WHO document, TRS 747. The GS was to be discussed at the World Health Assembly (WHA) in 2004. TRS 916 offended the sugar industry, and to a lesser extent the salt and palm oil producers. Norum wrote,

"Resistance against the GS was kept up until the last minute at the World Health Assembly in May 2004." [542]

---

[114] Also London School of Hygiene and Tropical Medicine, 2002-2013.

The palm oil industry's reactions led to some changes in the GS regarding saturated fat. The Salt Institute and the sugar industry protested in "concerted action". The GS was affected by this, as TRS 916 was the scientific document upon which the GS rested.

> "The sugar industry and its associations protested heavily, and wrote angry and threatening letters to Gro Harlem Brundtland, then Director General at the WHO."

The sugar industry wrote to the US Minister of Health, Secretary Tommy Thompson, requesting that the US not pay the contribution to the WHO if TRS 916 was published still suggesting intake of free sugars limited to 10% of daily energy intake. Norum said the sugar industry's claims – that TRS 916 was authored by "selected" experts, that the report was not peer reviewed, and that it had not been shown to industry for comments prior to publication – were dishonest.

That the WHO delegates were primarily from the health sector led to a lessening of their concern with things like "trade and price" policies, which were not dealt with in meetings. This lack of "general politicians" was "a problem" in the final development stages of the GS and the scientific authority of TRS 916, because it could have had "huge consequences" for countries like Brazil, regarding the "production of and trade in sugar."

Norum claims that WHO headquarters asked him to give an hour-long presentation on the TRS 916 regarding the development of the GS. Two days before the meeting in which he was preparing to speak, the Pan-American Health Organization (PAHO) told him to restrict his talk to 10 minutes only. This was because the "sugar issue" (Norum's emphasis) had been a focus of media attention,

> "... and delegates needed more time for questions, answers and discussion. Then, shortly before my scheduled talk, I was told that there should be no discussion afterwards."

Norum believed this was because the delegates, being from the health sector, were probably uncertain of how their governments wanted them to respond to "the content of the report" – primarily the "sugar issue" (Norum's emphasis).

> "The discussions were dominated by questions relating to trade and economics, not health issues, even though many of these countries, e.g. Mauritius and Brazil, had huge health problems with obesity and diabetes in their populations." [542]

What is the purpose of the World Health Organization? Most of us would answer this question in an obvious fashion – the purpose is to promote, recommend and help discover what makes people healthy. But most people are not economists or CEOs, and most people don't hold governmental purse strings that fund the WHO's endeavors in promoting health. Norum's paper is worth reading for anyone interested in food industry behaviour. The Sugar Association's letters to the WHO are available online [544].

What is the solution to this excess of sugar? Perhaps it will test the mettle of populations in terms of their self-control: simply don't buy it, and the food industry will have to change to foods people want. Yet herein lies the catch. While the wealthier middle class can afford the nutrient-richer foods, the poor cannot. And it is difficult (in Wellington, at least) to simply walk down the street without being reminded that tempting junk food is easily available everywhere. When the food industry claims that responsibility lies in consumption and not anywhere near their own doorstep, it is quite amazing that educated people can take them seriously. Yet in a business-run world, it is simply another example of the massive outreach of intellectual domination business has over not only those within their own rank and file, but those that seek to lead populations, and their advisors.

Politicians, intellectuals, health ministries and junk food companies use parents to scapegoat their own responsibilities. In many instances this is done without full knowledge of cause and effect – this ignorance being the end result of decades of industry's involvement with the intellectual community, so this argument has become part of the intellectual landscape with minimal criticism. It is no surprise that profits are more important. Yet everybody, including industry, benefits from healthy populations, so industry is undermining the health of its own work force.

If a drug dealer is selling to kids at the local high school shall we blame the school teachers or shall we arrest the dealer?

I don't like the food police any more that you do, I like the odd treat on a special occasion, but I dislike the way the corporate world has us exclusively blaming parents for junk food sales. Who has the most regulatory power out of parents, scientists, politicians, media and junk food corporations?

It is certainly not parents – yet according to experts in our media, in corporate press releases, the parents must take *total* responsibility for their children's eating habits – even though corporations do as much as possible to denigrate parental authority in the eyes of children, and politicians have the power to regulate businesses that advertise publicly, and scientists have the ability to issue prestigious press releases that the media can publicize. Parents obviously have much less time on their hands if they're busy raising children and working. Corporations and politicians interact heavily, so if there was one group that would be able to *help* parents restrict children's intake of junk foods it would be politicians. They are closer to seeing what really goes on behind the scenes as far as business is concerned than most parents are.

Yet *so much* of the responsibility goes to parents. I frequently see in Wellington huge billboards many stories high advertising junk food. I'm sure they're not (officially) *aimed* at children, but it's blatantly obvious children will see them. Parents, who did not put these things in place, did not ask for these things to be put in place, are expected to take near *total* responsibility for their effects.

An unpleasant aspect of the power dynamic in our lives is apparent here: that there's no money in working for the poor. Currently in New Zealand, unhealthy food is cheaper than healthy food. Yet every politician will tell us they care about the poor children [545]. When dentists recommend fluoridation, many of the intellectuals and politicians seem to get behind this and support it. Yet regulating the sugar industry is ignored, even when recommended by the same dentists.

In 1956, an editorial in the **New Zealand Dental Journal** claimed:

> "At present the truth is, of course, that some natural teeth for some people are worth saving. As for the other teeth in the jaws of the other people, their extraction has become almost a national custom or tribal initiation ceremony to be performed at adolescence or at the latest before marriage."

"... we are sometimes in the dangerous position of promising and attempting the impossible, even to the extent of bringing conservative dentistry into disrepute by our well-intentioned efforts against hopeless odds." [546]

In 2005, the New Zealand media printed a letter written by a lady who claimed her son needed 10 teeth out, but would have to wait at minimum a year because he was not in intense pain [547]. There was not enough staff to deal with the case.

In 2014, dentist John Twaddle was quoted as saying, regarding the removal of fluoridation:

"When you're dealing with it at the coalface you can see the benefits. And to be honest, we don't have the dental manpower to cope with the amount of decay if they took fluoride out." [548]

In 2017, another article discussed the terrible teeth of people living in fluoridated Porirua, near Wellington. The dentists were blaming the amount of easy-to-access sugary drinks available, cheaper than milk or fruit juice. [549]

It seems the "hopeless odds" that were discussed in 1956 are still with some of us. Seeing a speck of what goes on behind the scenes in the sugar industry, and in areas of dentistry, such results should not surprise.

In July of 2018, the Right Honorable Simon Bridges, leader of the New Zealand National Party, expressed his thoughts on his facebook page regarding the drop in business confidence since the 2017 election in which the coalition government had been in power.

He asked the camera rhetorically, what would his party do differently?

"We'd get out of business's way."

Whether small, medium or large, Mr. Bridges wanted to allow businesses to become

"... more efficient, more productive, and grow in what they do..." [550]

One can see that advertising and lack of food industry regulation has helped lead New Zealanders to compromising health in the name of benefits to business. Scientists seem unable at present to rectify or alter this with their own powers of persuasion. With all due respect to Mr. Bridges' knowledge and concern regarding the New Zealand economy, I would suggest that the businesspeople behind the companies discussed in this chapter ought to be faced with severe regulation, *not* more freedom, even if they go on to other enterprises and industries. Perhaps some even deserve incarceration [551]. They have shown their self-interest is prioritized over democracy. They often play the victim, but they are belligerent and cunning. One wonders how heavily their "work" and assets are taxed. Their use of front groups and public relations companies in media must be well-publicised and eliminated completely if we are to have an unbiased, democratic discussion around this issue.

Almost a hundred years ago, an American educator named John Dewey wrote:

"As long as politics is the shadow cast on society by big business, the attenuation of the shadow will not change the substance." [552]

The sooner that media and scientists in the field of public health realize their "battle" is not against weary parents, but against manipulative corporations and probably well-intentioned but economically inclined politicians, the sooner we may have results in this matter. But I think I'm saying something here everybody already knows.

I honestly think sugar taxes are a waste of time unless they are used to subsidize healthier foods. Perhaps corporations should be taxed for the amount of advertising they create, instead of the public for fulfilling the desires these businesses manipulate and exploit. The statement "parents ought to be responsible" makes perfect sense at first glance, but has a hidden meaning. Until healthy foods are not only cheaper than junk food, but *affordable* for the poor, the poor will be forced to eat junk – hardly fair to say "parents ought to be responsible" when the meaning of such a statement is "politicians, businessmen, scientists and media *don't* have to be responsible".

I have seen the occasional claim that advertising bans do not help reduce problems associated with sugar consumption. There are numerous reasons why. One is the amount of money given to universities and health-oriented organizations by the food industry, which must distort researchers' commitment to truth. A second may be that comfort foods can be habit-forming and breaking habits is difficult; a person goes from one unhealthy comfort to another. A third reason is simply that sugar is in many savoury foods as well as sweet foods, so we probably eat more than we bargain for or desire without even knowing it. A recent **New York Times** article discussed a European study which found parents underestimated the amount of sugar in children's food [553]. So even if parents *were* being responsible by their own standard, this study suggested their perception would in many instances be inaccurate.

There have been experiments and discussion on whether sugar is addictive [554].

If children have eaten sugar-laden food and drink for comfort for many years, ceasing the communication from the advertising industry will only be one step to greater health. A lot of advertising is about brand loyalty, getting consumers when they're young, ensuring their continuing consumption as they age[115]. Such a thing is worth contrasting with politicians' claims of caring about children, and politicians' attitudes to advertising.

This chapter about the sugar industry is a gateway in taking us from a strict questioning of a potential nutritional role for fluorine, yet is relevant to dental health. As already noted, the 2012 paper entitled *The Food Industry Is Ripe for Scrutiny* was the beginning of a series of articles on the food industry, authored by the editors of the **Public Library of Science Medicine** and written under the guidance of Marion Nestle[116] and David Stuckler[117] [487]. I will conclude by quoting a sentence from this article:

> "... the big multinational food companies control what people everywhere eat, resulting in a stark and sick irony: one billion people on the planet are hungry while two billion are obese or overweight." [487]

---

[115] I'm glad to see the New Zealand Dental Association has publicly called for more restrictions on advertising, *Dentists back calls for greater restrictions on junk food marketing*, NZDA Press Release, 2nd April, 2019.
[116] Department of Nutrition, Food Studies, and Public Health, New York University and Department of Nutritional Sciences, Cornell University, Ithaca, New York, United States.
[117] Department of Sociology, University of Cambridge, United Kingdom, Department of Public Health & Policy, London School of Hygiene & Tropical Medicine, United Kingdom.

5.8 The Concentration of Fluorine in the Hastings Water Supply 1953-1956, Private and Public Statements

This chapter looks at the concentration of fluorine in the water supply of the New Zealand (NZ) town of Hastings, the first city in this country to have fluoridation. The NZ Health Department archives (now on Mulgrave Street, Wellington) have been available to the NZ public since 1982. There are at least three files detailing the beginning of New Zealand's first Community Water Fluoridation program in Hastings in detail. More archival information on this topic is available from the National Library, also in Wellington.

In 1958 the **New Zealand Dental Journal** published a paper by T. G. Ludwig, the Medical Research Officer for NZ's Medical Research Council. Ludwig wrote:

> "During the period March, 1953 to September, 1954, a considerable proportion of the fluoride concentrations registered in the city's water supply were below the required optimal level. The solution-feeding equipment came into operation in September, 1954, and fluoride concentrations of 1 part per million were obtained soon afterwards in all sectors of the city." [555]

A 1987 paper authored by Peter B. Hunter[118] and E. Storey[119] focused on Hastings, and claimed:

> "During the period March 1953 to September 1954 a considerable proportion of the fluoride concentrations recorded in the city's water supply were well below 1 ppm with a few above that level." [556]

They gave no more detail, no numbers regarding concentration. People who support and oppose fluoridation alike may be aware of a claim made by Dr. John Colquhoun, and discussed in detail in his 1987 thesis [557]. Colquhoun claimed that the level of fluorine in the Hastings water supply in the early 1950s fluctuated rather drastically, mostly much below the desired 1 ppm, but as high as 8.0 ppm in at least two instances. Using documents from the Health Department archives, I will show evidence that there is accuracy in this claim.

In his first article in 1958, Ludwig did not mention that the concentration was high in some places, the implication being that it was always lower than, or at most, 1.2 ppm. I note this because I feel this perfectly demonstrates the fact that what we see in scientific literature and media available to the public is quite different to what goes on when we scratch beneath the surface. The experts felt they had justification to continue fluoridation even when there were problems in keeping the concentration between the desired levels of 0.8 – 1.2 ppm (nowadays the desired level in New Zealand is 0.7–1.0 ppm [558]). One can see from the following analyses (**Figures 50 – 54**) throughout the second half of 1953 that very few of the readings were within this range. I did not see any communication to the public via newspapers regarding these actual results.

---

[118] Principal Dental Officer (Research and Development), Department of Health, New Zealand.
[119] Professor, Department of Preventive and Community Dentistry, University of Melbourne, Australia.

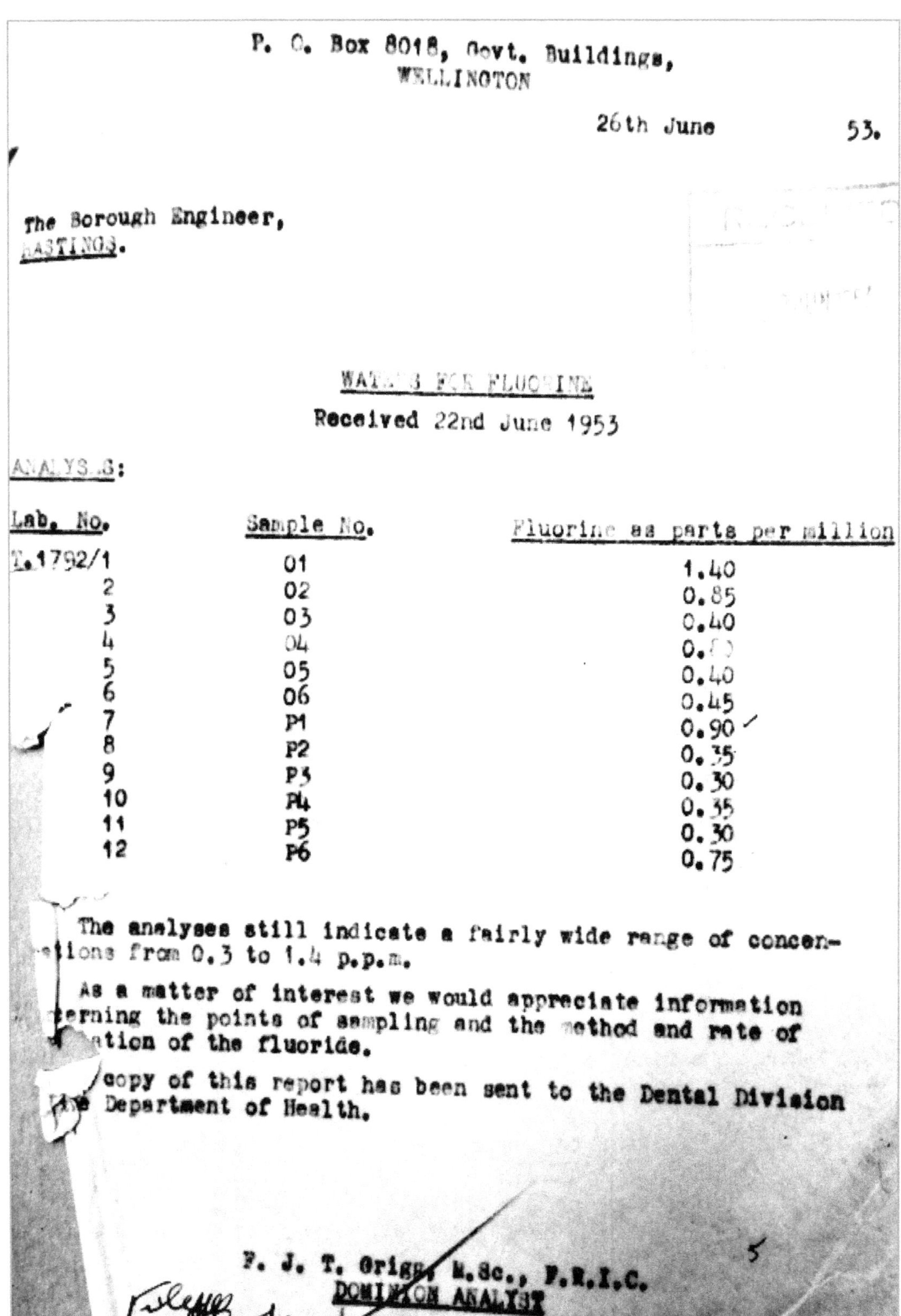

P. O. Box 8018, Govt. Buildings,
WELLINGTON

26th June   53.

The Borough Engineer,
HASTINGS.

WATERS FOR FLUORINE

Received 22nd June 1953

ANALYSIS:

Lab. No.	Sample No.	Fluorine as parts per million
T.1792/1	01	1.40
2	02	0.85
3	03	0.40
4	04	0.[illegible]
5	05	0.40
6	06	0.45
7	P1	0.90
8	P2	0.35
9	P3	0.30
10	P4	0.35
11	P5	0.30
12	P6	0.75

The analyses still indicate a fairly wide range of concentrations from 0.3 to 1.4 p.p.m.

As a matter of interest we would appreciate information concerning the points of sampling and the method and rate of application of the fluoride.

A copy of this report has been sent to the Dental Division of the Department of Health.

F. J. T. Griggs, M.Sc., F.R.I.C.
DOMINION ANALYST

Figure 50. *Waters for Fluorine, Hastings, 26.6.1953.* Source: 125/299/3 H1 Box 1704, available from Archives on Mulgrave Street, Wellington, New Zealand.

One sample exceeded 1.2 ppm fluoride.

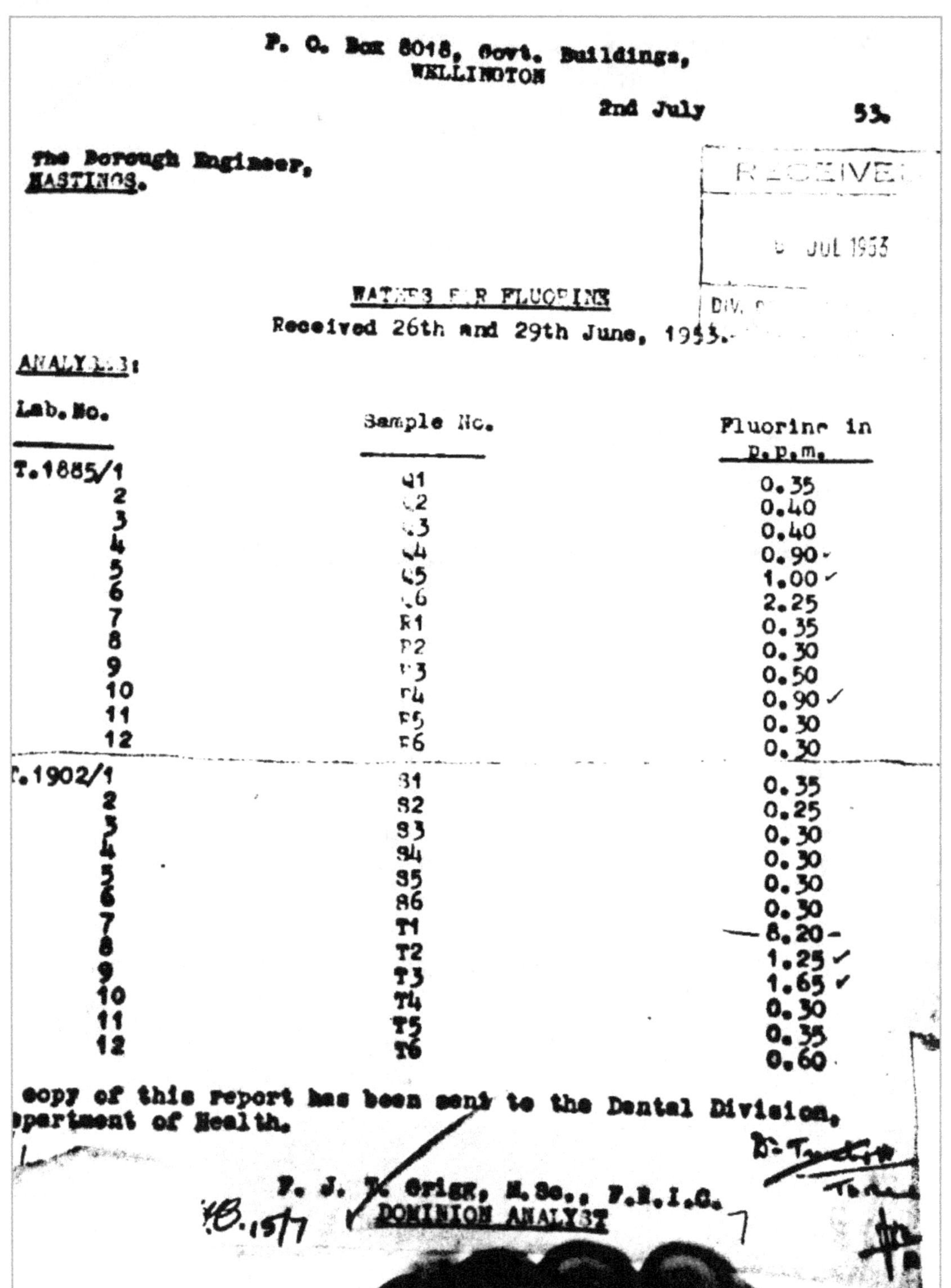

P. O. Box 8018, Govt. Buildings,
WELLINGTON

2nd July   53.

The Borough Engineer,
HASTINGS.

RECEIVED
6 JUL 1953
DIV.

WATERS FOR FLUORINE
Received 26th and 29th June, 1953.

ANALYSIS:

Lab. No.	Sample No.	Fluorine in p.p.m.
T.1885/1	Q1	0.35
2	Q2	0.40
3	Q3	0.40
4	Q4	0.90
5	Q5	1.00
6	Q6	2.25
7	R1	0.35
8	P2	0.30
9	P3	0.50
10	P4	0.90
11	P5	0.30
12	P6	0.30
T.1902/1	S1	0.35
2	S2	0.25
3	S3	0.30
4	S4	0.30
5	S5	0.30
6	S6	0.30
7	T1	8.20
8	T2	1.25
9	T3	1.65
10	T4	0.30
11	T5	0.35
12	T6	0.60

A copy of this report has been sent to the Dental Division,
Department of Health.

P. J. K. Grigg, M.Sc., F.R.I.C.
DOMINION ANALYST

Figure 51. *Waters for Fluorine, Hastings. Received 26 and 29.6.1953.* Source: 125/299/3 H1 Box 1704.

Four samples exceeded 1.2 ppm – one being as high as 8.2 ppm.

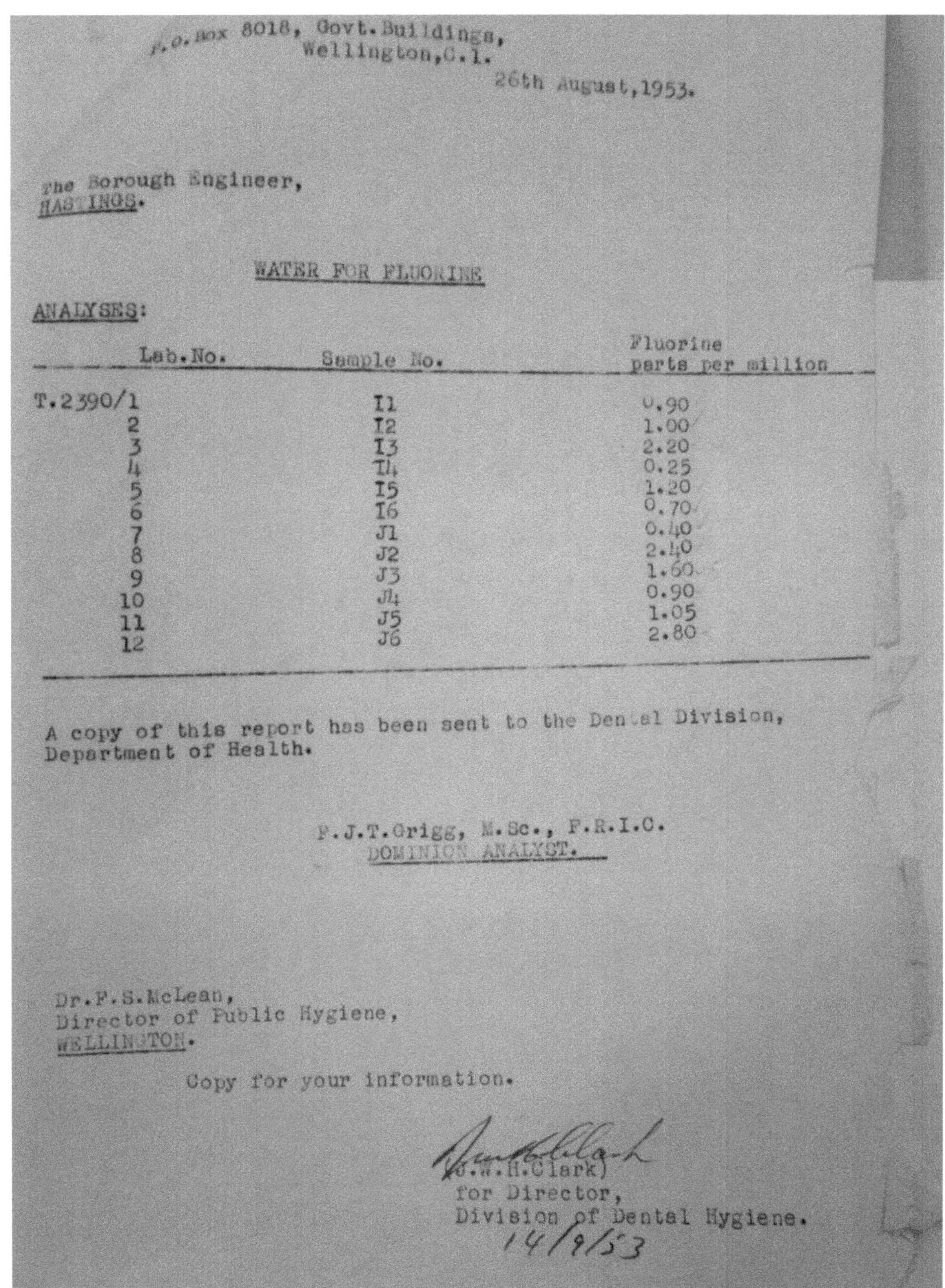

P.O.Box 8018, Govt.Buildings,
Wellington,C.1.

26th August,1953.

The Borough Engineer,
HASTINGS.

WATER FOR FLUORINE

ANALYSES:

Lab.No.	Sample No.	Fluorine parts per million
T.2390/1	I1	0.90
2	I2	1.00
3	I3	2.20
4	I4	0.25
5	I5	1.20
6	I6	0.70
7	J1	0.40
8	J2	2.40
9	J3	1.60
10	J4	0.90
11	J5	1.05
12	J6	2.80

A copy of this report has been sent to the Dental Division,
Department of Health.

F.J.T.Grigg, M.Sc., F.R.I.C.
DOMINION ANALYST.

Dr.F.S.McLean,
Director of Public Hygiene,
WELLINGTON.

Copy for your information.

(J.W.H.Clark)
for Director,
Division of Dental Hygiene.
14/9/53

Figure 52. *Water for Fluorine, Hastings, 26.8.1953.* Source: 125/299/3 H1 Box 1704.

Four samples exceeded 1.2 ppm fluoride, the highest being 2.8 ppm.

COPY.   T.2492

P.O.Box 8018, Govt.Buildings,
WELLINGTON,C.1.
9th September,1953.

The Borough Engineer,
HASTINGS.

WATERS FOR FLUORINE.

ANALYSES:

Lab.No.	Sample No.	Fluorine as parts per million
T.2492/1	M1	0.20
2	M2	0.30
3	M3	0.30
4	M4	0.55
5	M5	0.30
6	M6	0.50
7	N1	0.85
8	N2	0.70
9	N3	0.30
10	N4	0.80
11	N5	0.30
12	N6	0.65

A copy of this report has been sent to the Dental Division,
Department of Health.

F.J.T.Grigg, M.Sc., F.R.I.C.
DOMINION ANALYST

Dr.F.S.McLean,
Director of Public Hygiene,
WELLINGTON.

Copy for your information.

(J.W.H.Clark)

Figure 53. Waters for Fluorine, Hastings, 9.9.1953. Source: 125/299/3 H1 Box 1704.

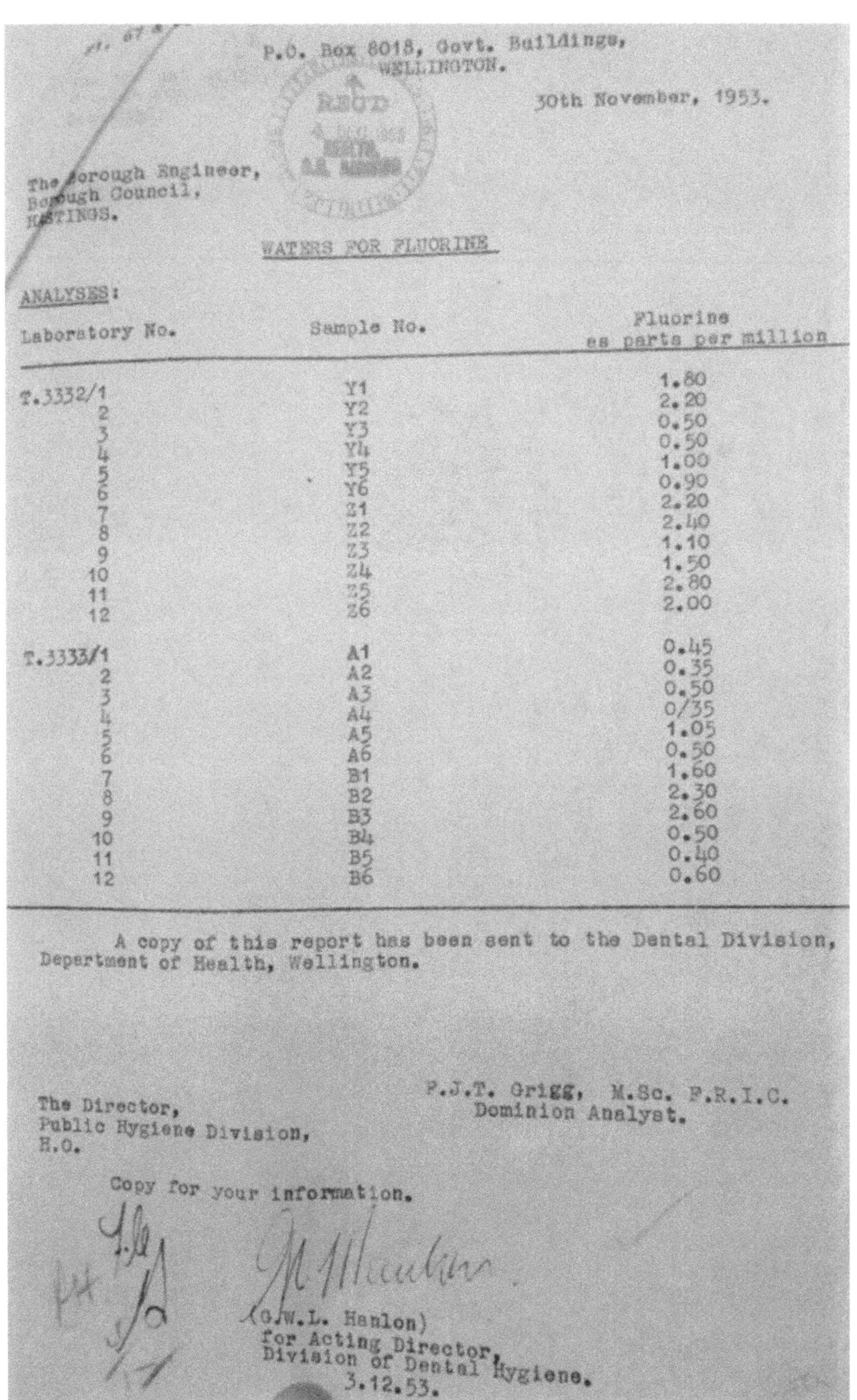

P.O. Box 8018, Govt. Buildings,
WELLINGTON.

RECD

30th November, 1953.

The Borough Engineer,
Borough Council,
HASTINGS.

WATERS FOR FLUORINE

ANALYSES:

Laboratory No.	Sample No.	Fluorine as parts per million
T.3332/1	Y1	1.80
2	Y2	2.20
3	Y3	0.50
4	Y4	0.50
5	Y5	1.00
6	Y6	0.90
7	Z1	2.20
8	Z2	2.40
9	Z3	1.10
10	Z4	1.50
11	Z5	2.80
12	Z6	2.00
T.3333/1	A1	0.45
2	A2	0.35
3	A3	0.50
4	A4	0/35
5	A5	1.05
6	A6	0.50
7	B1	1.60
8	B2	2.30
9	B3	2.60
10	B4	0.50
11	B5	0.40
12	B6	0.60

A copy of this report has been sent to the Dental Division, Department of Health, Wellington.

P.J.T. Grigg, M.Sc. F.R.I.C.
Dominion Analyst.

The Director,
Public Hygiene Division,
H.O.

Copy for your information.

(G.W.L. Hanlon)
for Acting Director,
Division of Dental Hygiene.
3.12.53.

Figure 54. Waters for Fluorine, Hastings, 30.11.1953. Source: 125/299/3 H1 Box 1704.

The analysis dated 30th November 1953 (**Figure 54**) shows 10 readings above 1.2 ppm fluoride.

On the 15th of April, 1954, Dr. Derek Taylor, the Medical Officer of Health, wrote to the Director-General of Health in Wellington (**Figure 55**). Taylor claimed Mr. Fish, the Borough Engineer, had said there were problems with the equipment, leading to underfluorination of water. Candy Filters, mentioned in this letter, was a company involved in the sale of fluoridating equipment to Hastings.

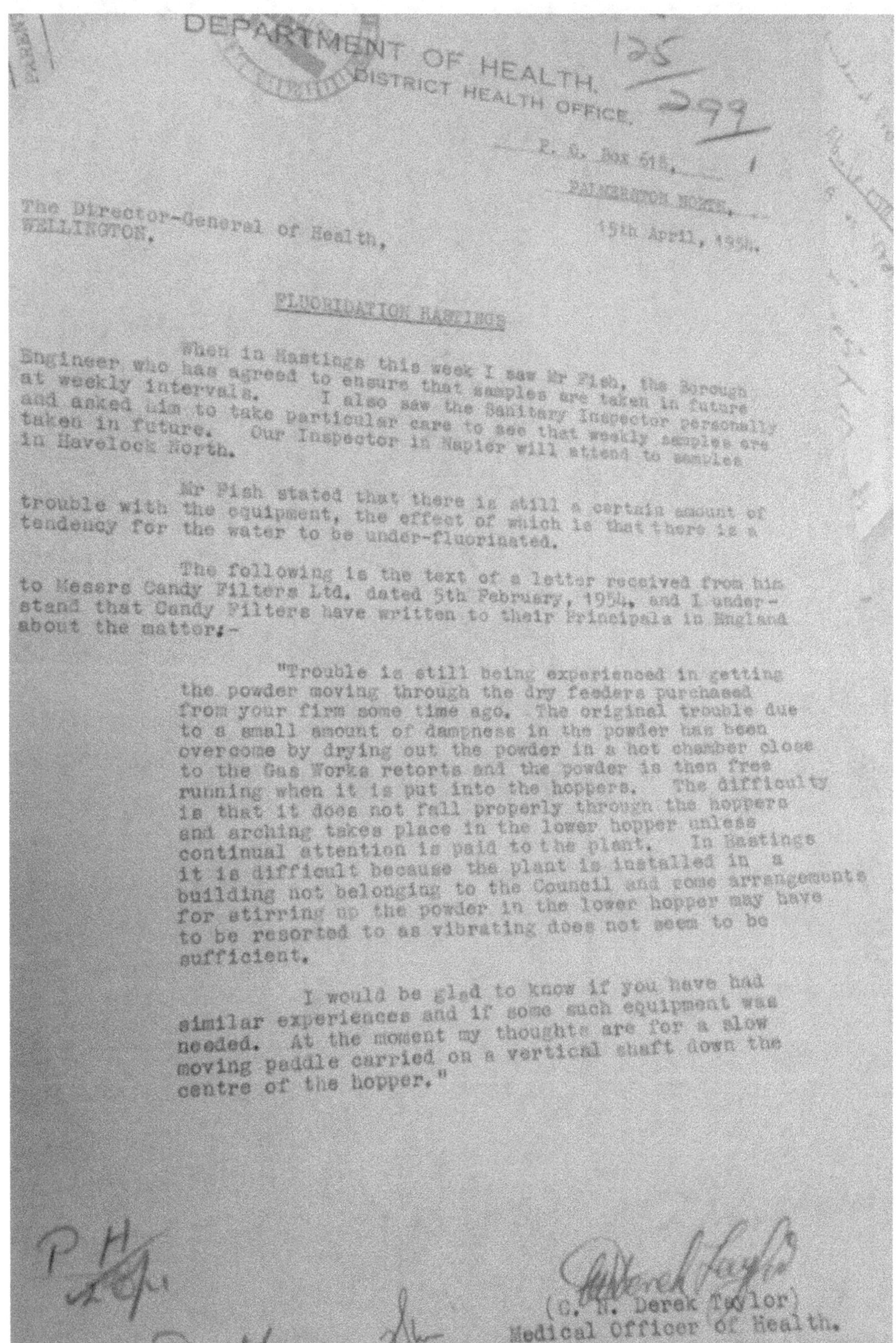

DEPARTMENT OF HEALTH,
DISTRICT HEALTH OFFICE.

125/299

P. O. Box 515,
PALMERSTON NORTH.

The Director-General of Health,
WELLINGTON.   15th April, 1954.

FLUORIDATION HASTINGS

When in Hastings this week I saw Mr Fish, the Borough
Engineer who has agreed to ensure that samples are taken in future
at weekly intervals.   I also saw the Sanitary Inspector personally
and asked him to take particular care to see that weekly samples are
taken in future.   Our Inspector in Napier will attend to samples
in Havelock North.

Mr Fish stated that there is still a certain amount of
trouble with the equipment, the effect of which is that there is a
tendency for the water to be under-fluorinated.

The following is the text of a letter received from him
to Messrs Candy Filters Ltd. dated 5th February, 1954, and I understand that Candy Filters have written to their Principals in England
about the matter:-

"Trouble is still being experienced in getting
the powder moving through the dry feeders purchased
from your firm some time ago. The original trouble due
to a small amount of dampness in the powder has been
overcome by drying out the powder in a hot chamber close
to the Gas Works retorts and the powder is then free
running when it is put into the hoppers.   The difficulty
is that it does not fall properly through the hoppers
and arching takes place in the lower hopper unless
continual attention is paid to the plant.   In Hastings
it is difficult because the plant is installed in a
building not belonging to the Council and some arrangements
for stirring up the powder in the lower hopper may have
to be resorted to as vibrating does not seem to be
sufficient.

I would be glad to know if you have had
similar experiences and if some such equipment was
needed.   At the moment my thoughts are for a slow
moving paddle carried on a vertical shaft down the
centre of the hopper."

(C. N. Derek Taylor)
Medical Officer of Health.

Figure 55. *Fluoridation Hastings, 15.4.1954.* Source: 125/299/1 H1 Box 1634.

On the 5th of May, 1954, the President of the New Zealand Dental Association wrote to Dr. Francis A. Arnold, the Director of the National Institute of Dental Research at the National Institutes of Health in Washington D. C. His letter claimed that the council was "under a certain amount of duress from anti-fluoride groups" and were "weakening in their attitude towards the project…" He wrote that the NZDA

"… feel it incumbent upon us to do all in our power to give them the support they so badly need."

"Recently the Hastings Junior Chamber of Commerce took up the cudgels on behalf of fluoridation, their object being to educate the public on the matter and refute incorrect or misleading press statements. Their knowledge and influence is of course limited but they are doing a grand job of work." [559]

He asked Arnold for help, saying:

"My committee feels that an outside authority such as yourself would do more to weigh the scales in favour of fluoridation … local efforts and it is to this end that we implore you to consider very seriously the possibility of your coming to Hastings to deliver a Public Address…"

"The Mayor and Councillors and all responsible public bodies would be specially invited to attend and the widest publicity possible give[n to] the address. It is sincerely felt by my committee that if fluoridation is rejected in Hastings it would indeed be difficult for another town in New Zealand to introduce it. If the Hastings project continues and succeeds, as it must, then the shocking dental state of New Zealanders may be reduced by its introduction throughout the country." [559]

He asked Arnold to consider the invitation earnestly, almost promising "every available means" to him. Another letter to Arnold followed the next day (6th May, **Figure 56**). It was from the Chairman of the Hastings Junior Chamber of Commerce Fluoridation Education Committee, who extended

"a very sincere invitation to visit Hastings…"

"My Committee was formed to combat incorrect misleading and scare-mongering propaganda being used by the anti-fluoridation group. The position is serious and we badly need expert opinion to convince the public of Hastings and the Borough Council of the benefits of fluoridation."

In May, 1954, newspapers announced that Dr. Arnold of the USA and Dr. Parfitt of the UK were to give a public talk on fluoridation. Both men had attended the recent World Health Organization dental seminar in Wellington, New Zealand's capital. One of the articles claimed:

"Dr. Arnold stated that no mechanical difficulties of any consequence had been encountered at Grand Rapids in keeping the fluorine content of the city's water supply to the specified concentration of one part per million…" [560]

This of course gave the impression to the people of Hastings that there was no problem in the mechanical aspects of the fluoridation of their own water supply. How could the media and the public know that this was true, when the mechanical difficulties in their own land were going undiscussed and uninvestigated by any third party?

An article with an advertising flavour appeared in one newspaper; the names of Arnold and Parfitt in large letters with their qualifications, referred to them as World Authorities.

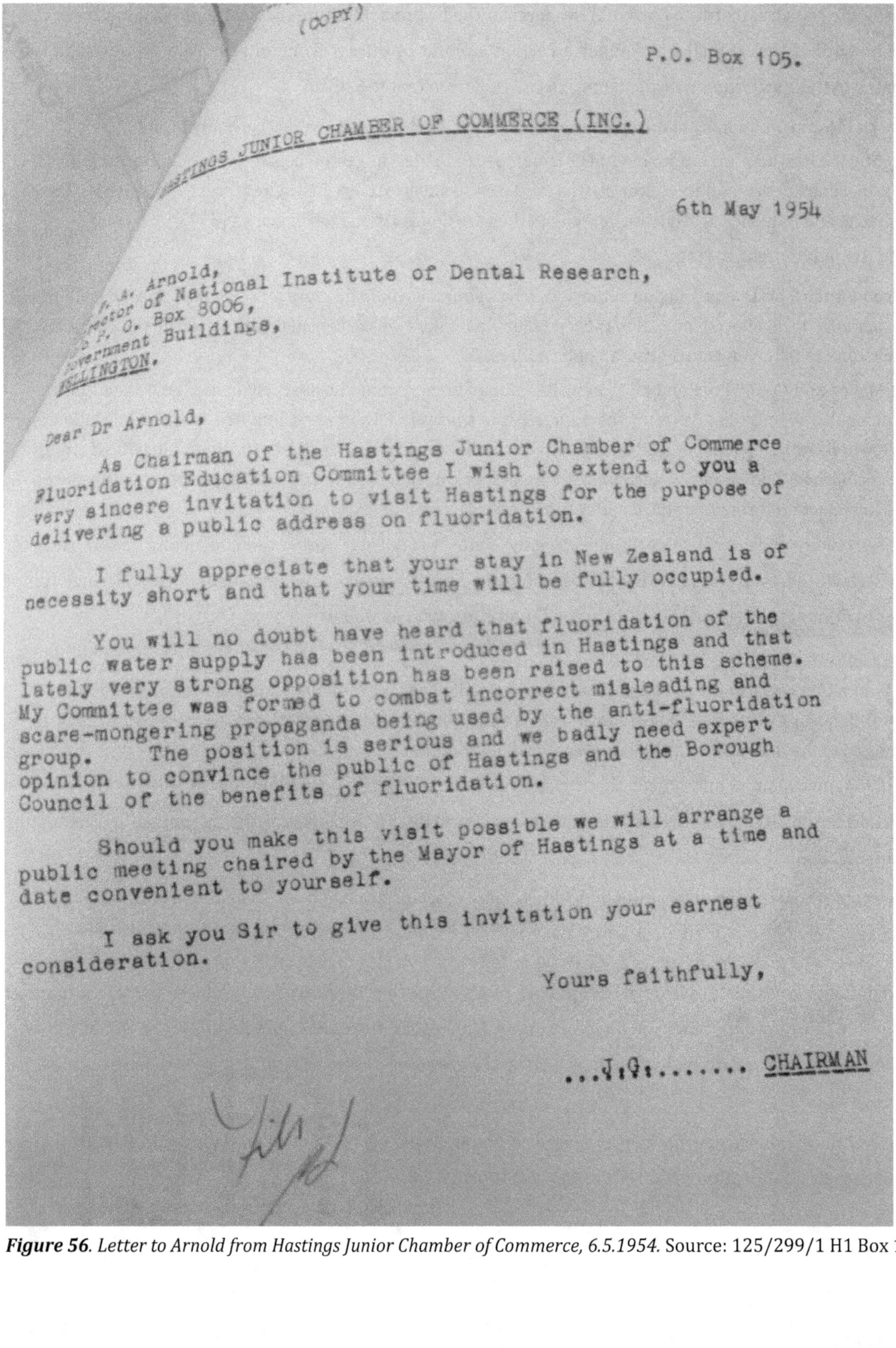

(COPY)

P.O. Box 105.

HASTINGS JUNIOR CHAMBER OF COMMERCE (INC.)

6th May 1954

Dr. A. Arnold,
Director of National Institute of Dental Research,
P. O. Box 8006,
Government Buildings,
WELLINGTON,

Dear Dr Arnold,

As Chairman of the Hastings Junior Chamber of Commerce Fluoridation Education Committee I wish to extend to you a very sincere invitation to visit Hastings for the purpose of delivering a public address on fluoridation.

I fully appreciate that your stay in New Zealand is of necessity short and that your time will be fully occupied.

You will no doubt have heard that fluoridation of the public water supply has been introduced in Hastings and that lately very strong opposition has been raised to this scheme. My Committee was formed to combat incorrect misleading and scare-mongering propaganda being used by the anti-fluoridation group.   The position is serious and we badly need expert opinion to convince the public of Hastings and the Borough Council of the benefits of fluoridation.

Should you make this visit possible we will arrange a public meeting chaired by the Mayor of Hastings at a time and date convenient to yourself.

I ask you Sir to give this invitation your earnest consideration.

Yours faithfully,

...J.G........ CHAIRMAN

Figure 56. *Letter to Arnold from Hastings Junior Chamber of Commerce, 6.5.1954.* Source: 125/299/1 H1 Box 1634.

On the 7th of May, 1954, a letter appeared in the **Hawke's Bay Herald-Tribune** written by P. T. Gifford, Member Jaycee of the Fluoride Education Committee. His letter began:

> "Mr. Editor – In the discussions on the fluoridation of our water supply it is apparent that the method by which sodium fluoride is put into the water is not fully appreciated." [561]

He then discussed how the Jaycee Fluoride Education Committee interviewed the town clerk and Mr. Fish the engineer, then "inspected the feeding mechanism." A few of his statements lend the reader to believe there would never be an irregularity in the feeding. Though *he* may have believed this, it was obviously untrue as demonstrated by the other documents (also consider this with regard to the meeting dated 30th June 1954 discussed later in this chapter). Once again, the information the public receives is different from reality. He claimed at least eight samples were taken weekly. He wrote of "several checks on the machines" daily. His letter ended with the words "there can be no possibility of danger."

Throughout the mid-1950s, the public were constantly reassured that there were no serious fluctuations in the concentration of fluorine above the level of 1.2 ppm. In his 1958 paper mentioned previously, Ludwig did admit the concentration was lower than 1.0 ppm until about September of 1954 [555]. In that paper he never discussed the fact that sometimes the concentration went far above 1.2 ppm. As far as I can tell, media never publicly asked the experts for any evidence or analyses.

On the 11ᵗʰ May, 1954 the fluorine concentration in 7 readings was less than 1.0 ppm with one reading of 6.4 ppm (**Figure 57**).

Figure 57. *Waters for Fluorine, Hastings, 11.5. 1954.* Source: 125/299/3 H1 Box 1704.

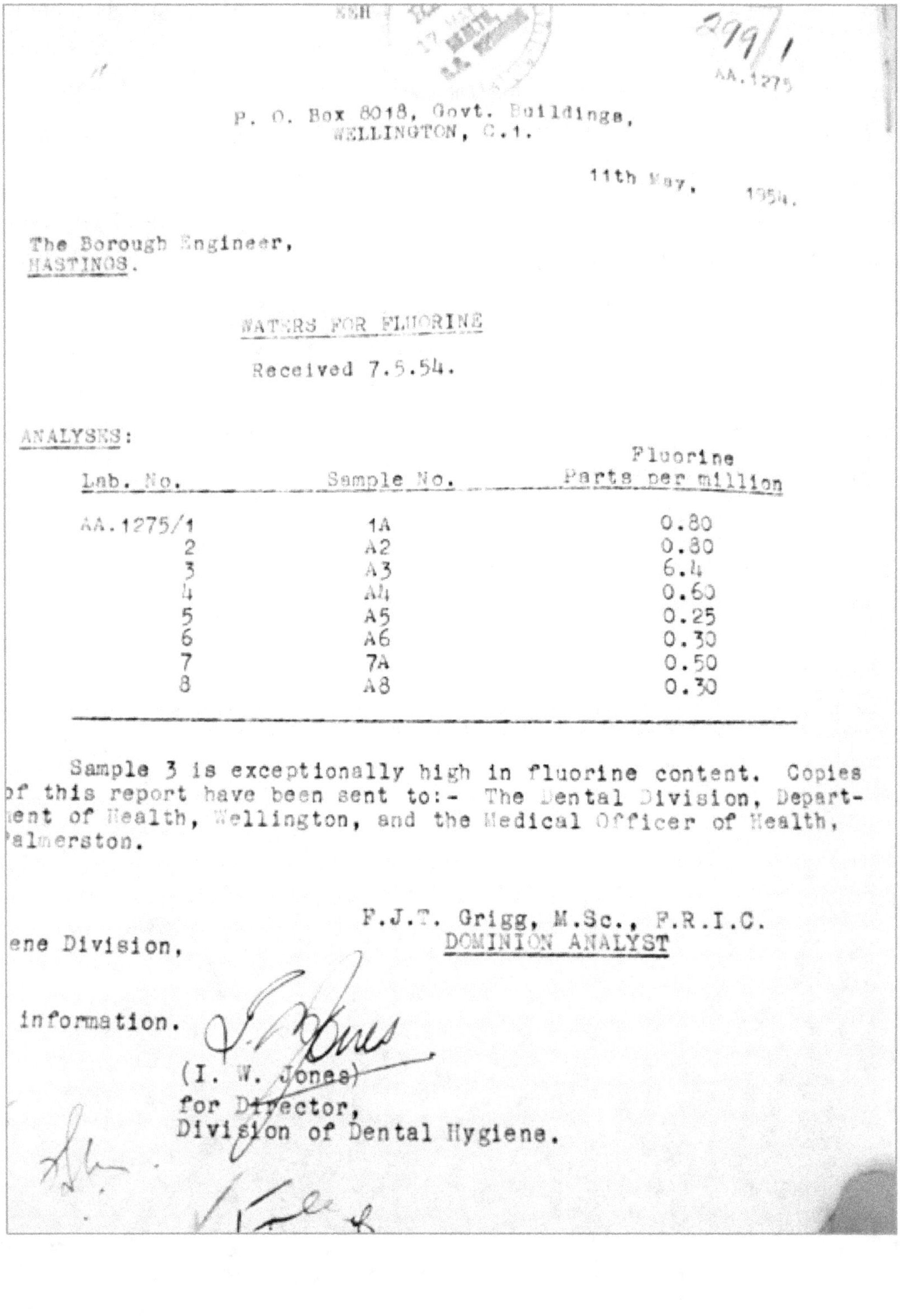

P. O. Box 8018, Govt. Buildings,
WELLINGTON, C.1.

11th May, 1954.

The Borough Engineer,
HASTINGS.

WATERS FOR FLUORINE

Received 7.5.54.

ANALYSES:

Lab. No.	Sample No.	Fluorine Parts per million
AA.1275/1	1A	0.80
2	A2	0.80
3	A3	6.4
4	A4	0.60
5	A5	0.25
6	A6	0.30
7	7A	0.50
8	A8	0.30

Sample 3 is exceptionally high in fluorine content. Copies of this report have been sent to:- The Dental Division, Department of Health, Wellington, and the Medical Officer of Health, Palmerston.

F.J.T. Grigg, M.Sc., F.R.I.C.
DOMINION ANALYST

ene Division,

information.

(I. W. Jones)
for Director,
Division of Dental Hygiene.

On the 15th of May, 1954, **The Daily Telegraph** published an ad by the Department of Health with the word *FLUORINE* in large, capital letters (**Figure 58**). Note the first sentence of the smaller print (bottom left of picture):

"The dose used is *one part per million*." (Their emphasis.) [562]

Also note the words "carefully controlled".

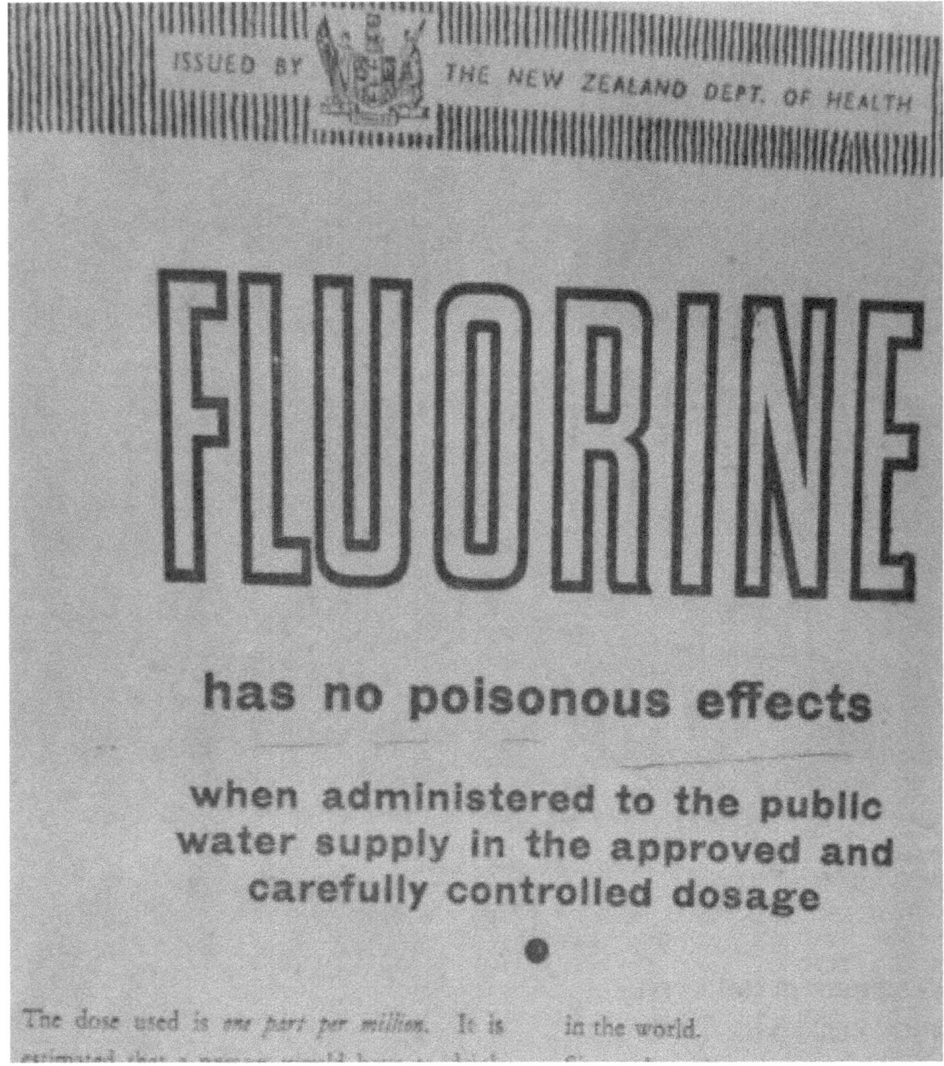

Figure 58. Fluorine has no poisonous effects. Source: **The Daily Telegraph**, 15th May, 1954 [562].

Three days later on the 18th of May, 1954, Dr. Taylor wrote to Dr. Maclean stating:

"You will have observed the high result of over 6 part per million of fluorine of one of the latest series of samples taken at Hastings."

Taylor claimed that when he mentioned this to Mr. Fish, the engineer had no idea how it could have happened.

"You will recall that the dosage is creating a problem in that there is a tendency for the material to stick in the hopper."

Taylor went on to say that while monitoring occurred in daylight hours, at night it was compromised. He claimed that Mr. Fish estimated the dose would be closer to 1 ppm than the test showed, based on Fish's observation of the amount of powder used. Taylor was to see Arnold and Parfitt at the plant, to obtain their guidance. He said there was an optimistic feeling among the supporters and very little to be heard from the opponents.

"However, the battle is far from won and the Jaycees realise this and are continuing their efforts to the full." [563]

As shown in a letter dated 18th of May 1954, (**Figure 59** and **60**) the engineer believed the concentrations were a little higher than what is shown here. This may have been the reason for the slow response on behalf of the experts when it came to addressing the problem, given that the majority of readings were much below the desired 1 ppm.

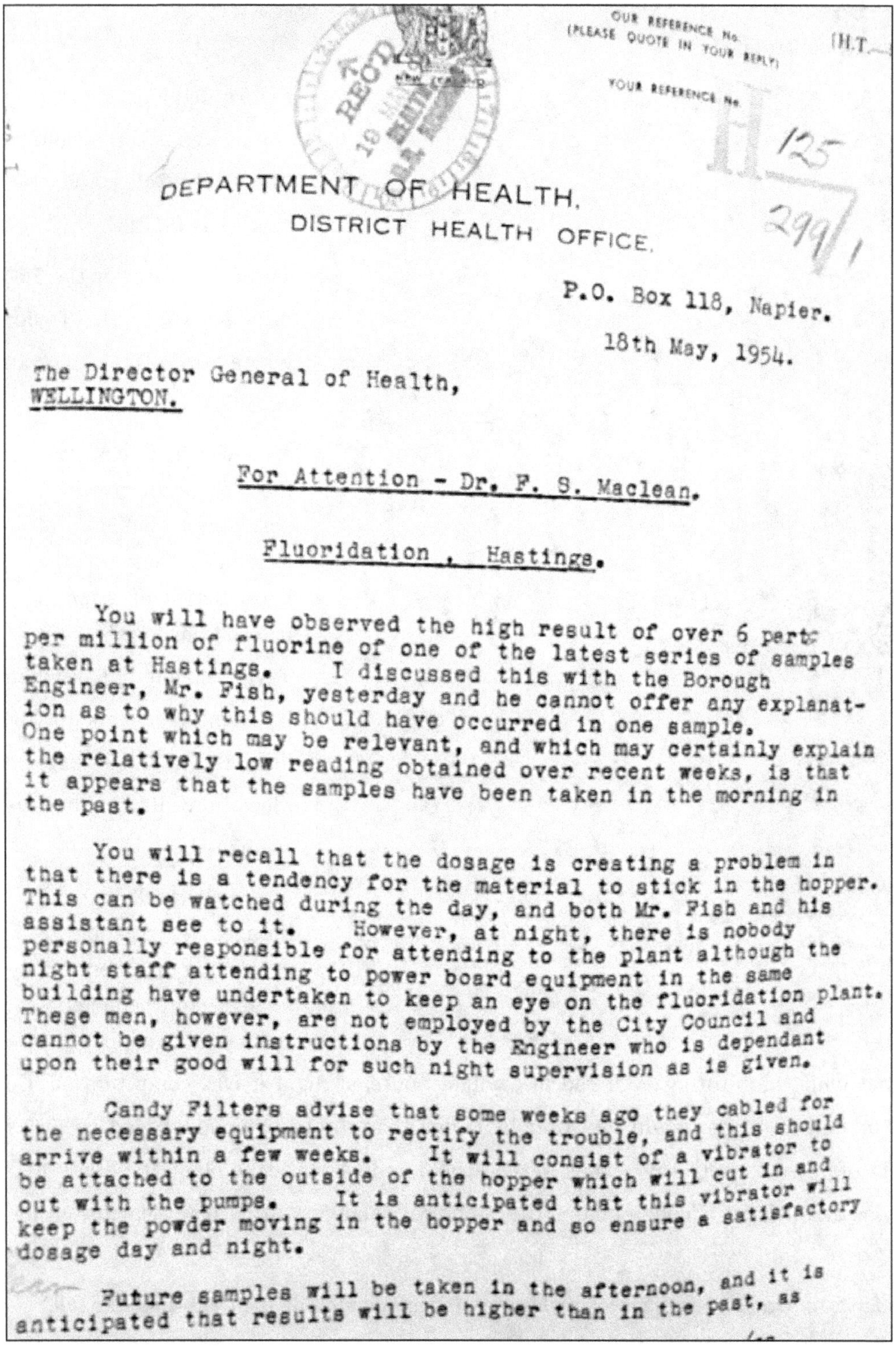

OUR REFERENCE No.
(PLEASE QUOTE IN YOUR REPLY)

YOUR REFERENCE No.

DEPARTMENT OF HEALTH.
DISTRICT HEALTH OFFICE.

P.O. Box 118, Napier.

18th May, 1954.

The Director General of Health,
WELLINGTON.

For Attention – Dr. F. S. Maclean.

Fluoridation , Hastings.

You will have observed the high result of over 6 parts per million of fluorine of one of the latest series of samples taken at Hastings. I discussed this with the Borough Engineer, Mr. Fish, yesterday and he cannot offer any explanation as to why this should have occurred in one sample. One point which may be relevant, and which may certainly explain the relatively low reading obtained over recent weeks, is that it appears that the samples have been taken in the morning in the past.

You will recall that the dosage is creating a problem in that there is a tendency for the material to stick in the hopper. This can be watched during the day, and both Mr. Fish and his assistant see to it. However, at night, there is nobody personally responsible for attending to the plant although the night staff attending to power board equipment in the same building have undertaken to keep an eye on the fluoridation plant. These men, however, are not employed by the City Council and cannot be given instructions by the Engineer who is dependant upon their good will for such night supervision as is given.

Candy Filters advise that some weeks ago they cabled for the necessary equipment to rectify the trouble, and this should arrive within a few weeks. It will consist of a vibrator to be attached to the outside of the hopper which will cut in and out with the pumps. It is anticipated that this vibrator will keep the powder moving in the hopper and so ensure a satisfactory dosage day and night.

Future samples will be taken in the afternoon, and it is anticipated that results will be higher than in the past, as

Figure 59. For Attention Dr Maclean, 18.5.1954. Source: HD 125/299/1. Page 1 of 2.

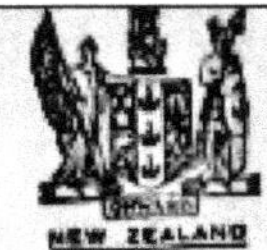

DEPARTMENT OF HEALTH,
DISTRICT HEALTH OFFICE,

P.O. Box 118, Napier.

18th May, 1954.

The Director General of Health.

For Attention – Dr. F. S. Maclean, (Cont'd).

Mr. Fish estimates that from the amount of powder that is being used, the dose must be closer to one part per million than tests indicated.

I am seeing Doctors Arnold and Parfitt at Hastings this afternoon, and they will be inspecting the plant, and will be speaking at the Public Meeting this evening.

The general feeling amongst the Fluoridation supporters in Hastings is optomistic, and very little is being heard of the Anti-Fluoridation Society. However, the battle is far from won and the Jaycees realise this and are continuing their efforts to the full.

(C. N. Derek Taylor).
Medical Officer of Health.

Figure 60. For Attention Dr Maclean, 18.5.1954. Source: HD 125/299/1 H1 Box 1634. Page 2 of 2.

On the 19th of May, 1954, the **Hawke's Bay Herald-Tribune** read: "VISITING AUTHORITIES UPHOLD FLUORIDE" in a headline regarding the talk by Arnold and Parfitt. About 150 people attended. Key claims were bullet-pointed at the start of the article, one read:

"Where the fluoride content was below 1½ parts in a million no mottling or staining of teeth occurred."

This implied that the concentration used was always less than 1.5 ppm.

Another article printed the same day in Napier's **Daily Telegraph** demonstrated the public's trust in their leaders:

"When a questioner began quoting 'human rights' and the rights of the minority, he was stopped by the mayor, but Dr. Arnold was loudly applauded when he declared the responsible duty of administrators in his country was to do that which was in the best interests of the community."

The Mayor spoke to this, claiming that the Director-General of Health had advised the council officially that it had the power to do what was necessary in the interest of public health.

"This announcement was greeted with renewed applause and cries of 'Good-o.'" [564]

On the 20th of May, 1954, Mr. Fish wrote to the Medical Officer of Health, claiming that members of the Hawke's Bay Electric Power Board were helping out in day time but not at night. Fish used the words "not operating continuously at night". He claimed this caused the fluorine content to be low, as it was measured in the mornings. He arranged for samples to be taken in the afternoons after this, so readings would be closer to the target of 1.0 ppm [565].

On the 21st of May 1954, the readings showed fluorine concentrations of 0.25 ppm to 1.1 ppm with an outlier of 9.0 ppm (**Figure 61**).

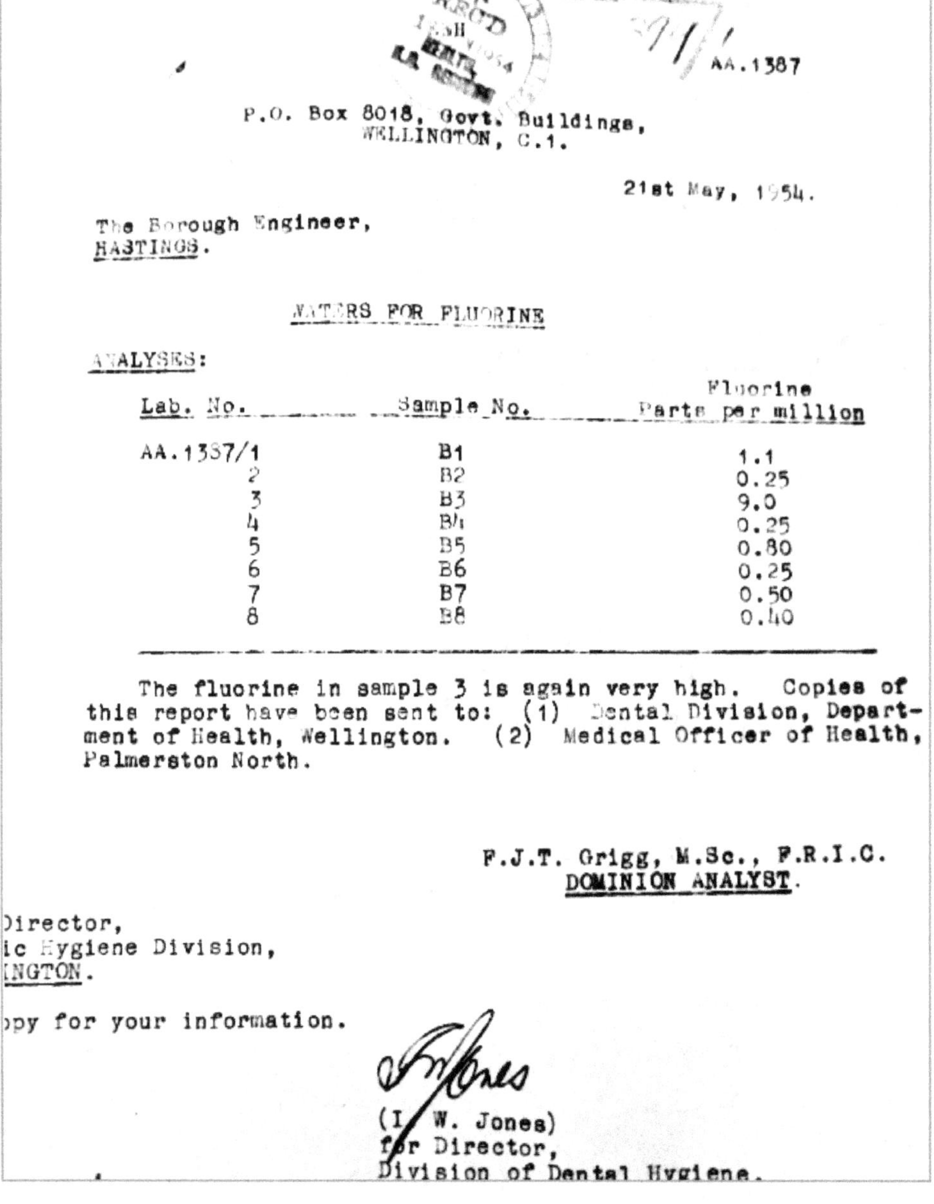

P.O. Box 8018, Govt. Buildings,
WELLINGTON, C.1.

21st May, 1954.

The Borough Engineer,
HASTINGS.

WATERS FOR FLUORINE

ANALYSES:

Lab. No.	Sample No.	Fluorine Parts per million
AA.1387/1	B1	1.1
2	B2	0.25
3	B3	9.0
4	B4	0.25
5	B5	0.80
6	B6	0.25
7	B7	0.50
8	B8	0.40

The fluorine in sample 3 is again very high. Copies of this report have been sent to: (1) Dental Division, Department of Health, Wellington. (2) Medical Officer of Health, Palmerston North.

F.J.T. Grigg, M.Sc., F.R.I.C.
DOMINION ANALYST.

Director,
ic Hygiene Division,
INGTON.

opy for your information.

(I. W. Jones)
for Director,
Division of Dental Hygiene.

Figure 61. *Waters for Fluorine, Hastings, 21.5.1954. Source: 125/299/3 H1 Box 1704.*

On the 4th of June, 1954, the Medical Officer of Health, C. N. D. Taylor, wrote to Mr. Fish about a higher level of fluorine in the water that was desired (**Figure 62**). The letter acknowledged that Dr. Maclean was "perturbed at the high result" – this was probably the 9.0 ppm reading in the analyses dated 21st May.

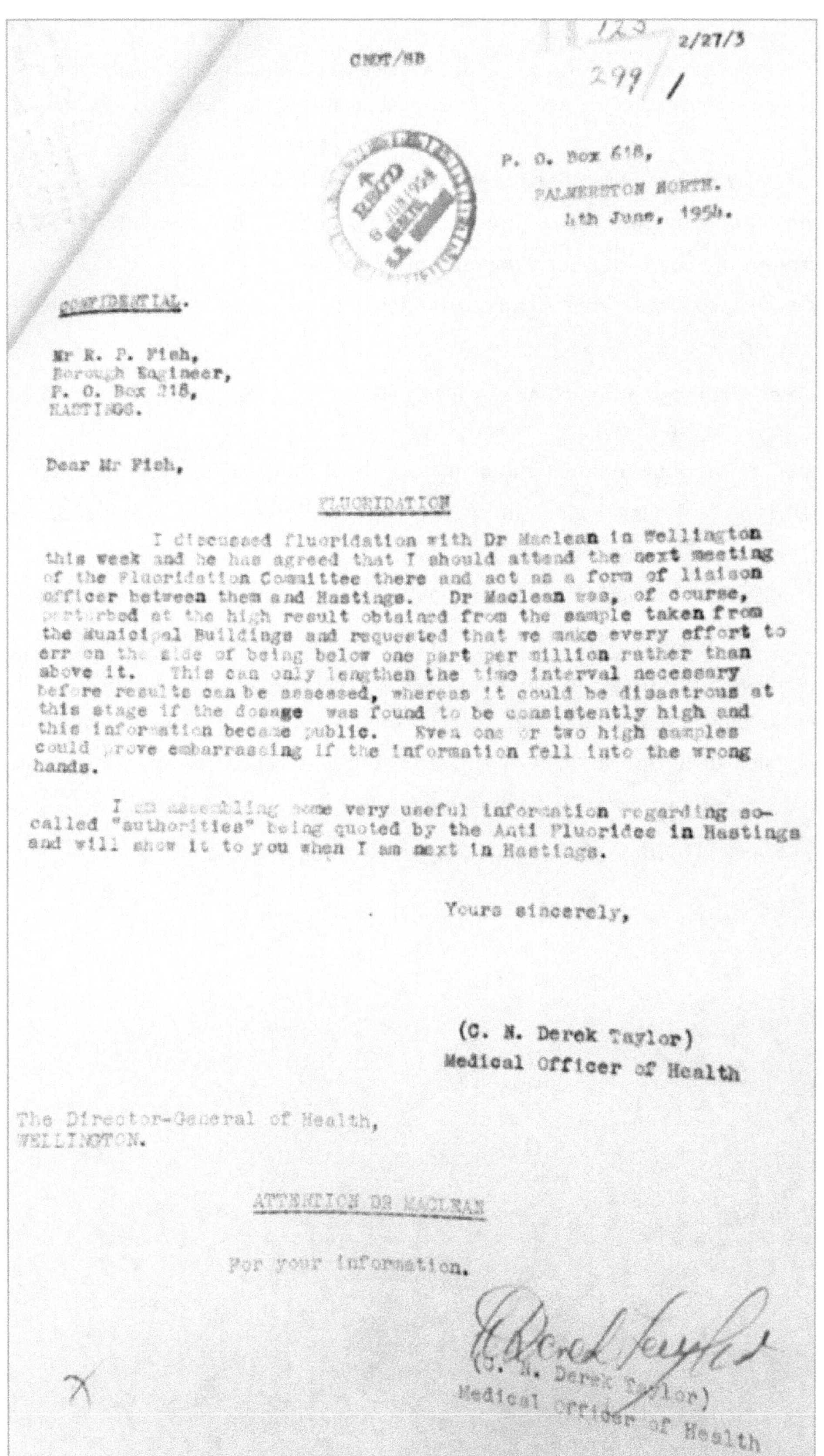

CMOT/HB

2/27/3

P. O. Box 618,
PALMERSTON NORTH.
4th June, 1954.

CONFIDENTIAL.

Mr R. P. Fish,
Borough Engineer,
P. O. Box 218,
HASTINGS.

Dear Mr Fish,

FLUORIDATION

I discussed fluoridation with Dr Maclean in Wellington this week and he has agreed that I should attend the next meeting of the Fluoridation Committee there and act as a form of liaison officer between them and Hastings. Dr Maclean was, of course, perturbed at the high result obtained from the sample taken from the Municipal Buildings and requested that we make every effort to err on the side of being below one part per million rather than above it. This can only lengthen the time interval necessary before results can be assessed, whereas it could be disastrous at this stage if the dosage was found to be consistently high and this information became public. Even one or two high samples could prove embarrassing if the information fell into the wrong hands.

I am assembling some very useful information regarding so-called "authorities" being quoted by the Anti Fluoridee in Hastings and will show it to you when I am next in Hastings.

Yours sincerely,

(C. N. Derek Taylor)
Medical Officer of Health

The Director-General of Health,
WELLINGTON.

ATTENTION DR MACLEAN

For your information.

Figure 62. Letter to Fish from Taylor. Fluoridation, 4.6.1954. Source: 125/299/1 H1 Box 1634.

Taylor cautioned Fish that

> "… it could be disastrous at this stage if the dosage was found to be consistently high and this information became public. Even one or two high samples could prove embarrassing if the information fell into the wrong hands."

Reading the letter you will see Dr. Maclean would rather have erred on the side of being below 1 ppm instead of above, so to say there was no concern for safety is not correct. There is a grey area here with regard to morality, in that the experts certainly did not want to hurt anyone, but they also did not want anyone to find their dishonesties – the times the concentration was significantly higher than 1 ppm. Note the following paragraph of the letter, about "authorities":

> "I am assembling some very useful information regarding so-called 'authorities' being quoted by the Anti Fluorides in Hastings and will show it to you when I am next in Hastings." [566]

On the 17th June 1954, Dr. Arnold of the United States' National Institute of Dental Research wrote to Dr. Saunders, the Director of the Division of Dental Hygiene in Wellington, with six criticisms of the Hastings fluoridation project. Arnold's complaints are summarized: Responsibility among staff on the project was unclear to him. Arnold believed both sources of water in Hastings should have been fluoridated; he claimed this was not done when he visited. He was concerned not with overdosing, but with underdosing, suggesting to Saunders that New Zealanders would not receive the benefit the Americans had. Arnold criticized the fact that sometimes weeks elapsed from the taking of a sample, and the reporting of a sample to the authorities; he claimed in America samples were taken daily. He also suggested involving the dental nurses more in the project, and complained that the water supply for the school was unfluoridated.

I have reprinted the letter from Dr. Arnold to Dr. Saunders in full (**Figures 63** and **64**).

DEPARTMENT OF HEALTH, EDUCATION AND WELFARE,
National Institutes of Health,
Betheada 14, Md.

June 17, 1954.

Dr. J.Ll.Saunders, Director,
Division of Dental Hygiene,
Wellington, N.Z.

Dear Mr. Saunders,

Now that I have finally returned from my World Cruise, I wish to take this opportunity to thank you and Mrs. Saunders for the many hospitable things you did to make my trip to New Zealand one of life's high lights. I also wish to take this opportunity to express my appreciation for the way you people organized the seminar. It was by far the best international meeting that I have ever attended. You and your staff are to be congratulated.

As I mentioned to you just prior to leaving, I should like to make a few remarks regarding my impression of the study at Hastings. As you know, following my visit to Hastings, I was somewhat concerned regarding this project and its future.

(1) I was quite disturbed regarding the supervision of this project. It appears to me that the responsibility for carrying out this study is not clear in the minds of the different people involved. I would think that if it were at all possible, somebody on your staff should be given complete responsibility for seeing that this project is effectively carried out.

(2) I was not at all happy to find that the control of fluoridation of the water supply at Hastings is not better supervised and carried out. It is my understanding that since the community actually can receive, at least at certain times, different sources of water; I believe that both sources of water should be fluoridated. This was not being done when I visited there.

(3) In discussing the fluoridation of the water supply with the gentleman who is in charge of this department in Hastings, I got the impression that the actual fluoridation of the water was not too carefully supervised. The equipment being used, while it is adequate to do the job, is not designed to indicate whether it is operating effectively. In this regard, would it be possible to obtain equipment such as we have used in this Country, in many cases, which will automatically record the fluoride addition and will automatically set up an alarm system when the machinery is not operating correctly.

I do not mean, in this regard, that I am worried about any danger concerning overloading the distribution system with too much fluorides. I am, however, concerned with the fact that too often people will be receiving water with much too low a concentration of fluorides. I can readily see the possibility that if this condition continues as in the past that you may not observe the same beneficial effects as have been observed in the various research studies here in this Country.

(4) From what I was told in Hastings, frequently a period of two to three weeks elapses between the time that a water sample is collected and the people are notified from the laboratories in Wellington regarding the fluoride content of that sample. In our studies here in the United States we make daily fluoride determinations of the water used by the respective communities. These determinations are done in the respective laboratories of the water works companies involved. In many cases, at specified

---

Figure 63. Letter to Saunders from Arnold, 17.6.1954. Source: HD 125/299/1 H1 Box 1634. Page 1 of 2.

intervals duplicate samples are also sent into the central State laboratories for check. I realize that this may not be practical in Hastings, but I do believe that <u>it is essential that more frequent analysis of the water be made, including samples taken at different times of the day.</u>

(5) I also think you should give some consideration to those factors related to your dental nurse program in Hastings. I think the study should be very carefully discussed with this group. As you realize, this program is doing a commendable job of treatment of the early stages of dental caries, particularly in the first molars. If the dental nurses are enthusiastic, which I am sure most are, there will be the tendency to place fillings, particularly on the <u>occlusals of first permanent molars on the basis of deep pits and fissures.</u> It has been our experience in fluoride areas that we find just as many deep pits and fissures as we do in non-fluoride areas. However, in fluoride areas these pits and fissures do not become carious to the same degree that they do in the non-fluoride areas.

(6) Another facet of this problem that concerns me in the Hastings study is the information that <u>the water supply for the school is not fluoridated.</u> Of course, you realize that this may or may not be a fact. However, if the water supply for the Hastings school is not fluoridated, I feel sure that steps should be taken to see that this condition is corrected. I feel so strongly about this point that if it is not possible to do this in Hastings, I would seriously consider changing the study to some other location.

I realize that I have brought up a number of points for your consideration and many of these points are based on information gained "second-hand", and thus may not be a true picture of the situation. I also hope you will appreciate the fact that I am making these comments to you for your personal information and I recognize that it would be impossible for me to fully evaluate the situation at Hastings during the short time I was there.

I would be very happy to receive your comments in this regard and if I can be of any further service to you, do not hesitate to write me.

Again, may I thank both you and Mrs. Saunders for entertaining me while in Wellington.

Sincerely yours,

F. A. Arnold, Jr., Director
National Institute of Dental Research.

Figure 64. Letter to Saunders from Arnold, 17.6.1954. Source: HD 125/299/1 H1 Box 1634. Page 2 of 2.

A sample of analyses taken on the 15th and sent on the 25th of June, 1954, showed readings between 0.25 ppm and 4.4 ppm (**Figure 65**).

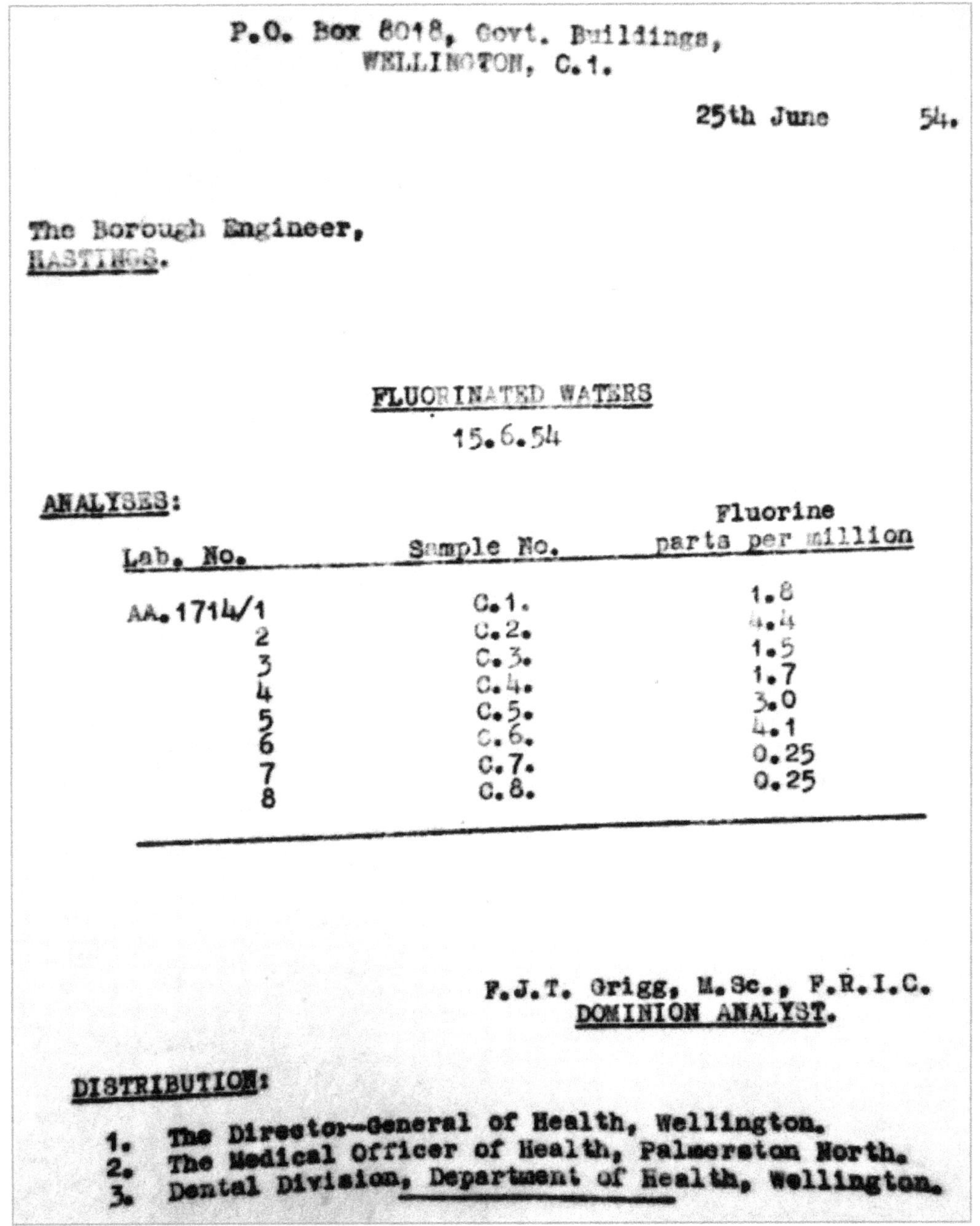

P.O. Box 8018, Govt. Buildings,
WELLINGTON, C.1.

25th June 54.

The Borough Engineer,
HASTINGS.

FLUORINATED WATERS

15.6.54

ANALYSES:

Lab. No.	Sample No.	Fluorine parts per million
AA.1714/1	C.1.	1.8
2	C.2.	4.4
3	C.3.	1.5
4	C.4.	1.7
5	C.5.	3.0
6	C.6.	4.1
7	C.7.	0.25
8	C.8.	0.25

F.J.T. Grigg, M.Sc., F.R.I.C.
DOMINION ANALYST.

DISTRIBUTION:

1. The Director-General of Health, Wellington.
2. The Medical Officer of Health, Palmerston North.
3. Dental Division, Department of Health, Wellington.

Figure 65. Fluoridated Waters, Hastings, 15.6.1954. Source: 125/299/3 H1 Box 1704.

On the same day, Dr. Maclean wrote to the Medical Officer of Health and Mr. Fish, the Hastings Engineer, claiming that (**Figure 66**):

> "The most recent analyses of the Hastings water suggests that a technical defect has developed in the dosage apparatus. I think that until this defect can be corrected and adjustments made the fluoridation should cease." [567]

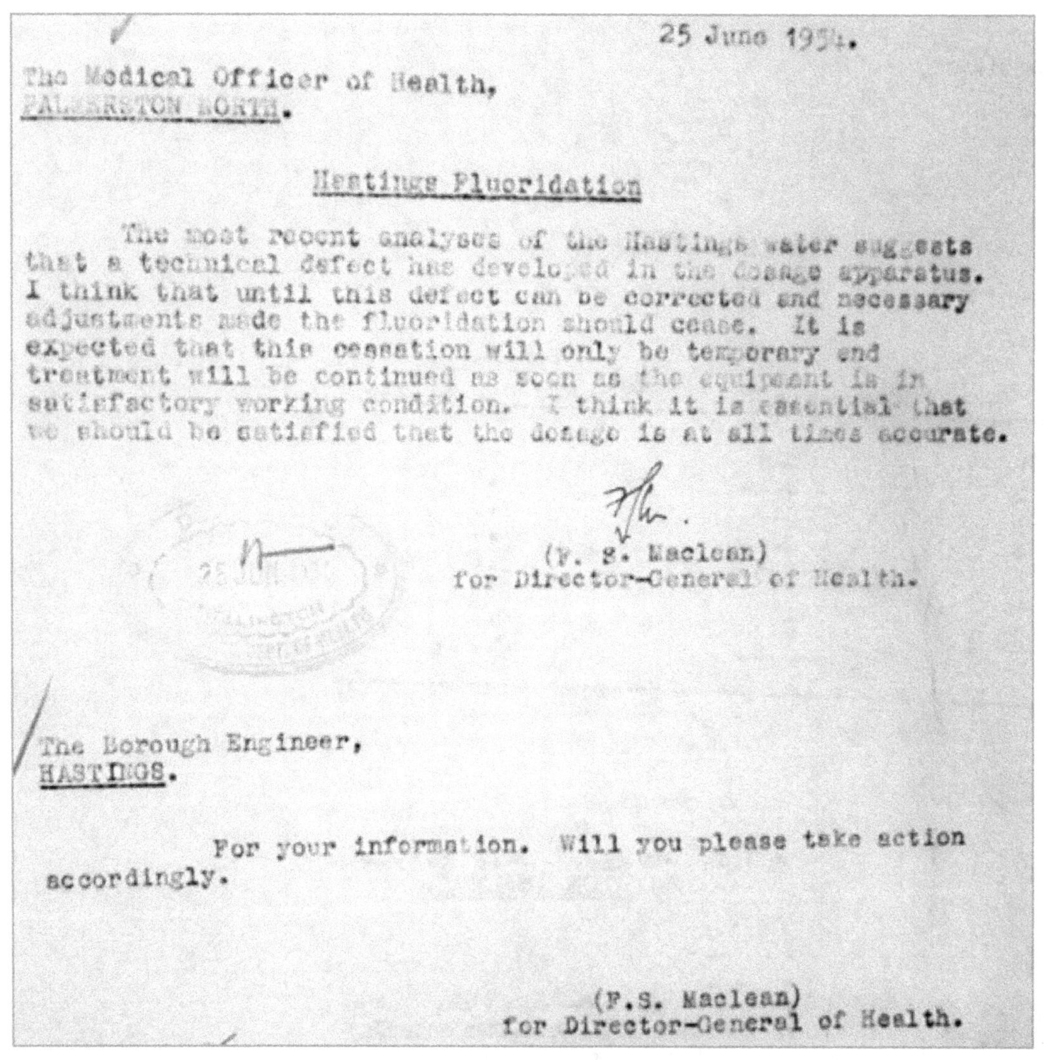

Figure 66. Hastings Fluoridation, by F.S. Maclean, 25.6.1954. Source: 125/299/1 H1 Box 1634.

This may have been the reason enthusiasm was waning for the project. The experts wanted the concentration to be accurate, and it was not.

On the very next day, the 26th of June 1954, the **Hawke's Bay Herald-Tribune** featured an almost full-page statement from the Mayors of Hastings (W. E. Bate) and Havelock North (J. J. Nimon) on the topic of fluoridation (**Figure 67**). One can see from the section pictured that the attitude favoured by the mayors was one of trusting the experts. They justified this by stating that the words of Sir Stanton Hicks had been misquoted by people opposed to fluoridation. Thus, Drs. Arnold and Parfitt were the appropriate people to go to for leadership. Trusting the authorities was emphasized.

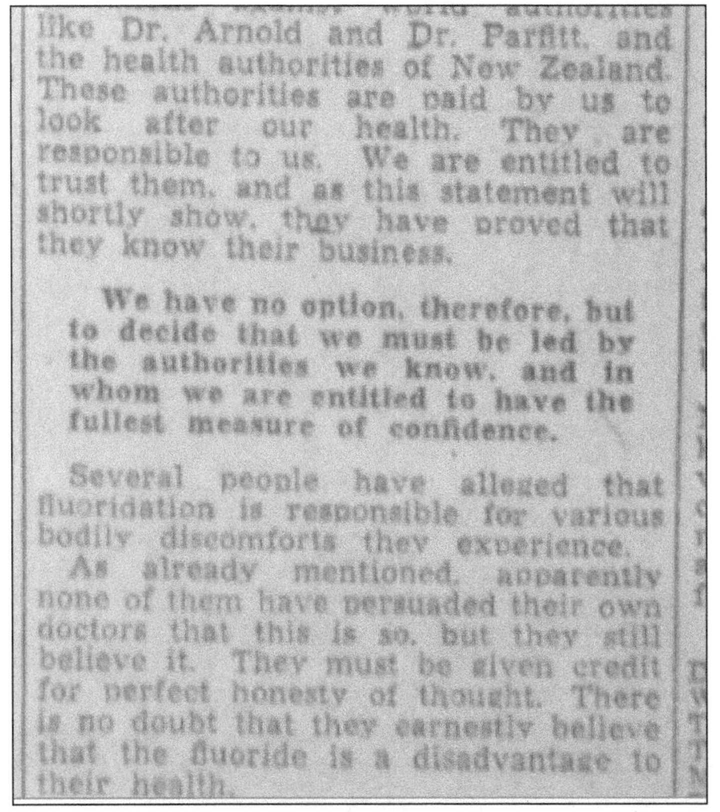

Figure 67. *Statement from two mayors.* Source: **Hawke's Bay Herald-Tribune**, 26th June, 1954 [568].

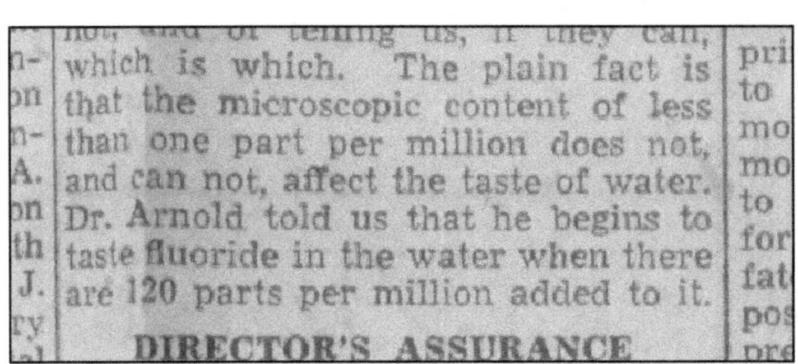

Figure 68. *Director's Assurance.* Source: **Hawke's Bay Herald-Tribune**, 26th June, 1954 [568].

This article claimed (**Figure 68**):

> "The amount put in the local water supply, which is less than one part in every million, is equal to approximately a pin's head in size put in a four-gallon tank."

> "The plain fact is that the microscopic content of less than one part per million does not, and can not, affect the taste of water." [568]

This again gave the public the impression that the experts were in control of the amount used.

You can see from the analysis dated 28th June 1954 (collected on the 22nd), that the concentration was sometimes much higher than one part per million (**Figure 69**):

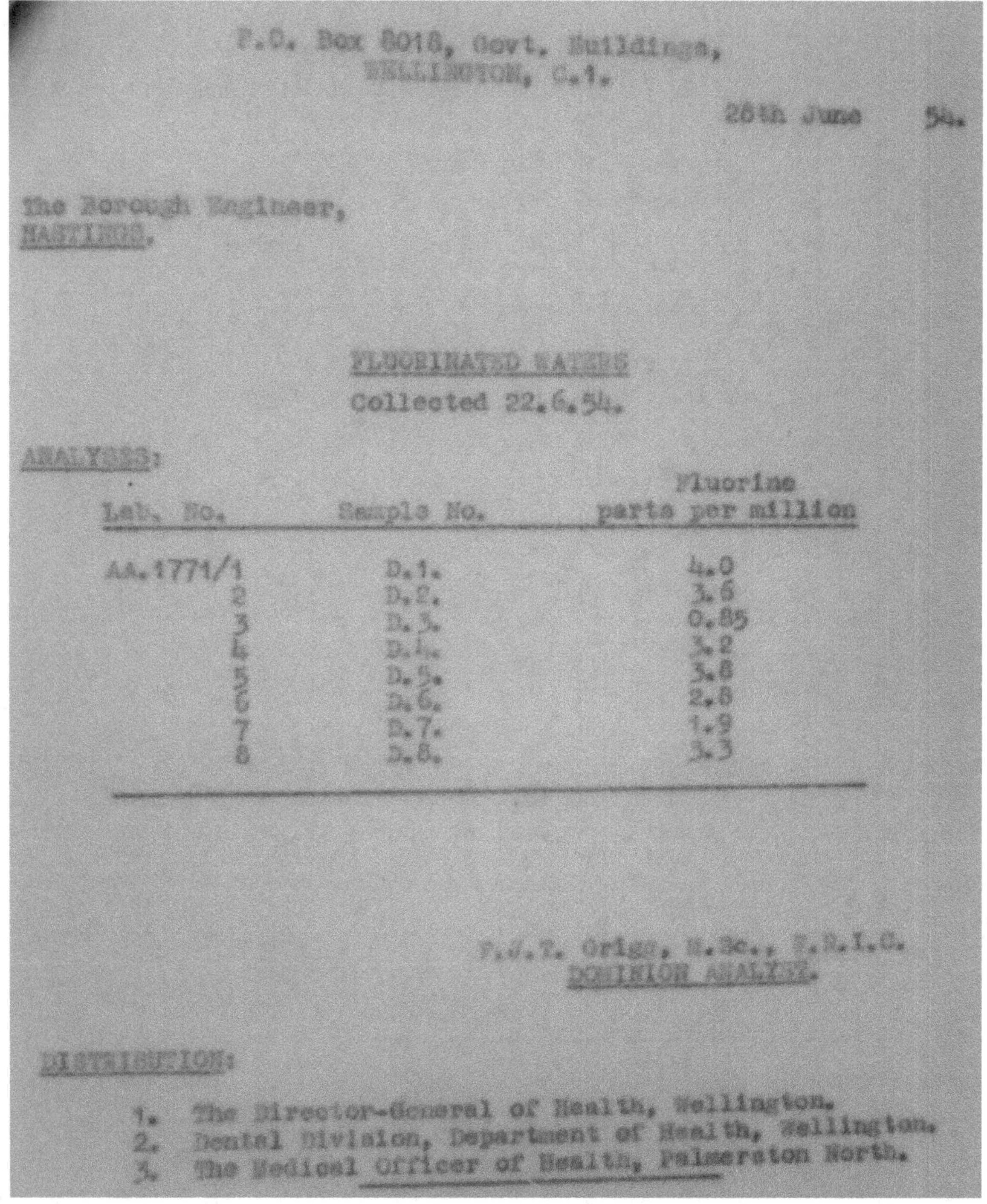

P.O. Box 8018, Govt. Buildings,
WELLINGTON, C.1.

28th June   54.

The Borough Engineer,
HASTINGS.

FLUORINATED WATERS
Collected 22.6.54.

ANALYSES:

Lab. No.	Sample No.	Fluorine parts per million
AA.1771/1	D.1.	4.0
2	D.2.	3.6
3	D.3.	0.85
4	D.4.	3.2
5	D.5.	3.8
6	D.6.	2.8
7	D.7.	1.9
8	D.8.	3.3

F.J.T. Grigg, M.Sc., F.R.I.C.
DOMINION ANALYST.

DISTRIBUTION:

1. The Director-General of Health, Wellington.
2. Dental Division, Department of Health, Wellington.
3. The Medical Officer of Health, Palmerston North.

Figure 69. Fluoridated Waters, Hastings, Collected 22.6.1954. Source: 125/299/1 H1 Box 1634.

The following summary is from the 15th January to the 11th June, 1954 (**Figure 70**). The concentrations ranged from 0.15 ppm to 9.0 ppm, very different from the public claims of 1 ppm.

HASTINGS

Fluorination of Water

SUMMARY OF FLUORINE ANALYSES 1954.

No.	Date	Batch	1.	2.	3.*	4.	5.	6.	7. (H.N.1.)	8. (H.N.2.)
AA. 82	15/1	A	0.15	0.20	0.25	0.35	0.20	0.20		
		B	0.20	0.80	0.50	0.95	1.25	0.85		
AA. 770	23/3	A	2.1	1.3	0.25	0.85	0.30	0.35	0.35	0.50
AA. 823	29/3	B	0.70	0.70	1.2	1.6	1.6	1.1	0.90	0.60
AA. 941	6/4		0.20	0.20	0.25	0.20	0.20	0.20	0.45	0.30
AA.1044	14/4	B	0.50	0.50	0.50	0.50	0.50	0.50	0.50	0.70
AA.1107	26/4	C	0.20	0.20	0.35	0.20	0.20	0.25	0.35	0.20
		D							0.25	0.95
AA.1213	3/5	D	0.30	0.25	0.90	0.30	0.25	0.85		
		E							0.25	0.30
AA.1275	7/5	A	0.80	0.80	6.4	0.60	0.25	0.30	0.50	0.30
AA.1387	17/5	B	1.1	0.25	9.0	0.25	0.80	0.25	0.50	0.40
AA.1434	21/5	C	0.35	0.40	0.45	0.35	0.50	0.65	0.25	0.45
AA.1499	27/5	D	1.5	1.0	0.80	1.0	2.4	1.1	0.95	1.9
AA.1582	9/6	A	2.4	3.0	2.6	1.1	1.4	2.8	1.9	3.6
AA.1633	11/6	B	2.4	0.45	0.40	0.40	0.45	0.35	0.25	0.25

* Hastings station.

Figure 70. Summary of Fluorine Analysis (part), Hastings, 15.1 – 11.6.1954. Source: HD 125/299/3 H1 Box 1704.

These analyses were problematic to the authorities, who met on the 30th June 1954, at Mr. Fish's office. In attendance were Dr. Maclean, Mr. Saunders, Mr. Hogg, Mr. Fish, Mr. Woods, Mr. Mansergh (of Candy Filters), Mr. Hassan (the Waterworks Engineer of Palmerston North City Council) and Dr. Taylor. The theme of the meeting was fixing the problems with the fluorine concentration. Of interest is the fact that Dr. Taylor stated:

"… that several well informed citizens in Hastings, including members of the Junior Chamber of Commerce, and dentists, who had been instrumental in saving the fluoridation survey, had heard that the equipment was not working satisfactorily and were anxious to be reassured that, having fought so hard, they were, in fact, fighting for something worthwhile." [569]

Some of the press releases, and the media statements of the experts, are shown and quoted in this chapter. I have reproduced the meeting in full here (**Figures 71 - 74**).

NOTES ON MEETING REGARDING FLUORIDATION,
HELD IN BOROUGH ENGINEER'S OFFICE, HASTINGS,
ON 30th JUNE, 1954.

PRESENT:-

Dr F. S. Maclean
Mr J. Ll. Saunders
Mr G. F. Hogg
Mr R. P. Fish
Mr H. J. Woods
Mr Mansergh (Candy Filters).
Mr Hassan (Waterworks Engineer, Palmerston North City Council).
Dr C. N. Derek Taylor.

DR TAYLOR opened proceedings and explained that Mr Hassan had attended with Mr Hogg to gain experience on fluoridation. He suggested that the problem we were faced with regarding the plant resolved itself into -

(1) Can the present dry feeder plant be improved to give satisfactory service?

(2) If not, what alternative plant can be adopted?

He suggested that nobody present was satisfied with the working of the present plant to date, and the inability to establish a constant concentration in the vicinity of one part per million, followed by the recent particularly high readings together with other inconsistencies, necessitated urgent attention being given to the experimental side of the fluoridation survey now that the principle that it be allowed to continue had been almost certainly established. He stated that several well informed citizens in Hastings, including members of the Junior Chamber of Commerce, and dentists, who had been instrumental in saving the fluoridation survey, had heard that the equipment was not working satisfactorily and were anxious to be reassured that, having fought so hard, they were, in fact, fighting for something worthwhile. When they had been informed that this meeting was to be held they had expressed their satisfaction. Dr Taylor then suggested that the engineers present discuss the problem and means of solving it.

MR HOGG suggested that the powder might not be getting sufficient mixing and that it might be settling in the suction chamber. Sodium fluoride or silico fluoride settled in this tank could lead to an uneven distribution through the mains. He suggested that more agitation may be necessary to give a better solution of the powder.

MR FISH suggested that the swirling motion caused by the pumps in the tank may be sufficient to cause adequate solution.

MR MANSERGH agreed with Mr Hogg.

MR WOODS, on a question from Mr Hogg, said that sodium fluoride was 4% soluble and it would be usual to work on 1% to give satisfactory results. Silico fluoride was .7% soluble and again one would work on one quarter of this.

MR MANSERGH suggested the concentration of fluorine may be higher after the pumps had been stopped for some time and then re-started as the slurry formed by the powder in the mixing chamber would have had a longer contact period in which to dissolve. He reiterated that most of the dissolving must take place in the tank (suction chamber).

MR FISH agreed with the above and added that the pumps are operated intermittently and particularly during the night. He considered that despite the question of the time it took the powder to dissolve, he was confident that the major problem was the feeder. He had found it impossible to control the dose satisfactorily because of the small amount required (1½ pounds an hour). From the outset the dosing had been irregular because the powder was constantly sticking in the bin and recently he had removed a stop nut to allow a freer flow of the powder. Even so, the bin had to be constantly knocked and shaken to maintain

***Figure 71**. Notes on Meeting Regarding Fluoridation, June 30th 1954. Source: 125/299/1 H1 Box 1634. Page 1 of 4.*

....flow of the powder, which was still sticking.   Conditions had
improved somewhat since the powder had been dried over retorts at the
gas works but it still packed hard together on occasions and would not
flow.   He said that silico fluoride was still being used but the supply
would be finished in about a fortnight when the change to sodium
fluoride would be made.

MR MANSERGH showed screenings of the sodium fluoride powder to be used
and suggested that some of the large particles which had been screened
out might interfere with the running of the machine.   They would also
take longer to dissolve.

MR FISH agreed and added that the cost of sodium fluoride would be
greater than silico fluoride.   The sodium fluoride delivered recently
would cost £789 for seven tons delivered (one year's supply).   Twelve
months ago a year's supply of silico fluoride cost £240 delivered in
Hastings (5 tons).

DR TAYLOR.   Can we at this stage decide that the dry feeder is not
satisfactory, and proceed to discuss alternatives?

MR MANSERGH.   The dry feeder certainly presents difficulties, particularly
in keeping the material in satisfactory form to pass through the feeder.
He stated that English manufacturers had had little experience with
fluorine equipment or with dry feeders.   They had no experience with
the practical application of dry feeders for fluoridation plants nor of
the gravimetric method used in the United States of America, as
observed by Mr Saunders in Grand Rapids.

MR SAUNDERS, MR FISH and MR MANSERGH agreed that from their study of the
literature the gravimetric method also had its problems, particularly
in towns the size of Hastings.

MR HOGG.   It seems that putting the fluorine in solution may be the
answer.   Hastings has a small population and with the amount of water
involved one cannot afford to have much variation in the fluorine added.
A wet method is easier to control.

MR MANSERGH agreed.   By the dry method we are down to adding in the
vicinity of half a teaspoon a minute.

MR FISH.   Over all we are not over dosing.   The supply of silico
fluoride just being finished was bought to last twelve months but has
taken sixteen months to be put into the supply.

MR WOODS.   Liquid feeders present their problems, such as corrosion, but
I agree that this seems to be the solution to the problem.

MR FISH.   Liquid feeder would also bring up the problems such as
obtaining building space, attention over the week-end, etc., but these
problems can be overcome.

MR HOGG.   We would need a trained man to do the mixing and the material
and the plant should be kept behind locked doors.   Logs should be kept
of visits to the plant, adjustments made, etc.

MR FISH.   The sewerage pump attendant could be utilized as he makes daily
visits and week-end visits to his pumps and could include the fluoridation
plant in his rounds.   The Borough turncock could be trained to do the
mixing.

DR TAYLOR.   Mixing in a small building such as would be necessary would
have to be particularly well supervised - protective clothing would have
to be worn.   He asked if the mixing would be a long process and whether
it would be highly specialised.

MR MANSERGH considered mixing would take about an hour a day and suggested
that plant which would take the sodium fluoride by the bag would eliminate
any necessity for re-weighing in the mixing process.   The mixing plant

...[sho]uld not be more than 50 or 60 ft away from the power house where, unfortunately, there was no room for equipment of any bulk. He agreed that the material was dangerous and should be isolated and locked.

MR FISH considered that it may be possible to get land adjacent to the power house belonging to the Power Board or, at the worst, a section over the road belonging to the Fire Brigade. This shed could be built on this. He said that two bags of sodium fluoride would be used some weeks and three bags on others.

MR MANSERGH. We would need then two tanks each of about 500 gallons – one in use while the powder was dissolving in the other. A cwt bag in a tank of this size would give approximately $\frac{1}{4}$ lb. to a gallon or a $2\frac{1}{2}\%$ solution. Cwt bags were not easy to handle but this could be overcome. The plant could be arranged to eliminate dust.

MR WOODS suggested $2\frac{1}{2}\%$ might be rather a high concentration and pointed out that in the United States a 1% solution was more common.

MR MANSERGH said that experiments conducted earlier this week showed that $2\frac{1}{2}\%$ solution with continual agitation by air dissolved in four to five hours.

MR HOGG. We would need, therefore, an air compressor.

MR WOODS. And a softener for the dilution water.

MR MANSERGH. A small base exchange softener on the feed line to the solution tanks would be best.

MR WOODS agreed and added that the dosing of the fluorine solution must be automatic and start when the pumps start and cut out with the pumps. The latter being particularly important as it must be impossible for the fluorine to continue to be added, due to some human error, when the pumps are not working.

MR MANSERGH agreed that this must be done. The matter of types of tanks, siting of tanks and chemical pumps and lining of tanks and type of piping to be used was discussed at some length. Mr Mansergh said he would prefer the pumps to be adjacent to the mixing tank so as to avoid air locks. If it was necessary to have the tanks sited some distance from the power shed there should be a visual pipe by the pumps in the power house to show that the solution is flowing. For the reasons stated, he was satisfied that this would be better than having the chemical pumps in the power house and so suck the solution over.

MR FISH said he would make every endeavour to get space for the new plant adjacent to the power house and once the distance the solution would have to travel was known, the question of whether it would be pumped or sucked could be discussed further.

MR MANSERGH. The flow would be at a rate of approximately nine gallons of the solution per hour. He added that the United States use Hydrofluorosilic acid in the wet plants.

DR MACLEAN confirmed this but it was agreed that it would be impractical to import this substance to New Zealand.

The matter of whether the plant should continue in operation in the meantime was discussed and Dr Maclean considered that in view of the recent high results, serious consideration must be given to keeping it closed down until the wet feeder was in operation. It was estimated that this might be a month from the time it was decided to go ahead. No decision was reached at the meeting but during a formal discussion it was decided it would be advisable to keep the plant working in view of the battle it had been to maintain fluoridation at all. A token addition of powder eliminated any possibility of rumours circulating in the town that the plant had been stopped, with the inevitable spate of inquiries and, more inevitable, improved health in the persons who had been claiming for so long that they had been suffering from the effects of fluoridated water.

All present stressed the necessity for keeping the amount well below one part per million and Mr Fish was confident that this could be done. It was thought that the removal of the stop nut a few weeks ago was probably responsible for the recent high readings and it was decided that the stop nut should be replaced.

MR WOODS was to advise Mr Fish and this Office by phone if any individual reading reached above 1.5 parts per million but Mr Fish was confident he could keep the proportion at .5 or even as low as .1 p.p.m.

MR MANSERGH suggested that the screening of the sodium fluoride to take up the larger particles, together with the fact that the dose per hour was larger to give the required one part per million, (2.3 pds per hour) might just enable the dry feeder to deliver a satisfactory dose.

This point was discussed but it was decided that in view of the uneven dosage to date it would be preferred to keep the dose low and to wait until the wet feeder was established before attempting an accurate dosage of 1 p.p.m. When this occurred Mr Woods would come to Hastings for a few days and take frequent samples so that these could be taken into consideration when adjusting the dosage. Once adjusted, sampling could be done less frequently.

DR TAYLOR advised that he had written to Dr Arnold in America for information regarding simple methods of making fluoride determinations by use of a comparator and that he would advise when further information was received. He suggested that if a suitable comparator could be obtained, daily estimations could be made in Hastings with samples sent two or three times weekly at first and later once a week to Mr Woods as a check. If the comparator suggested that any over or under dosing was occurring on any particular day then a sample would be sent immediately to Mr Woods.

MR WOODS agreed and suggested that once it was known regarding comparators it may be possible for him to evolve one in his laboratory.

MR FISH pointed out that to date Havelock North had not been considered in the discussion but he said that the pumps and equipment at Havelock North were old and that he personally considered the wells almost worked out. A geological survey at present being made will probably confirm this opinion and it is anticipated that within the next twelve months the Havelock North Borough Council will be approaching the Hastings Borough Council to undertake their water supply. When this is done Havelock North will be receiving the same water as Hastings except for rare occasions in dry summers when the Havelock North wells, which will be kept in reserve, may be brought into use for short periods.

It was agreed that no action be taken regarding fluoridation of Havelock North by wet feeders and that although Havelock North children may have to be omitted from the earlier part of the survey they could probably be included later when they receive fully fluoridated water. If it was found that in the meantime Havelock North was receiving reasonably highly fluoridated water (say .8 p.p.m.) then it was probable that an investigation could be done to see if this was giving any beneficial effects.

A general discussion was then held regarding costs of the proposed new method and approximate figures reached were as follows -

2 Tanks	£125
2 Chemical Pumps	£300
1 Shed (300 s.ft.)	£250 to £300.
Pipe Lines	£30
Water Softener	£100
Compressor	£75
Electrical installations, labour, etc.	£300

Total say £1,200 approx.

Figure 74. Notes on Meeting Regarding Fluoridation, June 30th 1954. Source: 125/299/1 H1 Box 1634. Page 4 of 4.

On the 2nd July 1954, Dr. Maclean, the Director-General of Health, received a letter from the City Engineer's Department in Palmerston North. I think it safe to assume it would be written by either Mr. Hogg or Mr. Hassan. The letter (**Figures 75 – 77**) criticized the fact that the water in Hastings was open to accidental or purposeful contamination, for instance during heavy rain, due to a difference in procedure with regard to water wells and their piping.

CONFIDENTIAL:

The Director General of Health,
WELLINGTON

Forwarded through M.O.H. Palmerston N.

Attention Dr. McLean:

Dear Sir:

Following our inspection of the water supply and fluoridation installation at Hastings, I would like to make some comments.

You will appreciate that from a professional etiquette point of view my comments on the general set up there must be of a confidential nature. In addition, it is important to retain the Borough Engineer's goodwill.

1.   GENERAL MECHANICAL SET UP OF PUMPS:

Whilst the general set up and location of the pumps is probably no concern of this Committee, there is one aspect which does concern us and your Department and that is that we ensure that we eliminate the possibility of the water being contaminated, either deliberately or accidentally.

Leaving aside for the moment the location and the accessibility of the fluorine dry feeders, there are two aspects which I feel should be investigated by your Department.

(a) There seems to be a potential serious source of contamination in the existence of the overflow from the suction chamber into the street channel.

The water from the wells will rise to a height five feet above ground and it is therefore necessary to provide for this. It could be looked after either by building into the top of the suction chamber at some convenient out of the way place, say a 6" or a 9" pipe, so that when the underground chamber became full the water would rise up the pipe to the static level of the wells and the flow would stop.   This pipe would also act as a "breather"; that is the inlet point for displaced air as the level in the chamber rises and falls.   This is normal procedure in pumping installations and ensures control of the open air inlet to the suction chamber.

In Hastings the above procedure is not used.   After the pumps are shut down the water in the suction chamber rises, and in order to provide an overflow, a pipe has been laid to the street channel on the opposite side of the road.   I am not sure whether the water flows continuously into the channel during the time the pumps are shut down, but it makes little difference to my comment.

Figure 75. Letter to Dr Maclean, 2nd July, 1954. Source: 125/299/1 H1 Box 1634. Page 1 of 3.

The pipe constitutes a direct connection with a foul water channel in that at some stage at any rate its outlet will be above the level of the water in the suction chamber and during periods of heavy rain the foul water in the street channel could enter this pipe and some of it at any rate could possibly find its way into the suction chamber.   I can envisage no satisfactory safe guard and even if a valve was provided on the overflow pipe line, water from the street channel could still lodge in the overflow.   I suspect this pipe also constitutes the "breather" for the suction chamber, in which case foul air and dust could be drawn into the chamber as the level in it dropped.

To some extent the above is guesswork on my part as this aspect only occurred to me since I returned to Palmerston North and I have had no opportunity of checking with the Borough Engineer.   It would be awkward for me to probe into this matter and I suggest it should be investigated by a member of your Department.

(b)   The loose plate in the floor of the workshop which gives direct access to the main suction chamber, can easily be lifted by unauthorised persons and should be bolted down against a rubber gasket.

2.   EXISTING DRY FEEDERS:

Although a decision has already been made to replace these, I would make the following comments which may be of use to you in your negotiations with Candy Filters as to what allowance they propose to make on them when they are taken out.

Although I have a very high opinion of Mr. Mansergh, the Managing Director of Candy Filters, I cannot understand why his Company should have allowed these feeders to be installed and used for the feeding into the system of such a potentially dangerous material such as sodium fluoride.   It was known to his Company that dry feeders in general, particularly for small additions, are unsatisfactory.   This was admitted by him during our conference on Wednesday last.   The fact that his Company has had little experience in the feeding of sodium fluoride has little bearing on the matter.

In the first place they knew that the amount to be fed in was only a fraction of that normally fed in by the machines supplied, and secondly they knew, or could have ascertained by simple experiments, that sodium fluoride was far more difficult to handle through the machines than lime.

The figure of £500 was mentioned by Mr. Mansergh as the possible salvage his Company would be prepared to pay for the existing machines.   In view of the fact that I consider they have supplied machines which were never designed for the purpose, I suggest that the Department takes up a strong attitude in this matter.   I do not consider the Borough Engineer can be criticised for accepting the installation in that it is doubtful whether he had had any experience in addition of chemicals in powder form to a water supply.

The location and accessibility to any of the workmen in the building or to the general public calls for some comment. The feeders are located just inside the roughly shuttered door, which is frequently left open.   Although during the greater part of the day some of the power board men would be in the vicinity there would be times during the morning and afternoon tea breaks and during the lunch hours when any person off the footpath would have direct access to the machines and the powder contained in them. From now until the time they are emptied, I suggest that padlocks be fitted to the covers over the hoppers.

Figure 76. Letter to Dr Maclean, 2nd July, 1954. Source: 125/299/1 H1 Box 1634. Page 2 of 3.

Figure 77. *Letter to Dr MacLean, 2nd July, 1954.* Source: 125/299/1 H1 Box 1634. Page 3 of 3.

3. CONTROL OF THE FLUORIDATION EXPERIMENT:

We were given to understand that the pumps and the dry feeders were mainly run at night and duringthese hours they were under the general supervision of the shift engineer on duty during that period. These shift engineers are not Council employees and the Borough Engineer has little or no authority over them. These men have no interest whatsoever in the experiment and their sole responsibility appeared to me to be to see that the pumps were run a sufficient number of hours to ensure an adequate supply of water. They appeared to have no interest in the efficient operation of the recording instruments or in the functioning of the dry feeders; for example the clockwork mechanism in connection with the level recorder of their reservoir had not been wound on the morning of our visit and had stopped. It appeared to me that this type of thing and the operation of the dry feeders was the sole responsibility of the Borough Engineer, who is I am given to understand, fairly busy in that he has other interests outside those of the Hastings borough, with the result that I could quite well envisage him being out of town or too busy on some days to give the equipment the attention it requires.

Seeing the decision has been made to only feed in a token amount of sodium fluoride from now until the wet feeders are installed, there does not appear to be any good purpose to be served in endeavouring to arrange some better method of supervision. As soon as the wet feeders come into operation however, I do suggest that the Borough Engineer be asked to exercise an overall supervision, but the detailed supervision of the dosing and preparation of the concentrated solution should if possible be made the responsibility of some other person. I suggest the Borough Sanitary Inspector could quite well carry out this.

4. RECORDS OF OPERATION:

It is essential if we are to be in the position to analyse and track down the origin of any possible troubles that accurate logs be kept, not only by the operators who start and stop the pumps, but also by those who visit and are responsible for the operation of the fluoride feeder. At a later date I will draw up a suggested log to be used in connection with the wet feeder. Had this been done in the past, I think your mind would have been relieved in that you would have been able to pin point the high readings and trace the origin back to the time the Borough Engineer removed the locking screw from the gate of the dry feeder.

I suggest that the Engineer be asked to keep a detailed log of all operations in connection with the dry feeder.

5. WET FEEDER:

I have had no experience in this type of feed. There are no great potential difficulties which could arise. The key to the efficient operation of these machines is in the use of the correct type of pump and in this regard the only difficulty which could arise is the action of the fluorine on the moving parts of the pump. Provided these are not of a material which will be affected they are simple and accurate. Mr. Mansergh assures me that the type of pump he proposes to supply has a rubber diaphragm and this would be the only part of the pump in contact with the fluorine. I suggest you ask for some guarantee from Candy Filters that the design of the pump to be supplied will be such that none of the moving parts will be affected by the action of fluorine on them.

The author suggested that this was his impression and while there was some uncertainty, the matter should be looked into by Dr. Maclean's department.

The author claimed to have a high opinion of the Managing Director of Candy Filters, yet suggested it was improper for the company to have

"... allowed these feeders to be installed and used for the feeding into the system of such a potentially dangerous material such as sodium fluoride."

The author claimed that it was known to Candy Filters that dry feeders were

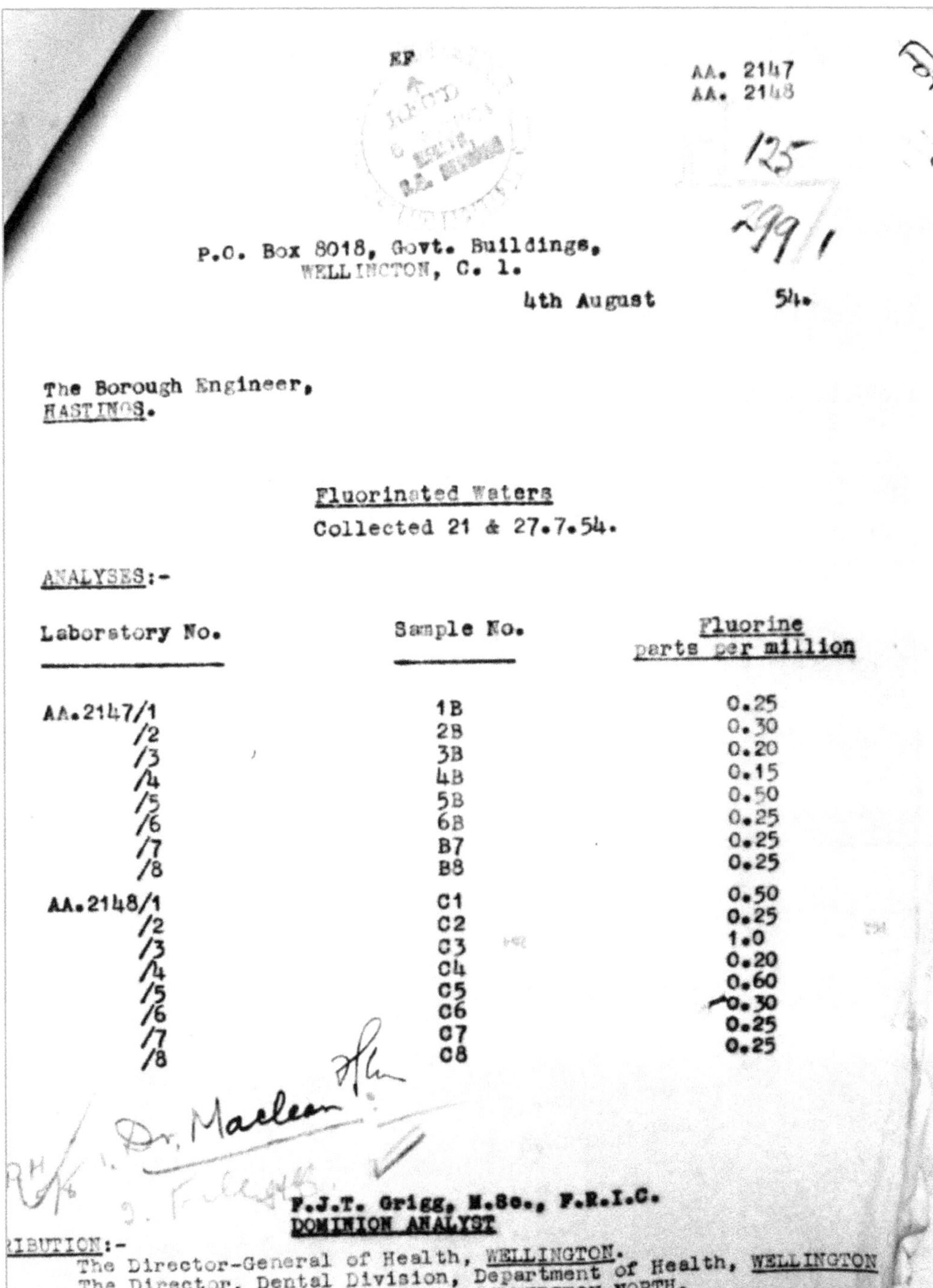

Figure 78. Fluorinated Waters, Hastings. Collected 21 and 27.7.1954. Source: 125/299/1 H1 Box 1634.

"... in general, particularly for small additions, are unsatisfactory. This was admitted by him during our conference on Wednesday last." (Both statements under section 2: Existing Dry Feeders) [570]

The author also criticized the fact that the building was left unlocked, so anyone could get inside, and suggested padlocks for the hopper covers.

The readings on the 4th and 18th of August, 1954, (**Figures 78** and **79**) show a much lower average.

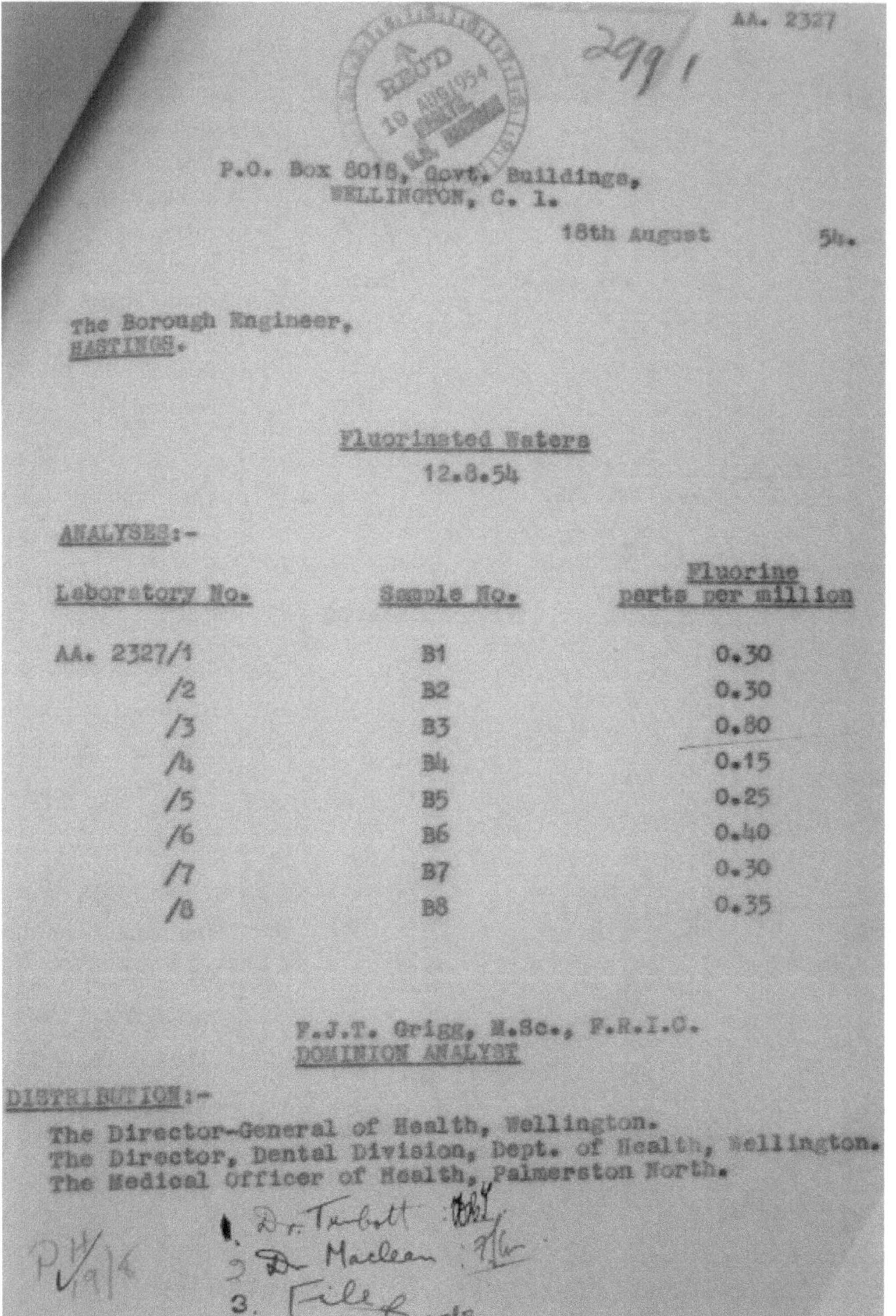

Figure 79.
Fluorinated Waters, Hastings, 12.8.1954. Source: 125/299/1 H1 Box 1634.

Here we see contradictions in the beliefs of the experts. In one file, there is a document called *Objections Raised by Dr. Eva Hill* which goes through a point-by-point refutation of Dr. Hill's objections to CWF. One such objection was that other methods such as tablets and fluoridated milk may be better in delivering the element. One response to this is:

> "It is almost certain that many children would receive their necessary fluoride in a haphazard and irregular manner." [571]

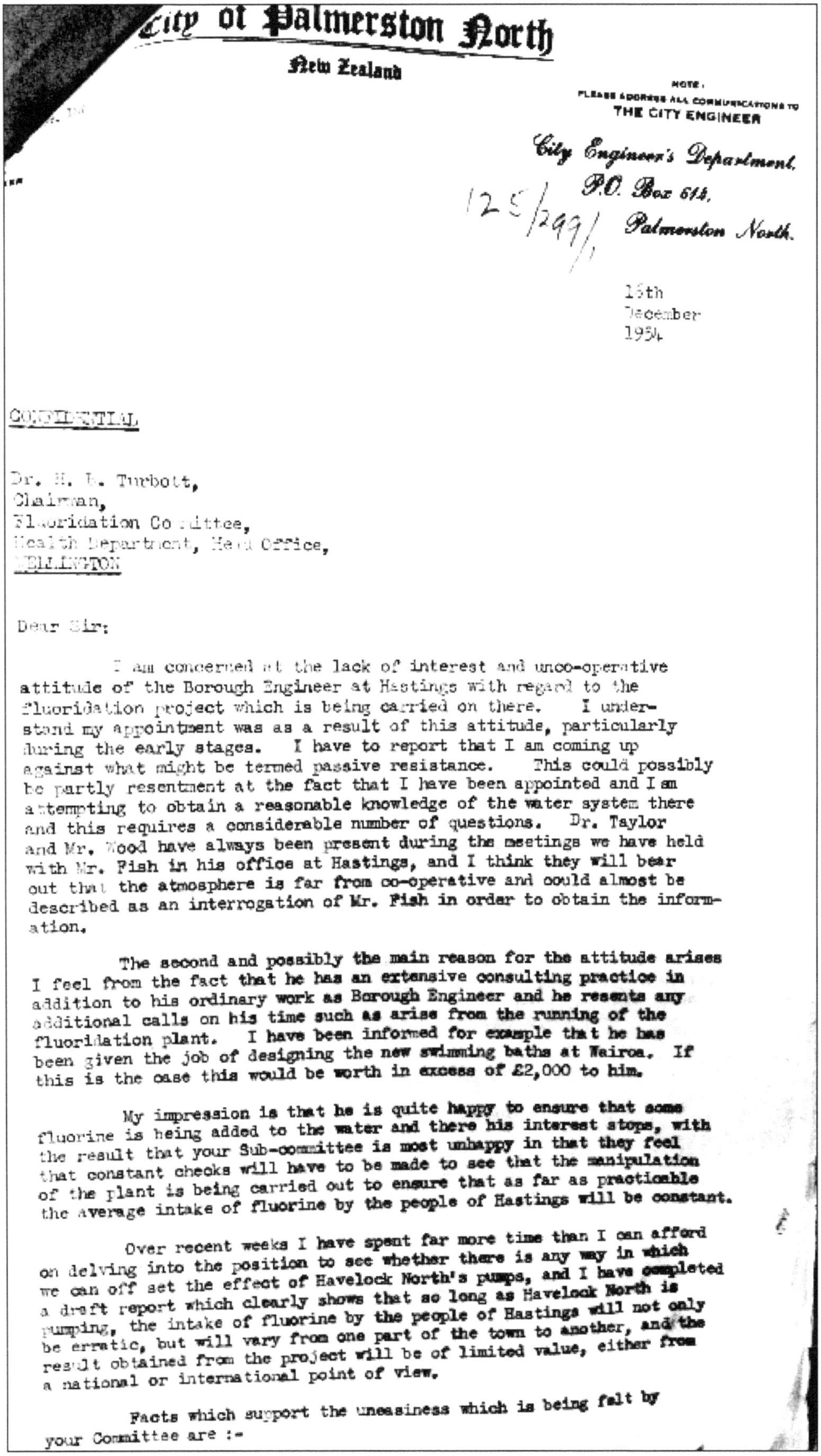

City of Palmerston North
New Zealand

NOTE:
PLEASE ADDRESS ALL COMMUNICATIONS TO
THE CITY ENGINEER

City Engineer's Department,
P.O. Box 614,
Palmerston North.

125/299/1

16th
December
1954

CONFIDENTIAL

Dr. H. B. Turbott,
Chairman,
Fluoridation Committee,
Health Department, Head Office,
WELLINGTON

Dear Sir:

I am concerned at the lack of interest and unco-operative attitude of the Borough Engineer at Hastings with regard to the fluoridation project which is being carried on there. I understand my appointment was as a result of this attitude, particularly during the early stages. I have to report that I am coming up against what might be termed passive resistance. This could possibly be partly resentment at the fact that I have been appointed and I am attempting to obtain a reasonable knowledge of the water system there and this requires a considerable number of questions. Dr. Taylor and Mr. Wood have always been present during the meetings we have held with Mr. Fish in his office at Hastings, and I think they will bear out that the atmosphere is far from co-operative and could almost be described as an interrogation of Mr. Fish in order to obtain the information.

The second and possibly the main reason for the attitude arises I feel from the fact that he has an extensive consulting practice in addition to his ordinary work as Borough Engineer and he resents any additional calls on his time such as arise from the running of the fluoridation plant. I have been informed for example that he has been given the job of designing the new swimming baths at Wairoa. If this is the case this would be worth in excess of £2,000 to him.

My impression is that he is quite happy to ensure that some fluorine is being added to the water and there his interest stops, with the result that your Sub-committee is most unhappy in that they feel that constant checks will have to be made to see that the manipulation of the plant is being carried out to ensure that as far as practicable the average intake of fluorine by the people of Hastings will be constant.

Over recent weeks I have spent far more time than I can afford on delving into the position to see whether there is any way in which we can off set the effect of Havelock North's pumps, and I have completed a draft report which clearly shows that so long as Havelock North is pumping, the intake of fluorine by the people of Hastings will not only be erratic, but will vary from one part of the town to another, and the result obtained from the project will be of limited value, either from a national or international point of view.

Facts which support the uneasiness which is being felt by your Committee are :-

Figure 80. Letter from Hogg to Turbott, 16 December 1954. Source: 125/299/1 H1 Box 1704. Page 1 of 2.

On the 16th December 1954, Mr. Hogg wrote to Dr. Turbott to complain about Mr. Fish (**Figures 80**, **81**). Hogg was to replace Fish as Borough Engineer, and was offended at what he called "passive resistance" – what I believe nowadays we call "passive aggression". Hogg commented that

"the atmosphere is far from co-operative and could almost be described as an interrogation of Mr. Fish in order to obtain the information."

1.   When the dry feeders were in operation, Mr. Fish removed the set screw which resulted in a very erratic feed of fluorine and he did not advise those who were testing that he had done this, with the result that we were unable to account for the erratic results which were being obtained at the time.

2.   Mr. Fish was asked to ensure that Havelock pumps were run as far as practicable at the same time as the Hastings pumps. Over a month later we found that no attempt had been made to carry this out.

3.   Again knowing that Havelock North water was diluting the amount of fluorine, he knowingly permitted Havelock to pump, using his own words - "considerably more, but they did not know it".

4.   In his latest letter, which consisted of his comments on my draft report, he stated that - "the large storage capacity of the pumping mains is significant and interesting and probably gives the answer to low tests of .6 p.p.m. which have been recorded." In the same letter he purports to give an analysis of his pumping for one particular day and concludes this by saying - "The present position has been followed in as much detail as possible but it is a time-consuming occupation which cannot be indulged in very often."

5.   With regard to the elimination of Havelock North pumps Mr. Fish appears to come out into the open when he stated in his letter dated 2nd December the following :-

"The Havelock North Borough Council has made its own decisions regarding its own pumping station and I doubt whether any approach now would cause them to change their minds. In my position as consultant to Havelock, I have my own opinion regarding the wisdom of their decision and also the future outlook regarding the possibilities of their pumping station but I would not like to be quoted by the Fluoridation Committee in this respect and any comments I made in Hastings recently should be considered as "in committee" only."

This in my opinion typifies his attitude, and that is he places his own interests ahead of his obligations to the Council which employs him and unless there is a change in this attitude, your Sub-committee will be faced with the responsibility of constantly checking his work - " a time consuming occupation which should not have to be indulged in very often ████" if Mr. Fish was doing his job.

Yours faithfully,

G. F. HOGG,
CITY ENGINEER

Hogg claimed that Fish resented being called to work at the fluoridation plant, due to Fish having "an extensive consulting practice" which involved baths at Wairoa, which Hogg claimed was worth £2,000 to Fish. Hogg also claimed to have written a draft report,

"… which clearly shows that so long as Havelock North is pumping, the intake of fluorine by the people of Hastings will not only be erratic, but will vary from one part of the town to another, and the result obtained from the project will be of limited value, either from a national or international point of view." [572]

Hogg's letter can be summarized by stating that he believed Fish placed his own interests above the interests of the fluoridation program and Hogg believed this may have caused or contributed to the erratic levels of fluorine in Hastings' water. We should not forget Fish's claim that there was "a tendency for the powder to stick in the hopper."

None of this prevented Mr. Fish from presenting the "technical aspects of fluoridation" to the committee in charge of authoring the 1957 Commission of Inquiry, on behalf of the Department of Health (**Figure 82**).

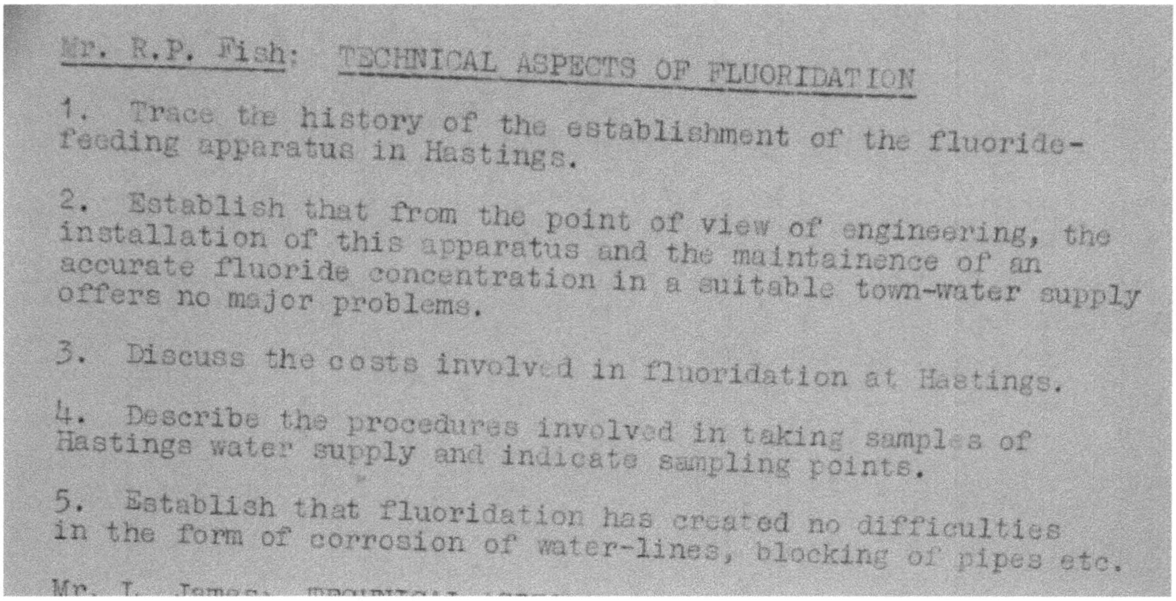

Mr. R.P. Fish: TECHNICAL ASPECTS OF FLUORIDATION

1. Trace the history of the establishment of the fluoride-feeding apparatus in Hastings.

2. Establish that from the point of view of engineering, the installation of this apparatus and the maintainence of an accurate fluoride concentration in a suitable town-water supply offers no major problems.

3. Discuss the costs involved in fluoridation at Hastings.

4. Describe the procedures involved in taking samples of Hastings water supply and indicate sampling points.

5. Establish that fluoridation has created no difficulties in the form of corrosion of water-lines, blocking of pipes etc.

Figure 82. Technical Aspects of Fluoridation (part) by R.P.Fish, Source: Evidence to be Presented by Department of Health Witnesses at Hearings of Commission of Inquiry on Fluoridation, p. 2. James Fuller MS-Papers-6167-09 General Files - Minutes of Meetings - Fluoridation Committee. Available at the National Library, Wellington, New Zealand.

There is an entire story that can be told regarding Hastings. The same is probably true in many cities where the subject of fluoridation was discussed heatedly. Here, I am omitting much.

The type of feeder used at the plant changed in September 1954. The experts wanted sincerely for fluoridation to bring about benefit to everyone, and for the equipment to function accurately. If their morality can be questioned, it is with regard to none of them informing the public of the higher concentrations.

On the 8th December 1954, the readings from 0.7 to 3.0 ppm can be seen in **Figure 83**.

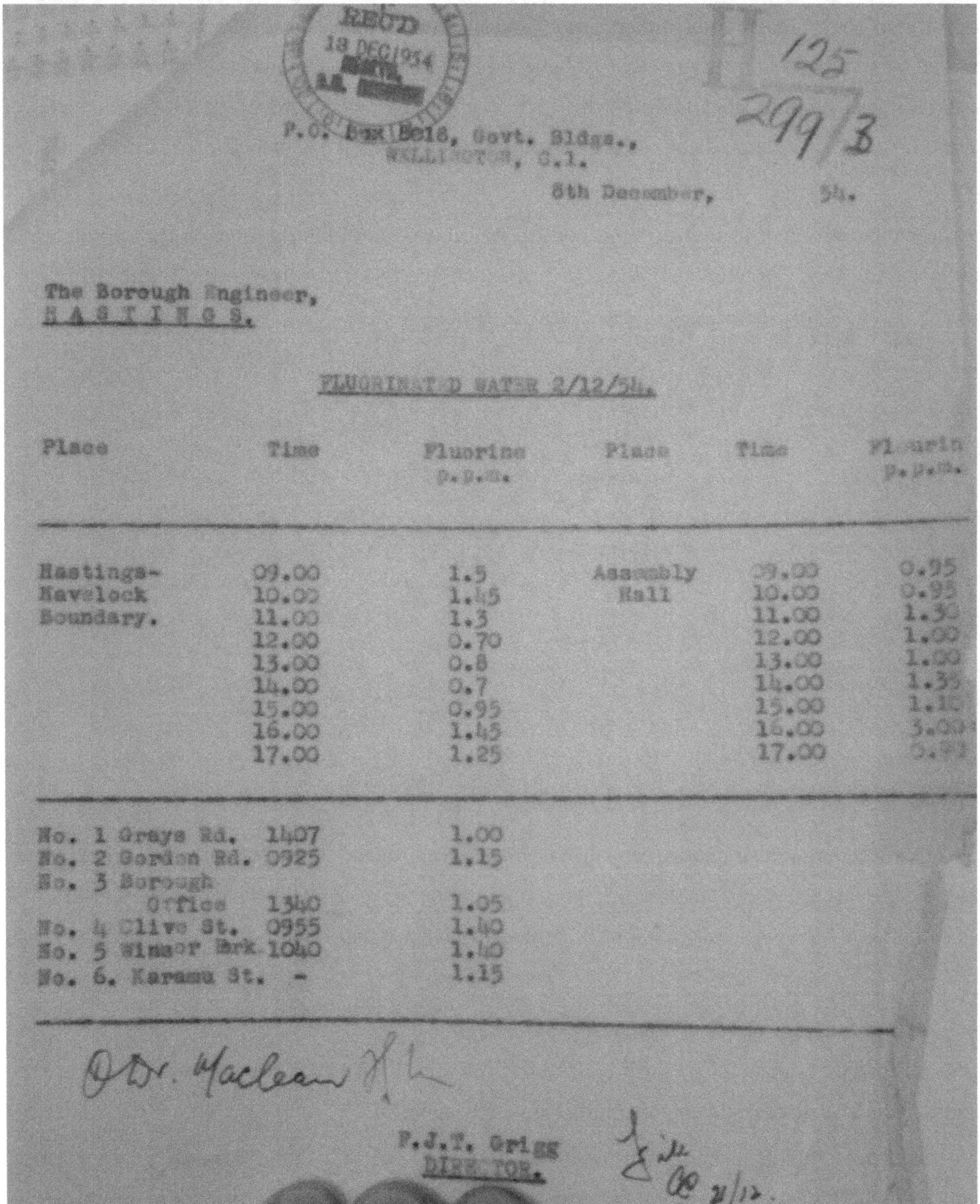

P.O. Box 8018, Govt. Bldgs.,
WELLINGTON, C.1.

8th December, 54.

The Borough Engineer,
H A S T I N G S.

FLUORINATED WATER 2/12/54.

Place	Time	Fluorine p.p.m.	Place	Time	Flourine p.p.m.
Hastings-	09.00	1.5	Assembly	09.00	0.95
Havelock	10.00	1.45	Hall	10.00	0.95
Boundary.	11.00	1.3		11.00	1.30
	12.00	0.70		12.00	1.00
	13.00	0.8		13.00	1.00
	14.00	0.7		14.00	1.35
	15.00	0.95		15.00	1.10
	16.00	1.45		16.00	3.00
	17.00	1.25		17.00	0.91

Place	Time	Fluorine p.p.m.
No. 1 Grays Rd.	1407	1.00
No. 2 Gordon Rd.	0925	1.15
No. 3 Borough Office	1340	1.05
No. 4 Clive St.	0955	1.40
No. 5 Windsor Park	1040	1.40
No. 6. Karamu St.	-	1.15

F.J.T. Grigg
DIRECTOR.

Figure 83. Fluoridated Water, Hastings, 2.12.1954. Source: 125/299/3 H1 Box 1704.

The second plant was slightly more accurate, as can be demonstrated from the following documents. The first gives a concentration range of 0.35-1.6 ppm, and the second a range of 0.5-1.45 ppm. (**Figures 84** and **85**).

... OF FLUORINE ANALYSES
HASTINGS SUPPLY
NEW PLANT IN OPERATION
SAMPLED IN ASSEMBLY HALL

	Date	Hrs.	p.p.m.	Hrs.	pp.m.
	20. 9. 54.	10.0	1.00	12.0	.55
	21. 9. 54.	10.0	1.00	12.0	.45
	22. 9. 54.	10.0	1.00	12.0	.50
2836	23. 9. 54	10.0	.95	12.0	.35
	24. 9. 54.	10.0	1.10	12.0	.30
	28. 9. 54.	10.0	1.00	12.0	.35
	29. 9. 54.	10.0	1.00	12.0	.60
2939	30. 9. 54.	10.30	.55	12.0	.70
	1.10. 54.	9.55	1.05	11.45	1.00
	5.10. 54.	10.0	1.05		.60
	6.10. 54.	[illegible].90	[illegible]		
	7.10.54.	9.40	.95		.60
3016	8.10. 54.	9.45	.95		-
	11.10. 54.	10.0	1.00		-
	12.10. 54.	10.15	1.00		1.00
	13.10. 54.	10.0	1.00	11.50	1.00
	14.10. 54.	10.0	1.10		-
3287	1.11. 54.			Noon	.80
	2.11. 54.	9.15	1.00		1.10
	3.11.54.			11.35	1.10
	4.11. 54.	10 [illegible]	1.05	Noon	1.05
	9.11. 54.			Noon	0.5
3388	10.11. 54.	9 [illegible]	.55	Noon	.55
	12.11. 54.	9 [illegible]	.85	Noon	1.0
	16.11. 54.	9.30	1.05	Noon	1.0
	17.11. 54.	9.30	1.0	Noon	1.0
	18.11. 54.	9.15	1.05	13.00	1.0
3525	19.11. 54.	8.55	1.00	11.55	1.05
	22.11. 54.	9.50	0.45	13.00	0.40
	23.11. 54.	10.30	1.0	13.00	
	24.11. 54.	10.00	0.95	13.00	
	25.11. 54.	10.00	0.90	11.30	0.95
	26.11. 54.	10.30	1.6	13.00	1.0
	29.11. 54.	10.15	1.0	13.00	0.95
		Reservoir		14.30	0.75
	30.11. 54.	10.45	1.05	13.85	1.0
*3586	2.12. 54.	10.00	0.95	13.00	1.0
3793	15.12. 54.	10.00	1.3	-	
	16.12. 54.	10.00	1.2		
	17.12. 54.	10.20	1.05		
	20.12. 54.	9.45	1.35		
	21.12. 54.	10.30	1.15		
	22.12. 54.	9.30	1.10		
	23.12. 54.		-	11.30	1.10

Figure 84*. Fluorine Analysis, Hastings Supply, 23.9.1954 – 23.12.1954 New Plant in Operation.* Source: 125/299/3 H1 Box 1835.

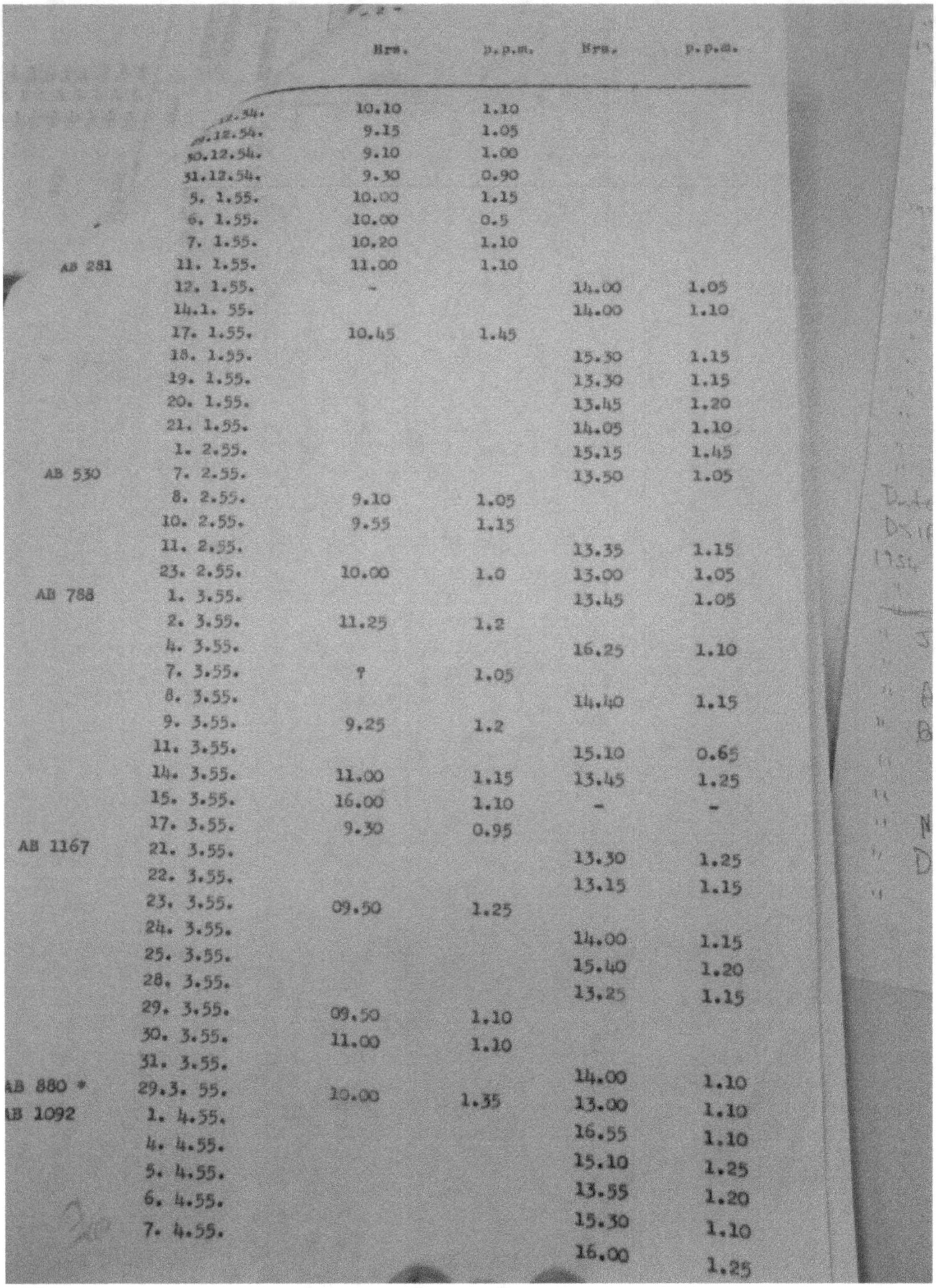

		Hrs.	p.p.m.	Hrs.	p.p.m.
	28.12.54.	10.10	1.10		
	29.12.54.	9.15	1.05		
	30.12.54.	9.10	1.00		
	31.12.54.	9.30	0.90		
	5. 1.55.	10.00	1.15		
	6. 1.55.	10.00	0.5		
	7. 1.55.	10.20	1.10		
AB 281	11. 1.55.	11.00	1.10		
	12. 1.55.	-		14.00	1.05
	14.1. 55.			14.00	1.10
	17. 1.55.	10.45	1.45		
	18. 1.55.			15.30	1.15
	19. 1.55.			13.30	1.15
	20. 1.55.			13.45	1.20
	21. 1.55.			14.05	1.10
	1. 2.55.			15.15	1.45
AB 530	7. 2.55.			13.50	1.05
	8. 2.55.	9.10	1.05		
	10. 2.55.	9.55	1.15		
	11. 2.55.			13.35	1.15
	23. 2.55.	10.00	1.0	13.00	1.05
AB 788	1. 3.55.			13.45	1.05
	2. 3.55.	11.25	1.2		
	4. 3.55.			16.25	1.10
	7. 3.55.	?	1.05		
	8. 3.55.			14.40	1.15
	9. 3.55.	9.25	1.2		
	11. 3.55.			15.10	0.65
	14. 3.55.	11.00	1.15	13.45	1.25
	15. 3.55.	16.00	1.10	-	-
	17. 3.55.	9.30	0.95		
AB 1167	21. 3.55.			13.30	1.25
	22. 3.55.			13.15	1.15
	23. 3.55.	09.50	1.25		
	24. 3.55.			14.00	1.15
	25. 3.55.			15.40	1.20
	28. 3.55.			13.25	1.15
	29. 3.55.	09.50	1.10		
	30. 3.55.	11.00	1.10		
	31. 3.55.				
AB 880 *	29.3. 55.	10.00	1.35	14.00	1.10
AB 1092	1. 4.55.			13.00	1.10
	4. 4.55.			16.55	1.10
	5. 4.55.			15.10	1.25
	6. 4.55.			13.55	1.20
	7. 4.55.			15.30	1.10
				16.00	1.25

Figure 85. *Fluorine Analysis, Hastings Supply, 28.12.1954–7.4.1955.* Source: 125/299/3 H1 Box 1835.

On the 19th January 1955, a selection of readings from late 1954 and early 1955 showed a concentration range of 0.5 to 1.4 ppm at the Hastings Assembly Hall and 0.4 to 1.8 ppm at the Hastings/Havelock North boundary [573].

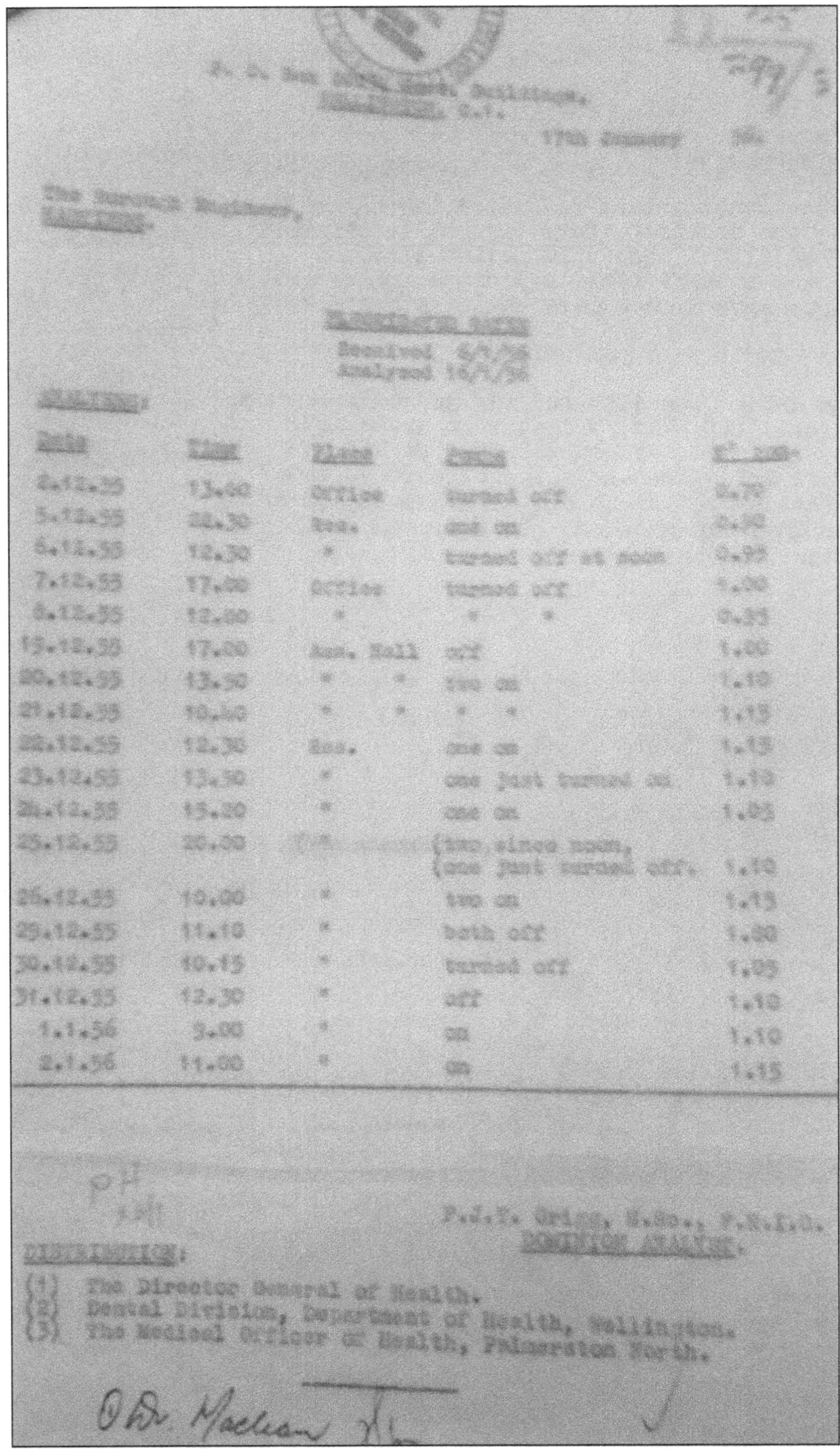

Throughout early 1955 the readings were much closer to 1 ppm, but were still a little erratic. By May 1955, they were consistently close to 1 ppm, with only the occasional reading lower (for instance the sheet dated 8th July shows 35 readings in total, with only one outside the range of 0.8-1.2 ppm; a single reading of 0.55 ppm). However in October 1955, there were a couple of samples showing 1.3 and 1.35 ppm.

On the 17th January 1956, there were a total of 18 readings sent to Mr. Fish from the Dominion Analyst. The readings were taken through December of 1955. Readings were between 0.7 and 1.15 ppm, except for one at 1.8 ppm. (**Figure 86**). This was after both pumps were on. Both were switched off, presumably in response to this.

Figure 86. *Fluoridated Waters, Hastings, Analysed 16.1.1956. Source: 125/299/3 H1 Box 1835.*

In February of 1956 one average was 0.913 ppm for one week [574].

The following document (**Figure 87**) was written in response to questions from Mr. E. D. Blundell Esq. of the Bell Gully & Company law firm, based in Wellington. It contains a statement regarding the "technical difficulties that were becoming apparent."

3.   Samples of analyst's reports:

Enclosed are two specimen samples, one dated 4th August 1954 which will indicate the unsatisfactory figures we obtained with the original dry feed plant. You will notice that the proportions of fluoride are insufficient to achieve the desired purpose. The other report shows a much more satisfactory result.

4.   When was the control committee expanded?

This was done round about June 1954 and was judged necessary on account of the technical difficulties that were becoming apparent. It will be appreciated, of course, that we had no first-hand knowledge of fluoridation and all published reports from America suggested that a continuous and accurate supply of fluoride was a simple engineering problem. This proved not to be the case and for that reason the control was intensified.

Figure 87.

Hastings Fluoridation, 26th April, 1956.
Source: 125/299/1 H1 Box 1704.

On the 26th of June, 1956, Dr. John Cairney, the Director-General of Health, was quoted in **The Daily Telegraph** (**Figure 88**):

Director-General Praises Accuracy Of Hastings Fluoridation Supervision

In a statement issued to-day, the Director-General of Health, Dr John Cairney, said that the Fluoridation Committee, which exercises general supervision over the fluoridation of water supplies, has written to the Hastings Borough Council congratulating its engineering staff on the very accurate and precise manner in which the technical aspects of the fluoridation of the water supply were being handled.

"Frequent sampling and analysis of the water is being made from day to day and the results achieved show that no greater degree of accuracy would be possible of attainment," said Dr Cairney.

"The Hastings people will therefore have the satisfaction of knowing that their interests are being carefully watched by highly skilled and conscientious officers," he added.

Dr Cairney recalled that fluoridation in reducing tooth decay.

An extremely painstaking investigation had also been made to ascertain whether any harmful effect on general health could possibly be attributed to the fluoridation. If anything, these investigations showed that the general health of the community receiving fluoridated water was superior to that of the corresponding community receiving ordinary water.

OPINION ABROAD

After Canada, New Zealand

"… the results achieved show that no greater degree of accuracy would be possible of attainment…"

"After a period of necessary technical adjustments, it may be said that the full amount of one part per million of fluoride has been added to the water since about April, 1954". [575]

You can see from the meeting pictured previously (30th June 1954 at the Borough Engineer's office, Mr. Fish's comment on the 2nd page) that a years' worth of compound had been used over sixteen months, meaning the concentration had been lower than one part per million from 1953–1954.

Figure 88. Director-General Praises Accuracy of Hastings Fluoridation Supervision. Source: **Daily Telegraph** (Napier), 26th June, 1956.

Yet sometimes the concentration was erratically elevated as can also be seen. I do not believe these elevations have been taken into consideration regarding the claims made of the Hastings experiment.

These exact words were sent to the editors of the **Daily Telegraph** (Napier) and the **Hawke's Bay Herald-Tribune** (Hastings) from the Director-General of Health [576]. One can see the **Daily Telegraph** has printed these words without showing the analyses to the public. The published statement reads exactly the same as Cairney's letter.

A letter dated 21st October 1958 (**Figure 89**) from K. E. Swann, the Secretary of the Fluoridation Committee, addressed to Mr. W. A. G. Penlington, one of the most persistent of the Hastings group opposed to CWF, claimed 66% of readings were below 0.9 ppm. This was probably accurate or very close, yet Swann did not mention the amounts that were above, nor acknowledge that any readings had been above 1.2 ppm. This is what sceptics refer to as "cherry-picking" – only showing what suits you so you don't appear wrong.

Officially the experts allowed for a +/- 0.2 ppm deviation from 1.0 ppm in concentration, meaning the highest tolerable concentration was 1.2 ppm, the lowest desired being 0.8. A table made in 1958 of fluorine content noted the variations, but the highest category was a concentration (in ppm) of 1.11+ (**Figure 89**).

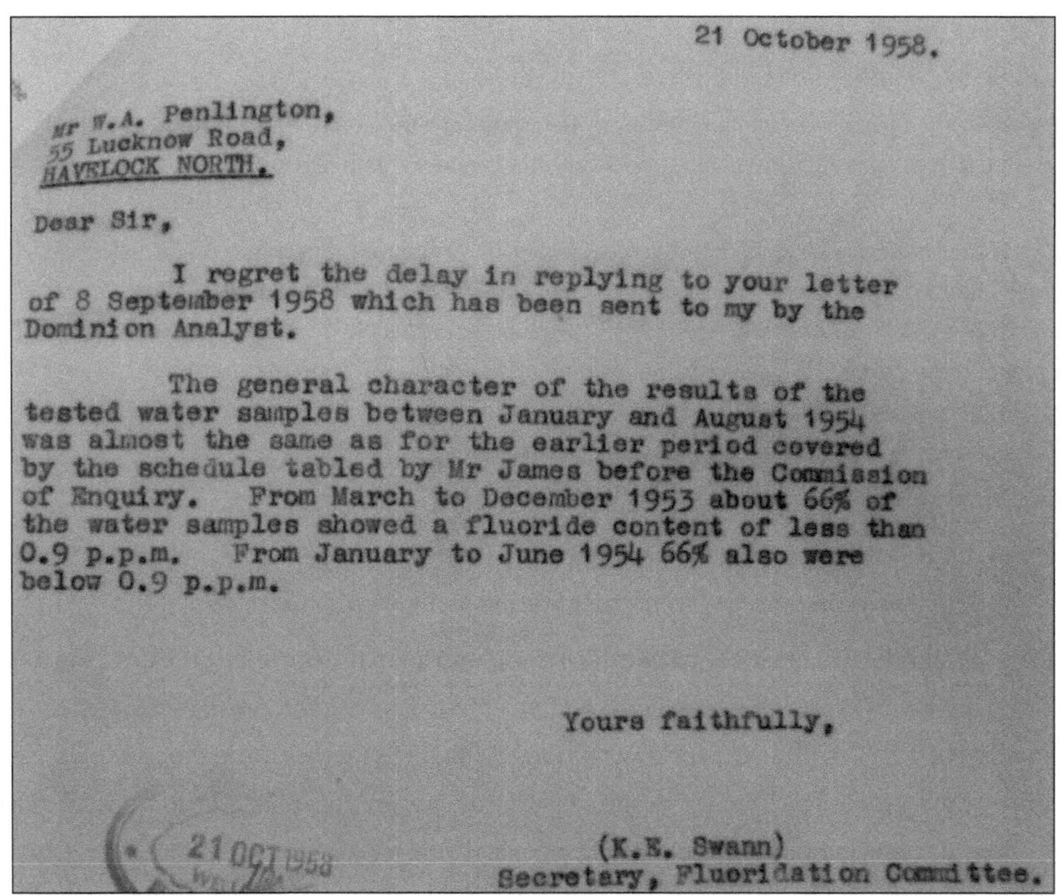

21 October 1958.

Mr W.A. Penlington,
55 Lucknow Road,
HAVELOCK NORTH.

Dear Sir,

I regret the delay in replying to your letter of 8 September 1958 which has been sent to my by the Dominion Analyst.

The general character of the results of the tested water samples between January and August 1954 was almost the same as for the earlier period covered by the schedule tabled by Mr James before the Commission of Enquiry. From March to December 1953 about 66% of the water samples showed a fluoride content of less than 0.9 p.p.m. From January to June 1954 66% also were below 0.9 p.p.m.

Yours faithfully,

(K. E. Swann)
Secretary, Fluoridation Committee.

Figure 89. Letter to Penlington from Swann, 21.10.1958. Source: 125/299/1 H1 Box 1766.

Note the "plus" sign. By categorizing the concentrations this way, the much higher concentrations were not specified.

TABLE 1

FLUORIDE CONTENT OF WATER – ANALYSES AT HASTINGS

(DRY FEED PLANT)

Fluoride Content	Mar. 1953 – Dec. 1953.		Jan. 1954 – June 1954.		Mar. 1953 – June 1954.	
	No. of Analyses	Per Cent of Total	No. of Analyses	Per Cent of Total	No. of Analyses	Per Cent of Total
0.00 – 0.50	163	48.95	74	55.22	237	50.75
0.51 – 0.75	43	12.91	8	5.97	51	10.92
0.76 – 0.89	13	3.91	7	5.22	20	4.29
0.90 – 1.10	30	9.0	12	8.96	42	8.99
1.11+	84	25.23	33	24.63	117	25.05
Totals	333	100.00	134	100.00	467	100.00

Note: The dry feeder was kept in operation until 9th August 1954 and the new liquid feed equipment came into operation 14th September 1954.

Figure 90*. Fluoride Content of Water Analyses at Hastings, March 1953 to June 1954.* Source: John Colquhoun MS-Papers-6670-81 Dept. of Health Research Papers available at the National Library, Wellington, New Zealand.

A ministerial statement dated 16th June 1959, began:

> "A spectacular increase in the number of young children in Hastings who are completely immune to dental decay has been noted in dental examination of 1,901 children there, said the Minister of Health, Mr. Mason, today."
>
> "The Minister said that the children examined had lived permanently in Hastings since fluoridation started, and were known to drink fluoridated water throughout this period. The examinations in 1954 showed that only 4 percent of the five-year-old children were completely immune to dental decay. In 1959 the proportion had risen to 23 percent. In the case of six-year-olds the proportion of completely immune children had risen from 3 percent in 1954 to 9 percent in 1959. The teeth of these children were generally well-formed and there was no sign of the unsightly appearance known as 'mottling' of the teeth." [577]

I did not find a published news article with the same words.

There is a whole story in the Hastings demonstration/experiment. I include this because I feel a duty to the people of this country, who have been discouraged from participation in the fluoridation issue.

The examples from Hastings shown here illustrate the weaknesses of human nature including the desire to not be proven wrong. They demonstrate that when people have a position of power and prestige, they want to justify maintaining and exerting it. The experts probably believed with sincerity they were doing something helpful for the future of New Zealanders' dental health. This is an obvious justification to conceal the information presented here from the public – the anti-fluoride people would have been correct at least as far as some of their accusations of administrator incompetence, justified in some of their claims of nausea and sore stomachs, and this possibly would have ended fluoridation in New Zealand or at least postponed it for a great many years.

Many of the experts, including the analysts in Wellington, knew about the problems in keeping the concentration accurate, yet none spoke publicly. None wanted to jeopardise the fluoridation program. This brings us to the question why… an answer is difficult to come by, because I have never seen it admitted that this actually happened. Again we must bring up a point of lying to protect public health: how much lying is acceptable? You can see here this is not a question that can be publicly discussed, because one of our presuppositions is that experts have not lied.

It may be rewarding to scour the literature on CWF, and see if Dr. Arnold had mentioned any of the problems in Hastings in his published writings on the subject. I have not done this, but the impression I have is that everyone has spoken highly of the Hastings experiment.

This chapter also demonstrates another key feature of this strange topic of a need for fluorine: that what we get in public is almost in total contrast to what we get when we dig deeper – in this case, government archives available to the NZ public since 1982.

Throughout the writing of this book I have come to the conclusion that the public relations industry needs to be regulated if we are to get close to an accurate picture of the world out to the public. This is particularly important given the environmental and wealth inequality issues the current youth will face as they age. Yet such regulation may be very difficult to implement and have little effect at first given the past century spent training people to tilt claims and public statements in favour of organizations and systems that cause environmental problems and wealth inequality. As well as this, we face the unpleasant reality that lying or simply turning a blind eye to save our product's reputation, job, etc – what public relations companies may call "crisis management" is all too human. Modern communication means anyone can spin, yet it would be so much better for us if this did not exist as a paying industry.

Many of the experts in Hastings were aware of fluctuating concentrations of fluorides in the water, yet none of them became whistleblowers. I found no letters or communications between experts admitting dishonesty in writing, though such feelings are probably not expressed in official channels, if at all. It did appear that before the visit from Drs. Arnold and Parfitt in mid-1954, the City Council and others were losing enthusiasm, though this may have been because of the constant arguing, undermining of claims, nit-picking and general animosity and divisiveness the subject brought with it to the town. It looked to me as though in the 1960s the problems with fluctuating concentrations were fixed, and most analyses were between 0.8 and 1.2 ppm. This is based on a cursory, not a detailed examination, of readings between 1961 and 1967. I spent many hours studying the files from the 1950s. Hastings was the first city in New Zealand to be fluoridated, at least according to the official record[120]. It's impossible to say what would have happened had the public known the concentrations were at least on one occasion, as high as 9.0 ppm.

In 1956, it was thought by the experts that a Commission of Inquiry be used to address all of the charges for and against CWF. This was to impress expert opinion upon leading intellectuals and the media, who may have been influenced by the claims of activists and the public. Regarding the concentration of fluorine in the Hastings water supply, the authors wrote:

> "As is mentioned in paragraph 433, the dry feeder caused slight variations in the supply and, for this reason, the concentration of fluoride in the water was kept below the optimum level. When the liquid-type feeder was introduced at the end of 1954 the reason for these slight variations was removed, and since that time the concentration of fluoride in the water has been maintained at 1 ppm as is established by the water analyses. Confirmation of this is contained in the results of the analyses of certain 24-hour urine specimens taken from six adult subjects in 1955. These gave values lying between 1.18 and 1.49 milligrams of fluorine for daily excretion in urine. These values are slightly above 1 ppm because, of course, the excretion includes fluorine originally absorbed from food and tea. The samples show clearly that these subjects were ingesting the desired amount of fluoride from all sources." [578]

Paragraph 433 concludes:

> "Mr. Fish … informed us that the material was inclined to clog in the hopper and, for this reason, it was difficult to keep a uniform flow. During this period the quantity of fluoride introduced into the Hastings water supply was kept below the proposed or optimal level."

People had complained of adverse reactions to the fluoridation scheme in Hastings, they wrote many letters and drafted a petition of over 4,000 signatures, these were treated with great scepticism. Complaints of reactions like stomach aches and rashes were submitted to the 1957 Commission of Inquiry, and dismissed [579]. The concentrations over 1 ppm in the official borough engineer analyses sent to the government were not mentioned in the Inquiry. While the authors of the Inquiry did address the readings under 1 ppm, they did give readers the impression of accuracy:

> "The process of fluoridation involves no new or unusual problems in water-works engineering."

> "Apparatus capable of mixing the fluoride in water supplies with precise and unvarying accuracy is readily available." [580]

One of the principal promoters of CWF in New Zealand was Brigadier Ferris Fuller, a dentist who had served in WWII. Fuller made mention of the Hastings project in a chronology of his life he had written, available for reading in the Katherine Mansfield room of Wellington's National Library. Fuller wrote of "an inexperienced team tackling a new technical operation" and that

---

[120] In 2013 the US National Academy of Sciences wrote about one expert who engaged in "tiptoe" fluoridation – persuading city officials to fluoridate without the public knowing; this way debate is avoided (see **Oral Health Literacy**, pp. 49-52, 2013). This is not a new idea; in 1951 C. S. Hercus, Professor of Public Health at Otago University, New Zealand, suggested an area in Auckland be fluoridated without the public knowing, in order to obviate complaints (17th December, 4th paragraph, HD 125/299 H1 Box 1615). Also see Dr. John Colquhoun's 1987 thesis, Chapter 12.

"... fluoride levels were inconsistent and irregular, delivered to some points and not to others, in some places too low and in others alarmingly high..." [581]

This document is dated October-December 1997.

Fuller wrote to R. Harvey Brown, BDS, DDSc., then editor of the **New Zealand Dental Journal**, explaining why it had taken him such time to send his memoir to Brown:

"I promised to send you an account of the errors and omissions at Hastings when the fluoridation trial began as revealed to me by Arnold and Parfitt in May 1953 and the steps then taken to rectify..." [582]

In 1989 the **New Zealand Dental Journal** printed Fuller's retirement speech in the January and April issues. He said nothing about the excess of fluorine in Hastings' water. To my knowledge Dr. Brown has said nothing about the occasional excess in concentration in issues of the **Journal** after 1997, though I will stand corrected if I've missed them. In another letter from this collection Fuller told Brown of "notes on faults at Hastings recorded on 28 May..." Dentists in New Zealand will get a different picture of the Hastings experiment/demonstration depending on whether they read Fuller's speech in the **Journal** or whether they read Fuller's memoirs in the National Library. Councillors and the public will get a different picture depending on whether they listen to activists who've read Fuller's memoirs and Colquhoun's thesis, or dentists who read the **Journal.** And why would dentists feel the need to read much more? The **Journal** is written by presumably hard-working, intelligent people they probably know, trust, respect and care about. People opposed to fluoridation will know that the United States has often held the precautionary principle in some contempt; this is the inevitable consequence of being a business-run society [583].

In the discussion of his first paper on Hastings mentioned at the start of this chapter, Ludwig wrote:

"The fluoride concentrations registered in the city water supply during this period [1953-1954] were generally below an optimal level." [555]

That sometimes concentrations were far *above* an optimal level was not mentioned by Ludwig. Perhaps it needed no elaboration – after all, it took sixteen months to use twelve months of compound from early 1953 [569].

The media never publicly asked for the analyses when they printed the claims and implications that the concentration was a steady 1 ppm, never more. They simply accepted the press releases and claims made by authorities. They also published a lot of opinion pieces and letters from people opposed to fluoridation. Such a thing matters little given that they avoided showing analyses, which would have been much more powerful than protest.

Peter B. Hunter and E. Storey's paper is described as a "detailed critique" of a study by Dr. John Colquhoun and Robert Mann that appeared in **The Ecologist** in 1986 [584]. This 1986 study did not mention the excesses in concentration in 1953 and 1954, but did discuss a different set of archived files a little. Regarding the amounts of fluorine in the water supply, Hunter and Storey's critique claims:

"The equipment proved unsuitable and was operated only intermittently until September 1954 when it was replaced with apparatus feeding sodium fluoride in solution. During the period March 1953 to September

1954 a considerable proportion of the fluoride concentrations recorded in the city's water supply were well below 1 ppm with a few above that level. Following the installation of the solution feeding equipment in September 1954 fluoride concentrations of 1 ppm were obtained in all sectors of the city and maintained with only minor variations." [556]

The Health Department archives have been available to the New Zealand public since 1982. In 1987, Dr. John Colquhoun, former Dental Officer for Auckland, published his thesis in which he cited many of the documents and letters you have just read regarding the fluctuating concentrations of fluorine in the Hastings water supply [557]. His work contained reference to a letter from the New Zealand Police to the Health Deparment in response to questions regarding whether people involved in opposition to CWF had links to the (NZ) Communist Party; the Police replied in the negative [585] (and see Appendix 3). In 1990, this letter was mentioned in an article on fluoride with a heavy focus on Colquhoun [352] (discussed a little in Chapter 5.5), though the media did not say where they obtained the letter from – his thesis, or the Department archives. Though if they had read his thesis, surely they would have read the claims about the concentration of fluorine in Hastings' water? Surely the media would have pursued this in the 1980s, given that the files had been available since 1982…? Is this too much to ask given that the Dominion Building is only a half hour's walk from the archives?

This is the only mention of something from the archives I have ever seen in New Zealand media regarding CWF. The letter from the NZ Police could have got to the media through a completely different channel. Also, the media may have discussed the fluorine analyses from the archives in articles I have never read, although I doubt this as I have never seen this mentioned in the claims of New Zealand activists, even on the internet. Colquhoun's presence is consistent in NZ newspapers in the late 1980s.

Two weeks after the article featuring Colquhoun was published [352], **The Evening Post** allowed Peter B. Hunter, at this time Manager of the Health Department's Dental Health Unit, a right of reply. His article was half a page; he stressed the safety and effectiveness of CWF. He did not mention the archived information at all [586].

The media may claim to have thoroughly represented both sides of the fluoridation issue; a claim that makes very good sense at first, and if we confine our research strictly to media – as many *opinions* are presented. Yet such a claim is made on a flimsy foundation when we consider Colquhoun's claim of excessive concentrations of fluorine in Hastings' water during the first couple of years of the trial was based on real evidence, not just idle speculation or paranoia. For those who don't spend hours going through the archives – almost all of us – the media's claim will appear true. One probably would never know the archived files existed unless one had read Colquhoun's thesis. This is why in polarizing issues, it is so important to read the literature presented by each group and to pay attention to details and evidence, not just claims and counter-claims. Very few people opposed to CWF discuss or even mention this thesis in detail (the book by Connett *et al.* is one exception to this [149]). As well as this, much reporting has been (in my opinion) of variable quality and detail – some excellent, some terrible, most in between.

The 1990 **Dominion Sunday Times** article discussed some of the ways in which "the anti-fluoride campaign looks set to demand fresh attention." Yet such fundamentally powerful evidence, that can be seen in the government's own archive, was ignored, except for one letter, which amounted to very little (see Appendix 3).

Professors Herman and Chomsky's propaganda model suggests that the media must have some pretense of antagonism towards power, because their presumed societal purpose would obviously be farcical if they did not show some antagonism towards power. No doubt much of this is very sincere. Given that I know nothing of how the media obtained the letter regarding the NZ Police's investigation of the anti-fluoride activists, I feel a little presumptuous making the following suggestion. Sharing the information found in the Health Department files would of course be "ammunition for antifluoridationists" – even if modern equipment and modern concentrations could be guaranteed and shown to be very accurate. Yet mentioning the letter regarding the Police investigation that amounted to nothing helps make the fluoridation issue look a little eccentric, perhaps makes the NZ Health Department look a little silly, but does almost nothing to resolve the back-and-forth arguments around Hastings. Thus, the media's antagonism towards power is fulfilled, without creating a "crisis of democracy" [315]. Believing that one's own professional purpose is antagonistic to power is a self-serving belief – if journalists are "fighting the power" they don't need to be *more* antagonistic because to be *more* antagonistic would make them crazy.

The 1990 article mentioned that arguments raged over Hastings even thirty-something years later. This was the same article that quoted a dentist as claiming people opposed to CWF were as bad as child molesters. In 1999, Colquhoun co-wrote on the topic of the Hastings demonstration with Bill Wilson. This was published in the journal **Accountability in Research** [587]. They mentioned how poorly the information in the Health Department archives had been discussed. This has knock-on effects for our future too: American or overseas audiences may be sceptical of my claims, and fair enough. Without an official (government, expert or media) verification of the claims made in this chapter, the strength of this particular argument is compromised.

John Colquhoun (now deceased) and myself are the only two people on the planet that to my knowledge, have independently shown that the concentrations of fluorine in Hastings were much higher than publicly claimed in 1953. By the passivity of New Zealand journalists, and by the refusal of experts to acknowledge these analyses and the numbers recorded, journalists and experts have allowed a lie to perpetuate.

You may also remember the New Zealand Health Department document from 1956 mentioned in Chapter 3.1, claiming

> "... administration in the water supply is a method far surpassing any other methods in safety, economy and consistency of dosage." [183]

Such a phrase is incredible when compared with the archived findings.

The Minister of Health (Mr. Ralph Hanan) was quoted in 1957 in **The Evening Post** as describing "... the [1957 Commission of Inquiry] report said the results of the Hastings experiment had been 'very, very favourable.'" [588]

6.   Relating Animal Work to Humans, Research on Humans, and a Bigger Picture of Tooth Decay

I am simultaneously appreciative of the precision and uniformity capable in experiments on rodents or other animals in laboratory conditions, and sceptical of their applicability to humans in non-laboratory conditions.

Not mentioned in the experiments cited in Chapter 1 are the molecular or anatomical differences in the biology of human and rodent teeth. If one had not studied such a topic, one would simply have to guess at the likenesses and differences between human and rodent dentition, and how relevant rodent experiments are to humans.

I have included many rodent experiments, yet for these to have any practicality to us, we need to see healthy humans. There is so little discussion that links the two groups together, though it appears molecular biology has come closer than anatomical and physiological writings that I have seen. This may be indicative of the available literature, however I have not found more of such work.

For the years I spent working on this investigation, my wonder grew – when was I going to find work discussing the relation of rodent to human dental research? I looked and looked, and came up almost empty-handed. As I looked and read through the research on deficiencies in rats' teeth I felt a gnawing tension – the relevance of my research was suffering because there was so little written on applying results to humans. What was the purpose of studying rats, if this was not it? What was the 'bigger picture' reason of creating a rat with healthy dentition? If such a thing is of only theoretical or conversational relevance to our own teeth, then why waste so much time and effort?

I have also been unable to find any discussion by experts on *defining* fluorine deficiency as a *different deficiency* in specific symptomology to deficiencies in calcium, vitamin D, and other necessities or beneficial compounds. Fluoride, so abundant, in this way becomes so solitary.

Why were the SCHER, the EFSA and the WHO not rebuked in the dental literature and corrected in media when they claimed no real fluorine deficiency existed? Perhaps this is answered by the subservient importance of the topic of a nutritional role when the answer is given in the negative – given here by groups with some clout and prestige. One may think their contradiction of expert claims on this point are painful, but if this is so it is not voiced anywhere I've seen.

A 2009 paper looking at dental evolution and the importance of oral health in structure of dentition claimed:

> "The favored animal model for such studies is the common laboratory mouse, since teeth development in mice is similar to that of man." [589]

We may recall the World Health Organization's 1970 monograph, *Fluoride and Dental Health*:

> "Where fluoride data for man are unavailable, corollary studies on experimental animals are presented." [590]

It was not until I read the 1925 McCollum experiment [55] that I read that rodent incisors grow so quick. This was not mentioned in any of the other experiments, which is unfortunate because it is probably very important.

It may have a small part to play in rodent tolerance for fluorine. The element is attracted to calcium, and finds its way into the teeth. The chewing of the rodent wears the teeth down. This attrition (meaning stress and compression) involves the loss of small tooth particles, meaning that fluorine and other components of teeth can be 'recycled' simply as a normal facet of rat growth.

Rats have an enormous tolerance to fluorine – much rodent food is between 20-60 ppm [29, 34].

I wrote to the current (2018) New Zealand Health Minister, the Right Honorable David Clark, to ask if he had any information regarding the similarities and differences between rodent and human teeth. My email was forwarded to the office of the Minister of Research, Science and Innovation. The answer was in the negative.

I wrote to the publisher of many science journals, Elsevier. I was given the email of a man who could supposedly help me. He suggested I contact a librarian regarding my research. The National Library did contatin one book on rodents which was not of much use. I have also contacted the National Academy of Sciences regarding this question of rodent vs human requirements.

I have no real issue with claims for a beneficial nature of naturally occurring levels of fluorine (often 0.05-0.1 ppm), yet I feel the element has taken much credit for the effects of other elements. Fluoride is often called a mineral, and this is true when it is bound to a cation (a positively charged ion like calcium). Yet what gets no credit in these instances is the cation – the calcium, the magnesium, the iron or other transition metal or element involved. Bear in mind there is no 'semantics' in calcium's essentiality, no need to argue over definitions here.

The reader may feel some scepticism and ambivalence toward experiments carried out decades ago; I think this is only fair. I can only say I am unaware of any studies looking at a precise, controlled use of fluorine with an emphasis on abundant amounts of other dietary factors after 1976, though there have probably been many that were not relevant to the question of essentiality. Controlling the concentration of fluorine in water is not the same as controlling the amount that goes into an experimental subject's body.

In the following chapters more recent studies are mentioned. The work of doctors Steven Levy and Johnathan Featherstone are discussed as well as historical work regarding nutrition, which will aid somewhat in understanding why the direction of our studies moves in the direction it does.

The speed at which rodents mature has been compared with humans, and differs for such parameters as sexual maturation, lifespan, protein turnover, and more [591].

Rodents have a great convenience for the scientist. Upkeep is minimal when compared with larger animals and humans. Procedures can be more invasive, leading to information unobtainable from humans, for ethical reasons. One can observe many generations of rats in a few human years. Rats are quite hardy. As early as 1931, experiments with x-rays demonstrated the ability of rats' teeth to grow, even after small doses of radiation that had initially inhibited growth by disturbance to the cells in contact with the dentin (odontoblastic layer). The growth after disruption appeared normal [592], though we must consider microscopes in those days were inferior.

There have recently been problems with applying research on rodents to humans, but this has largely focused on genetic and pharmaceutical work [593].

A recent claim is that mice are more stressed if handled by men, not women. Some have argued that this may impact results of drug use, but such things are possibly less applicable to deficiency studies [594]. I would suggest it obvious that we know more about human than rodent psychological factors that influence dental health.

A 2010 study from Johns Hopkins University in Baltimore looked at "fat rats" and the way they may distort results. The researchers suggested that rats stuck in a cage become lazy and are often overfed [595].

However in deficiency studies, the opposite is quite possibly true, at least in regard to the issue of weight gain. Of the studies from Chapter 1, McClendon's and Schwarz's rats seemed to be the sickest, probably because of nutritional or lifestyle reasons, but there is little to go on. The Wuthier and Phillips rats died after a year, but the claim of illness here was one of infection or virus.

In a 1944 study that is briefly discussed in Chapter 6.4, researchers claimed:

> "The evidence emerging as the result of much painstaking animal experimentation, despite its early promise, proved to be extremely disappointing and inconclusive. Moreover it is always difficult to evaluate the results of animal experimentation with regard to their application to the human subject in view of the differences in metabolism, in the morphology of the teeth, and in the type of lesion produced." [596]

In 1955, a study published in the ADA's journal discussed malformations of the skeleton of rats, including a shortness of the jaw which inhibited the growth of the dentition. Feeding the mother rat pig livers led to the prevention of the condition in young. This was concurrent with diets deficient in riboflavin (a vitamin B analogue). Addition of riboflavin had the same preventive effect as pig liver.

The author writes:

> "Needless to say, conclusions drawn from animal experiments should always be applied to human conditions with caution and restraint." [597]

The distilled water scientists use in the laboratory may be less applicable to humans and water fluoridation, as city drinking water goes through entirely different processes.

In the application of these experiments to humans, every city's water supply is probably different, none (or very few) of us drink distilled, or deionized water, which is what is often used in laboratory conditions. This may be another factor that renders rat experiments less than perfect.

Why, if a deficiency of this element is so difficult to prove – to the point of being near-impossible, does this element have such a beneficial effect upon teeth? When one considers the huge claims in reduction of decay – 40%, 60%, 80%, one could be very forgiving of the experts for claiming fluorine deficiencies exist, even if there was little known as to how or why such a thing could play out at a molecular level.

I have thought perhaps fluoridation's benefit occurred due to fluorine's ability to mask the symptoms of nutritional deficiencies in teeth. This may be similar to the way coffee may mask the symptoms of a weak adrenal gland – the underlying problem still exists, but we're less aware of it.

Studies that look at teeth and diet are problematic in inconvenient ways. Perhaps a tooth is going to decay and rot regardless. We may supply abundant calcium, phosphorous, fluoride and everything else we think or know to be important, and the tooth goes anyway. Experiments looking at nutrition often do so with an exclusive nature. Without looking at examinations of nerve function, blood flow, and many other things that may impact tooth health, we may inhibit our understanding.

For now, I do not have definite answers to this question that I will set in stone. One must always consider what one is *not* aware of, difficult when one is not aware of it. Expert claims of a nutritional role appear so well-justified given the supposed decay-reducing ability of the element. Yet why do we still read so much of children with terrible teeth, as we did in the 1950s, given our slowly increasing abundance of fluoride rinses, mouthwashes, toothpastes, and CWF? The following chapters will examine some possible answers.

6.1 A Logical Hypothesis Following from the Observations Made in this Investigation

"What the people want they get: making them feel a real need is the difficulty; when it is a matter of their children's well-being parents respond as they will to no other stimulus. Mix these chemical ingredients together – and the explosive compound will be known by the symbol PTA."

- Henry F. Helmholz, M.D., *Views of the National Congress of Parents and Teachers in Regard to Fluoridation*, **American Journal of Public Health**, p. 884, July, 1954 [598].

"The quality of research studies is critical."

- Dr. Ken Perrott, *Is fluoride an essential dietary mineral?* 16th June, 2013 [152].

In 1953, **Chemical Week** reported that the Surgeon General of the United States Public Health Service, Dr. Leonard Scheele, claimed:

"The epidemiological studies of fluorine in natural water supplies and artificial fluoridation have been classics."

Dr. Scheele went on to say:

"We in the Public Health Service have every reason to be proud of the work of some of our men in this field. Time will prove that this single discovery and development has been one of the great contributions to human health." [599]

In the 1954 article quoted at the start of this chapter, Henry F. Helmholz, M.D., wrote:

> "Applied in scientific studies in a number of American cities, it has been proved beyond any doubt that about 1 part in a million of fluoride added to water supplies will reduce dental caries, without any other measure, by from 50 per cent to 65 per cent." [598]

In 1956, Dr. Prothro, Public Health Director at Grand Rapids, Michigan, claimed:

> "80.7 per cent fewer children of five had dental caries after eight years of fluoridation in Grand Rapids than were found in children the same age in Muskegon, where fluoridation was not introduced until 1951." [600]

Grand Rapids was the first city in the world to be fluoridated officially. In November of 1962, Samuel L. Andelman, Chicago's Commissioner of Health, claimed:

> "No longer can anyone with a scientific background doubt the efficacy of the fluoridation of the water supply in preventing dental caries." [601]

In 1974, **The Daily News** (Port Angeles, Washington) interviewed Dr. Vincent L. Shoemaker, assistant supervisor for the dental health unit of the state Department of Social and Health Services:

> "Dr. Shoemaker said extensive research on fluoridation has shown that nothing reduces decay as much as fluoridated water."

Dr. Shoemaker spoke of the 190 letters he had received from citizens, most of which were critical:

> "'Thirty people thought fluoride was a poison, 36 said it was harmful, and 17 said it was a form of mass medication,' he said. Nothing has been as extensively researched as fluoridation, he said, and fluoride is 'definitely a nutrient.'" [602]

Since the early 1950s the experts have been strong and confident in their claims. New Zealand health professionals were no doubt swayed by the certainty of the American experts. As well as this, experts here did not want to set up animal experimentation due to cost and time factors, while the public suffered a lot of tooth decay. Experts here looked to the confident claims of Americans with trust. For this certainty to exist, the quality of studies must have been good – or *believed* to have been good.

More statements regarding such certainty are readily available at a glance toward history. I have wondered so many times over the course of this investigation why studies show so much benefit from Community Water Fluoridation (CWF), when clearly the necessity of the element fluorine has been so exaggerated, or claimed with such little acknowledgement of contradictory research.

Great confidence in these incredible ranges of benefit induces confidence in some, scepticism in others. When you're trying to find out what is true, investing exhaustive hour after hour, it can be very frustrating, so I empathize with people who end up walking away from an issue.

Perhaps the experts could argue that the exaggerations of a nutritional role were 'good lies' because they helped lead to adoption of fluoridation programs, which were of so much benefit. But if the much-used claim that fluoridation corrected a deficiency is either false, biased, or grotesquely misleading, then why does so much research conclude that this element does so much good for our teeth?

A logical hypothesis that follows from the observation that fluorine's *essentiality* has been exaggerated for decades by experts, is that the *benefits* have also been exaggerated. In conjunction with this is the hypothesis that the benefits or necessities of other elements involved in dental health have been somewhat downplayed. This chapter will focus on the first part of this theory. The impact of other elements is discussed in more detail in subsequent chapters.

The word exaggeration is an understatement. Consider that this bias is almost *total* – the only public deviations still manage to make fluorine appear necessary in some way, or that we're missing out on it [158, 178]. Much evidence demonstrates that the opposite is true, so if the experts were really interested in being accurate about this topic of a nutritional role for fluoride, we'd *at least* see some deviation and disagreement, with some experts citing literature claiming a non-essential role, instead of this public uniformity.

On the Ministry of Health webpage *Effective and Safe*, the University of York's Report that was published in 2000 is quoted as suggesting just under 40% less tooth decay (figure calculated by Sapere Research Group) [603].

It is no wonder people get put off this issue. Ben Goldacre's book that looked at science and journalism, *I Think You'll Find it's a Bit More Complicated Than That*, claimed the York Review suggested 15% more caries-free children in fluoridated areas,

"… but the studies generally couldn't exclude other explanations for the variance." [604]

These are obviously two different categories of measurement – *total tooth decay* and *caries-free children* in a town or city. One can find a bigger or smaller percentage depending upon which measurements are taken, and this can sometimes be a little confusing.

Turning to a 2007 article authored by Trevor Sheldon[121], K. K. Cheng[122] and Iain Chalmers[123], we find the claim of a 15% increase in children without decay:

"Estimates of the increase in the proportion of children without caries in fluoridated areas versus nonfluoridated areas varied (median 15%, interquartile range 5% to 22%). These estimates could be biased, however, because potential confounders were poorly adjusted for.[124]" [605]

Such a sentence about poor adjustment for confounding factors can be compared with the 1953 statement of Dr. Scheele quoted earlier. Sheldon chaired the advisory board of the York Review [606].

The report from Sirs Gluckman and Skegg called the York Review inclusion criteria of studies "stringent" but did not go into detail [607].

Of 3,246 studies available, only 254 met the York Review's inclusion criteria. A commentary of the York Review authored by 6 of the 10 authors of the review claimed the following, with regard to the studies on CWF:

"The difference in the number of children found to be caries free in fluoridated and non-fluoridated areas ranged from -5.0% to 64% with a median of 14.6% in the 19 included analyses."

---

[121] Professor and pro-vice chancellor, Health Services Research, University of York.
[122] Professor of epidemiology, Public Health Building, University of Birmingham.
[123] Editor, James Lind Library, Oxford.
[124] The York Review [606] is cited here by Sheldon *et. al.*

"The most serious defect of these studies was the lack of appropriate analysis. Many studies did not present an analysis at all, while others only carried out simple analyses without attempting to control for potentially confounding factors. While some of these studies were conducted in the 1940s and 50s, prior to the common use of such analyses, studies conducted much later also failed to use methods that were commonplace at the time of the study." [608]

In 2013, Dr. Felicity Dumble from Waikato, New Zealand, claimed a 10% reduction in dental caries from fluoridation [609]. She probably meant *at least* 10%.

In 1997, the Lord Mayor of Brisbane, Australia, organized a taskforce to appraise evidence on fluoridation. Some of the statements of the taskforce are appropriate here:

"It was recognised that computerised databases such as Medline do not cover all the scientific literature, e.g. some studies published in non-English languages were not included. The literature in these databases may also be subject to a degree of professional bias." (page 12)

"Broad agreement was reached by the two sides of the debate on the following aspects:

• there have been large reductions in dental caries in both fluoridated and unfluoridated communities in the developed world since the 1960s;

• many early fluoridation research studies had flawed methodologies and their findings have proved to be unreliable;

• factors other than fluoride (water or other sources) have contributed to the decline (Dr Clutterbuck[125] favoured changes in diet, general health, and immunity as contributing factors, while Dr Walsh[126] referred to an increase in anti-bacterial agents).

Dr Clutterbuck and Dr Walsh disagreed on the extent of the benefits from water fluoridation - Dr Clutterbuck agreed with Prof Diesendorf[127] (Chapter 7 refers) that the benefits were marginal, had been exaggerated by the pro-fluoridationists... Dr Walsh acknowledged that the absolute benefits of fluoridation, in terms of numbers of teeth saved, had declined in recent decades but still considered that the benefits were significant, particularly for adults." (page 30)

"It is widely acknowledged that the quality of studies from about 1980 onwards has been better than earlier studies[128]." (page 35)

"even if current caries data did exist, it would be extremely difficult to separately identify benefits attributable to water fluoridation alone;"

"the skewed nature of the distribution of dental caries (e.g. 23% of children have 72% of the dental decay problem - Appendix 6, p9) meant that statistical averages of reductions can be misleading." (page 36)

"The Taskforce recognised that there were differences in the quality of statistical recording between [Australian] states, and that dental statistics were not specifically intended to be used to make comparisons between fluoridated and unfluoridated areas." (page 44)

---

[125] Dr. Fred Clutterbuck, Australian College of Nutrition and Environmental Medicine.
[126] Dr. Laurence Walsh, School of Dentistry, University of Queensland, Australia.
[127] Diesendorf's work was his famous paper *The Mystery of Declining Tooth Decay*, published in **Nature**, Vol. 322, 10th July, 1986.
[128] Here the taskforce cites Public Health Commission, *Water Fluoridation in New Zealand*, 1994.

"Taskforce members were generally agreed that the literature showed that many fluoridation studies prior to 1980 had employed unsound methodologies or had omitted relevant factors. More recent studies had employed more rigorous and defensible methods." (page 46)

"A number of Taskforce members considered that the use of percentages to record the effectiveness of water fluoridation was misleading, in the light of relatively low and declining levels of decay. The majority of the Taskforce found it surprising that the concern about the lack of research in Australia expressed in the 1991 NHMRC Report 21 (Section 8), and the call for an effective monitoring and research program in relation to Australia's water fluoridation policy, appeared to have gone largely unheeded." (page 47) [610]

Compare the claim of Dr. Scheele regarding the quality of early studies with the claim of "flawed methodologies" in this Australian document.

The Cochrane Collaboration is one group of experts who have claimed to be more neutral than others. However, their reviews look at studies others have performed so while Cochrane may be less biased or closer to unbiased, the work they look at may be biased. The *about us* page on the Cochrane website claims:

"We do not accept commercial or conflicted funding. This is vital for us to generate authoritative and reliable information, working freely, unconstrained by commercial and financial interests." [611]

To quote from Cochrane's 2015 review of 20 studies regarding the benefits of CWF and 135 studies on dental fluorosis:

"Other, more recent studies comparing fluoridated and non-fluoridated communities have been conducted. We excluded them from our review because they did not carry out initial surveys of tooth decay levels around the time fluoridation started so were unable to evaluate changes in those levels since then."

"Our review found that water fluoridation is effective at reducing levels of tooth decay among children. The introduction of water fluoridation resulted in children having 35% fewer decayed, missing and filled baby teeth and 26% fewer decayed, missing and filled permanent teeth. We also found that fluoridation led to a 15% increase in children with no decay in their baby teeth and a 14% increase in children with no decay in their permanent teeth. These results are based predominantly on old studies and may not be applicable today.

"Within the 'before and after' studies we were looking for, we did not find any on the benefits of fluoridated water for adults.

"We found insufficient information about the effects of stopping water fluoridation.

"We found insufficient information to determine whether fluoridation reduces differences in tooth decay levels between children from poorer and more affluent backgrounds.

"We assessed each study for the quality of the methods used and how thoroughly the results were reported. We had concerns about the methods used, or the reporting of the results, in the vast majority (97%) of the studies. For example, many did not take full account of all the factors that could affect children's risk of tooth decay or dental fluorosis. There was also substantial variation between the results of the studies, many of which took place before the introduction of fluoride toothpaste. This makes it difficult to be confident of the size of the effects of water fluoridation on tooth decay or the numbers of people likely to have dental fluorosis at different levels of fluoride in the water.

"There is very little contemporary evidence, meeting the review's inclusion criteria, that has evaluated the effectiveness of water fluoridation for the prevention of caries.

"The available data come predominantly from studies conducted prior to 1975, and indicate that water fluoridation is effective at reducing caries levels in both deciduous and permanent dentition in children. Our confidence in the size of the effect estimates is limited by the observational nature of the study designs, the high risk of bias within the studies and, importantly, the applicability of the evidence to current lifestyles." [612]

Critiques of the review can be found online [613]. Relevant here is the "high risk of bias" regarding benefit, which has been demonstrated in the appraisal of a nutritional role in public.

The following does not appear immediately relevant to CWF, but of concern to all interested in evidence-based medicine. On the 13th of September 2018, Cochrane fired one of its founders, Peter Gøtzsche. I write this as events unfold. Four other members resigned in solidarity. Legal details are not in the public domain [614].

One critique of Cochrane's 2015 work on fluoridation was published in the **British Dental Journal** [615]. It acknowledged the words of the American Academy of Pediatrics, which was that the Cochrane review had excluded 97% of the evidence.

In 1991, the Australian National Health and Medical Research Council discussed the issues surrounding studies that observe differences in human populations when a change in only one variable is desired.

"In principle, this approach should entail the random allocation of communities, from among two or more other equivalent communities, to receive either fluoridated drinking water (the 'intervention') or non-fluoridated water (the 'control'). The phrase 'otherwise equivalent' refers to similarity in other factors (that is, potential confounding factors) that affect the occurrence, the detection or the reporting of dental caries."

"In practice, the quality of the early intervention trials was generally poor, when judged against the above ideal. Random allocation was usually not possible and the choice of 'control' populations was often inadequate; insufficient baseline data were recorded to allow for adjustment between compared populations; there was a lack of 'blinding' of observers in the recording of dental health outcomes; and detailed and critical statistical analyses were often lacking."

To have said such things in the 1950s would possibly have meant professional suicide or public ridicule. Compare these statements with the Surgeon General's, quoted at the beginning of this chapter.

"It is relevant to note that such departures from idealized experimental design are commonplace in epidemiological research into the efficacy of preventive intervention. The limitations and deficiencies in research design and implementation reflect the social, political, and ethical realities of the circumstances in which the public health intervention is introduced. While this does not make for high-grade science and unambiguous results, the problem is not peculiar to research in relation to water fluoridation. Because of these research limitations and shortcomings, it is necessary to examine critically the totality of evidence available and to proceed cautiously in the drawing of inferences." [616]

Grand Rapids, Michigan, was the first city to ever be officially fluoridated. Regarding the Grand Rapids and Muskegon trial, the NHMRC claimed that deficiencies in the study became "apparent from the reported findings after ten years." Here they cite Arnold, Dean, Jay and Knutson's 1956 study [617].

The NHMRC discussed their issues with the trial:

"... there were some marked differences in the number of children examined from year to year. In some years, only a very small number of children were examined (for example, 3 children aged 16 in Grand Rapids during 1946)[129] with the consequences that the estimated mean DMFT[130] must be regarded as very unreliable. This is also reflected in some irregular fluctuations in the overall rate of caries decline in Grand Rapids. For example, in some periods, it is apparent that the sampling procedure resulted in findings of biologically implausible DMFT rates. In 1946 the 10-year-old DMFT in Grand Rapids was 3.70 (based on 109 examinations) but in 1947 the 11-year-old DMFT was 3.56 (based on 18 examinations). The 11-year-olds should be representative of the same group (or birth cohort) of children who, one year earlier, were aged 10. Since it is impossible to experience a real reduction in the DMFT index (which is cumulative in nature), it is clear that the observed reduction from 3.70 to 3.56 represents some form of error." [616]

The above may be one factor in explaining the attitudes regarding exclusion of public opinion in CWF [310-313] (see Chapter 5.4). I have thought that the reduction in DMFT from 3.70 to 3.56 may have occurred due to a different set of children being observed. Whether such a thing is acceptable in statistics is beyond my knowledge. If the children were the same, the implication here is that caries have healed, regrown, regenerated. If this were true, then poor people from fluoridated areas would consistently have less tooth decay than rich people who drink fluoride-free water. Yet the poor consistently have worse teeth than the rich [618].

Therefore I think a far more realistic explanation for the drop in DMFT here is that the caries were not counted.

After this small critique, the NHMRC wrote:

"However the Working Group considers that there is consistency in the full series of findings from the Grand Rapids – Muskegon trial."

Such a statement will elicit differences of opinion in many, as will the observation of 3.7 to 3.56 (which can be confirmed by looking at the study by Arnold *et al.* [617]). If the experts were willing to use what we might call "impossible data" once, then they may have used *near*-impossible data on other occasions. I have not set my own opinion in stone based on what is presented here. I am not the only one who is sceptical of the incredible claims attributed to the addition of this element alone. It seems to have superseded the need for elements that are *definitely* essential, like calcium. Do not think I am refusing to accept that fluorine may be of benefit in certain circumstances.

There is one more fascinating piece of information regarding this Australian document. I wrote to the NHMRC for a copy of the document after seeing it cited in other work, and I received a reply with the 2017 report attached. The Water Team of the NHMRC told me:

"The National Health and Medical Research Council (NHMRC) advises on water fluoridation and human health. Please find attached NHMRC's *Public Statement 2017: Water Fluoridation and Human Health in Australia (2017 Public Statement)*, which contains NHMRC's recommendation on community water fluoridation, and a range within which NHMRC supports Australian states and territories fluoridating their drinking water supplies. More information is available on the NHMRC website here - https://www.nhmrc.gov.au/health-topics/health-effects-water-fluoridation.

---

[129] Only one 16-year-old was examined in non-fluoridated Muskegon in 1946 [617].
[130] DMFT: Number of decayed, missing or filled teeth per individual.

> "In regards to your question about the '1991 fluoridation document,' previous versions of NHMRC's water fluoridation advice have been rescinded and are now no longer available to the public.
>
> "I hope you find this information helpful." [619]

I interloaned a copy from Otago University. I asked the NHMRC why the 1991 document was rescinded, no reply was forthcoming.

The Lord Mayor of Brisbane's taskforce was organized in January of 1997, and reported to the Mayor in October. The 17 members of the taskforce (excluding the Lord Mayor and officials) were from a variety of backgrounds and affiliations. At the start of the project, 9 members were confirmed as 'committed' because they had expressed strong views, or their views were known because of their professional affiliation. The other 8 were classified 'uncommitted' because their position was unknown at first. Surveys were taken at the project's initiation, which showed a total of 10 members in support, 5 opposed and 2 uncertain.

> "Of those 8 Taskforce members regarded as 'uncommitted' at the start of the Taskforce process, 3 members had changed from 'strongly support' to 'oppose', while 1 member changed from 'uncertain' to 'oppose'. Another member switched from 'uncertain' to 'support' for fluoridation."

The following is one reason of many given for the people who changed their opinion from 'strongly support' or 'uncertain' to 'oppose':

> "reference was made to the apparent manipulation of statistics by the pro-fluoride side to support its case." (page 81) [610]

One wonders if the arguments used in the letters of Dr. Herschel Horowitz and Dr. Howard Greene mentioned in Chapter 5.7 that were applied to the cereal experiment published in 1974 could also be applied to some of the CWF experiments. Obviously I am impressed by the concerted efforts of public health officials to address issues. Yet I think the lack of focus on diet and dietary history of many generations, and the fact that fluorine in water is the only monitored factor, slightly casual. It may appear similar to "cherry-picking" to some people. I have not seen mentioned if calcium and magnesium intake, both necessary in enamel formation, are constant throughout CWF experiments, or constant in city drinking water.

The impact of more knowledge in nutrition, hygiene and sanitation has not lifted the dental health of all (see the article at the end of this chapter. 'Confounding factors' are not considered if the only thing we do is measure the fluorine concentration of the water supply and count teeth, and holes in them.

The following is taken from a newspaper in 1954:

> "**Progress of System**: Mr. [J. Llewellyn] Saunders [Director of Dental Hygiene, New Zealand Department of Health] said that as a result of the use of school dental nurses, toothache, broken-down teeth and septic mouths, which were commonly seen [sic] among children 30 years ago, were unheard of to-day. In 1921, the first year of operation of the dental nurse system, 114 teeth were extracted for every 100 filled. As the service was extended this figure had steadily dropped to 6.3 in 1946 and had remained at that low level ever since." [620]

CWF began in New Zealand in the early 1950s. The article noted that "for some years now school dental nurses had been applying fluoride solution to the teeth of their patients." It did not say how many years. I believe the government increased the amount of milk drunk by children in the early 1940s (Muriel Bell's idea, though some American dentists in the 1940s were also claiming it to be an important source of calcium and vitamins).

This lessening of decay from WWI to the 1940s was no doubt the end result of one or many 'confounding factors'. Yet we can empathize with the experts in their excitement about CWF. Consider the article quoted here and the dates it discusses with Muriel Bell's 1944 claim in **The Listener** that in New Zealand the amount of fillings in teeth, and the number of false teeth were

"probably greater than anywhere else in the world." [191]

Even if such a statement was an exaggeration – and I'm not saying it was – we can still understand and appreciate the concern. The experts were excited about fluoridation, and the American researchers they knew, trusted and looked up to were claiming huge benefits. Perhaps this can be understood in light of the end of WWII with the USA not only demonstrating their superior technology in the form of the atom bomb, but coming to the aid of New Zealand's allies.

In late July of 1955, Colonel Fuller wrote a confidential letter to the New Zealand Dental Association (**Figure 91**) in which he claimed the equipment at Hastings had been working perfectly "for the last six months", giving less variation than what the USA experiments allowed, a margin of 0.2 ppm above or below 1.0 ppm. He also claimed that Dr. Ludwig would re-perform the baseline examinations of children's teeth, because:

"... he could not calibrate his dental examinations alongside those of Dr. Hewat. Accordingly the base line examinations of Hastings and Napier children have been completely re-done by Mr. Ludwig whose standard is in line with that used in fluoridation studies in the U.S.A. These base line re-examinations were completed towards the end of June." [621]

In his paper on Hastings published in a 1958 issue of the **New Zealand Dental Journal**, Ludwig wrote:

"Commencing immediately on the author's arrival in New Zealand, baseline dental examinations of 1,869 children were carried out in Hastings between September and November, 1954." [555]

I am uncertain if this is good practice in statistics, but it is noteworthy to see that Fuller did not want the public to know about it. Over sixteen months, only twelve months' supply of fluorine was used in Hastings in 1953-1954, yet results were, according to experts, excellent. The claim was made on a televised debate in 2008 [446] that the Hastings trial was one of the best, with about an eighty percent reduction in decay, by lay fluoridation supporter Mark Miller and Dr. Dorothy Boyd, Specialist in Children's Dentistry and Senior Public Health Dentist of the Otago District Health Board. Yet if less than the desired amount of fluoride was used, it may be possible that some of the alleged benefit was caused simply by confirmation bias or a change in criteria for what constituted decay, or some other reason. From what was admitted by Mr. Fish shown in Chapter 5.8, it appears that the desired amount was only below throughout the first year, yet an analysis by Ludwig suggests a small percentage of readings below 0.76 ppm even as late as 1956 (**Figure 92**).

PROSTHETIC DENTISTRY EXCLUSIVELY

TELEPHONE 40-707

J. FERRIS FULLER, B.D.S., F.D.S.R.C.S. (EDIN.)
DENTAL SURGEON
KELVIN CHAMBERS 16 THE TERRACE
WELLINGTON, C.1

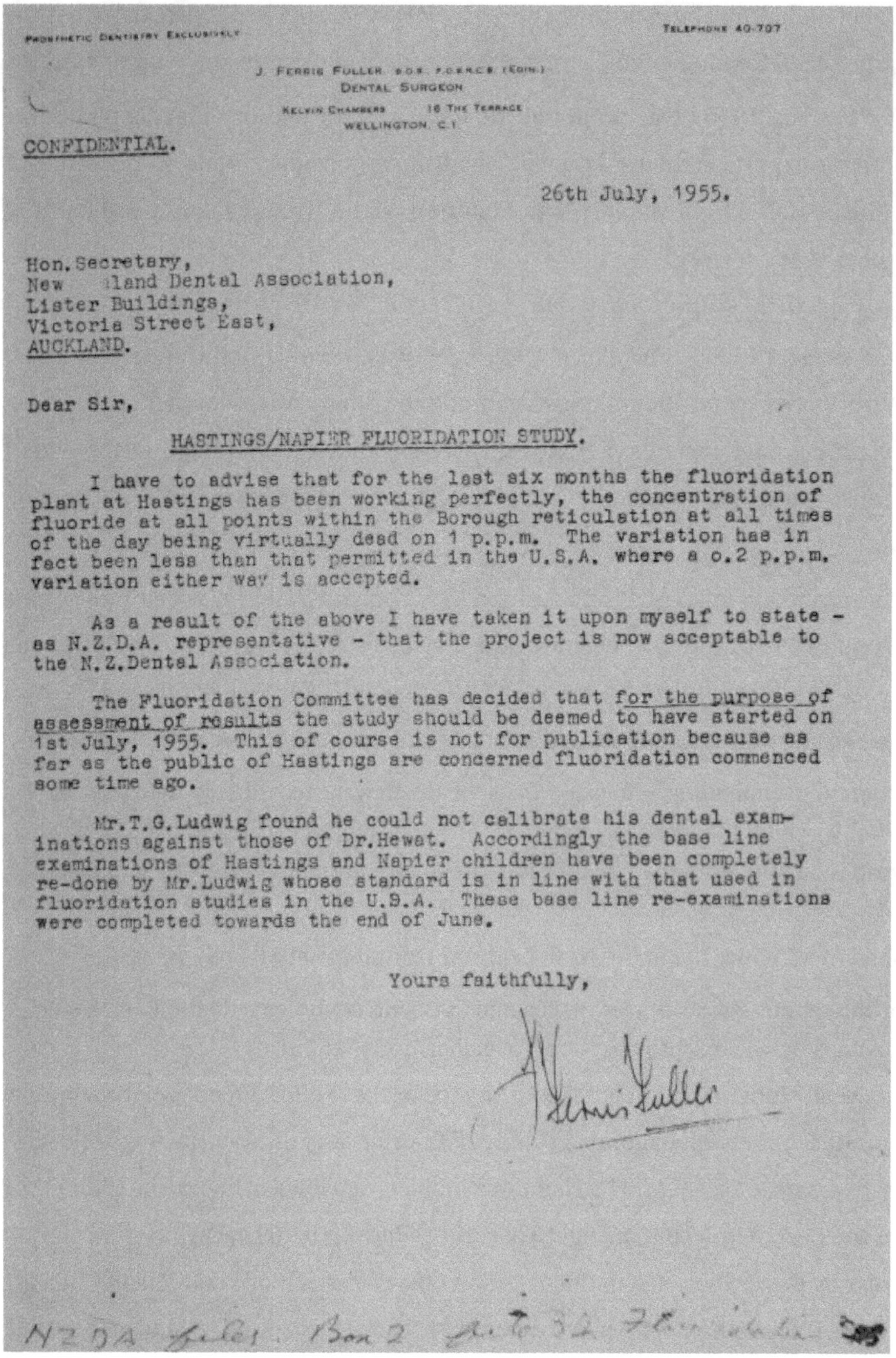

CONFIDENTIAL.

26th July, 1955.

Hon. Secretary,
New Zealand Dental Association,
Lister Buildings,
Victoria Street East,
AUCKLAND.

Dear Sir,

HASTINGS/NAPIER FLUORIDATION STUDY.

I have to advise that for the last six months the fluoridation plant at Hastings has been working perfectly, the concentration of fluoride at all points within the Borough reticulation at all times of the day being virtually dead on 1 p.p.m. The variation has in fact been less than that permitted in the U.S.A. where a o.2 p.p.m. variation either way is accepted.

As a result of the above I have taken it upon myself to state - as N.Z.D.A. representative - that the project is now acceptable to the N.Z.Dental Association.

The Fluoridation Committee has decided that for the purpose of assessment of results the study should be deemed to have started on 1st July, 1955. This of course is not for publication because as far as the public of Hastings are concerned fluoridation commenced some time ago.

Mr.T.G.Ludwig found he could not calibrate his dental examinations against those of Dr.Hewat. Accordingly the base line examinations of Hastings and Napier children have been completely re-done by Mr.Ludwig whose standard is in line with that used in fluoridation studies in the U.S.A. These base line re-examinations were completed towards the end of June.

Yours faithfully,

J. Ferris Fuller

NZDA files. Box 2 File 34 Fluoridation

Figure 91. Letter from Fuller, Hastings/Napier Fluoridation Study, 26.7.1955. *Source: John Colquhoun MS-Papers-6670-81 Department of Health Research Papers, available at the National Library, Wellington, New Zealand. Marked "NZDA files. Box 2. File 34 Fluoridation." [621]*

TABLE 2

FLUORIDE CONTENT OF WATER - ANALYSES AT HASTINGS
(LIQUID FEED EQUIPMENT)

Fluoride Content	Oct. 54 - Dec. 54		Jan. 55 - Dec. 55		Jan. 56 - Dec. 56		Jan. 57 - Dec. 57		Jan. 58 - June 58		Oct. 54 - June 58	
	No. of Analyses	Per Cent of Total	No. of Analyses	Per Cent of Total	No. of Analyses	Per Cent of Total	No. of Analyses	Per Cent of Total	No. of Analyses	Per Cent of Total	No. of Analyses	Per Cent of Total
0.00-0.50	3	5.17	1	0.42	-	-	-	-	-	-	4	0.48
0.51-0.75	5	8.62	7	2.97	7	4.19	1	0.36	2	1.94	22	2.62
0.76-0.89	2	3.45	15	6.36	3	1.80	-	-	25	24.27	45	5.34
0.90-1.10	43	74.14	169	71.61	130	77.84	224	80.58	68	66.03	634	75.29
1.11+	5	8.62	44	18.64	27	16.17	53	19.06	8	7.76	137	16.27
Totals	58	100.00	236	100.00	167	100.00	278	100.00	103	100.00	842	100.00

Figure 92. Fluoride Content of Water, Analyses of Hastings, Liquid Feed Equipment, October 1954 to June, 1958.
Source: John Colquhoun MS-Papers-6670-81 Dept. of Health Research Papers available at the National Library, Wellington, New Zealand.

Ludwig claimed:

> "The solution feeder has operated continuously since September, 1954, so that children examined in 1957 have been exposed to a continuous optimal level of 1 ppm of fluoride for 27 to 30 months *longer* than the children examined in 1954." [555] (His emphasis.)

His data are shown here. A small percentage of readings were still below 0.76 ppm. The possibility of exaggeration regarding this one experiment is potentially thwarted by the accuracy of later readings.

In 1997, the Lord Mayor of Brisbane's task force claimed:

> "World War 2 triggered a greater interest in dental health in Australia and elsewhere because of the large number of potential recruits who were found to be unfit for service because of their level of dental decay. The post war rationale for water fluoridation in Australia rested on the poor dental health of Australian children, where an average 12-year-old [sic] might have a decayed, missing or filled tooth (DMF index) for every year of his/her life, i.e. as many as 10 – 12 affected teeth at age 12." (page 17) [610]

A year after Dr. Scheele, the U.S. Surgeon General claimed the early studies were regarded as "classics", the **American Journal of Public Health** published a study funded by the Sugar Research Foundation. The study was performed by a dentist and a doctor from the Department of Pediatrics, College of Medicine, and the Department of Pedodontics, College of Dentistry, at the State University of Iowa. Doctors Boyd and Wessels looked at progression of dental caries in selected individuals. This study pointed to the "variability of caries progression from individual to individual" as well as changes in the mouths of subjects. Relevant here are their points on examiner variation:

> "Even criteria for the diagnosis of dental caries are inconstant. There may be widespread disagreement among examining dentists as to whether or not a specific dental lesion is carious."

> "Serial examinations of the same tooth, even though made by the same examiner at different times, may result in different interpretations from one examination to another as to whether a break in the continuity of the enamel represents the early stage of a cavity or whether it is a developmental defect. When a series of examiners is used and each employs his own criterion of judgment and technique of examination, the results for the total caries score for a given mouth may differ by as much as 100 per cent.[131] In serial examinations, cavities once described may disappear from record, due to a change in interpretation."

Boyd and Wessels claimed most examiners had made no distinction between incipient (beginning) cavities and those that are unmistakable.

> "Consideration of affected tooth surfaces or of individual caries lesions is more reliable as an estimate of caries progression than is the limitation of attention to the number of affected teeth."

Boyd and Wessels suggest "serial study of specific teeth" may yield less interpretative errors. They claimed:

> "When it is possible to express results clearly and individually for respective teeth, this seems a better statistical approach than to lose identity of teeth or even of subjects through the merging of data in terms of group averages." [622]

The Grand Rapids study is still cited in the literature as a successful demonstration of CWF. One example is a 2005 article on the history of CWF in the **British Dental Journal**:

> "The early studies reported reductions in decay experience of the order of 50% or more. That was at a time when fluoridated water offered the only significant source of fluoride." [623]

---

[131] Here the authors cite Dunning, J. M. *Variability in Dental Caries Experience and its Implication upon Sample Size.* **Journal of Dental Research** 29:541 (Aug.), 1950.

Such a statement is laughable when compared with statements regarding food fluoride levels (found in Chapter 4) made by supporters of CWF. Nothing is quoted by those opposed.

A group of researchers from the Department of Nutrition at the University of East Anglia, Norwich, examined studies from January 1990 to March 2011 to find Dietary Reference Values for fluoride, for the European Food Safety Authority. They concluded that many studies suffered from a high risk of bias:

> "Few studies were identified which met the study inclusion criteria and the majority were assessed as being at high risk of bias. Overall, there was a lack of high quality evidence upon which DRVs may potentially be based for fluoride. However, data was suggestive of a protective role for fluoride in the reduction of dental caries." [624]

In 2012, Professor Murray Thomson, Otago University head of dental public health, was quoted in Wellington's **Dominion Post** as saying the following:

> "'Parents' lack of education, the inability to access dental services, no fluoridation in water, and poor tooth brushing contributed to bad oral health,' he said. 'It's just another marker of poverty really.'"

You will note calcium, phosphorous and other nutritional factors are not mentioned; it is assumed that everybody has enough of them – though perhaps this comes under "parents' lack of education". I should say it is quite normal in New Zealand to respect parents' freedom in nutritional choices for children, though recently some discussion has centred on the fact that unhealthy food is cheaper than healthy food. The article then discussed dental examinations and the District Health Board. Professor Thomson did not speak specifically on the subject of Porirua, a town near Wellington which has been the focus of much discussion regarding health. Quoting the article:

> "A Pacific health advocate in Porirua said the shake-up of services did not go far enough to reverse the 'horrendous' oral health rates.
>
> 'I think there needs to be more integration with the community about how to improve these rates,' Utulei Anitpas said.
>
> 'There will be no children in Porirua with any lower teeth soon, the way it's going.'" [625]

Porirua has been fluoridated since 1965 [626].

This was not mentioned in the article. It is quite a relevant piece of information.

6.2 An Optimal Level?

"This is, therefore, a beneficial physiological effect of fluoride which merits unquestionable authority and acceptance."

> - Dr. Frank McClure, *Water Fluoridation: The Search and the Victory*, p. 111, 1970.

"Although fluoride should probably be regarded as essential, there is no evidence so far from human studies that overt clinical signs of fluoride deficiency exist. No specifically diagnostic clinical or biochemical parameters have

been related to fluoride inadequacy. The Expert Consultation was therefore unable to specify a minimum desirable intake. However, in view of the toxicity associated with excessive fluoride ingestion from a variety of sources, recommendations for maximum safe intakes are required. For this purpose, dental mottling may be taken as a definitive indication of toxicity."

- World Health Organization, *Trace Elements in Human Nutrition and Health*, p. 192, 1996 [105].

"... the same range of fluoride intakes is associated both with reductions in dental caries and fluorosis."

- National Academy of Sciences, **Guiding Principles for Developing DRIs Based on Chronic Disease**, p. 284, 2017. DRIs are Dietary Reference Intakes.

This chapter will begin with a study from the 1960s and move chronologically forward to very recent work. Some of the statements in this chapter will be discussed a little more in Chapter 6.5.

It occurred to me that when experts discuss deficiencies of fluorine, they may perhaps mean a sub-optimal amount. "Sub-optimal" and "deficient" sound similar enough to not matter at a casual glance, yet deficiency states of nutrients are not described as "sub-optimal", they are simply referred to as what they are – deficient. Therefore I think the terms used *do* matter, assuming a scientific discussion should be precise.

I have not found any real discussion on this, though some may exist. The experts seem to be more interested in changing the definition of nutritional essentiality and applying this to fluorine – yet experts are certainly not conscientious in letting the public, or even researchers, know the definition has changed. That they do this quietly in their own works instead of communicating defined parameters that distinguish between their own ideas and standard biochemistry, is an interesting testimony to a self-justifying or group mentality. That the majority involved have good intentions and concern for the most vulnerable helps protect such imprecise communication from criticism.

Given a presupposed benefit from ingesting fluorine, the 'optimal' intake refers to the amount of fluorine that can aid in strengthening enamel without causing the disfiguration of dental fluorosis to a visibly unpleasant degree. What constitutes unpleasant is decided upon by CWF-supporting experts, not the public (discussed in Chapter 6.5). For decades, the optimal level of fluorine in water was thought to be 1.0 part per million, within the range of 0.8-1.2 ppm.

Note that this is the 'optimal level in water' not the 'optimal level in a body or tooth'.

In 1967, the **Journal of Postgraduate Medicine** published a study by Dr. Jean Mayer and Dr. Mark Hegsted of Harvard University [627]. I did not discover this study until mid-2018, when I had nearly finished writing the first draft of this book. Had I found it earlier, I would have included it earlier. There is of course the possibility that it was mentioned in some of the research cited in Chapters 1 or 2, but if this is the case, I did not see it.

Some will argue that the age of this work makes it less relevant, but it is the only study I have ever seen that has positively claimed a deficiency role for fluorine in humans. To my knowledge, it has never been verified.

This study began by discussing an abstract of a paper[132] that looked at levels of osteoporosis in Framingham, Massachussetts, compared with two Texas communities. In Texas the fluoride concentration was about 8 ppm in the water, in Massachussetts, 0.4 ppm.

Mayer and Hegsted believed the Leone study (see footnote) required confirming with populations that were similar; they claimed Texas and Massachussetts were too different to warrant a definite conclusion. They picked "small towns in farming areas" of North Dakota. They obtained over 1,000 x-rays from adults over 45 years of age. Medical and dietary histories were obtained. A radiologist who was ignorant of the areas of subject origin interpreted the x-rays.

Relative bone density decreased with age, as expected. In the low-fluoride (0.15-0.3 ppm) areas, the percentage of women with low bone density were: 45-54 years, 22%; 55-64 years old, 64%, over 65 years old, 85%. Women in high-fluoride (4-6 ppm) areas had half these rates of low bone density. There were larger differences in the percentage of women with collapsed vertebrae, which Mayer and Hegsted called "a more objective measure of osteoporosis than evaluation of bone density". Of the women over 65, 34% of the low-fluoride area, and only 10% of the high-fluoride area were affected. Mayer and Hegsted claimed that calcification of the aorta was between 2 and 3 times as prevalent in low-fluoride areas.

"Limited data were obtained on the consumption of milk and cheese."
But no differences were found between those who claimed to eat, or not eat, these two foods. They did suggest the disease was caused by a calcium deficiency, as calcium resorption was, in their eyes, compromised.

"The subjects must be in a negative calcium balance."
This means the bone is losing more mass than it is forming. It is typical among the elderly. Mayer and Hegsted wrote:

> "Certain limitations of the study are evident. The subjects were not a random sample of the population, the dietary information was inadequate, and the evaluation of bone density was subjective. Other important differences in these populations may also bear on the problem. Until such differences have more experimental support, however, it seems reasonable to conclude that fluoride deficiency is an important etiologic factor in the development of osteoporosis." (page A-51)

These limitations may explain why I did not find this study until I had almost finished writing this book. I had not seen it mentioned in any of the research I had looked through regarding an essential or nutritional role, though perhaps it had been mentioned in sections on bone that I in my exclusive approach, did not investigate.

Mayer and Hegsted discussed two other researchers who had looked into calcium retention and deficiency, and pointed to the temporary nature of calcium retention in treatments. The study that found increased retention

---

[132] N. C. Leone, C. A. Stevenson, B. Besse, L. E. Hawes, and T. R. Dawber, *The effects of the absorption of fluoride II. A radiological investigation of five hundred and forty-six human residents of an area in which the drinking water contained only a minute trace of fluoride.* **AMA Archives of Industrial Health**, 21: 326, 1960.

found little radiographic evidence of bone remineralization[133]. The other found no help from fluoride in calcium retention[134]. This study, according to Mayer and Hegsted:

"re-emphasized the probability that much of the calcium balance data is not trustworthy."

A third study[135] discussed was

"unable to demonstrate any significant relationship between the calcium intake, as revealed by dietary history, and the extent of osteoporosis."

Regarding method, they suggested epidemiological studies were possibly more useful in discerning etiologies (causes, beginnings of disease) than metabolic studies. They claimed dietary histories could be misleading without precision, a fair point.

"A rather difficult problem will be posed if the fluoride requirement for the prevention of osteoporosis in adults is substantially higher than that required for the prevention of dental caries."

"The data available to date appear to warrant the conclusion that fluoride is the most important etiologic factor in osteoporosis."

This study may explain where Dr. Fredrick Stare got the claim he made in **Nation's Business** (a publication of the USA Chamber of Commerce) in 1967:

"... I think that fluoride deficiency, lack of fluoride, is probably the most prevalent nutritional deficiency in this country. We know fluoride has something to do with lessening tooth decay. We know it has something to do with preventing and it can be useful in treating osteoporosis, a decalcification of the bones. And we think it may have something to do with preventing hardening of the arteries."[136] [628]

Dr. Stare also told New Zealanders through **The Evening Post** (Wellington) in 1967 that

"the mineral nutrient called fluoride not only lessens tooth decay but also lessens the development of a condition of the aged called osteoporosis." [198]

Mayer and Hegsted concluded:

"Considering the estimates of the number of adults in our aging population with severe demineralization and assuming, according to the data from North Dakota, that appropriate intakes of fluoride can cut this number in half, fluoride deficiency is probably the primary nutritional deficiency in the United States. If one includes any estimate of the benefit derived from fluoride in preventing dental caries, there is no doubt of the truth of this statement." [627]

This study has been cited by three subsequent articles, one of which was published in the Journal of the American Dental Association in 1968. Funded by the bureau of medicine and surgery, U.S. Navy. Robert Van Reen, Ph.D., began by discussing the importance of parathyroid hormone (PTH) in calcium metabolism. He

---

[133] B. E. C. Nordin, *Calcium balance and calcium requirement in spinal osteoporosis*, **American Journal of Clinical Nutrition**, 10: 384, 1962.

[134] G. A. Rose, *The study of osteoporosis and osteomalacia*, **Postgraduate Medicine**, 40: 158, 1964.

[135] R. W. Smith and B. Frame, *Concurrent axial and appendicular osteoporosis: its relation to calcium consumption*, **New England Journal of Medicine**, 273: 73, 1965.

[136] Ten years later, in 1977, the 4th Edition of Underwood's *Trace Elements in Human and Animal Nutrition* would claim that between 5 and 64% of infants were found to have iron deficiency (page 36). Regarding adults, Underwood wrote that "Iron deficiency is probably the most prevalent deficiency state affecting human populations today."

discussed radiographs of the lateral lumbar area of women from high- and low-fluoride areas, concluding that women in low-fluoride areas had more osteoporosis[137] (high and low were not specified in concentration in Van Reen's paper). Van Reen claimed that work was encouraging regarding the use of sodium fluoride in osteoporosis treatment. He mentioned the Mayer and Hegsted study only once, in the final sentence of his paper:

"A recent review of the relationship of fluoride deficiency and osteoporosis was made by Hegsted." [629]

The other two studies that cited Mayer and Hegsted's work do not appear related to a nutritional role for fluorine[138].

I wrote to Harvard University and the journal that published the paper to ask if there was much feedback from readers, from other scientists or anything else relevant to the study. It seemed very strange that I had seen so little of it. I received an email from the Office of the Dean at Harvard, which claimed that my request had been forwarded to a faculty member. This person was unaware of anything specifically related to the 1967 study, but did quote a few paragraphs from question 16 of the 1999 edition of *Fluoride Facts* authored by the American Dental Association. I do not have this document but I have quoted what was sent to me in the email. Citations were included in the original communication and are included here. I have not altered or edited the words in any way.

> "The second major area of study regarding fluoride and bone health is the role of fluoride in strengthening bone and preventing fractures. For nearly 30 years, fluoride, primarily in the form of slow-release sodium fluoride, has been used as an experimental therapy to treat osteoporosis, a condition characterized by a reduction in the amount of bone mass. Individuals with osteoporosis may suffer bone fractures as a result of what would be considered minimal trauma. Sodium fluoride therapy has been used in individuals in an effort to reduce further bone loss, or add to existing bone mass and prevent further fractures [630]."

> "The results of the clinical trials have been mixed as noted in the two following studies. The need for further research is indicated."

> "In 1995, the final report of a four year study was published demonstrating the ability of fluoride to aid in an increase in bone mass[139].

> "The study examined females with post-menopausal osteoporosis who took slow-release sodium fluoride (25 mg twice a day) and calcium citrate (400 mg twice a day) for four years in repeated 14 month cycles (12 months receiving treatment and 2 months not receiving treatment). The study concluded this treatment was safe and effective in reducing the number of new spinal fractures and adding new bone mass to the spine." (Citing Pak *et al.* here, see footnote.)

---

[137] D. S. Bernstein, and P. Cohen, *Use of Sodium Fluoride in the Treatment of Osteoporosis*, **Journal of Clinical Endocrinology**, 27: 197, 1967.

[138] W.H. Allaway. 1968. *Agronomic Controls Over the Environmental Cycling of Trace Elements*. **Advances in Agronomy**, pages 235-274. Richard F. Mattingly, Wei Y. Huang. (1969) *Steroidogenesis of the menopausal and postmenopausal ovary*. **American Journal of Obstetrics and Gynecology** 103:5, pages 679-693.

[139] Pak CY, Sakhaee K, Adams-Huet B, Piziak V, Peterson RD, Poindexter JR. *Treatment of postmenopausal osteoporosis with slow-release sodium fluoride: final report of a randomized controlled trial*. **Ann Intern Med** 1995;123(6):401-8.

> "In a six year clinical trial in 50 postmenopausal women, treatment with sodium fluoride and supplemental calcium was not effective in the treatment of osteoporosis[140]." [631]

Searching Harvard's library for "Hegsted 1967" resulted in one hit: the Jean Mayer papers, 1953-1975. Thirteen boxes of Mayer's work exist, Mark Hegsted and Fredrick Stare are listed as subjects.

> "Mayer corresponded regularly with a variety of scientists and researchers, including D. Mark Hegsted, the United States Army, the World Health Organization, and the Monsanto Corporation, as well as from private individuals seeking advice or medical assistance with issues of diet or weight control. The remainder of the records reflect Mayer's work as a Professor in the Department of Nutrition at the Harvard School of Public Health, his involvement with professional associations, and his international consulting work, including the 1969 White House Conference on Food, Nutrition, and Health." [632]

They are not available online.

Perhaps it can be argued that Dr. Stare and Dr. Mayer in the 1970s were differing in their conclusions regarding a nutritional role for fluorine because of their own research done at Harvard. This would mean they were "cherry-picking" or playing favourites with research because they had still not publicly discussed research others had, but this is partially forgiveable – who better to discuss Mayer, Hegsted and Stare's research than Mayer, Hegsted and Stare? The media publicized their work a lot. In their syndicated columns they capitalized on the rodent experiments that concluded fluorine essential, and ignored those experiments that concluded otherwise.

There are many factors involved in structurally weak bone. A 2014 textbook on nutrition claims that a deficiency that takes 30 years to show symptoms is a deficiency nonetheless, and no less important in rectifying than a deficiency that is obvious in infancy. Vitamin C and copper help in the cross-linking of collagen fibrils that are necessary for structurally strong bone. Zinc has been shown important as an enzyme catalyst, an "integral part of proteins and nucleic acids", and a requirement in cell proliferation.

Nonprimate animals have shown skeletal deformities from manganese and magnesium deficiency. Vitamins D and K are also important in calcium absorption and bone proteins respectively. Calcium and phosphorous are extremely important in bone maturation and osteoblast (bone cell) mineralization [633].

> "Fluoride supplementation, either in short- or long-acting forms, is not approved by the US Food and Drug Administration for the prevention or treatment of osteoporosis. [634]

We can see an interesting aspect on the topic of fluorine's essentiality in this textbook. This is especially relevant when we consider statements like "all the experts agree". Let's imagine we're biased toward a conclusion of non-essentiality. So let's turn to page 766:

> "Fluorine has not been proved an essential element for humans, but it has a role in bone mineralization and hardening of tooth enamel. Areas with low fluorine content in the water supply have high rates of dental caries. Fluoridation of the water or use of supplemented tooth paste is associated with a significant fall in dental caries rates." [635]

---

[140] Riggs BL, O'Fallon WM, Lane A, Hodgson SF, Wahner HW, Muhs J, Chao E, Melton LJ III. *Clinical trial of fluoride therapy in postmenopausal osteoporotic women: extended observations and additional analysis.* **J Bone and Min Res** 1994;9(2):265-75.

Now let's imagine we're biased toward a claim of essentiality. In this case we look within the chapter on Nutrition and Dental Medicine, page 1019, and point to the table of *Nutrient Deficiencies on Tooth Development*, where fluoride is listed due to its function regarding stability of enamel crystal (formation of enamel), inhibition of demineralization, stimulation of remineralization, and inhibition of bacterial growth. This table also pointed to mottling as an effect of excess [636].

From this table, nutrients necessary for the building of teeth are listed: Protein has roles in tooth size, eruption time, enamel insolubility and salivary gland function. Vitamin A influences epithelial tissue, tooth morphogenesis, odontoblast (tooth cell) differentiation; deficiencies lead to enamel hypoplasia (underdevelopment). Vitamin D, calcium and phosphorous are necessary for tooth integrity, eruption patterns, and plasma calcium. Ascorbic acid deficiency leads to dental pulp and dentin changes, odontoblast degeneration, though deficiency is not claimed to result in caries (but no human data were available). Iodine deficiency is claimed to delay tooth eruption, alter growth patterns, and lead to malocclusion, but is not implicated in caries directly. Iron deficiency leads to slow growth, loss of tooth integrity, and salivary gland dysfunction (but no human data were available) [636].

Regarding malocclusion and caries, there has been at least one suggestion of a link in adolescents [637].

This 2014 textbook did not include fluorine in the "trace elements" section. The introduction to that section begins:

> "Elements ingested in milligrams or less per day are referred to as trace elements[141]. Chemists originally used the term trace to indicate that concentrations were lower than the detectable limits of the analytic procedure in some of their samples. Statistical analysis cannot use words, so the practice was changed by replacing 'trace' with an estimated number, often the midpoint between [sic] the lowest detectable limit and zero." [638]

I should add that just because a *textbook* is written recently, this does not mean the studies used to write it have been carried out recently. There is no doubt in my mind that fluorine can be beneficial. About twenty-five years ago here in Wellington, nuclear scientists examined the distribution of fluorine and calcium in teeth. Nuclear scientist Dr. Graeme Coote worked with scientists from the Dental Research Unit. They found fluoride levels in the outer enamel of New Zealanders' teeth have barely changed over the years.

> "Significantly, they discovered that in a decayed part of a tooth, fluoride moves in to form a more stable mineral structure. It appears that the tiny amount of fluoride in mouth saliva – whether from fluoridated water, toothpaste or natural sources – is critical to repair the decay." [639]

It's great that fluorine has a role in helping our teeth, regardless of where it is from. If calcium was important, it was not mentioned in the article beyond the sentence claiming Dr. Coote examined its distribution.

Dental fluorosis or 'mottling' is characterized by chalky white spots on tooth enamel. It is classified according to various levels, from the barely visible to the extremely dark. It creates a hypomineralization of tooth enamel, which initially makes teeth harder, yet as teeth become more fluorosed, they become softer. The experts

---

[141] Here the authors cite the textbook by O'Dell and Sunde [89].

ultimately want to balance the maximal preventive ability of teeth with a cosmetically acceptable level of fluorosis.

In 2002, the WHO claimed:

> "Based upon the studies conducted by Dean and colleagues five decades ago, the 'optimum' level of fluoride in drinking-water, associated with the maximum level of dental caries protection and minimum level of dental fluorosis, was considered to be approximately 1 mg/litre."

> "In human fluorotic teeth, the most prominent feature is a hypomineralization of the enamel. In contrast to many animal species, fluoride-induced enamel hypoplasia (indicating severe fluoride disturbance of enamel matrix production) seems to be rare in fluorosed human enamel. The staining and pitting of fluorosed dental enamel are both posteruptive phenomena (i.e., acquired after tooth eruption and occur as a consequence of the enamel hypomineralization). The incorporation of excessive amounts of fluoride into enamel is believed to interfere with its normal maturation, as a result of alterations in the rheologic[142] structure of the enamel matrix and/or effects on cellular metabolic processes associated with normal enamel development[143]."

> "Unlike skeletal fluorosis, which is considered to be a marker of long-term exposure to fluoride (due to the ongoing process of bone remodelling), dental fluorosis is considered to be indicative of the level of exposure to fluoride only during the period of enamel formation." [640]

In 1995, an article in the **Journal of the American Dental Association** by Dr. Steven Levy, Professor and Graduate Program Director at the Department of Preventive and Community Dentistry at the University of Iowa; along with four colleagues, made an interesting claim about the recommended "optimal" intake:

> "Some children had estimated fluoride intake from water, supplements and dentifrice that exceeded the recommended 'optimal' intake (a level that has yet to be determined scientifically)."

> "The optimal level of fluoride intake has never been determined scientifically and has been used only in general terms." [641]

In the 1999 paper discussed below, Levy and Chowdhury claimed the optimal level was derived empirically – meaning through observation and experience, as opposed to reasoning and calculation under stricter laboratory conditions.

In 1997, the Brisbane Lord Mayor's Taskforce claimed:

> "There are no definitive limits in the scientific literature concerning safe and unsafe doses of fluoride. Responses can vary considerably between individuals depending on a range of factors, including age, body weight, nutritional status, etc." (page 42) [610]

Statements like these are quite fascinating when compared to the certainty with which the experts have consistently spoken, when they discuss the optimal amount. Statements regarding the certainty of the experts are given here.

---

[142] Rheology: "science dealing with the flow and formation of matter", Oxford Illustrated Dictionary, 1962.
[143] Three papers are cited here: WHO Technical Report Series 846; T. Aoba, *The effect of fluoride on apatite structure and growth*, **Crit Rev Oral Biol Med**, 8: 136–153, 1997; and G. M. Whitford, *Determinants and mechanisms of enamel fluorosis*, **Ciba Found Symp**, 205: 226–245, 1997.

The November, 1962 issue of the **Journal of the American Dental Association** quotes the 1957 Commission of Inquiry from New Zealand:

> "Fluoride is beneficial in proper amounts and the optimal level in drinking water can be established with certainty." [642]

Consider this statement with regard not only to the inability of the Hastings experiment during 1953 and 1954 to actually *attain* the 'optimal' level (thought then to be 1 ppm) consistently, but also the multitude of problems Dr. Arnold wrote to the Health Department about regarding the Hastings experiment (his letter shown in Chapter 5.8).

The same 1962 article quotes many people and commissions. All agree on the safety and effectiveness of CWF. Toxicologist Robert Kehoe claimed:

> "The evidence as a whole is consistent. It offers assurance that bringing the fluoride concentration in communal supplies to that level known to be optimal for dental health is an effective preventive public health measure which has an ample margin of safety." [643]

Note "... that level known to be optimal...". The word "known" here is not indecisive.

Dr. David Ast[144], D.D.S., M.P.H., and Bernadette Fitzgerald[145], B.A., authored a paper in 1962 in which they claimed:

> "The evidence today is overwhelming that ingested water fluoride at the optimum concentration during the years of tooth development will definitely reduce the incidence of dental caries." (page 587) [408]

This issue also contained a paper on the Aurora-Rockford, Illinois study, which claimed in the summary:

> "The prevalence and severity of periodontal disease, of oral hygiene status and dental caries experience were compared for young adults who were lifetime residents in a city supplying water containing an optimal concentration of naturally occurring fluoride and in a fluoride-deficient city." (page 620) [409]

(This paper also suggested a link between osteoporosis and low-fluoride areas, citing the same Leone study that Hegsted and Mayer cited.) Note that in these studies the word 'optimal' is used decisively. Compare this with the words of Dr. Muhler in 1970:

> "It is also possible that our present state of knowledge concerning optimal levels and essential functions may be quite inadequate, and with additional investigations it might well be demonstrated that the microquantities normally present in most commonly eaten mixed diets and water supplies are not fully 'adequate'." [102]

Dr. Muhler was voicing the possibility that people needed more fluoride. The only other reference relevant from the 1995 Levy *et al.* study was an offhand comment regarding the complexities involved with determining the appropriateness of fluoride supplementation for children. The authors remarked that one of the factors was

> "... the role of systemic fluoride understood to be less important than previously believed..." [641]

---

144 Director at the Bureau of Dental Health, New York State Dept. of Health, Albany.
145 Senior Biostatician, Division of Special Helath Services, New York State Dept. of Health, Albany.

Such a phrase is fascinating again from the perspective of expertise – the experts in the earlier years of fluoridation were not uncertain at all, and as can be demonstrated by multiple examples in media, seriously concerned with fluorine deficiency (see Appendix 1).

Levy *et al.* pointed to a paper that was at the time awaiting publication in the **Journal of Public Health Dentistry**, that addressed the issue of an 'optimal' level [644].

This 1999 paper, also co-authored by Levy, is concerned with problems of a non-optimal amount. Levy and Chowdhury write of the 12,300 ppm fluoride gels used by dentists:

> "... unclear whether they influence fluorosis risk." (page 218) [644]

Such information is useful for parents and caregivers. Since the beginning of fluoridation, the experts have claimed certainty. Yet one can see the experts quoted here are looking at the amount in water. This has been a consistent point of contention. The few times this topic is aired, the people opposed to CWF point to the fact that the experts have never fronted up with an actual demonstration of fluorine deficiency ensuring all other nutritional bases are covered. From the expert point of view, the benefit attributable to CWF is enough to warrant fluorine's place next to calcium and vitamin D and so on. A "calcium deficiency" refers to an insufficient amount of calcium in one's body, and can be confirmed in repeated experimental demonstrations. A "fluoride deficiency" refers to the amount in soil, in water, etc, *not* to the amount in one's body.

Talk of an 'optimal' amount had always seemed to be independent of fluorine's status as a nutrient. There is a reason for this; it is that traditionally, 'optimal' referred to the concentration in water, not in a body or tooth. The 1999 paper by Levy and Chowdhury attempted to ascertain an optimal intake based on a total daily intake.

Levy and Chowdhury looked at work done previously that suggested daily fluoride intake in children should not exceed 0.1 milligram per kilogram (mg/kg) of body weight daily. They also suggested 0.05-0.07 mg/kg of body weight as an 'optimal intake', based on much of the work they investigated. They commented that there was insufficient evidence regarding 'optimal' levels of intake.

> "Because detailed data are not available from comprehensive, individual studies concerning the distribution of total fluoride intake from multiple sources, determination with any precision of the relative proportional contribution from each of these sources on a population basis is very difficult." (page 221) [645]

In the 1995 study Levy and his team suggest manufacturers of juices, bottled waters, soft drinks and infant formula be made to label the fluoride levels of their products:

> "Practitioners should estimate fluoride ingestion from all these sources if considering systemic fluoride supplementation." [641]

Levy and Chowdhury's 1999 paper suggested that

> "... if current recommended 'optimal' levels, which have been derived on an empirical basis, are actually lower than what has been quoted in the literature, then more children could be ingesting excessive amounts of fluoride, which could increase their risk of developing objectionable dental fluorosis. The variation and complexity of fluoride ingestion from all sources should be considered in the evaluation of recommendations for use of dietary fluoride supplements." [644]

J. Moorhouse, a general practitioner from England, wrote a letter to the **British Dental Journal** claiming that due to the small window of possibility that a child has of developing dental fluorosis, children should receive no supplements before 26 months of age.

"It is therefore essential that a child receives no fluoride supplement at all before 26 months with the exception of a carefully controlled optimum dose via the water supply." [646]

Unfortunately, Dr. Moorhouse did not tell readers exactly how much an optimum dose was, but we can tentatively assume one of the Levy studies would be relevant.

In 2016, the WHO stated:

"It is important that fluoride exposure be known and health administrators be made aware of exposure before the introduction of any fluoridation or supplementation programmes for prevention and dental caries." [211]

The Cochrane review briefly mentioned in the previous chapter, claimed (after looking at 135 studies on dental fluorosis):

"Overall, the results of the studies reviewed suggest that, where the fluoride level in water is 0.7 ppm, there is a chance of around 12% of people having dental fluorosis that may cause concern about how their teeth look.

"There is a significant association between dental fluorosis (of aesthetic concern or all levels of dental fluorosis) and fluoride level. The evidence is limited due to high risk of bias within the studies and substantial between-study variation." [612]

Regarding fluoride toothpaste, the Cochrane Collaboration carried out another investigation on 25 studies:

"There is weak unreliable evidence that starting the use of fluoride toothpaste in children under 12 months of age may be associated with an increased risk of fluorosis. The evidence for its use between the age of 12 and 24 months is equivocal. If the risk of fluorosis is of concern, the fluoride level of toothpaste for young children (under 6 years of age) is recommended to be lower than 1000 parts per million (ppm)."

"More evidence with low risk of bias is needed." [647]

Looking in my local supermarket in Wellington, the toothpastes contain between 1,000 to 1,450 ppm fluoride.

In 2000, the **Journal of the American Dental Association** published an article by Dr. John M. B. Featherstone, M.SC., Ph.D. The article was the cover story of the July issue. Dr. Featherstone began his article by stating that dental caries is a "bacterially based disease" and that prevention of caries involves a balance between protective and pathological factors. He gave an explanation of how fluoride interacts with calcium and phosphorous to create a less soluble enamel.

"Only when fluoride is concentrated into a new crystal surface during remineralization is it sufficient to beneficially alter enamel solubility. The fluoride incorporated developmentally – that is, systemically into the normal tooth mineral – is insufficient to have a measurable effect on acid solubility[146]." (page 890)

"Fluoride incorporated during tooth development is insufficient to play a significant role in caries protection. Fluoride is needed regularly throughout life to protect teeth against caries." (page 891) [648]

---

[146] Two studies are cited here by Dr. Featherstone: ten Cate JM, Featherstone JD. *Mechanistic aspects of the interactions between fluoride and dental enamel.* **Crit Rev Oral Biol Med** 1991;2(3):283-96. And Fejerskov O, Thylstrup A, Larsen MJ. *Rational use of fluorides in caries prevention. A concept based on possible cariostatic mechanisms.* **Acta Odont Scand** 1981;39(4):241-9.

Featherstone claims fluorine in teeth attract calcium in saliva, this brings in phosphorous from the saliva, which leads to a "veneer" on the teeth of approximately 30,000 ppm fluoride. It is compositionally between hydroxyapatite and fluorapatite. He discussed the "weak, pre-eruptive effects" of fluoride. This refers to the use of fluoride supplements for pregnant women, which supposedly help form healthy teeth in children, though as you can see there are conflicting beliefs around this.

In December of 2000, a letter was published rebuking Dr. Featherstone's words regarding the lack of ability of fluoride to have a pre-eruptive effect on teeth.

Quoting Dr. Glenn's letter:

> "Scandinavia's small countries are admirably advanced in many areas but they are officially antifluoridationist, as are the Netherlands and most of England. Their legislated antifluoridation proved increasingly embarrassing to their dentists, especially at International Association of Dental Research meetings."

> "In this country [the USA], there is no money to be made in fluoridation, and F supplements are not patentable, but there are billions to be made from proprietary posteruptives. The torrent of money from that industry is now driving our academic dental research centers."

No evidence was given on this statement, but one is reminded of Jennifer Washburn's work [261]. The next sentence in Dr. Glenn's letter:

> "With Hersch Horowitz retired, and National Institute of Dental and Craniofacial Research declaring premature victory over caries and turning fluoride policy over to the Centers for Disease Control and Prevention almost a decade ago, there may be no one left who can keep F, officially recognized as an essential nutrient for 32 years, from being turned into just a topical agent."

Regarding "nutritional fluoride", Dr. Glenn claimed:

> "Here, there is cause for optimism as the Food and Nutrition Board in November 1999 published in final form its new dietary reference intakes for mineralized tissue nutrients. Fluoride garners 35 pages as an essential nutrient, with recommendations as the minimum for adequate intakes, or AI, of 0.05mg/kg/day for infants and children over six months and 3 mg/day for women, including during pregnancy. Men's AI is 4 mg/day. Adult upper limit, or UL, is 10 mg/day (Standing Committee on the Scientific Evaluation of Dietary Reference Intakes, Food and Nutrition Board, Institute of Medicine. Dietary Reference Intakes for Calcium, Phosphorus, Magnesium, Vitamin D, and Fluoride. Washington, D.C.: National Academy Press; 1999)." [649]

I believe Dr. Glenn has mistakenly attributed this publication to the wrong year, as a document with this name was released in 1997, discussed in chapter 2.1 [71].

In 2017, the NAS released their **Guiding Principles for Developing DRIs Based on Chronic Disease**, which listed the DRI-related documents. This confirmed that 1997 was the only year such a document had been produced, though there is a chance that Dr. Glenn was referring to an update or press release that I am unaware of, dated November, 1999.

This document claimed that "Upper Limits have been identified for some essential nutrients" and included fluoride in the list. An explanation was given a few pages later. Regarding "indicator review and selection" the NAS used various indicators which may "reflect a desirable or undesirable outcome" – examples given were tissue saturation or high blood pressure. Indicators may also demonstrate functional outcomes related to a chronic disease or a "physiological effect". The example given here is "dental caries are a clinical outcome, where risk is increased by inadequate fluoride intake". I reiterate that no fluorine deficiency had been demonstrated in humans [105, 116, 119], not discussed here by the NAS who claimed:

> "chronic disease endpoints have been used as the indicator to establish a Dietary Reference Intake (DRI) for six nutrients: calcium, fluoride, potassium, sodium, total fiber, and vitamin D. AIs were set for fluoride, potassium, sodium, and total fiber, and Estimated Average Requirements (EARs) were set for calcium and vitamin D." [650]

A table is given titled "Current DRIs Linked to Chronic Disease and/or Surrogate Endpoints" in which fluoride's reference value is AI. The footnote attached here reads:

> "An EAR could not be established for any of these nutrients due to inadequate data. SOURCES: IOM, 1997, 2002/2005, 2005, 2011."

In the table, the indicator is given as "prevention of dental caries", the "biomarker of Nutrient Adequacy" is given as "fluoride balance", and the "Surrogate Endpoint" is "bone mineral content".

Regarding the Upper Limit (UL) the NAS claims:

> "UL for infants and children ages 0-8 years is based on risk of enamel fluorosis (two studies from 1937 and 1942)."

The age of these studies is incredible. They were both performed before Community Water Fluoridation officially began. The "biomarker of Nutrient Adequacy" is "Enamel fluorosis". [650]

It appears that the NAS had not moved on from the 2008 report, in which Dr. Miller suggested that AIs were,

> "developed primarily as 'placeholders' because no other data were available to allow a recommendation to be made." [95]

The 2008 report is cited consistently in the 2017 document. Consider the World Health Organization's 1996 claim with regard to the term 'Adequate Intake':

> "No specifically diagnostic clinical or biochemical parameters have been related to fluoride inadequacy." [105]

In Appendix B, the NAS inform readers:

> "The relation between the risk of dental caries and fluoride intake appears to have an inflection point and a critical value for statistically detectable risk reduction (dental caries prevention), but the range of intakes associated with benefit overlaps with the range of intakes associated with harm (fluorosis)[147]." [650] (page 281)

In 2010, Peter Cressey, a researcher from the Department of Environmental Health in Auckland, carried out an investigation of dietary fluoride and fluorosis levels in Auckland. Cressey prepared infant formula according to manufacturers' specifications with optimally fluoridated water. Mean content was 0.069 mg/L. A 'stochastic' or random model was used to estimate distribution patterns. He claimed:

---

[147] Here, the NAS cite the 1997 document discussed [71].

"At water fluoride concentrations of 0.7 and 1.0 mg/L the UL would be exceeded 30 and 93 percent of the time, respectively." [651]

Regarding the 'optimal' amount of fluorine, it is easy to confuse *dosage* with *concentration*. For instance, Dr. John Dodes, D.D.S., claimed in an interview in 2011:

"Fluoride given at the proper dosage which is one part per million..." [652]

A *concentration* is an amount of a substance in a medium, for instance part per million is a concentration. One part per million fluorine in water means one fluorine ion for every 999,999 water molecules. Suggesting that a person use water fluoridated at a specific part per million does not tell us how much of that water this person is drinking, therefore we have no idea how many fluorine ions this person has as their intake. Part per million refers to an amount *in solution* not an amount given to a person. A *dose* is an amount given to a person. For instance a tablet with one milligram of fluorine is a *dose*. The amount of fluorine relative to what else may be *in this hypothetical tablet* is a *concentration*.

On this note, consider the words of the New Zealand Health Department document from 1956 mentioned in Chapter 3.1, claiming

"... administration in the water supply is a method far surpassing any other methods in safety, economy and consistency of dosage." [183]

On the 6th of June, 2015, the American Academy of Pediatrics updated their webpage healthychildren.org regarding the amount of fluorine appropriate for babies:

"Babies should not receive fluoride supplementation during the first six months of life, whether they are breastfed or formula-fed. After that time, breastfed and formula-fed infants need appropriate fluoride supplementation if local drinking water contains less than 0.3 parts per million (ppm) of fluoride." [653]

In 2015, a group of experts from the American Dental Association announced proudly that 0.7 ppm was no doubt the optimal amount of fluorine in a water supply:

"The American Dental Association (ADA) today commended the Department of Health and Human Services (HHS) for announcing the final recommendation for the optimal level of fluoride in community water systems. The recommended ratio of fluoride to water, newly calibrated at 0.7 parts per million, results from years of scientifically rigorous analysis of the amount of fluoride people receive from all sources." [654]

In New Zealand, the Ministry of Health adjusts fluoridated water supplies to between 0.7 and 1.0 ppm [558].

Simply eliminating the detrimental from our diet is not enough to jolt us back to good health. Restoring the beneficial that has been absent must also take place. Realistically, this may take generations. Are the soils where we grow our food rich in minerals? Are the animals we keep and eat as healthy as we ourselves want to be? Evolutionary science suggests we come from nature, how far from nature does refining, freezing, packaging, fumigating, irradiating, transporting and the like take our foods from biological compatibility?

A far more sensible study than attempting to ascertain potential harm from the individual aspects of our food industries might be "who had the healthiest, happiest children, and what did *they* do?"

6.3 The Possibility of Perfection

"Trifles make perfection. But perfection is no trifle."

- Michaelangelo.

"Although no race may be said to be absolutely immune to dental caries, yet in some races – namely, the Esquimaux and the Maori – it is so extremely rare, compared with the enormously high incidence amongst European races, that a practical immunity may with reason be claimed."

- Dr. Henry Pickerill, M.D., Ch.B., M.D.S., L.D.S., Professor of Dentistry and Director of the Dental School of the University of Otago, New Zealand, *The Prevention of Dental Caries and Oral Sepsis*, 2nd Edition, p. 309, 1914.

"In an examination of 260 Maori skulls – all from an uncivilized age – I found carious teeth present in only two skulls, or 0.76 per cent."

- Dr. Henry Pickerill, *The Prevention of Dental Caries and Oral Sepsis*, p. 11, 1914.

"Since the discovery of New Zealand the primitive natives, the Maori, have had the reputation of having the finest teeth and finest bodies of any race in the world. Only about one tooth per thousand teeth had been attacked by tooth decay before they came under the influence of the white man."

- Dr. Weston Price, *Nutrition and Physical Degeneration*, 6th Edition, p. 207, 1998 (first published in 1939).

"The rapid degeneration of the Australian Aborigines after the adoption of the government's modern foods provides a demonstration that should be infinitely more convincing than animal experimentation."

- Dr. Weston Price, *Nutrition and Physical Degeneration*, 6th Edition, p. 182, 1998.

This investigation has focused on fluorine's role in teeth and nutrition, and while such a study is fascinating for many reasons, the more practical question of how an individual or population may obtain and maintain excellent dental health has not been addressed from a picture incorporating many variables.

In asking "is this element or compound beneficial or essential for teeth?" we exclude many other elements and compounds. From the perspective of wanting to prevent tooth decay, it is more sensible to ask "who had or has the best teeth in the world, and what did they do nutritionally?"

This question is limiting in scope as well, for it excludes the rest of the body, mind and social order. Yet it is a sensible step toward a bigger picture.

I must advise that sometimes different measurements of data are used. One is the percentage of total individuals with dental caries in a community. Another is the number of carious teeth per mouth. A third is percentage of total teeth in a community. These differing measurements do not make a significant difference to the principles expressed, but they are something to be aware of.

In the 1930s, a dentist by the name of Weston Price travelled the world, and looked at teeth belonging to many tribes and societies in many different countries. His work took him to every continent. He examined the foods the inhabitants ate and the way they lived. Dr. Price was in a position to observe what occurred when isolated tribes, for centuries untouched by technology or modernized refined foods, began integration with the Caucasians, who *did* use refined foods, foregoing natural methods of preparation.

He found a consistent pattern: after the cessation of natural, often wildly grown foods and the introduction of refined foods like white flour, sugar, margarine and canned foods, changes in health took place among isolated peoples. Children were born with not enough room in their mouth for all their teeth, and their teeth decayed quickly. Children who ate refined and processed foods, and children born to parents who ate these foods, had many of the same cranial deformities as the Caucasians – cleft palate (incomplete roof of mouth formation), harelip, torus palatinus (sunken roof of the mouth), narrowed nasal passages, occlusion (teeth growing in front of each other) and impaction (teeth pushing into each other). As well as these basic skeletal and dental problems, there were others: degenerative disease occurred more frequently, as well as mental problems such as delinquency, mental retardation, and insanity. If only one parent switched to refined foods before conception, these problems still occurred.

One African tribe spent six months providing excellent nutrition for couples preparing to conceive a child. After couples married they were given the most precious and rare foods by the rest of the tribe to ensure the health of their children [655].

Within one generation of the switch from traditional diets to refined foods, these problems went from being the exception to being the norm. Females conceived by a parent eating refined foods found much more difficultly in giving birth when they matured, due to a narrowing of the pelvic structures caused by the consequences of malnutrition. Dr. Price wrote:

> "One of the most important developments to come out of these investigations of primitive races is the evidence of a rapid decline in maternal reproductive efficiency after an abandonment of the native foods and the substitution of foods of modern civilization." [656]

These problems and deformities that were the exception in societies that obeyed fundamental principles of nutrition, became the norm when these cultures ceased the dietary practices that had been their tradition for hundreds, sometimes thousands of years.

Dr. Price's work is meticulously documented in his book *Nutrition and Physical Degeneration*. The Price-Pottenger Foundation, named after Dr. Price and Dr. Francis Pottenger, keeps the work of Dr. Price relevant to the modern world [657].

All of the theories in the world are useless to us beyond academic interest if they do not produce results.

Here I will outline some of Dr. Price's observations regarding native New Zealanders (Māori) and Indigenous Australians. I recommend his work to the aspiring parent, or the sincere student of nutrition.

Dr. Price quotes Dr. Pickerill of New Zealand's Otago University. Pickerill had authored a book called *The Prevention of Dental Caries and Oral Sepsis* [658].

> "By taking the average of Mummery's[148] and my own investigations, the incidence of caries in the Maori is found to be 1.2 per cent in a total of 326 skulls. This is lower even than the Esquimaux, and shows the Maori to have been *the* most immune race to caries, for which statistics are available."

> "Comparing these figures with those applicable to the present time, we find that the descendants of the Britons and Anglo-Saxons are afflicted with dental caries to the extent of 86 per cent to 98 per cent; and after examining fifty Maori school children living under European conditions entirely, I found that 95 per cent of them had decayed teeth." [658] (p. 201)

Compare this with rates claimed in 1976 by Dr. Jean Mayer (see Chapter 5.2) published in the **New York Times**: 98% of American children had tooth decay, and about half the population of America had no teeth by age 55. Their source:

> "... in the 1960s, a U.S. Government agency compared the results of more than 100 international surveys of the prevalence of tooth decay in different populations. Except for the fluoride content of the water supply, the consumption of sugar was the only consistent relationship between nutrition and tooth decay." [659]

In this column Dr. Mayer was opposing sugar; with regard to current (1976) research, he wrote:

> "... not only are excessive caloric intakes undesirable but where the calories come from is important."

He was commenting on the food industry's use of terms like "the body's need for sugar" which helped the industry justify selling high-sugar cereals to children.

Some people are very black and white in their thinking, and when they hear about Weston Price's work they think it is claiming that *all* indigenous people in the world had near-perfect teeth and health until they began consuming refined foods. This is *not* what Weston Price concluded, and I would encourage the sincere reader to investigate slowly and with patience. Even those that Price and others claimed to have the best teeth, the Māori, still had small amounts of decay and other health problems.

Price confined his investigation to the North Island of New Zealand. In comparing Māori, he wrote:

> "Detailed examinations including measurements and photographic records were made in twenty-two groups consisting chiefly of the older children in public schools. In the examination of 535 individuals in these twenty-two school districts their 15,332 teeth revealed that 3,420 had been attacked by dental caries or 22.3 per cent. In the most modernized groups 31 to 50 per cent had dental caries. In the most isolated group only 2 per cent of the teeth had been attacked by dental caries." [660]

In many modernized groups living with Caucasians and eating the refined, canned, processed food, Price placed the amount of dental arch deformity at between 40 and 100%. He said many of the older Māori who had grown up on traditional foods retained perfectly formed facial structures, yet their children "showed a much higher percentage of deformed dental arches." [660]

---

[148] Dentist and Microscopy enthusiast Dr. John Howard Mummery, author of *The Microscopic Anatomy of Teeth*, 1919. Mummery held the office of President of the British Dental Association and of the Sixth International Dental Congress in London in 1914.

In the Pukerora Tubercular Sanatorium forty native Māori lived; they were mostly young men and women. They ate the modernized foods given to them by the colonists.

"Their modernization was demonstrated not only by the high incidence of dental caries but also by the fact that 90 per cent of the adults and 100 per cent of the children had abnormalities of the dental arches." [661]

Similar findings were seen at Hukarera College for Māori girls in Napier. The Māori living on the Mahia Peninsula however, had stayed eating an abundance of sea foods and native, or traditional Māori foods. One group of children,

"... had only 1.7 per cent of their teeth attacked by dental caries." [661]

Price claimed that consistently, while on their traditional foods, Māori had mouths with enough room for all thirty-two adult teeth, and the absence of dental deformities such as overcrowding, impaction and occlusion. Here, we can see four Māori faces, that Price described as "typical" (**Figure 93** – Price's Figure 69).

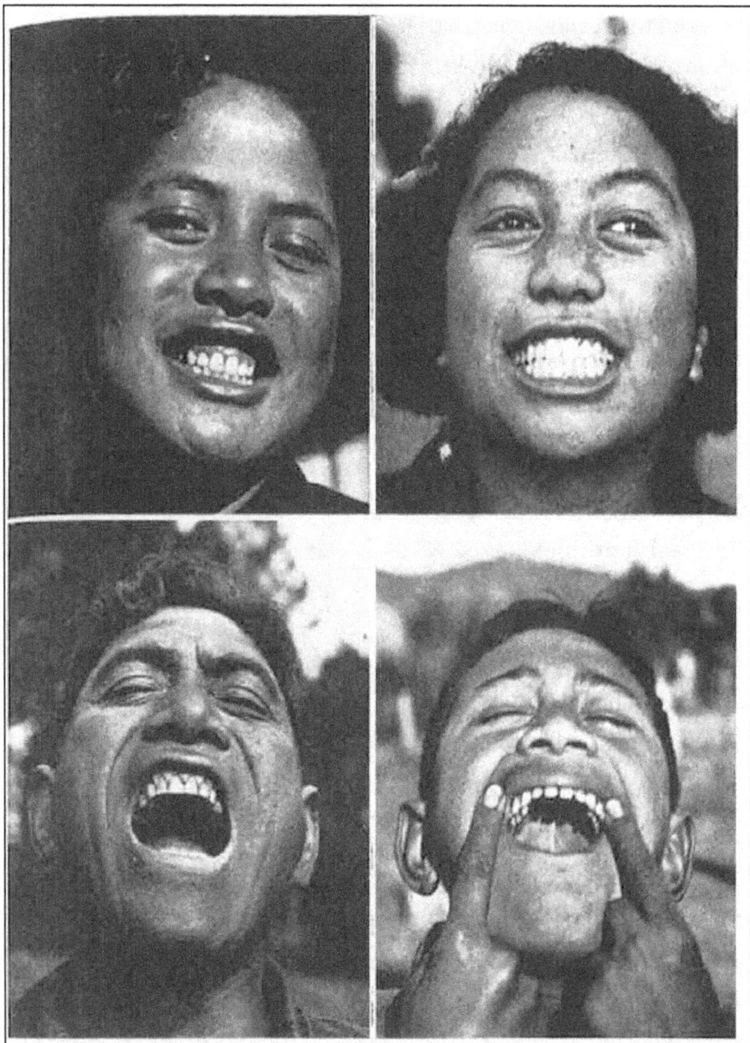

FIG. 69. Since the discovery of New Zealand the primitive natives, the Maori, have had the reputation of having the finest teeth and finest bodies of any race in the world. These faces are typical. Only about one tooth per thousand teeth had been attacked by tooth decay before they came under the influence of the white man.

Figure 93. Growing up with traditional foods. Source: Weston Price, Nutrition and Physical Degeneration, 6th Edition, p. 207. Pictures reprinted with permission. © Price-Pottenger Nutrition Foundation, Inc. All rights reserved. www.ppnf.org.

Dr. Price's work may help us to explain why some arguments opposed to Community Water Fluoridation are emotional:

> "The reputation of the Maori people for splendid physiques has placed them on a pedestal of perfection. Much of this has been lost in modernization." [662]

> "The Maori men have great physical endurance and good minds. Many fine lawyers and government executives are Maori. The breakdown of these people comes when they depart from their native foods to the foods of modern civilization, foods consisting largely of white flour, sweetened goods, syrup and canned goods. The effect is similar to that experienced by other races after using foods of modern civilization." [662]

In the 2013 Hamilton City Council Tribunal, Dr. Price's work was mentioned a few times by people opposed to CWF. It was never mentioned by the supporters of CWF during the four days.

Price looked at the skulls of Māori from generations before, and claimed the wonderful health they held had lasted for many generations [663]. Only one parent needed to give up the traditional food and take up the refined food, for children to be born with *dental* deformities. Children conceived by parents eating the modernized diet, and growing up with the modernized diet, are shown in **Figure 94** (Price's Figure 72).

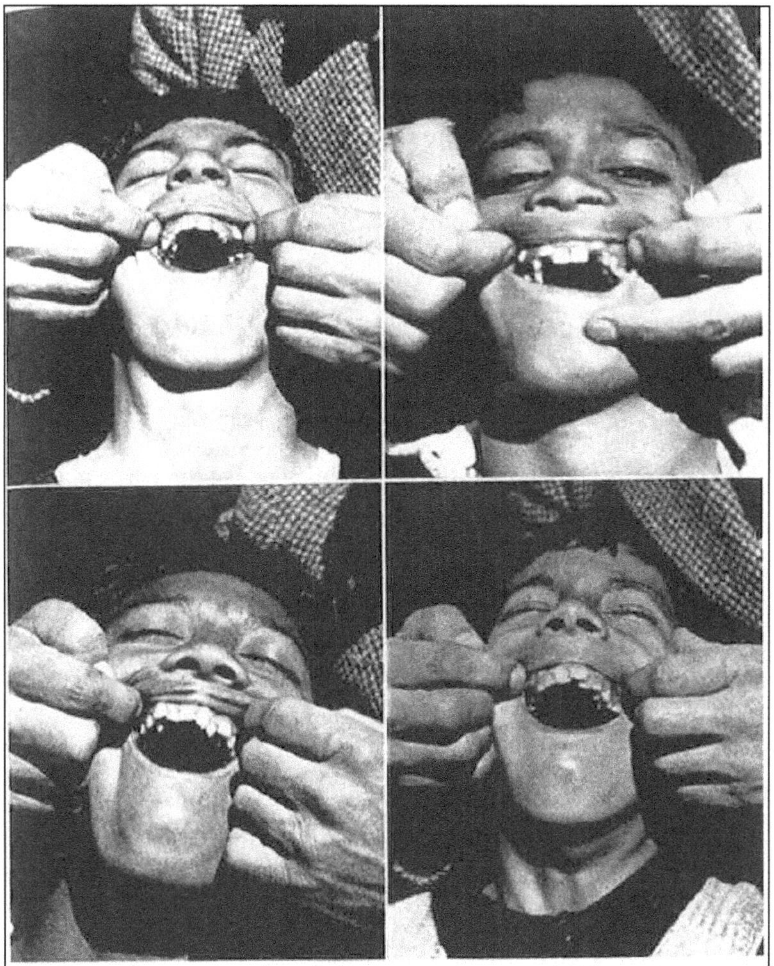

There are many people who have claimed New Zealand soil and water to be deficient in important nutrients [664, 665], and it is obvious this research contradicts that claim somewhat. Yet the land has undergone vast changes – eradication of much wildlife and native forest, introduction of other plant and animal species, more population, etc, so there may be some truth to these claims in a modern context.

FIG. 72. In striking contrast with the beautiful faces of the primitive Maori those born since the adoption of deficient modernized foods are grossly deformed. Note the marked underdevelopment of the facial bones, one of the results being narrowing of the dental arches with crowding of the teeth and an underdevelopment of the air passages. We have wrongly assigned these distorted forms to mixture of racial bloods.

Figure 94. *Growing up with a modernized diet. Source: Weston Price, Nutrition and Physical Degeneration, 6th Edition, p. 211. Pictures reprinted with permission.* © *Price-Pottenger Nutrition Foundation, Inc. All rights reserved. www.ppnf.org.*

Some things fundamental to nutrition can be said here. One is that soil microbes provide a role in the mineralization of plants. While much of our modern insecticides and herbicides may kill insects that harm the economic aspects of food production, these compounds may also destroy soil microbes, rendering their role in plant mineralization compromised. If soils have abundant minerals, these are rendered less available by an absence of microbes.

In their book *The Survival of Civilization* Don Weaver and Jon Hamaker conducted an experiment using extremely fine rock dust in soil, comparing food grown in this freshly mineralized soil, and food grown using conventional methods. The freshly mineralized soil contained more phophorous, potassium, calcium and magnesium [666]. Another, more extensive experiment demonstrated conventional chemical methods caused foods to have a much lesser mineral content:

> "... in a four-year study in which 1,000 crop samples were taken from farms in eleven midwestern states, samples were analysed for their levels of calcium, phosphorous, potassium, sodium, magnesium, iron, copper, zinc and manganese. The following year, 1,000 new crop samples were taken and analysed. This procedure was repeated again for the next two years. When the data from the four-year study were tabulated, there was an unmistakable decline in the trace mineral contents. To illustrate, in corn, calcium dropped 41%, phosphorous 8%, potassium 28%, sodium 55%, magnesium 22%, iron 26%, copper 68%, zinc 10% and manganese 34%." [667]

In the 1930s, work on minerals was presented to the United States Congress, which claimed that around 99% of Americans were deficient in minerals [668].

We mainly eat the muscle meat of animals. Conversely, many of the tribes that Dr. Price investigated consumed organ meat. Typically in healthy animals this is higher in fats, vitamins and minerals than muscle meat. Price found a much greater content of required mineral elements in the foods of the healthiest people:

> "... foods of the native Eskimos contained 5.4 times as much calcium as the displacing foods of the white man, five times as much phosphorus, 1.5 times as much iron, 7.9 times as much magnesium, 1.8 times as much copper, 49.0 times as much iodine, and at least ten times that number of fat-soluble vitamins." [669]

I found no mention of Price's work in the Health Department archives beyond newspaper clippings and occasional letters. In the 1950s people consistently wrote letters asking why New Zealand authorities in government and medicine believed populations needed CWF when Māori had excellent teeth before introduction to modernized life. While some authorities believed junk food to be an impossible problem to fix without policing food, I found one person (a Jaycee) pointing to another answer. It was that only coast-dwelling Māori had superior teeth to inland Māori due to fluorine in seafood; other minerals were not mentioned. [670]

The claim was made that the Otago University Dental School had proven this, but no citation or reference to any document was given so finding such work would involve a lot of searching. I am currently looking for it, but without even a study or author name to go with, I'm not hopeful. This is the problem faced by casual or professional researchers when people don't provide adequate citations in their statements. There is obviously the possibility the letter's author misread work which was saying something else. Media are in a position to help here by replying to authors asking for clarification of their statements before printing.

Nevertheless the statement that fluoride is abundant in fish is true, but so are many minerals, as well as fats and oils. Inland South Island was heavily populated with sea birds, no doubt also abundant in fluoride and other minerals.

Price showed the path he travelled in New Zealand's North Island in his book. He was consistently near the coast, though inland west of Hawke's Bay and south of Auckland. There is nothing in his book about inland vs coastal Maori being different in the quality of their dentistry. From what I can tell the same is true of Pickerill's work, though I will stand corrected if I've overlooked something. Inland New Zealand was abundant in its bird population prior to modern times, and Maori ate many of them. I do not believe there has been much recent interest in Price's work as far as New Zealand's education system and government has been concerned. Price wrote,

> "In anticipation of making these studies I had been in correspondence with the officials for over two years."
> [671]

Price claimed Colonel Saunders, Director of Oral Hygiene in NZ's Department of Public Health met him and his co-workers at Auckland to offer assistance. It seems the government of the time was interested in this work. Price wrote highly of the NZ government, they seemed to care for people, with an active, socialized, dental program. For whatever reason (I have found nothing beyond the obvious), Price's work has been ignored.

Dr. Henry Pickerill was Professor of Dentistry and Director of the Dental School of Otago University, New Zealand. The second edition of his book *The Prevention of Dental Caries and Oral Sepsis* appears to have more information on Māori than the first. Pickerill wrote in the introduction that it included "… my own investigation into the cause of immunity in less civilized Maori children."

Pickerill disagreed with Dr. Mummery's claim that the races most immune to dental caries were those who ate the most meat. His investigation of Māori lifestyle and diet holds Māori in honour and esteem. Pickerill claimed Mummery attributed Māori excellence to cannibalism, to which Pickerill disagreed:

> "The consumption of human flesh occurred only on more or less rare occasions after a war-party had returned home with prisoners, and then not all the prisoners were eaten; a large number were always reserved as slaves. But, most important of all from our present point of view, the consumption of such food was confined almost entirely to the warriors. Human flesh was strictly *tapu – i.e.,* forbidden – to women, and only the elder boys were allowed a very small portion. Yet, as a matter of fact, both women and children had just as good teeth as the men. This disposes completely of any theory that the Maori [sic] owed their immunity to caries to cannibalism." [672]

Pickerill also pointed to other highly carnivorous races mentioned in Dr. Mummery's work, like the South American Guachos, with the highest rates of caries Mummery found (20.8% of individuals with carious teeth). Reasons given were a distaste for cultivation and even simple agriculture, flavourless cassava bread, and a complete lack of salt (minerals) [673].

Pickerill claimed Māori ate birds and fish in varying amounts. Sharks were an occasional delicacy. Meat and vegetables were often cooked together, with food covered in leaves, earth and mats, to keep in flavour.

"The leaves having once been opened, the food was either eaten or thrown away; no food was ever recooked or touched a second time upon any consideration whatever."

"The Maori was allowed to exercise his idiosyncrasies of taste, and was not bound by any custom or law to eat what he did not relish; he simply stated that he was 'wainamu' for certain food – even human flesh in many instances – and that wish or declaration was accepted by parent, host, or guest, without demur." [674]

Price claimed very few, if any, native races practiced regular cleaning of teeth. In many instances he had to remove debris in the mouth to examine the quality of teeth.

Pickerill claimed he had

"been unable to gather any evidence either from the Maori [sic] themselves or from other observers that they ever practiced cleaning the teeth by any artificial means." [674]

Though he did point to other races using sticks to clean their mouths.

In 1934, a small book by R. M. S. Taylor, a dentist from New Zealand, was published. It focused on Māori foods. While Taylor's beliefs were different to others, he too held Māori health in high regard:

"As regards their dental conditions, it is certain that the comparison [to the 'average colonial of today'] is overwhelmingly in favour of the Maori."

"... the old-time Maori attained a degree of intelligence and physical perfection that might well be the envy of our present-day folk who boast the advantages of civilization." [675]

Like Price, Taylor agreed that the skulls of old Māori gave proof that foods required much mastication. However, his work on the Māori diet was different to Price's or Pickerill's.

"... the outstanding feature of the average Maori diet in the old days would appear to be its simplicity. Water was the only beverage, and the variety of foods consumed at any one time was small. The staple foods were starchy, and though fat and oily foods were favoured, flesh of any kind was often absent from the diet. Mastication was vigorous and efficient. Digestive organs had periods of rest. On account of these facts, or perhaps in spite of them, the old-time Maori attained a degree of intelligence and physical perfection that might well be the envy of our present-day folk who boast the advantages of civilization." [675]

Taylor's book is only nine pages, incapable of the detail of Price's or Pickerill's. Taylor's claim of animal flesh being "often absent" is in some contrast to claims of the other two.

Incidentally, a recent argument expressed against the use of fluoride tablets is:

"They need to be taken daily and chewed, which is difficult for children." [676]

I worked in a seafood bar once. We served New Zealand mussels (*Mytilidae* family) to tourists from all over the world. I worked mainly in the kitchen so my customer contact was minimal; though I remember one customer complaining that mussels were too difficult to chew. Yet this is a blessing, as it gives the muscles of the lower face a workout, with possible far-reaching consequences. Dr. Pickerill believed modern people suffered because of their penchant for soft foods. The masseter muscle joins the corner of the mandible (jaw) to the zygomatic bone (the bone around the outer part of the eye). The temporalis muscle attaches to the coronoid process at the upper mandible, and has attachments to the frontal, parietal, and temporal bones (these bones make up most of the upper skull), and to the two greater 'wings' of the sphenoid, the bone that spans the width of the head between the temples. The lateral and medial pterygoideus muscles attach from the corner of the mandible to the pterygoid plate of the sphenoid. The buccinator muscle has attachments to the alveolar processes of the maxilla and mandible (upper and lower jaw) near the molars, and to the muscles on the lip [677].

The point I want to make here is that muscles atrophy if they're not used. I would suggest that eating soft food which seldom requires energetic chewing does for our facial structure (and our dentition) what lack of exercise does for the rest of our body.

And as the junk food industry can tell us, exercising is important.

Pickerill believed that "'stagnation' within the oral cavity" – meaning lack of use of the facial muscles in chewing – led to facial deformities as aging occurred over time:

He wrote of the "general 'softness'" in the refined foods,

> "resulting in a lack of sufficient stimulus to the jaw-bones – therefore in a crowded and irregular state of the teeth, and hence a predisposition to caries." [678]

He believed that the removal of fibre from foods, which is what we get in refined flours and sugars, disabled "their detergent action upon the teeth". He also claimed large amounts of cellulose were not necessarily a security against caries.

He pointed to the blandness, neutrality, and "comparative non-sapidity[149]" of refined foods. Also to their "alkaline reaction, and their general uniformity" which he believed were shown to not stimulate the salivary glands enough to keep the mouth free from fermenting food debris.

> "... paradoxical as it may seem, modern communities have acquired or developed a 'taste' for tasteless things." [679]

He felt this tendency for bland foods was entrained over many years, more in adults than in children. He pointed to the amount of sour fruit schoolboys would eat, "within the knowledge of all".

Pickerill claimed in a modernized community in which there was almost no poverty, to have found carious teeth in over 90 percent of children. He also believed the tutu berry[150] kept Māori salivary glands in a state of excitation, which helped with tooth remineralization. It appears varieties of berry differ in their tendency to cause harm, so I am certainly not recommending anyone start using these.

Regarding bacteria of the mouth, Pickerill wrote about his comparison between carious and non-carious individuals:

---

[149] 'Sapid' means to have an agreeable taste; not bland.

[150] According to Andrew Crowe's book *A Field Guide to the Native Edible Plants of New Zealand*, the tutu (*Coriaria arborea* and *Coriaria sarmentosa*) have berries that are really "swollen flowers" when observed closely. "Part eaten: the soft succulent petals and their dark purple juice. **Every other part of these two plants is highly poisonous, including the tiny seeds enclosed in the 'fruit'**. Children should be warned to leave the plant alone, and adults are well advised not to experiment." Crowe warns that "death and serious illness have occurred" as a result of including seeds in beer and pie made from tutu. He claims the tāpia (*Tupeia antarctica*) has edible berries that were eaten by the Tūhoe Māori.

"... there exists no great difference between the oral flora of immune and of susceptible individuals, and that *freedom from caries in such children is not due to the absence of those organisms which are usually regarded as causal factors.*" (His emphasis) [680]

This is possibly one thing that caused others to ignore his work (though his work had been mentioned in the **New Zealand Dental Journal**, which also printed an obituary for him). In 1968, the **New York Times** reported that it had been known for 20 years that bacteria was an essential factor in tooth decay.

"Decay could not be produced in animals that were bacteria-free." [681]

The article discussed a task force headed by the National Institutes of Health that would focus on microbes in the mouth. "If tooth decay becomes completely preventable in the 1970s..."

Dr. Weston Price found the Aborigines of Australia succumbed to the distorting effects of the modernized foods within a generation, as with races from every continent. Before their incorporation into the modernized world, their health was glorious. Dr. Price commented:

"They have been able to build good bodies and maintain them in excellent condition in a country in which the plant life, and consequently the lower animal life can be maintained at only a very low level because of the absence of rain. Over half of Australia has less than ten inches of rain a year. It is significant that the natives have maintained a vigorous existence in districts in which the white population which expelled them is unable to continue to live." [682]

"Little baldness was seen even in the very old." [683]

Typical deformities are shown (left and bottom) in **Figure 95** (Price's Figure 54), compared to a woman who had followed a traditional diet since her childhood (top right).

At one reservation, 47.5% of Indigenous peoples' teeth were carious and 40% of dental arches were disfigured or "abnormal". Of the women, 81.3% of teeth were carious, in men, 60.4%, and in children, 16.5%. Every individual in this reservation where the government provided processed food – sugar, flour, margarine – had some dental decay.

The native Australians knew that they suffered once they were colonized. Dr. Price wrote:

"As we had found in some of the modernized islands of the Pacific, we discovered that here, too, discouragement and a longing for death had taken the place of a joy in living in many. Few souls in the world have experienced this discouragement and this longing to a greater degree."

"This [degeneration of the facial pattern that occurs so often in our modern civilization] has its expression in the narrowing and lengthening of the face and the development of crooked teeth. It is most remarkable and should be one of the most challenging facts that can come to our modern civilization that such primitive races as the Aborigines of Australia, have reproduced for generation after generation through many centuries – no one knows for how many thousands of years – without the development of a conspicuous number of irregularities of the dental arches. Yet, in the next generation after these people adopt the foods of the white man, a large percentage of the children developed irregularities of the dental arches with conspicuous facial deformities. The deformity patterns are similar to those seen in white civilizations." [684]

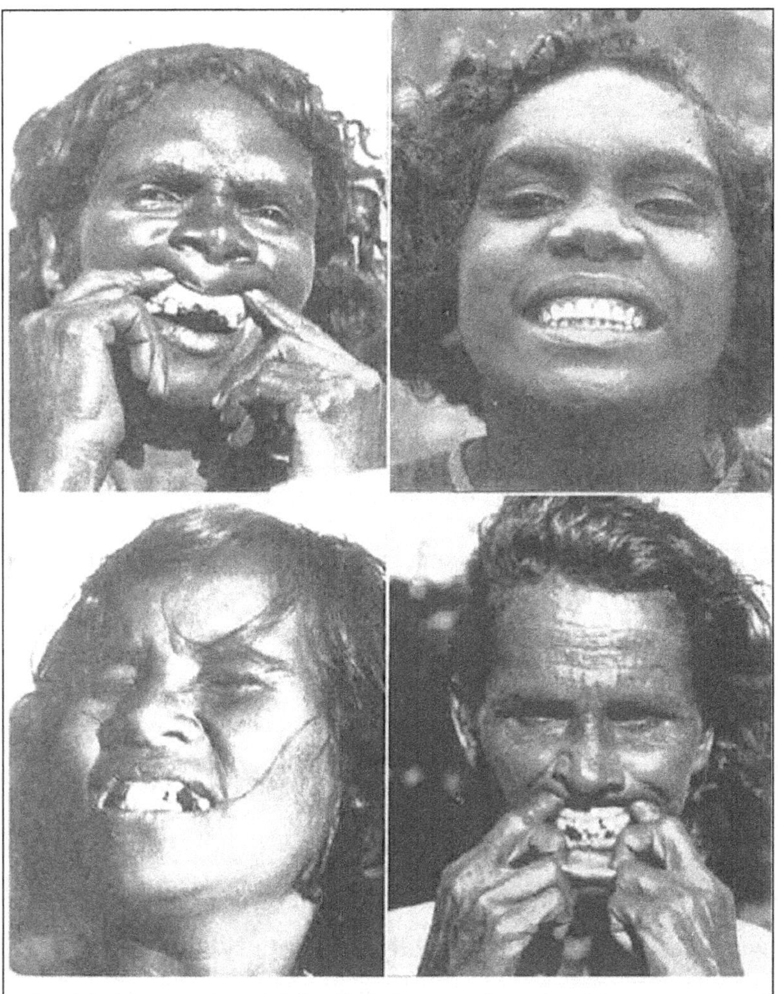

FIG. 54. Wherever the primitive Aborigines have been placed in reservations and fed on the white man's foods of commerce dental caries has become rampant. This destroys their beauty, prevents mastication, and provides infection for seriously injuring their bodies. Note the contrast between the primitive woman in the upper right and the three modernized women.

Figure 95*. Indigenous Australians' Teeth – Contrast in Diets. Source: Weston Price, Nutrition and Physical Degeneration, sixth Edition, p. 173. Pictures reprinted with permission. © Price-Pottenger Nutrition Foundation, Inc. All rights reserved. www.ppnf.org.*

At Cape Bedford, Dr. Price looked at a small group of Indigenous Australians that were no longer partaking of the traditional diet their ancestors used:

> "Of the eighty-three individuals, 48.1 per cent had been affected by dental caries. Many of the adults in this group had been born on plantations under the influence of the modern nutrition, and many of the children had been born in the mission. For the adults, 46 per cent had abnormally formed dental arches, and for the children, 41.6 per cent. We were advised that deaths occurred very frequently from tuberculosis. This reservation does not provide the natives with natural hunting grounds capable of providing the people with animal life for food." [685]

> "While the coast is well supplied with a variety of deep-water fish the natives have practically no equipment for obtaining them, a condition which restricts them very largely to the use of the imported foods supplied by the officials."

> "Our next stop, using the special aeroplane, was at Lockhart River, which is about four-fifths of the way up the east coast of Australia. Here again we were able to land on the beach near a large group of primitive Aborigines. The isolation here is so nearly complete that they are dependent upon the sea and the land for their foods. This

part of Australia, namely, the York Peninsula, is still so primitive that there has been very little encroachment by the white population. It will be remembered that in this area there are no roads, the country being a primitive wilderness. Of fifty-eight individuals examined, their 1,784 teeth revealed that only 4.3 per cent had been attacked by dental caries. For the women, this amounted to 3.4 per cent; for the men, 6.1 per cent; and for the children, 3.2 per cent. Some of these men had at some time worked on cattle ranches for the white men. Of the children, only 6.3 per cent had abnormal dental arches, and of the adults, 8.7 per cent. In this group, therefore, 91.4 per cent of all ages had reproduced the typical racial pattern as compared with 56 per cent of the group at Cape Bedford, 62 per cent of the group at Palm Island, and 60 per cent at LeParouse. At Lockhart River, 32.7 per cent of the individuals had dental caries."

"One can scarcely visualize, without observing it, the distress of a group of primitive people situated as these people are, compelled to live in a very restricted area, forced to live on food provided by the government, while they are conscious that if they could return to their normal habits of life they would regain their health and again enjoy life."

"In their native life where they could get the foods that keep them well and preserve their teeth, they had no need for dentists." [685]

"The rapid degeneration of the Australian Aborigines after the adoption of the government's modern foods provides a demonstration that should be infinitely more convincing than animal experimentation. It should be a matter not only of concern but deep alarm that human beings can degenerate physically so rapidly by the use of a certain type of nutrition, particularly the dietary products used so generally by modern civilization." [686]

That the bodies and character of people can be maintained to such a near-flawless state in such an inhospitable environment where water, meat and plant are so scarce is perhaps an unpleasant reality for us to face when we look at our own deformity and sickness in a world that stands on the shoulders of a century of scientific genius and invention.

Price told us:

"This group provides evidence of exceptional efficiency in obeying the laws of Nature through thousands of years, even in a parched land that is exceedingly inhospitable because of the scant plant foods for either men or animals. While the Aborigines are credited with being the oldest race on the face of the earth today, they are dying out with great rapidity wherever they have changed their native nutrition to that of the modern white civilization. For them this is not a matter of choice, but rather of necessity, since in a large part of Australia the few that are left are crowded into reservations where they have little or no access to native foods and are compelled to live on the foods provided for them by our white civilization. They demonstrate in a tragic way the inadequacy of the white man's dietary programs." [687]

For those interested in other aspects of the native Australians, journalist John Pilger has recently (2013) made a documentary called *Utopia*. It is one of many documentaries he has made on Australia's indigenous people. In New Zealand it has aired on Māori TV, but not the more mainstream TVNZ [688].

Below are shown Indigenous Australians who were *not* raised on the modern civilization's food (**Figure 96** – Price's Figure 53). Note the straightness of teeth, spacious nature of the mandible and upper dental arch.

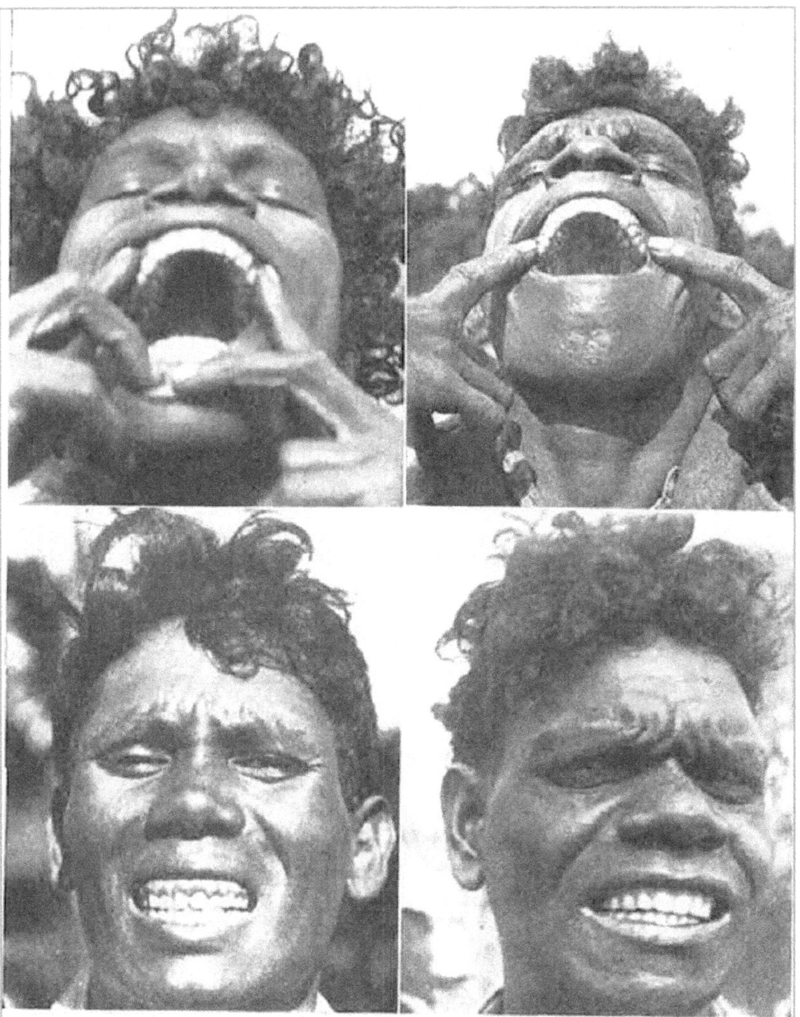

FIG. 53. No other primitive race seems to deserve so much credit for skill in obeying nature's laws as these primitive Aborigines because of the perpetual drought hazards of much of the land they live in. Half of Australia has less than ten inches of rain per year. Note the magnificent dental arches and beautiful teeth of these primitives. Tooth decay was almost unknown in many districts.

Figure 96. *Indigenous Australians' Teeth on a Traditional Diet. Source: Weston Price, Nutrition and Physical Degeneration, 6th Edition, p. 172. Pictures reprinted with permission. © Price-Pottenger Nutrition Foundation, Inc. All rights reserved. www.ppnf.org.*

"Tooth decay was almost unknown in many districts." (page 172)

In the islands of the Torres Strait (north of Australia), Dr. Price found some very healthy natives, and very unhealthy Caucasians.

Children typical of the native upbringing and traditional foods are shown in his work. Well-formed dental arches and excellent teeth were also a feature of adulthood. Modernized Torres Strait islanders conceived by parents living on foods provided by modern civilization suffered the same dental problems as the colonizing, white race. Price wrote of these white immigrants:

"They are within reach of some of the best foods to be found anywhere in the world and yet do not use them; a typical characteristic of modern whites." [689]

He wrote of the traditional inhabitants:

"It would be difficult to find a more happy and contented people than the primitives in the Torres Strait Islands as they lived without contact with modern civilization. Indeed, they seem to resent very acutely the modern intrusion. They not only have nearly perfect bodies, but an associated personality and character of a high degree of excellence. One is continually impressed with happiness, peace and health while in their congenial presence."

"Their home life reaches a very high ideal and among them there is practically no crime."

"The sea foods include large and small fish in great abundance, dugong, and a great variety of shellfish. These foods have developed for them remarkable physiques with practically complete immunity to dental caries. Wherever they have adopted the white man's foods, however, they suffer the typical expressions of degeneration, such as, loss of immunity to dental caries; and in the succeeding generations there is a marked change in facial and dental arch form with marked lowering of resistance to disease." [689]

It's more revolting to think that the poorest layer of civilized society are the people who need nature the most, as nature, if governed sanely, charges not one cent for an abundant harvest [690]. Yet in our market-driven economy – "the only way the financial system could work" – the poorest are those who are *least* able to obtain organic, pesticide-free foods that are the closest we now have to the nutrient-abundant foods used by more primitive people. (These may be the best foods we can create today, however I am not suggesting they are the same as people ate hundreds of years ago.) We claim to care so much for the health of the poor, how shameful that our system almost forbids them from making healthy purchases. The result of some policies is to decrease the price of unhealthy foods, and increase the cost of healthier food [488]. This is one (unspoken) reason why the rich consistently have better dental (and overall) health than the poor [618, 691].

Tobacco companies are possibly to blame for many dental caries in Asia. Professor Chomsky discussed a 1993 British study in which it is estimated that about 50 million Chinese will die from tobacco-related deaths as a result of the American government's demand that the Chinese market be open to Big Tobacco, and argues that this should be considered violence [692].

What can Dr. Price's work tell us about fluorine? For one thing, the element was acquired in seafood. All the indigenous races made great effort to eat food from the sea. This is reason for us to treat our seas with reverence, assuming we care about our own bodies and minds.

We get abundant fluorine in our modern world, yet suffer much greater dental caries than the indigenous people who were, to paraphrase Dr. Price's words "obedient to nature's laws". This is probably one reason why his work is ignored by mainstream dentistry, though his work is featured in the early 20th century issues of the **Journal of the American Dental Association**.

Regardless of the quality, veracity and lessons in Dr Price's work, I believe the New Zealand and Australian public may be interested in it. Mainstream dentistry has stumbled and fallen in its understanding of fluorine's non-essentiality, vastly exaggerating the importance of the element to the point of almost completely ignoring the dental effects of elements that *are* essential. The people of New Zealand and Australia ought to pursue avenues of research beyond the narrow foci of experts. To this end I submit what are important aspects of heretofore ignored dental success. We may not be able to recreate the conditions of the pre-civilization people given that our free market ideologies prevent us from putting environmental protection before profits and the externalities required to maximise them, but we may be able to begin having slightly less deformed offspring. Minerals in the soil in which we grow our food would be a good step in this direction. It may take a few generations before any improvements become apparent. Our race's degeneration could be slowed by putting a tax on heavily refined flours, sugars and oils, and subsidizing foods closer to nature. *Regeneration of our bodies* and minds is, I believe, more in the hands of individuals, though no doubt bolstered and strengthened by policy decisions.

The NAS, in 1989 discussed Aristotle's idea in the fourth century B.C. that sweet figs may cause dental caries due to their tendency to stick to teeth. After telling us that, they say:

"However, as McDonald[151] points out, even after 23 centuries we know only a little more than Aristotle about the relative cariogenicity of foods." [693]

This is reason enough to go back and consider Māori and Indigenous Australian diets, and our ability and willingness to replicate them.

The same document also states:

"Although the increased consumption of dietary sugars has led to increases in dental caries prevalence internationally, World Health Organization data indicate that caries is decreasing in Western countries and increasing in developing countries."

As part of "development" these poor countries need their economies opened up to foreign investors, notably corporations like Coca-Cola and the tobacco companies. [692] According to a 1964 **Pensacola News** article, an American government researcher, Dr. Albert B. Russell of the US National Institute of Dental Research, claimed that white people in Baltimore had teeth *worse* than people in Ethiopia. He spoke of

"a study of tooth decay showed white people in Baltimore rank almost as poorly as the urbanized Aleuts of Alaska's National Guard. The Aleuts have a record of missing and filled teeth about 60 times worse than people in Ethiopia." [694]

Dr. Russell presented this study at an international meeting of scientists (of the AAAS), and said that Baltimore was a reasonable representation of the US as a whole. (He also told the **News** that there is no single explanation for tooth decay.) Baltimore was fluoridated in 1952, according to a 1969 article in the Evening Post archive in Wellington's public library:

"Dr. H. Berton McCauley, director of dental care in the city health department, estimated that decay reductions of up to 60 per cent have been observed among children who have been raised on fluoridated water... As a result, Baltimore's fluoridation programme has sparked wide interest and Dr. McCauley points to a 3-inch stack of correspondence, much of it from Canada and Britain. A 1960 survey of 2,139 Baltimore School children 6, 3 and 10 years of age found tooth decay reductions of 70, 50 and 30 per cent respectively." [695]

Though this article was written in December of 1969, more recent research was not mentioned.

Given this kind of result in their own people, it seems distasteful that American experts can champion their own claims to nutritional authority in other people's countries with such certainty and confidence.

Dr. Price wrote of the Indigenous Australians:

"Their fertility has been so greatly reduced that the death rate far exceeds the birth rate." [687]

---

[151] McDonald, J.L., Jr. 1985a. *Cariogenicity of foods.* Pp. 320-345 in R.L. Pollack and E. Kravitz, eds. *Nutrition in Oral Health and Disease.* Lea & Febiger, Philadelphia.

It is worth noting that Armstrong *et al.* pointed out in 1972, that infertility is a "relatively common manifestation of deficiency" of elements like manganese, copper, zinc, iodine and selenium [28].

In 1974, Nielsen and Sandstead wrote in their review that the American diet contained a high amount of empty calories, and that excess junk food may "contribute to the occurrence of deficiencies" [27].

In 1984, the **Wall Street Journal** wrote

> "In recent years, infertility specialists have seen a marked increase in the number of couples unable to conceive... At the same time physicians note, the average sperm count among men is decreasing. Toxic environmental pollution is thought to be a culprit." [696]

Pollution is no doubt part of it. I believe nutritional deficiencies are another part. **The Guardian** recently published an article discussing research from the Hebrew University of Jerusalem, which claimed:

> "sperm counts among men in the west have more than halved in the past 40 years and are currently falling by an average of 1.4% a year." [697]

The article discussed different perspectives from scientists, and different reasons for such results, including methodological reasons regarding data selection. There was one very interesting sentence in the article:

> "And why do men outside the western world appear not to be affected?"

The purity of certain elements comes at the expense of others. Consider that a pure chemical used for food in an experiment is hugely different from normal, natural food, which is essentially plant and animal cells. Simple biology textbooks tell us that cells, the fundamental building blocks of life, have a huge variety of compounds and elements within them. Thus, purified chemicals, though they may be essential to nutrition, are not representative of normal diets, that are basically made of cells.

Dr. Price found that in European, Arabian and some other groups the sources of fats, protein and minerals were from dairy products. In the Americas, organ meat from buffalo and similar animals was used, as well as eggs from wild and domesticated birds. Another source of fats, protein and minerals was food from the sea, the importance of which Dr. Price emphasized [698]. If modern politicians want to ensure the health of future populations they will start prioritizing environmental issues above corporate profits. This means getting "in the way" of business.

Seafood has been considered an essential food for humans in at least one article published in the **Global Journal of Health Science** [699]. The authors of this article also stress the importance of one burden the Māori and other native populations did not feel the effects of hundreds of years ago – pollution.

> "Fish consumption, however, also carries certain risks associated with exposure to environmental toxicants." (page 77)

Assuming our current health, and the health of future generations is of any importance at all, we had better treat the seas, and the life in them, with reverence. This would mean a very strict attitude to over-fishing, pollution, and the usual excesses associated with our profit-driven culture.

In relating Dr. Price's work to the modern world, a few things become immediately apparent. The native people Dr. Price studied were hunter-gatherers, foragers, sometimes farmers, though they had no advanced technology helping them. The foods were not produced in order to satisfy shareholders or markets, rather they were produced as a result of the abundance of nature.

Modern agricultural practice, for better or worse, has given us mass-produced food. Part of the evidence that this food is mineral deficient is that we do not conceive healthy children, as did the native people Dr. Price studied.

Dr. John Yudkin was one scientist who cautioned the world in the 1970s regarding hazards of refined sugar. A paper comparing work he did with more mainstream work was published in the **Journal of Dental Research** in 2009. Dr. Yudkin's claims are being taken more seriously nowadays, particularly after Kristin Kearns' findings, and the increasing popularity of the work of Dr. Weston Price.

This paper also suggests dental disease may be a "canary in the coal mine" so to speak – a precursor or indication of destructive lifestyle choices:

> "Possibly, when it comes to fermentable carbohydrates, teeth would then become to the medical and dental professionals what they have always been for paleoanthropologists: 'extremely informative about age, sex, diet, health[152]'" [700]

In her 2015 book, Dr. Marion Nestle wrote about Dr. Karen Sokal-Gutierrez, who visited Ecuador in the 1970s as a Peace Corps volunteer.

> "The children, who had little or no exposure to sodas and sugary snacks, had beautiful teeth and lovely smiles. Twenty years later... she was shocked to see that many children had rotted and eroded teeth. Heavily advertised sodas and other commercial sweetened products had taken over local markets and replaced traditional foods." [701]

I am not a doctor or medical professional. The information shared here is for academic interest. I believe it to be true. A little knowledge is a very dangerous thing. When we are highly compulsive and polarized in our thinking it is very easy for us to do more harm than good to others and ourselves. I would encourage readers to seek out a copy of *Nutrition and Physical Degeneration* for contemplative inquiry.

As far as politicians and policy is concerned, I am surprised Dr. Price's work is not taught in schools. We are already close to halfway there, at least in attitude: Dr. Rob Beaglehole of the New Zealand Dental Association has for some years now been encouraging schools in this part of the world to go without soft drink and confectionary. The other half of a simplified nutritional picture is food grown in healthy soils, organs from healthy animals, healthy seas, and other fundamentals outlined in Dr. Price's work. I would also point out that the native populations with excellent teeth were not subjected to food advertising. They had more freedom when it came to listening to their own bodies.

---

[152] Here the authors cite Johanson DC, Edgar B (2006). *From Lucy to language*. Rev., updated, and expanded ed. New York: Simon and Schuster.

Our natural world now is heavily polluted, and we almost certainly face the fact that the diets examined in the work of Doctors Pickerill, Price, Taylor and others a century ago, are incapable of being perfectly recreated unless we can improve our environmental conditions. We will require governments and organizations that have the willingness to stand up to, and regulate the business community's greed.

However, there are some things we can take from this work. A healthy diet contains:

- Sources of raw protein
- Sources of fats and oils
- Minimal refined and processed foods
- Abundant and various minerals
- Facial deformities can develop if the chewing muscles are not used in childhood.
- The use of healthy, mineral-rich soil in which to grow food is tantamount.

Dr. Price did not find any race creating healthy children with excellent dentition on vegan or vegetarian diets, though some races ate only small amounts of animal meat.

Not only would sharing Price's work give children reason to avoid the worthless food in so many of our shops and supermarkets, it would also potentially demonstrate that every race can hope not only to survive, but to excel.

Price's work has been a consistent feature of an undercurrent of the literature opposed to fluoridation. It can partially explain why elements of the movement were passionate in some of their arguments, and cared little for claims of progress in public health. The neglect of his work may have been partially due to the enticing American influence. In the early parts of last century, before the 1940s, researchers in the US had made small claims regarding the prevention of tooth decay using dietary factors – vitamins from milk, cod liver oil, and the like. Dr. Price himself had much published in the American Dental Association's journal. This research was not abundant in studies, but it was there. Compiling such work is interesting for the detail-oriented academic yet impractical for the citizen, perhaps irrelevant in the light of the work shown in this chapter.

It is obvious why the pre-1940s papers do not mention fluorine[153] much more than in passing – it had never been claimed to be an essential factor (until 1944, the year before CWF began), and success in reducing caries had been achieved by dietary methods alone in *some* instances. Roholm's work on fluorine was published in 1937, and the profession was possibly more concerned with excess fluorine than with 'sub-optimal' levels.

In papers published by the American Dental Association's journal in the 1930s, food quality – concentration of nutrients in food – was seldom discussed, though it was no doubt forefront in the minds of some researchers. Effects of deficiency states, both direct and indirect were considered. Salivary glands were claimed to atrophy

---

[153] A search of the **Journal of the American Dental Association** issue archive on 8th July, 2018, for "fluorine diet", "fluoride diet" and "fluoride nutrition" revealed that the vast majority of papers were post-1940s. For instance, "fluoride nutrition" yielded 1,258 results, only 8 of which were from the 1930s.

in a vitamin deficient diet in 1931 [702]. A dentist named Sigmund Franken quoted Professor McCollum: "The American people are starving themselves on a full stomach." Franken claimed improvements regarding tooth sensitivity in 17 patients were brought about primarily by adding vitamin A and calcium to their diets for months. These were given via raw greens, fresh vegetables only lightly cooked and served with their juice, liberal eggs, milk and cheese [702].

Much work was performed on animals - vitamin C deficiencies led to soft teeth in guinea pigs, who like humans, do not store it. One researcher claimed there was some evidence that vitamins A and B were also important in "tooth formation and preservation". He discussed a study wherein dogs were fed white bread and lean meats; in which the researchers "observed a rampant disintegration of the crowns" – odontoclasia [703].

In 1938, Dr. Butler of Oak Park, Illinois, wrote:

> "We agree that a diet of adequate caloric value, containing liberal quantities of milk, vegetables and fruit, together with meat, eggs and wholegrain cereals, and supplemented with cod-liver oil or other vitamin concentrates, should furnish the building materials for proper tooth growth and development. Many groups of children maintained on such a diet have shown a low incidence of caries and developmental defects, and others on deficient diets have shown arrest of disease and improvement when changed to such a régime." [704]

Dr. Butler pointed to hyperthyroidism as a co-factor in decalcification.

A doctor named Philip Jay wrote an article on sugar's role in the cause of carious teeth, published in 1940. He discussed the formation of hypoplastic (underformed) teeth in dogs when fed diets low in vitamin A and D, though the teeth were not more carious than normal. Similar experiments on children but in the opposite direction – with fortified vitamin A and D – resulted in reduction in caries. From this work it was concluded that these two factors were necessary not only in the formation of teeth in the protection of teeth against caries [705].

In 1940 Jay mentioned the work of McCollum, who claimed to see carious teeth in rodents denied phosphorous. This had led to the "widespread" use of dicalcium phosphate as a means of preventing caries, though Jay claimed there was no clinical evidence of its value.

> "It was assumed, then, that these procedures necessarily prove that the structure of the tooth determines its susceptibility to caries and, secondly, that the structure of the erupted tooth can be influenced through nutrition. Both of these assumptions are debatable."

Jay claimed there was "even less evidence" that the structure of enamel could be changed after the initial calcification.

> "Despite these inconsistencies, it is unquestionably true that caries activity has been reduced in children through dietary management." [705]

By the 1940s the American Dental Association was heavily critical of the idea of healing, or preventing caries with foods.

If refined sugar is as bad as some would say, one reason for our failure to reap maximum benefit from our foods may be found in Jay's paper. He claimed Bulgarians at the time were consuming 10 pounds of sugar per capita annually, compared with 110 pounds in America.

In 1948, the **Journal of the American Dental Association** published *The Michigan Workshop on the Evaluation of Dental Caries Control Technics*. The paper discussed research of a gathering of 114 dental and medical educators, who were to investigate "the mechanism of the caries process," "systemic conditions" and their relationship to caries, dentifrices and prophylaxes, vitamin and mineral use, various types of diets, and fluorides as possible/probable preventive measures. The educators divided into groups to study these topics. The workshop ran for a week. Funders were not mentioned, but can probably be deduced. The workshop coordinated the School of Public Health with the School of Dentistry and W. K. Kellogg Foundation Institute for Graduate and Postgraduate Dentistry, to "appraise critically the present status of the various control measures" available.

In an outlining statement, the second committee claimed:

> "A careful review of scientific reports reveals that sickness, general health or nutritional status has no significant bearing on the caries process. In fact, several scientific reports reveal that malnourished persons have a decreased incidence of dental caries." [706]

This was discussed by the committee that looked at nutritional factors.

The claim made was that in a study that looked at 7 children with rickets born to women with severe osteomalacia in North India, only 2 of 144 teeth were carious. There was nothing said in the ADA's Journal about the diet of these people. We can probably assume it had much less sugar and refined food than the standard Western diet of the time. Nor was anything said about what happened to these children's teeth once they had aged, or the teeth of the elderly where they lived. North India and Pakistan used to be famous in natural health circles for having highly mineralized waters that run down from the mountains.

The study showed pictures of Indians, adults and children, with bowed legs, hunched backs, yet good teeth. One is reminded of pictures of skeletal fluorosis. A potential explanation was found in a 2014 nutrition textbook, though it is unknown whether this affected Indians in the 1940s.

> "Nearly three fourths of poor pregnant women living in villages in Northern India who consume monotonous diets suffer from concurrent iron and zinc deficiency." [707]

Zinc is an important element in enzyme function. One symptom of zinc deficiency is 'photophobia' – meaning an aversion to sunlight, which may lead to vitamin D deficiency; vitamin D has (arguably) a necessary role in bone formation [708].

However, I feel I have presented a "bottom line" that I think ought to cut through the errata: if we want to learn about health, let's look at healthy people, and not only what occurred in one moment or for one generation, but what had brought them to, and kept them at, that level of health. This assumes that we're people capable of receptivity and perception.

Regarding vitamin and mineral supplementation, the Michigan committee set out a premise:

> "Any effects derived from the ingestion of vitamins and minerals must be considered intrinsic in character and manifested, in their relation to dental caries, as (1) variations in the structure, form or composition of the teeth, produced during the period of tooth formation, or (2) variations in the saliva or other factors comprising the environment of the teeth, produced during any period of life."

Their claims are different to the previous research mentioned here. They claimed:

> "There is no conclusive evidence to indicate that there is any significant difference in the caries attack rates of patients who receive vitamin D from sunshine, cod-liver oil or irradiated ergosterol." [706]

Dr. Price's name did not appear in the paper, and none of his work appeared in the references. Philip Jay's paper was mentioned, though his claim that vitamin A additions prevented caries in children may not have met the strict requirements of the committee, that a change in tooth morphology be demonstrated. Consider that prevention of caries attack does not show up as any change, as the tooth simply stays the same.

Dr. Price's claim that more modern, processed foods had from a tenth to a quarter of the nutritional value of more natural food [709] was ignored, as was McCollum's small critique, that Americans were "starving on full stomachs." Incidentally, the word "Maori" only showed one result in the journal archives [710], a 1981 study that cited a study from New Zealand with the word "Maori" in the title.

That our experts in this part of the world were so quick to do whatever the American researchers said, is quite tragic considering what was right under their noses. Such an opinion is mostly held by non-experts.

The committee summarized:

> "Although the committee found no conclusive evidence that an adequate, optimal or balanced diet as outlined by the Food and Nutrition Board, National Research Council, would influence the caries attack rate, it is imperative that a diet conducive to individual health be advocated." [706]

The researchers looked at many dental journals of the time; **Dental Cosmos, Journal of Dental Research, Journal of The American Dietetic Association, American Journal of the Diseases of Children, Journal of Biological Chemistry**, the **Journal of the American Medical Association**, and more.

I have limited my search here to the **Journal of the American Dental Association**. A paper published six months after the summary of the meeting in Michigan also mentioned the studies on Indian children. Again it was mentioned that "in spite of marked rickets" teeth were less carious than in American children.

> "Why these poorly fed children should have so much less decay is worthy of extended consideration. Although they may have protective factors which control caries, the important point in this consideration is that caries is controlled to a greater extent in India than in America despite a diet that admittedly is grossly deficient." [711]

Again, no details on the diet were given, and no details on sugar or fluoride levels were given (this was written 4 years after the initial commencement of CWF). The phrase "grossly deficient" is interesting when we consider Dr. Price's work regarding the poor quality of refined foods in use in the west in the first half of the 20th century.

We read this work not knowing *why* it was grossly deficient. The author had previously suggested fluoride as a mineral should be investigated. The author concluded:

> "Good nutrition is important for general well-being and health, but neither good nutrition nor freedom from systemic disease offers any substantial assistance in prevention of dental caries." [711]

A modern quote from the American Dental Association is justified. The ADA's *Policies and Recommendations on Diet and Nutrition* is available on their website. The first part of their statement begins:

> "... oral health depends on proper nutrition and healthy eating habits, and necessarily includes avoiding a steady diet of foods containing natural and added sugars, processed starches and low pH-level acids..." [712]

Nutrition is a field that can go on forever, it seems. We have incredible numbers of studies and tests, much of which are conflicting. Our knowledge is vast in scope, yet we seem to create the same degenerative conditions generation after generation, often earlier and earlier. No doubt people will argue about it getting better or worse. We did not have children with cancer until a few decades ago; nowadays whole organizations devote themselves to preventing such occurrences. One is reminded of the phrase "learning and learning yet never coming to a knowledge of the truth." [713]

Being bogged down in details is sometimes appropriate for clarification of technicalities and fine-tuning one's diet to one's lifestyle. A look at larger principles is more fitting when so many of us have the same underlying illnesses. A look at nutrition is not intended to diminish the relevance of factors like genetics, evolution, climate and technology.

Following the simple principles presented in Dr. Price's work would require a much more environmentally conscious society, something notoriously bad for corporate profits. Independence and freedom in lifestyle were no doubt also factors in the happiness Dr. Price observed in the more nature-oriented races; such things are probably not in line with the business community's employment goals [530, 618]. Business lore alone would be enough to disqualify not only Dr. Price's work, but the consequences of our collective meditation upon such work.

6.4 How Much Fluoride is too Much? What do the Experts and Media Say?

"Certainly it seems on the basis of the evidence and opinions herewith presented – evidence and opinions supplied by leaders in preventive medicine, public health, biologic research and general medical practice – that no one, except the most biased, could question the safety of water fluoridation."

- Lon W. Morrey, D.D.S., Editorial, **Journal of the American Dental Association**, Vol. 49, No. 3, p. 365, September, 1954.

"Seven respondents opposed to water fluoridation also referred to indemnification, suggesting that if water fluoridation was so safe, why was there a need for local authorities to be indemnified against legal action."

- Brisbane Lord Mayor's Taskforce, p. 77, 1997. One example of legal protection can be given. *Health: Protecting Fluoridators*, **The Bulletin**, pp. 7-8, 24th August, 1963. I have not looked for recent work on this topic.

"There are no definitive limits in the scientific literature concerning safe and unsafe doses of fluoride. Responses can vary considerably between individuals depending on a range of factors, including age, body weight, nutritional status, etc."

- Brisbane Lord Mayor's Taskforce, p. 42, 1997.

"Water fluoridation is a population-level caries preventive strategy. Therefore, the appropriate method of measuring effectiveness is to look at the population level effect rather than look at the effect on any given individual."

- Professor Jason M. Armfield, *Debate: When public action undermines public health: a critical examination of antifluoridationist literature*, **Australia and New Zealand Health Policy**, 2007, 4: 25, p. 6.

This will show some of the differing statements expert Community Water Fluoridation (CWF) supporters have made on how much fluorine is harmful, and highlight some of the communication issues involved. The focus is more on historical than recent statements. I will remind the reader that expert literature often relies on very old research, for instance the 2005 textbook citing the 1950 study with regard to unsubstantiated claims of fluorine deficiency [87, 91]. Another example is the more recent National Academy of Science (NAS) document using studies from 1937 and 1942 with regard to fluorosis in children, mentioned in Chapter 6.2. Another example is given in this chapter.

In looking back through the history of CWF, I have found that many experts supportive of the practice have expressed quite contradictory statements regarding exactly how much fluorine is harmful. That the media have not seen or spoken on this is a testament to their lack of knowledge on the matter. Again we can see a failure of memory. Media believe experts (supporters) and opponents of CWF are highly contradictory in their statements, and this is true. Also true is that experts are highly contradictory themselves in their statements. The same is true for people opposed in various areas, but this is not surprising given the variety of people who oppose CWF. Yet we hear many times that 'all the experts agree'. Undoubtedly there is agreement on the issues of safety and benefit, yet when one looks at details, differences emerge. The unity we see in media is sometimes only in media, as the topic of a nutritional role can demonstrate.

Because the experts have a bias toward exaggerating the necessity of fluorine, they almost certainly have a bias towards minimizing harm and accentuating benefits from CWF, so it is probably extremely difficult to find studies in academic literature that suggest harm from CWF and are well-known. Experts by and large do not even want to accept fluorine is non-essential, how then are they capable of objectively investigating and appraising research discussing harm?

The matter of safety is complicated by discussing parts per million in water as a *concentration*, versus the amount of fluorine taken into the body, as a *dose*.

In September of 1943, the **Journal of the American Medical Association** published an editorial which read:

> "Distribution of the element fluorine is so widespread throughout nature that a small intake of the element is practically unavoidable. Fluorides are general protoplasmic poisons, probably because of their capacity to modify the metabolism of cells by changing the permeability of the cell membrane and by inhibiting certain enzyme systems." [714]

> "The sources of fluorine intoxication are drinking water containing 1 part per million or more of fluorine, fluorine compounds used as insecticidal sprays for fruits and vegetables (cryolite and barium fluosilicate) and the mining and conversion of phosphate rock to superphosphate, which is used as fertilizer."

> "The known effects of chronic fluorine intoxication are those of hypoplasia of the teeth, which has been called mottled enamel, and of bone sclerosis. The classic epidemiologic studies of McKay clearly demonstrated the relationship of the fluorine content of the domestic water supply to the anomaly of mottled enamel of the teeth. The condition is now known to be endemic in isolated communities on every continent."

> "Dean and McKay succeeded in the unique epidemiologic experiment of arresting the production of the endemic mottled enamel at Oakley, Ida., Bauxite, Ark., and Andover, S. D., by changing the common water supply from one containing amounts of fluorides toxic to calcifying dental enamel to one the fluoride content of which does not exceed the permissible maximum, i. e. 1 part per million. Children using domestic waters containing as little as 1 part per million of fluorine experience only a half to a third as much dental decay as comparable groups using fluoride-free water, such as the Lake Michigan or the Mississippi River waters. The same inverse relationship has been observed in England, South India and North Africa. Apparently teeth require traces of fluorine for optimum dental health, although excessive amounts may result in the disfiguring condition known as mottled enamel."

Regarding anemia in one population exposed to excessive cryolite dust, the editorial claimed that fifteen years exposure brought about the observable symptoms of the condition.

> "The incidence and severity of the disease had a definite relationship to the economic and nutritional status of the community. A pronounced deficiency of the vitamin C factor in the diet was especially associated with a severe incidence of the disease. Factors other than the amount of fluorine in the water supply may assume a contributory role in the development of chronic fluorine intoxication." [714]

In August of 1944, Dr. Muriel Bell authored an article published in New Zealand's **The Listener**, which read:

> "... the presence of more than one or two parts of fluorine per million parts of water in the reservoirs serving certain areas was attended by an ugly mottling of the enamel; the teeth became pitted and discoloured, and in severe cases dental decay occurred in these teeth." [191]

This changed, and by 1958 she wrote in a letter to a newspaper editor that fluorine was almost harmless in concentrations as high as 14 ppm (naturally occurring), excepting fluorosis, which she claimed did not occur at 1 ppm [196]. This change in opinion was caused by her studies in America in the early 1950s; in her paper *Medical and Nutritional Aspects of Fluoridation* she discussed work done in Bauxite, Arkansas, claiming that American doctors would have noticed any adverse effects from people who were using 14 ppm fluoride in water [715]. There was no mention of her **Listener** article in this paper.

In October of 1944, an editorial appeared in the **Journal of the American Dental Association** that claimed:

> "We do know that the use of drinking water containing as little as 1.2 to 3.0 part per million of fluorine will cause such developmental disturbances in bones as osteosclerosis, spondylosis and osteopetrosis, as well as goiter, and we cannot afford to run the risk of producing such serious systemic disturbances in applying what is at present a doubtful procedure intended to prevent development of dental disfigurements among children."
> [716]

I read about this editorial in Donald McNeil's 1957 book *The Fight for Fluoridation* (pages 74-75). McNeil claimed readers of the **Journal** had written after its publication, saying it promoted "alarm". McNeil accurately cited the editorial in his references (and the apology that followed in the December issue, yet still claimed more research was needed – fluoridation began in January 1945), but only quoted the last part of another sentence: "... the potentialities for harm far outweigh those for good."

It is commendable that McNeil quoted what he did, yet we don't see any discussion of bone disturbances, any detail. Harold Hillenbrand (mentioned briefly in Chapter 5.5), and L. Pierce Anthony, DDS, were editors of the **Journal** in 1944.

I wondered if the chapter *'Battle-Axe Bell': The Fight for Fluoridation* in Diana Brown's book [186] was homage to McNeil's work of the same name, (Brown told me it wasn't). Both omitted detail regarding ideas on concentrations thought to be excessive from 1944. Discussion of fluorine deficiency in Brown's book is present. This is understandable given that she kept purely to Dr. Bell's research, writing and opinion; and it is so easy to find conflicting claims in scientific literature. So I don't blame Brown for avoiding modern statements. I must point out that in her work there is no discussion on recent or current claims regarding the words of bodies such as the EFSA or SCHER disagreeing with Dr. Bell's claims of a nutritional role for fluorine. In one sense this is fair enough as it would have detracted from her focus on Dr. Bell. Brown told me she carried out her research in 2005. Yet the modern reader is rescued from the discomfort of contradiction. I believe a resourceful researcher like Brown would not have missed these comments *if* the New Zealand media had publicized them. Regarding promotion, a one-sided approach is most apparent on page 115, when we read the claim that "contemporary observers found that 'the pattern of opposition [to fluoridation] ... was almost identical with overseas experience.'" An absolutely true, yet rather audacious statement when given without its counterpart: that New Zealand promoters were also heavily influenced by American and British experts; Drs. Arnold and Parfitt, Captain Losee, Dr. Wallace Armstrong[154], and of course Dr. Bell's own admiration of Professor McCollum[155] [715] and Dr. Fredrick Stare (McCollum and Stare are mentioned in Brown's book). Although New Zealand experts (as did most American experts) jumped on the claim that fluorine was a nutritional essential and refused to publicly deviate, even when the American research they claimed to admire so much told an opposite, or more confusing story.

In many other ways Diana Brown's book is excellent and I recommend it.

This editorial [716] also discussed the work of Margaret and H. V. Smith that was published in the September, 1940 issue of the **American Journal of Public Health**. The Smiths reported on a community which had a water supply with between 1.6 and 4.0 ppm fluorine. They wrote that while fluorine seemed to yield a protection from bacteria, the teeth were "structurally weak" (according to the ADA editorial). To quote the Smiths:

> "Very rarely, adults were found whose teeth, though mottled, were free from caries."
>
> "It would appear therefore, that even though fluorine ingestion during the period of tooth formation may produce teeth which offer more resistance to bacterial invasion, the disadvantage of the resulting poorly constructed, internally weak, mottled teeth may far more than offset the advantage of a greater resistance to external invasion by bacteria."
>
> "Cox[156] makes rather sweeping conclusions and very broad recommendations for the application of his findings made on rats to the dental ills of the human race. He goes so far as to state that addition of fluorides to community water supplies provides an 'attractive means of mass reduction of dental caries; that prophylactic measures through other media such as bottled water, milk supply, and fluorine containing medicinals are feasible; and that means of control of fluorine in the whole dietary of children should be undertaken.' To one who is familiar with the disfiguring dental defect known as mottled enamel which affects the teeth of every person who drinks water containing as little as 1 p.p.m. of fluorine during the years of tooth formation, this recommendation seems, to put it mildly, unsafe." [717]

The statement from the **Journal of the American Dental Association** [716] ("We do know that..." quoted previously) was quoted *exactly* on the back cover of Anne-Lise Gotzche's 1975 book that was critical of fluoridation, but not mentioned in two reviews of her book [718, 719].

It is quite possible that the Smiths were discussing the effects of excess fluorine *and* malnutrition without knowing it. It appears that as a person becomes more malnourished, the threshold at which amounts of fluorine become toxic is lowered.

This was discussed in 1952 by two dentists, Drs. Maury Massler and Isaac Schour in the **Journal of the American Dental Association**:

---

[154] See a letter from K. E. Swann of NZ's Fluoridation Committee to Dr. Armstrong dated 12th December, 1958, HD 125/299/1 Box H1 1766, 1958-1961.
[155] Though McCollum did not appear in Diana Brown's index.
[156] The Smiths cite Cox, G. J., *et al.* **J. Dent. Research**, 18:469, 1939.

"The data from this and other investigations suggest that malnourished infants and children, especially if deficient in calcium intake, may suffer from the effects of water containing fluorine while healthy children would remain unaffected." [720]

They suggest mottling caused by excessive fluoride may be caused by deficiencies of calcium, and would not occur if these were non-existent.

"Thus low levels of fluoride ingestion which are generally considered to be safe for the general population may not be safe for malnourished infants and children."

"Nutritional studies should be included in any comprehensive program of fluoridation of water with special attention to chronically ailing infants and children."

This is one reason why I have advocated the subsidization of healthier foods. Given that many working people have barely enough money after their bills to buy even cheap foods, I think this would be a helpful social policy if we care about the poor.

"The poorer the nutritional status and the lower the calcium intake, the more prevalent and more severe the mottling." [720]

This has the added convenience of allowing supporters of fluoridation to abdicate responsibility for the mottling of children's teeth in fluoridated areas – because the responsibility of calcium intake and the like are ultimately shouldered by parents and caregivers, sometimes schools and governments.

Three issues later in the same journal, the editor made the statement:

"Cox and Ast[157] point out that even in the case of gross negligence it would require more than four tons of sodium fluoride per million gallons of water processed to produce a concentration of 450 ppm fluorine – sufficient to produce salivation and vomiting – and such a concentration they point out is not possible in any program of water fluoridation." [721]

The article was responding to claims that fluoridation was a bad idea because compounds at waterworks sites could be overfed by military enemies into the supply. I have no comment here on the relevance or realism of such a statement.

Bernard and Judith Mausner responded to the same claim in their article published in **Scientific American** in 1955:

"Enormous amounts of fluoride, more than is ever normally stored at a water-treatment station, would be required to produce a concentration high enough even to mottle the teeth." [722]

The Mausners probably meant in terms of concentration, *not* a cumulative dose. The statement ought to be compared with the NAS' 1951 statement on mottling:

"At approximately 1.0 ppm, less than 10 per cent of children [158] show the least detectable evidence of disturbance in enamel formation, which are not visible except to the trained eye of the examining dentist.

---

[157] Charles R. Cox and David B. Ast, *Water Fluoridation – a Sound Public Health Measure*, **Journal of the American Waterworks Association**, Vol. 43 (August), p. 641, 1951.

[158] "The epidemiological studies of Dean (1942), based upon examination of 5,824 white children in ten states, showed direct correlation between severity of the manifestations of mottled enamel and the increasing fluoride content (up to 5 ppm) of the

Beginning at about 2 ppm, an increasing proportion of children have mottled enamel of a grade that is easily apparent. While such teeth are caries-resistant, they are esthetically objectionable." [74] (page 25)

Again, we are not dealing with an amount in a human body, but a concentration in water. The Mausners' article ends with the sentence:

"However, an attempt, at least, to understand anti-intellectualism and to meet it on its own ground should make it easier to defeat." [722]

In 1957, the Commission of Inquiry from New Zealand quoted Sir Charles Hercus of Otago University. Sir Hercus quoted a letter from Professor Sosman, Emeritus Professor of Radiology at Harvard. The excerpt quoted reads:

"In summary I would say that from my study of the material I would conclude that fluorine of 8ppm in the drinking water has no deleterious effect on the individual living in the area and drinking that water. In fact there may be a slight benefit in the sense that it keeps the bones from softening as the patients grow older." [723]

In 1959 the experiment by Wuthier and Phillips was published in the **Journal of Nutrition**. I mentioned in Chapter 1 that this experiment was not cited anywhere near as frequently as other experiments. I believe the reason for this was the first sentence:

"There is a paucity of data on the long-term effects of the intake of small amounts of fluoride on experimental animals, despite the consensus of opinion to the contrary." [18]

The word 'paucity' means 'a very small amount'.

In 1989, the National Academy of Sciences claimed in **Diet and Health Implications**:

"A fluoride concentration of 4 ppm has been associated with an increased incidence of caries[159]." [80]

Note that this is a concentration, not a dose. In the 2002 textbook *Essentials of Human Nutrition*, Stewart Truswell and Marion Robinson authored the section on fluoride. Regarding the upper limits, they wrote:

"... toxic effects start at about 10 mg/day." [125]

Other research claiming lower amounts of fluoride harmful were not mentioned. The authors cite the 1980 and 1989 US **Recommended Dietary Allowances**, from the NAS. The **Diet and Health Implications** that was also published in 1989 was not mentioned.

The 1989 **Recommended Dietary Allowances** claimed:

"The estimated range of safe and adequate intakes of fluoride for adults is 1.5 to 4.0 mg/day. This takes into account the widely varying fluoride concentrations of diets consumed in the United States and includes both food sources and drinking water. For younger age groups, the range is reduced to a maximal level of 2.5 mg in order to avoid mottling of the teeth. Ranges of 0.1 to 1 mg during the first year of life and 0.5 to 1.5 mg during the subsequent 2 years are suggested as adequate and safe." [724]

---

water supplies upon which they were dependent." H. T. Dean, *The investigation of physiological effects by the epidemiological method*, in *Fluorine and Dental Health*. F. R. Moultin ed., pub. No. 19, A. A. A. S., Lancaster, Science Press, pp. 23-31, 1942.

[159] The NAS cites: Ericsson, S.Y. 1977. *Cariostatic mechanisms of fluorides: clinical observations*. **Caries Res**. 11 Suppl. 1:2-41, and Jenkins, G.N. 1978. *Fluoride*, pp. 466-500 in *The Physiology and Biochemistry of the Mouth*, 4th ed. Blackwell Scientific Publications, Oxford.

The fact that the 1989 document claimed 4.0 mg/day may cause an increase in caries was not mentioned. The following statements are from *Essentials of Human Nutrition*:

"The skeleton is affected by chronic high levels of fluoride intake as from drinking water with 4-12 ppm fluoride. This may cause dense bones and joint abnormalities; skeletal fluorosis occurs in parts of India, China and South Africa. Large doses of fluoride have been used in the treatment of osteoporosis, but the bone quality tends to be poor, fractures may increase, and there are doubts about the safety of such treatment." (page 184)

"It is widely agreed that fluoridation of drinking water to a level of 1 ppm F has no known adverse health effects. There is no good evidence that fluoridated water is associated with allergic reactions and hypersensitivity..." (page 185)

"The issue of fractures remains unresolved; if there is an increased risk of hip fractures, it is likely to be very slight." (page 185) [125]

The 1996 World Health Organization document cited in Chapter 2.3 claimed:

"There are indications that susceptibility to the dental mottling of fluorosis is increased by generalized malnutrition[160]. In the absence of malnutrition dental mottling has been reported very occasionally when the fluoride content of drinking-water has exceeded 0.8 mg/l. However, it is rarely significant from the age of 4 years onwards unless fluoride intake from the diet plus drinking water exceeds 2 mg/l or the intake from water alone exceeds 1.5 mg/day." [105] (page 192)

Note that in 1996, a study from 1948 can be cited without comment from experts, the WHO loses not a whit of credibility or prestige, and the reason more recent studies are not cited is not an issue.

In 1997, the Brisbane Lord Mayor's Taskforce claimed:

"The Taskforce were aware from the literature that chronic fluoride intake of 1-2 ppm can lead to dental fluorosis, while intake of 4 ppm could lead to skeletal fluorosis (though some reports have indicated that skeletal fluorosis can occur in people exposed to fluoride levels as low as 0.7ppm)[161]." [610] (page 42)

Again, we are looking at concentration in water, not an amount going into one's body accumulating over time. One would think a public health policy given with such confidence would have engendered more precision. No doubt the experts will point to the words of Professor Armfield quoted at the beginning of this chapter.

In 2002 a WHO committee wrote:

"There is clear evidence from India and China that skeletal fluorosis and an increased risk of bone fractures occur at total intakes of 14 mg fluoride/day and evidence suggestive of an increased risk of bone effects at total intakes above about 6 mg fluoride/day." [725]

I will remind the reader that the fluorine concentrations in food cited by the WHO and NAS are at the lower end of the spectrum. European and Asian work has been largely excluded here.

---

[160] Murray MM, Wilson DC. *Fluorosis and nutrition in Morocco; dental studies in relation to environment.* **British Dental Journal,** 1948, **84:** 97-100 is cited here.

[161] Here, the taskforce cited the 1991 Australian National Health and Medical Research Council study *Effectiveness of Water Fluoridation.* I discussed this 1991 document a little in Chapter 6.1. This 1991 document overwhelmingly claimed CWF safe and effective. The studies in question were A. Singh and S. S. Jolly and B. C. Bansal, *Skeletal fluorosis and its neurological complications,* **The Lancet,** Vol. 1, pp. 197-200, 1961; and U. K. Misra, M. Husain, G. Newton, D. Nag and P. K. Ray, *Endemic fluorosis and presenting as cervical cord depression,* **Archives of Environmental Health,** Vol. 43, pp. 18-21, 1988.

A 1953 article from a Delaware newspaper claimed:

"Actually there is no such thing as 'artificial fluoridation.' Fluorides are always added to water, generally being picked up by the water running through underground passages and crevices where the ground contains various fluoride compounds. In this process, man has no control over the concentration. The same results occur whether the fluoride is added in controlled amounts or whether added by nature, except that safety is assured when fluoride is added in controlled amounts."

The article also addressed the possibility of harm from overdosing:

"Engineers of the American Water Works Association report that equipment used for adding fluorides to water is accurate within 5%. The amount of fluorides added to water is so small that it would be impossible, even with gross negligence, to increase the concentration to a dangerous or harmful level." [726]

The "accurate within 5%" claim is surprising in light of what was happening in our own city of Hastings in 1953 and 1954.

In 1980 the **Journal of Nutrition Education** reported that of eight people

"... undergoing renal dialysis in an Annapolis, Maryland hospital became ill during or within 12 hours after completion of dialysis. One patient died, and 5 others were hospitalized and recovered." [727]

The article claimed that the tissue and serum concentrations of fluoride were "generally high in those samples measured" (no numbers given).

The death occurred on the 12th or 13th of November, 1979.

A worker at the water plant left a valve open, which caused an overdose of fluoride. The **Baltimore Sun** reported that

"Dr. Sorbey [Chief of Maryland's Division of Communicable Diseases] said yesterday that the fluoride level in the Annapolis water supply may have been as high as 36 ppm November 13. A sample taken the next day by state health investigators showed levels of 23 ppm."

"The fluoride level in the Annapolis water supply may have been even higher than first announced, state officials said." [728]

A report co-written by Sorbey, appearing in the Center for Disease Control's journal **Morbidity Mortality Weekly Report**, and discussed in the **Journal of Nutrition Education**, reported in 1980 that the highest level of fluoride in Annapolis' city drinking water was 7.5 ppm:

"This spill apparently reached the public water supply, although the maximum concentration measured was only 7.5 ppm, considerably lower than that in the dialysis fluid." [727]

This figure of 7.5 ppm came from the CDC's journal:

"Subsequent investigation by the Maryland State Department of Health and Mental Hygiene revealed that on November 11, 1979, a technician at the Annapolis water treatment plant had failed to close a valve to stop the flow of 22% hydrofluosilicic acid from a 4,000-gallon storage tank to a 50-gallon fluoride feed container. One thousand gallons of the acid overflowed into drains leading to sand-filter-backwash and sludge-decant tanks from which decanted liquid was recycled as raw water. The accident had not been reported to the health officials. Daily water samples were routinely tested for fluoride level by the treatment plant personnel using a colorimetric dye method capable of measuring up to 1.6 ppm[162]; during the 2 days following the accident, fluoride levels were at least 1.6 ppm. On November 14, through serial dilutions made with commercial distilled water, a water sample was measured at 7.5 ppm fluoride." [729]

The spill occurred on the 11th of November, measurement was made three days later on November 14. It is very important to see that the maximum amount of fluoride capable of measurement was 1.6 ppm, before dilution. The **Journal of Nutrition Education** pointed out neither of these.

The **Baltimore Sun** also reported that

"Even though state and county health officials had learned of the spill nine days after it occurred, no public announcement was made and the Annapolis City Council was not told of the situation for six more days, according to accounts from officials involved."

'We didn't want to jeopardize the fluoridation program because it has been so good for children' explained Charles M. Yost, a deputy to the county health officer. 'You have to wait until you're really sure there is a problem before you go out and panic people.'" [728]

This was reported on the 28th November, 1979. Consider Mr. Yost's final statement in relation to the precautionary principle [583].

The wife of the 65-year-old dialysis victim took the city to court. The **Sun** reported:

"Judge Martin A. Wolff ruled the city was acting as a business by supplying customers with water and is 'liable in the same manner as any corporation.' An autopsy showed the spill was a 'contributory' factor in his death." [730]

Dr. Sorbey's report pointed out, contrary to what Judge Wolff had said about the autopsy:

"Although it is certainly possible that the fluoride spill contributed to the illness of 7 and death of 1 person undergoing dialysis for end-stage renal disease, this report does not provide cause-and-effect evidence." [727]

I use the word 'contrary' because we've gone from a "contributory factor" to "certainly possible that the fluoride spill contributed..." If the word 'possible' was in the autopsy, the newspaper did not use it, and Sorbey and co-authors did not discuss it. I've been unable so far to obtain the autopsy.

It appears that the media were unaware of what was written in the **Journal of Nutrition Education** regarding the change from a "contributory factor" to "certainly possible that the fluoride spill contributed..." and perhaps never asked for a death certificate or autopsy report to show to their critically thinking audience. So people received different information depending on whether they read the newspaper or the journal.

The experts support the program so I would expect them to minimize any claim of harm it may cause even in extreme cases like this. It would not be in their interests to do otherwise. This may explain why experts sometimes get offended by media in this issue. This example demonstrates that those who read academic literature will believe the fluoridation programs are safer than those who read more public media, and may help to explain scepticism from the public.

---

[162] Bellack E. *Fluoridation Engineering Manual.* Washington, DC: Environmental Protection Agency, 1974. (EPA publication no. EPA-502/9-74-022).

Three years later, it was announced that Pepsi-Cola, who had to destroy 4,600 cases of their product due to excessive fluoride levels, also sued the city in a $1.6M suit. Both parties settled out of court.

"Mr. Sussman [City Solicitor] would not comment on reports that [widower] Mrs. Blake received less than $100,000 in the settlement…"

Mrs. Blake's suit was for $1.5M.

"He also would not discuss the amount paid to Pepsi-Cola. Mrs. Blake also declined to say how much money she received in the settlement, but she expressed dissatisfaction with the amount. The settlement was agreed to only to avoid a lengthy trial and publicity, she said." [730]

The **Journal of Nutrition Education** reported that

"Locally bottled soda had as high as 30 ppm of fluoride the day after the fluoride spill; the report does not mention whether or not the bottling company used fluoride compounds for sanitation purposes, although this has been the case in this industry." [727]

A statement from *Fluoridation Facts: Answers to Criticisms Against Fluoridation*, published by the American Dental Association, April, 1956, responded to the assertion that "An accident in the water plant might cause over-dosage and severe harmful effects":

"Acute morbidity manifested by increased salivation and vomiting may be caused by ingesting 0.25 grams sodium fluoride. This quantity in an 8-oz glass of water represents 1,000 ppm sodium fluoride, or about 450 ppm fluorine. To obtain this concentration, it would require more than four tons of sodium fluoride per million gallons of water processed which is obviously not possible in a program of water fluoridation, even if gross negligence occurred." [731]

In 2016, the **British Dental Journal** echoed the words of Professor Armfield:

"Water fluoridation is not a clinical intervention done to an individual. It is a population level intervention and should be judged as such." [732]

There were ten studies cited in support of this sentence. This approach of looking at a 'population' rather than 'individuals' takes no account of the range of impacts on those individuals.

The 2005 article mentioned in Chapter 6.1 from the **British Dental Journal** discussed the York Review:

"The question of the safety of water fluoridation has been investigated time and time again by a variety of national and international commissions, most notably in recent times by the NHS Centre for Reviews and Dissemination in 2000 (the York Review). This was a Systematic Review – which means that all relevant studies in all languages and in all publications were searched for and critically evaluated using validated guidelines. Over 3,000 studies relevant to dental and general effects of water fluoridation on humans were identified. York's main conclusion was that there was no clear evidence of any adverse effect from water fluoridation other than staining of enamel (dental fluorosis)." [623]

Quoting the York Review:

"214 studies met full inclusion criteria for one or more of the objectives."

This was 214 out of 3,246.

"Given the level of interest surrounding the issue of public water fluoridation, it is surprising to find that little high quality research has been undertaken."

"The evidence of a benefit of a reduction in caries should be considered together with the increased prevalence of dental fluorosis. The research evidence is of insufficient quality to allow confident statements about other potential harms or whether there is an impact on social inequalities. This evidence on benefits and harms needs to be considered along with the ethical, environmental, ecological, costs and legal issues that surround any decisions about water fluoridation. All of these issues fell outside the scope of this review." [733]

In discussing what has been said about how much fluorine is harmful, we must acknowledge a complication regarding the relationship between the public and the media. The book recommended to us by Dr. Fredrick Stare in 1981, authored by Drs. Stephen Barrett and Sheldon Rovin, suggested how campaigners for CWF should act if their local paper suggested CWF was harmful, or published the writings of people who did so:

"If the editor agrees to help you, your political action subcommittee should generate letters congratulating him on this decision. If he does not, and letters are published which claim that fluoridation is dangerous, the newspaper should be bombarded with a steady stream of letters (not for publication) suggesting that irresponsible claims should be curbed. In addition, at every contact between committee members and reporters, a plea should be made to ignore anti claims of dangerousness when writing news reports." (page 74) [291]

Regarding rat experiments cited here, I find fluoride levels in rodent food of interest. The United States Public Health Service quoted Schroeder *et al.* as claiming fluorine harmless in mice at 10 ppm:

"In no way are these data to be construed as recommending actual limits. They merely show which elements showed recondite toxicity in small mammals in the doses given and which did not, as far as could be ascertained." [170]

"Mice fed [10 ppm] fluoride [in water] and antimony survived as well as their controls."

"According to measured life spans, male mice fed fluorine lived longer than their controls by 29 to 60 days at 3 intervals, whereas females did not." [30]

Perhaps the third statement can be explained by the pharmacological effect observed in the 1976 experiments.

Compare the 1954 and 1957 experiments [13, 17] – one found a seventy-eight percent reduction in dental caries from fluorine addition (10 ppm to a diet certainly lacking in other factors), the other found the fluorine (2 ppm) and non-fluorine (<0.007 ppm) groups "indistinguishable". These results suggest a potential benefit from fluorine if the mineral aspects of diet are compromised. The matter is complicated by the fact that rodents have a much higher tolerance for fluorine than humans. Also consider the 1952 study by Massler and Schour, demonstrating poorer nutrition lead to an increased susceptibility to detrimental effects of excess fluorine [720]. In Dr. Armstrong's experiment, we read:

"... commercial rodent food contains 40-60 p.p.m. F." [29]

Ophaug and Magil wrote:

"In addition to the experimental groups of animals, a control group was fed commercial rat chow (Purina Laboratory) containing 200 ppm of iron, 8 ppm of copper, and 20-60 ppm of fluoride." (page 414) [34]

I have seen very little work on particle size of naturally-occurring fluoride salts.

I suspect differing particle sizes of naturally-occurring fluorides is a possible reason why such a wide range of 'harmful' and 'safe' concentrations have been claimed.

Obviously a fluorine ion with its small size and negative charge is easily absorbed into the body. A larger particle made of thousands of ions, positive and negative – literally a tiny lump of rock – probably has very different behavior in the body. In this hypothetical instance, I would suggest much less fluorine is absorbed because it is already bound to a cation in a particle. Natural water from rivers without industrial influence is probably very different to city drinking water in terms of its particulate composition. Even though a fluorine ion is a fluorine ion is a fluorine ion, I do not think it entirely accurate to claim CWF 'natural' for this reason. Free-floating fluorine ions are possibly quite different in their absorption into the mammalian body compared with fluorine already bound to fine dirt particles and sediment found in natural water. In 1954, we read in the midst of the Hastings fluoridation experiment:

> "To the letter of Mr. A. N. S. Moore, one short answer suffices: Millions of people in the United Kingdom and United States have lived for many generations on water supplies containing one part per million and more than this, with no ill-effects..." [734]

The paragraph continues: "... and their teeth are infinitely superior to those of peoples living in areas with water supplies deficient in this trace element." If there is occasional truth to this, perhaps it is due to particles in naturally occurring water being quite different to what we get in city water. This is obviously complicated by pollution. Underwood discussed particle size in 1971:

> "Under most conditions the more soluble forms of fluorine, such as sodium fluoride, are more toxic per unit of fluorine than are the highly insoluble compounds, such as calcium fluoride."

> "Particle size may also have a bearing on toxicity. The finer the particle size the more nearly the toxicity of cryolite approaches that of sodium fluoride[163]." (page 388)

> "Sodium fluoride or cryolite provided in the drinking water promotes greater fluorine retention in the rat than a dry diet supplying the same intakes of those compounds[164]. Further, NaF given in milk to young rats in relatively low concentrations is less available than when similarly administered in water[165]." [735]

I must apologize that I have not found more work on this that is both recent and detailed. Experts claim CWF to be natural and that is that [726, 736]. This is an interesting view given so much technology must be involved.

I often wonder if we are giving credit or blame only to an anion when a cation may also have some influence[166]. Could this explain not only the existence of some of our high percentages, but the incredible *range* of percentages?

---

[163] Underwood cites M. Lawrenz and H. H. Mitchell, **Journal of Nutrition**, Vol. 22, pp. 451 and 621, 1941; and K. Roholm, *Fluorine Intoxication*, Lewis, London, 1937.

[164] Citing M. Lawrenz, H. H. Mitchell, and W. A. Ruth, **Journal of Nutrition**, Vol. 19, p. 531, 1940, Vol. 20, p. 383, 1940; and D. A. Weddle and J. C. Muhler, **Journal of Nutrition**, Vol. 54, p. 437, 1954.

[165] D. A. Weddle and J. C. Muhler, **Journal of Nutrition**, Vol. 55, p. 347, 1955.

[166] The **Auckland Star** reported that calcium fluoride was to be used for CWF in 1965 (14th December).

6.5 The Current State of Affairs Regarding a Nutritional Role for Fluorine

"There's been more research on fluoride than on any other essential element. It is an essential element. You couldn't live without fluoride."

- Dr. John Dodes, D.D.S., Quoted in *The Tooth About Dentistry* hosted by Karen Stollznow, available from *Point of Inquiry with Paul Fidalgo*, http://www.pointofinquiry.org/john_dodes_the_tooth_about_dentistry/ (about 6½ minutes into the interview), 5th September, 2011.

"No signs of fluoride deficiency have been identified in humans... caries is not a fluoride deficiency disease... Fluoride is not an essential nutrient."

- *"Scientific Opinion on Dietary Reference Values for Fluoride*, **European Food Safety Authority Journal**, Vol. 11, No. 8, 3332, p. 10, 2013.

"... fluoridation is not medication – it just simply corrects a deficiency."

- Dr. Ken Perrott, Science Advisor of Making Sense of Fluoride, *Fluoridation – Topical Confusion*, (comments section, 17th July, 2013), 10th July, 2013 (article publication date). https://openparachute.wordpress.com/2013/07/10/fluoridation-topical-confusion/.

"The purpose of water fluoridation has never been intended to be to correct any sort of fluoride deficiency."

- Dr. Steve Slott of the American Fluoridation Society, *Dr. Paul Connett Gets Schooled*, 26th April, 2015, Making Sense of Fluoride website, http://msof.nz/2015/04/dr-paul-connett-gets-schooled/.

"If you ever want something put out on your work or whatever, just email it to me and I'll put it in front of three hundred thousand dentists for you."

- Dr. Howard Farran D.D.S. to Dr. Ken Perrott, *Fluoridation: My Podcast with Howard Farran*, posted on 31st March, 2016. https://openparachute.wordpress.com/2016/03/31/fluoridation-my-podcast-with-with-howard-farran/.

All of the people quoted at the start of this chapter support and advocate for community water supplies to be fluoridated.

Beyond those already given, there is another way in which fluoride is different to normal nutritional components. The World Health Organization (WHO) claimed in 1996:

"... dental mottling may be taken as a definitive indication of toxicity." [105]

In 2002 the WHO claimed:

"In children, intakes of fluoride associated with beneficial effects on dentition overlap with those that lead to an increased prevalence of dental fluorosis." [737]

Calcium's 'optimal range' – an amount in between 'not enough' and 'too much' – is not harmful. The same can be said for iodine, magnesium and other nutritional factors. Yet the range of intake for fluoride that apparently leads to increased caries prevention *is* harmful, in the sense that it causes dental fluorosis. I suggest this is a powerful argument that fluorine not be considered a nutritional essential. Iodine does not damage a thyroid in correcting iodine deficiency.

Regarding bone, in 1970 the WHO claimed:

"Fluoride is not deposited uniformly throughout a given bone and may be related to the rate of growth and the degree of vascularization in various parts of the same bone." [738]

Fluoride migrates to the ends of bone, the joints. Another possible argument against fluorine's essentiality has to do with its excretion. In 1996, the WHO claimed:

"Individuals living in endemic, high-fluoride areas have been shown to have positive fluoride balances, but these change to negative ones when they are withdrawn from environmental exposure. However, they continue to excrete abnormally large quantities of fluoride long after their removal from such areas."

This document discusses the amount in water:

"Long-term exposure to high levels of fluoride leads to dental destruction. As drinking-water fluoride increases above 1 mg of fluoride/L, a variety of clinical symptoms of toxicity may develop. The blood concentration of fluoride increases from the value for normal blood fluoride of 0.04, µg/ml to values as high as 0.5-8.0, µg/ml, which have been reported in patients exhibiting clinical signs of fluorosis. The term fluorosis covers a wide spectrum of clinical manifestations related to fluoride toxicity. Fluoride is a cumulative toxin." (page 189) [105]

In New Zealand, the Ministry of Health adjusts fluoridated water supplies to between 0.7 and 1.0 ppm [558]. The problem for us is that 0.7-1.0 mg/Litre is a concentration in *water*, not an amount in *our body*. If we were to drink the Ministry of Health's recommended 8 glasses of water per day, we would be drinking between 1.4 and 2 mg fluorine per day. Add to this an unknown amount in our food, drugs and consumer products. The National Academy of Sciences claimed 4 ppm fluorine is associated with an increase in caries, but did not state how much of this water was consumed. It is worth remembering the experts are probably very biased against any conclusion from harm occurring among populations using water fluoridated at 0.7-1 ppm. When they look at effects, they claim it is on populations, not individuals [732, 418 (page 6)].

The fact that fluorine is not required in any metabolic or biochemical pathways, that it is not only very abundant but accumulates throughout life [296], and the fact that the body excretes it, demonstrates that supplementing this element is probably unnecessary and wasteful, not to mention burdensome for many.

Also of consideration here is the work of Dr. Price, who found every healthy culture went almost out of their way to get seafood, no doubt abundant in many mineral salts, fluorides included. Note that Māori in Dr. Price's investigations did not suffer the prevalence of goiter, so their iodine was sufficient.

I find the National Academy of Science's term 'Adequate Intake' quite inappropriate and grossly misleading when no symptoms or clinical signs of inadequacy can be identified, as the World Health Organization has pointed out [105]. Such contradiction is never brought before the NAS, or held next to the NAS' words in public, and never pointed to in the writings of official experts.

Yet here we come to the fact that the experts see CWF as a necessity; the public suffers *without* it. This may help us to understand the compliance of the experts when words like 'adequate' and 'deficiency' are used.

All of the experts quoted at the start of this chapter advocate Community Water Fluoridation (CWF). With regard to Dr. Perrott's statement about correcting a deficiency quoted at the start of this chapter, one is reminded of his claims regarding the Li *et al.* study [153] discussed briefly in his debate with Professor Connett [146], and mentioned in Chapter 2.7. Beyond this study and a German study[167] it cites, as well as the work discussed in Chapter 6.2, it appears the whole subject of hip fractures is generally treated at an arm's length to the topic of a nutritional role. I've only seen the gentlemen from Harvard and Dr. Perrott bring the two subjects together, though others may have. A recent example can be given involving the likening of fluorine to iodine. Here, the deficiency apparently applies to us not water. Quoting Dr. Perrott:

> "[Professor Paul] Connett attempts to raise ethical questions by defining water fluoridation as medication. But the correction of a mineral deficiency is not medication. Use of fluoridated water to correct a fluoride deficiency is like the use of iodized salt to correct iodine deficiency. That is something we are all used to and accept." [739]

This example shows how quickly things are forgotten, and how easily contradictions are made. This is possibly a consequence of the staggering amount of information available to us. Dr. Perrott had quoted on his own website in September 5 years previously [154], the Scientific Committee for Health and Environmental Risks (SCHER), who had claimed:

> "… [fluorine] is not an essential element for human growth and development." [116]

Note that iodine *is* an essential element – with no need for us to change the meaning of words, or to use benefit as a criterion for its essentiality. This may explain why much of the public has a scepticism toward the experts. There is a misleading consequence when experts discuss fluorine-deficient waters and soils. *Obviously* if the public believes they are drinking fluorine-deficient water, and eating food grown in fluorine-deficient soil, it follows as *perfect logic* that the public would then become fluorine-deficient.

The use of the term 'fluoride-deficient' for six or so decades has no doubt subtly influenced many a textbook author, and provided an easier inclusion of fluorine into a nutritional category. That most of these people don't comment on the fact that the experts mean deficient *water* or *soil* is probably not noticed by the majority. "Fluoride-deficient" by definition has for decades in scientific literature [130-132, 165, 390] meant water with a concentration less than 1.0 ppm fluorine; the experts have consistently failed to mention there are no symptoms associated with absence of fluorine in the human body [103, 105, 116-119].

---

[167] R. Lehmann, M. Wapniarz, B. Hofmann, B. Pieper, I. Haubitz, B. Allolio, *Drinking water fluoridation: Bone mineral density and hip fracture incidence*, **Bone**, Vol. 22, pp. 273–278, 1998.

Experts around the world that advocate for CWF are to my knowledge silent on this while discussing claims of deficient soil and water. It is only fair to expect the experts to have refuted such claims of no real fluorine deficiency in humans given how long they have claimed a nutritional role, but it has gone ignored. Sirs Gluckman and Skegg's report only used the term 'deficiency' with regard to iodine. Fluorine's abundance is also relevant here. One would think it relevant that biochemists could not create a diet with absolutely zero fluorine, even over many years of experimentation, but this too is seldom discussed in media.

On the 24th of January, 2016, a dentist and supporter of CWF from the American Fluoridation Society named Dr. Steve Slott left a comment on an online forum in response to a claim of 'medical sensitivity' to fluoride:

> "If you expect credence for your claim that you are 'medically sensitive' to fluoride then you will have to produce that documentation you claim to exist. Otherwise all you have is an anecdote." [740]

I share this to relate Dr. Slott's desire for documentation because I have seen so few people ask experts to demonstrate the existence of a fluoride deficiency, when experts have claimed such a thing to be real for so many decades in media.

In the multitudinous thousands of studies demonstrating a benefit, a reduction of decay is used as a criterion for essentiality. If experts want to use benefit as a criterion for essentiality they ought to make this very clear. In scientific literature I have never seen the charge of "semantics" levelled at even one expert, though such a thing is no doubt appropriate.

One of Professor Jason Armfield's criticisms of people *opposed* to CWF is "moving the goalposts" [418] (page 9). Perhaps the same criticism can apply to experts who have ignored standard criteria for essential element categorization, with so few public explanations.

Would the peer that publishes or reviews the work of a young aspiring expert be willing to accept evidence that peers had exaggerated? Even if it makes that peer's own work look bad? History is perhaps the only thing we have to go by, and if patterns are to repeat the answer is no. Yet patterns and habits can be changed and broken. A couple of the Australian documents cited here [610, 616] have given examples towards acknowledging a possible exaggeration of benefit, or at least allowing such a thing to be part of the discussion around CWF.

In this investigation I had not included social media in the analysis. Judging from what I've seen it's simply more of the same or worse (at least there is editing and some filtration in newspapers, biased though it no doubt is). I was more interested in the history. Yet I have followed a few online comments of some New Zealanders and the American experts they associate with. To further illustrate this point about water being considered deficient, a guest post by Gordon Burnside[168] discusses the superior health of his childhood neighbour's bulls, and his own bulls. His neighbour added selenium to the soil, as Mr. Burnside claims to nowadays. I find Mr. Burnside incorrect on two counts – one being that he has not pointed out that death from lack of selenium *has* been observed while death from lack of fluorine has *not* been verified beyond the occasional refuted rodent experiment, none of which he discussed. The second fault being that he has simply *claimed* fluorine to be a trace

---

[168] From New Plymouth and a **Taranaki Daily News** columnist.

element. Pointing to another element's behavior and saying "fluorine is like that" does not meet any requirement as far as proof is concerned, it is not even a first step to verifying a result with repeated experimentation. But because everyone else says it, the need for peer-reviewed evidence is relaxed. He wrote on the Making Sense of Fluoride (MSOF) website:

> "Similarly fluoride is a trace element, naturally occurring in balanced quantity over much of the inhabited world, but deficient in most of New Zealand. Our teeth in particular suffer as a result since its a vital building and maintenance block for our teeth.
>
> What else in our bodies require it is unknown to me but I'm not a scientist or naturopath. What is known is that despite countless scientific research tests, trials, surveys, study of statistics, no professional, without any financial interest in his own outcome, has been able to discover or demonstrate any reason whatsoever why the fluoride element should not be added to water to bring levels to normal. On the other hand, Fluoride is cheap to buy, it's not from some massive secretive industry with unlimited funds to bribe its way into use, its cost is a nothing. Every world health and dental health agency in the world recommends its addition via the water supply in areas deficient like ours." [741]

Mr. Burnside is claiming the *country* not the *people* are deficient. The term 'trace element' goes undefined here - this is normal. There is nothing insidious about this, but the term does mean different things to different people. To some the element is necessary, to others not.

New Zealand is a country in which animals outnumber humans many times over, yet animals have no need of fluorine supplementation, even with New Zealand's soil and water.

On 17th July, 2013, Dr. Perrott wrote:

> "... fluoridation is not medication – it just simply corrects a deficiency. Moves the F concentration from around 0.3 to 0.7 ppm. This has beneficial effects." [158]

Some of Dr. Perrott's previous claims of deficiency can be found in the 2014 debate he had with Professor Connett that was discussed in Chapter 2.7 [146] and see [158]. On the Making Sense of Fluoride website, Dr. Steve Slott, D.D.S., is quoted as saying:

> "The purpose of water fluoridation has never been intended to be to correct any sort of fluoride deficiency. It is simply to provide additional strength..." [742]

Yet we find so many instances of the term "fluoride-deficient" waters going back many decades in the work of the American Dental Association [130-132, 165, 390]. Media examples are given in Appendix 1. More can be found [129, 140].

Again, you can see that the experts do not correct each other when their statements contradict and do not pester each other for citations. In this case Dr. Perrott's claims of deficiency – or Dr. Slott's claim of CWF's purpose not being the correction of a deficiency – go by unchallenged. Remember this website is called Making *Sense* of Fluoride. Though the ability to back them up is negligible, these claims suit CWF programs, and so the desire for the scientific method, for near-definite proof, can be momentarily slackened.

In this instance, Dr. Slott was critiquing Professor Paul Connett's response to an article in the **Boston Globe**. Obviously Professor Connett had seen claims of a nutritional role for fluorine, perhaps not in the **Globe** itself, but he had no doubt seen such claims over his years of research.

If, as Daniel Ryan claims, Dr. Steve Slott is a "mythbuster" then Slott is in partial agreement with Professor Connett and a great deal of people opposed to CWF on this point – that fluoride should *not* be considered a nutrient (this little agreement is discussed nowhere). To my knowledge there is no evidence of Dr. Slott ever correcting Dr. Perrott or anyone else on this (Slott has left many comments on Perrott's website). Dr. Slott's comment that CWF was never intended to correct a deficiency demonstrates an ignorance of history, as the following shows:

> "The Hastings water supply is deficient in fluorine and by adding this element in the form of fluoride this deficiency is corrected." [743]

This is from a New Zealand newspaper article found in the 1954-1955 Health Department archives, discussing claims made by the Hawke's Bay branch of the New Zealand Dental Association. Similar statements have been made in American (see Chapter 5.2), Australian and New Zealand newspapers (see Appendix 1).

In the comment quoted, Dr. Slott seemed oblivious to the fact that the experts have constantly claimed a nutritional role for fluorine going back many decades. As Professor Brian Martin and Dr. John Colquhoun pointed out, the experts present a united front even when they disagree about details. I don't know if experts consider this deceptive or not because I have never seen it discussed. For all their condemnation of misinformation, it seems a double standard that experts don't see their own disagreement and contradiction is misinforming to the rest of us. I want to make it clear I'm *not* interested in undermining people's character or integrity, but in shedding light on some of the trends and behaviours that people have. Motivations of people are nearly impossible to see.

Everybody knows CWF and fluoride treatments are not a cure-all. Yet fluorine has taken the position of greatest importance in dental health, usurping the role of calcium and probably a great deal of other important and useful compounds and elements. Often other factors are acknowledged, though this appears token and ineffectual; only CWF, toothbrushing and stepping away from sugar (a parental responsibility) is recommended by the mainstream. Reevaluating social policy to be less market-oriented is beyond debate (even more so than CWF), even though poverty is probably the most-recognized contributor to poor overall health (a study on this is discussed later). The overarching emphasis on fluoride is detrimental to a recognition of other factors.

Recall Professor Broadbent's statement about fluoride's availability being a human right, quoted at the start of Chapter 4. If we care so much about the dental health of poor people, why not make calcium a human right? After all, calcium is *definitely* a nutritional essential, with no need for semantics, changing criteria, public relations and advertising, or ignoring the research that we don't like in public.

The Jaycee mentioned in Chapter 6.3 wrote in his letter that due to faulty eating habits,

> "... every action must be taken to supplement the supply of deficient elements." [670]

Such a statement compels us to consider not only the content of teeth, but the question of modern malnutrition, discussed in previous chapters. Who has ever advocated the addition of calcium, magnesium and the like to our water supplies? Why not just turn the food industry to public ownership and make healthy food a right?

Dr. Price's work is echoed in the animal kingdom. Animals are not used to eating purified diets, they are used to natural or "wild" foods produced by interactions of geological, evolutionary and other forces.

As early as 1916, Professor McCollum pointed to experiments which had demonstrated diets of polished rice had caused polyneuritis (disorder of the peripheral nerves) in birds[169].

> "The studies of a number of investigators have now fully established the fact that animals cannot grow when limited to rations of carefully purified proteins, carbohydrates, fats, and salts.[170]" [744]

This experiment [744] and another using rats showed the importance of animal and plant-based fats in securing growth [745]. These were substances like milk, butter, eggs and wheat.

A 2013 experiment investigating iron in rodent dentition claimed the element's importance was not understood, however it pointed to the staining characteristic in rodent tooth enamel that was caused by iron, the content of which is less than half a percent.

One way the body copes with excess iron is to increase expression of the iron storage protein ferritin, this appears true for humans and rodents. Ferritin and iron level were found to be correlated throughout the "developmental course of the rodent incisor" [746].

The researchers discussed a study on butterflyfish teeth which found more iron in the teeth of fish that fed on harder-bodied prey, which the researchers considered suggestive of a role for iron in the strengthening of teeth[171].

They cited two studies from about 50 years ago that suggested iron and calcium could substitute for each other in hydroxyapatite[172]. Dentin is largely collagen, the development of which requires iron [747].

They said nothing about applying their work to humans, yet claimed their work supported the idea of a necessary role for iron in tooth development. They pointed to a 1984 experiment that claimed not only a decrease in this typical pigmentation, but enamel hypoplasia (underdevelopment) in the incisors of rodents fed an iron-deficient diet for six months [748].

---

[169] Eykman, C., **Arch. Path. Anat.**, 1897, cxlviii, 523; cxlix, 187; **Arch. Hyg.**, 1906, lviii, 150. Suzuki, U. Shimamura, T., and Odake, S., Biochem. Z., 1912, xliii, 89. Funk, C., **Ergebn. Physiol.**, 1913, xiii, 125, "gives an extensive resume of the literature relating to the so-called deficiency diseases, together with a complete bibliography of the older literature." Funk, **Z. physiol. Chem.**, 1914, lxxxix, 374.

[170] Hopkins, F. G., **J. Physiol.**, 1912, xliv, 425. Hopkins, F G., and Neville, A., Biochem. J., 1913, vii, 97. Funk, C., and Macallum, A. B., **Z. physiol. Chem.**, 1914, xcii, 13. Stepp, W., **Z. Biol.**, 1913, lxii, 405.

[171] Motta PJ: a quantitative analysis of ferric iron in butterflyfish teeth (*Chaetodontidae Perciformes*) and the relationship to feeding ecology. **Can J Zool** 1987, 65:106–112.

[172] Brudevold F, Soremark F: Chemistry of the mineral phase of enamel. **Structure and Chemical Organization of Teeth**, 1967, **2**:247-290. Hales A: Effect of dietary iron deficiency on the pigmentation and iron content of rat incisor enamel. **Scand J Dent Res** 1973, **81**:319-334.

Hypoplasia in most instances refers to the number of cells that make up the enamel. These researchers also found aplasia (lack of development) in the rats' teeth. We may want to consider these findings with regard to Dr. McClendon's rats on a vegan diet.

The following dental roles of other elements and compounds are taken from the 2014 textbook *Modern Nutrition*: Protein has roles in tooth size, eruption time, enamel insolubility and salivary gland function. Vitamin A influences epithelial tissue, tooth morphogenesis, odontoblast (tooth cell) differentiation; deficiencies lead to enamel hypoplasia (underdevelopment). Vitamin D, calcium and phosphorous are necessary for tooth integrity, eruption patterns, and plasma calcium. Ascorbic acid deficiency leads to dental pulp and dentin changes, odontoblast degeneration, though deficiency is not claimed to result in caries (but no human data were available). Iodine deficiency is claimed to delay tooth eruption, alter growth patterns, and lead to malocclusion, but is not implicated in caries directly. Iron deficiency leads to slow growth, loss of tooth integrity, and salivary gland dysfunction (but no human were data available) [636].

Many of these elements or compounds are *definitely essential* – yet are almost never mentioned in discussions around CWF or dental health. A factor being in our diet does not guarantee assimilation and digestion of that factor.

Dr. John Howard Mummery, President of the British Dental Association, claimed in 1919 that calcium phosphate and fluoride make up 89.82% of enamel (with fluoride contributing 2%), and calcium carbonate taking up 4.37%. The rest were from magnesium phosphate at 1.34%, other salts at 0.88%, cartilage at 3.39% and fat with 0.2% [749].

In 1946 Dr. W. Armstrong gave figures of 35.35% calcium and 17.43% elemental phosphorous (not including oxygen, contained in *phosphate*), 3% carbon dioxide and 0.3% magnesium, and 0.0111% fluorine [59]. These were figures from the 'sound teeth' group. This work was discussed in Chapter 1.2.

A 2018 paper in the **Journal of the American Dental Association** investigated molar hypomineralization (MH). Seventy-five prevalence studies had been carried out, none of which originated in the US[173]. The author, Dr. Hubbard of the Faculty of Medicine, Dentistry and Health Sciences at the University of Melbourne, Australia, argued that addressing this medicodental issue was long overdue. Dr. Hubbard claimed MH is

"the most common manifestation of what are popularly termed chalky teeth…" [750]

Hubbard claims that a "perplexing diagnostic feature" is the way in which MH does not affect teeth uniformly or evenly. Up to 4 molars may be affected, though other teeth may also succumb to the condition, which is called "molar-incisor hypomineralization".

"The above criteria distinguish MH from the classic D3s (fluorosis, enamel hypoplasia, amelogenesis imperfecta) and early caries in enamel (white-spot lesions)."

---

[173] Cited is a website where these studies can be seen, http://www.thed3group.org/prevalence.html.

Confusing these symptoms clinically is easy, according to Dr. Hubbard. One wonders if prioritizing economies over health has caused MH to become a factor in lives worldwide, since

"… it now appears certain that MH manifests similarly in the Americas as the rest of the world."

Dr. Hubbard claims that severely under-mineralized molars may face "more than 10-fold higher risk of developing caries". He points to a lack of desire for research:

"First, the problem is diluted over a broad sector, which raises questions about who should own it academically."

Billions of dollars has been spent on health-related research in the last hundred years. This is one thing we have to show for it. The second issue was the existence of an "educational deficit" regarding the attention MH receives worldwide, this depending on myriad factors.

"Third, MH is clinically obscure for many. From the medical perspective, pathologic onset happens invisibly within the jaw long before tooth eruption."

One is reminded of Dr. Glenn's claims (Chapter 6.2). This is why I think we ought to regulate the business community's propaganda efforts through advertising and public relations. The impact such lack of regulation has had on health can be seen here.

"Orally, some see MH but misname it (usually as hypoplastic molars), others look but erroneously see it as caries, and many others have little opportunity to look." [750]

This after six or so decades of fluoride's "enamel remineralization". Dr. Hubbard recommended the The Chalky Teeth Campaign [751].

This group recommends:

"fluoride-based prevention – fluoride-containing toothpaste, professional fluoride treatments."

"Casein phosphopeptide–amorphous calcium phosphate (CPP-ACP) preventives – avoid fluoridated formulation in under-10 y.o." [752]

These are thought to help with remineralization, Dr. Featherstone's work published in 2000 mentioned in Chapter 6.2 discussed this. From 2009-2012, The Chalky Teeth Campaign had funding from Colgate [752].

This focus on calcium and phosphate appears to me to be a step in a positive direction. For a long time, we have known that both calcium and phosphorous make up the largest percentage of dental enamel [59, 749, 753].

We see how often fluorine is likened to iodine. There is a possibility fluoridation may have taken some of the credit due to iodisation of salt, when we see iodine has positive effects on teeth. Iodine is a necessary component of hormones in the thyroid gland, which have regulatory effects on calcium [754]. Iodine has been added to salt in New Zealand since 1924 [755].

In 2016, two researchers from Department of Pediatric and Preventive Dentistry, Vokkaligara Sangha (VS) Dental College in Bangalore, India, claimed to find developmental defects of enamel (DDE) scores higher (5.0 to 1.5 DDE score) in 100 children with hypothyroidism than 100 children without [756].

The earliest work on the impact of the thyroid gland on enamel formation and health is probably a little outdated and imprecise, but recent work has verified the importance of the gland on tooth health.

In 1914, Dr. Henry Pickerill claimed rabbits with thyroid glands removed had much more calcium in their faeces than normal. His conclusion was quite tentative based on his work. He claimed their teeth were normal, yet without the yellow staining and tiny black blemishes that were considered normal in rodents and rabbits "(and also in many cases on human teeth immune to caries)". Pickerill found 2.1% less calcium in thyroidectomized teeth than control animals' teeth. Similar was true for saliva, 0.0220% in controls and 0.0206% post thyroidectomy. Pickerill thought the alkaline salts had lessened in production: he found the animals did not salivate any more in terms of quantity to make up for this. Quoting Pickerill:

> "From clinical evidence I am inclined to think that there is an association between that condition seen in children which is now diagnosed as 'thyroid insufficiency' and the presence of dental caries. This, however, is an exceedingly difficult matter to decide definitely: there are so many concomitant circumstances relating to habits and to food which require to be considered and eliminated." [757]

Pickerill was hesitant to read too much into this small work, but pointed out that it showed the impacts of thyroidectomy all move in one direction: "that which would lower the resistance of the teeth to disease."

In 1973, researchers from Cornell University in New York performed thyroidectomies in 6 yearling grade horse colts, and compared them with 5 controls for a little over a year (67 weeks).

Animals were examined in four five-week periods during the experiment. There was a lowering of serum calcium after thyroidectomy. The researchers described the thyroidectomized animals as "docile and lethargic". Their coats of hair were "dull" and "coarse." I was reminded of Schwarz's rats. The skeletal growth of these horses was stunted. The researchers believed there were not enough horses in their sample to make definite conclusions, but they did point to other research similar. [758]

In 1995, the journal **Connective Tissue Research** published the first part of a study on the effects of thyroidectomies on the growth of dentin in rat incisors. They found defective mineralization as a result of calcium loss [759].

In 1996, the journal **Cell Tissue Research** published an experiment on the effects of thyroidectomies on rat incisors. The word "perturbations" (meaning disturbances, agitations, confusion) was used to describe the effect on enamel mineralization. The researchers pointed to the reduction in calcium as a causative effect [760].

In 2002, the **Journal of the American Dental Association** published an article which looked at the clinical management of patients with hyper- (overactive) and hypo- thyroidism (hypo- meaning underactive). The symptoms of hypothyroidism were delayed dental eruption and compromised periodontal (gum) health – delayed bone resorption. The symptoms of hyperthyroidism were increased susceptibility to caries, periodontal disease and accelerated dental eruption [761].

Regarding prevention, we seem to have gone full circle. Dr. Helmholz's article in the **American Journal of Public Health** claimed:

"The greatest advances in medicine have been made by the prevention and not by the cure of disease." [598]

In 2013, we read:

> "A paradigm shift is emerging in dentistry and dental treatments are now aimed at maximum conservation of tooth structure. It is nowadays considered an ethical duty of a dentist to provide their patients with minimally invasive treatment. Remineralization therapy is preferred in cases, where there is a chance of gaining success by preventive methods." [762]

Perhaps it could be considered an "ethical duty" of politicians and the business community to make healthy food not only cheaper than junk food, but affordable for the poor. If such a circumstance does not develop, the desire and work of dentistry will continue being an uphill battle, whether we are doused in fluorides or not.

The media and some intellectuals are correct in noticing that in some aspects the underlying ways of approaching fluoridation are totally different depending on whether one supports or opposes the programs. This leads to points being unaddressed, arguments passing each other like ships in the night, and endless accusations of selectivity, cherry-picking and favouritism.

In dental fluorosis, we come to one of these divergences. One can see why the experts believe dental fluorosis to be a necessity in maximizing tooth strength. In Chapter 6.2 I quoted the NAS, who had claimed that there is an overlap between small amounts of fluorosis and maximum benefit in prevention.

> "... the same range of fluoride intakes is associated both with reductions in dental caries and fluorosis." [763]

Here is the same statement, though from the WHO in 2002:

> "In children, intakes of fluoride associated with beneficial effects on dentition overlap with those that lead to an increased prevalence of dental fluorosis." [737]

A 1957 statement from a couple of people opposed to CWF regarding dental fluorosis is this:

> "The determination of whether damage resulting from dental fluorosis is 'objectionable' is a matter for the person whose teeth are affected and not for the arbitrary assertion of public officials." [764]

With dental fluorosis, we see it is the experts who will decide what is an acceptable level of fluorosis in your smile, my smile, all of our smiles. A citizen is not supposed to decide this because a citizen is not an expert.

The people opposed to CWF want to be free to decide the level of fluorosis that suits them, and the experts feel a professional, societal and moral obligation to help the population attain the 'mild' or 'very mild' levels of dental fluorosis that they believe help maximize resistance to tooth decay. This ties in with the conceptions of democracy – should the public decide what is in their best interests or not? Such a state is a "crisis of democracy", as discussed in Chapter 5.4. One can understand the experts' distaste for such things – many of us are carefree, appearing even self-destructive in our approach to our lifestyles. Dental fluorosis is pictured in **Figure 97**.

The WHO wrote in 2014:

> "... public health administrators should assess the total fluoride exposure of the population before introducing any additional fluoridation or supplementation programmes for caries prevention." [214]

In Chapter 6.3 I discussed how dentistry's workload was at its limit in the 1950s, and at its limit in some ways nowadays. In discussing fluorosis, we must wonder how many people have looked at strange marks on their teeth, and felt they should go to a dentist. Is this administration of fluorides to nearly all of us counterproductive?

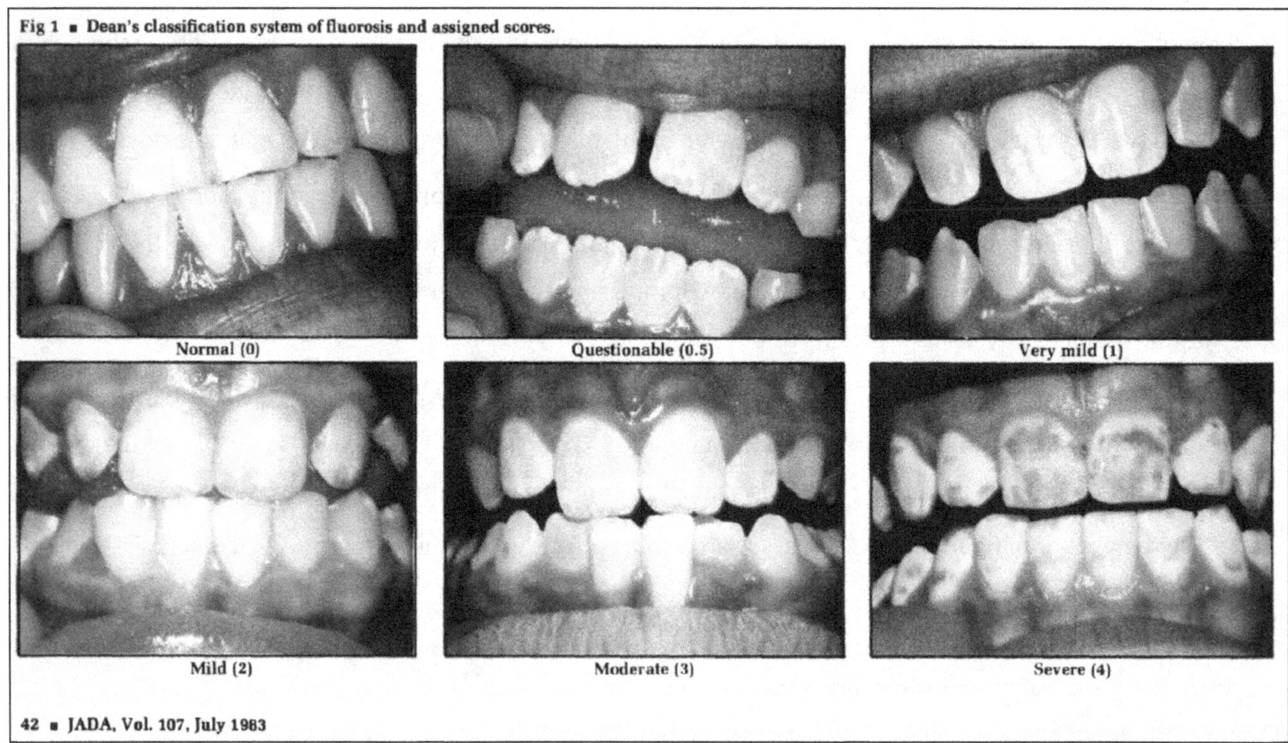

Figure 97. *Dean's classification system of fluorosis and assigned scores. Source: Driscoll et al., Prevalence of dental caries and dental fluorosis in areas with optimal and above-optimal water fluoride concentrations, **Journal of the American Dental Association**, Vol. 107, p. 42, July, 1983.*

In 2013, dentist Dr. Steve Slott left the following comment on a **Guardian** article:

> "Fluoride is not a drug, and it is not 'forced' upon anyone. Fluoride is a mineral which the FDA must classify as a drug for the sole reason of its stated use in water as a therapeutic rather than as a disinfectant. No other reason. As the EPA regulates all mineral additives to water, it is the EPA, not the FDA, which controls and regulates fluoride in water. Fluoridated water meets all NSF Standard 60 certification requirements as mandated by the EPA. There are no dosage requirements for fluoride, nor is there any need for such, any more than is there any need of dosage requirements of chlorine in water." [765]

Recently in New Zealand, the Supreme Court has ruled on CWF [766]. Taranaki District Council was taken to court by a group called New Health New Zealand Inc. This was covered a little on the TVNZ show Q+A, featuring Sir Peter Gluckman, who was asked about the polarization of scientific opinion, and "science denial" that was discussed in a recent EPA report [767]. These deniers opposed fluoride, 1080, vaccinations, glyphosate and the like, on "the unmoderated milieu of the internet…"

It is unfair to blame people for going online partly due to the fact that it is *convenient* to go online and we are *encouraged* to go online and use technology. People are almost forced to go online to learn about a subject if experts and media refuse to quench an intellectual thirst for *details*.

To quote a couple of sentences from Sir Peter, on Q+A:

> "There are people that are going to come at it and say whatever the science says I'm not going to change my views that it's medicalization of the water supply and I object to that on philosophical grounds."

> "I think it is tragic that we cannot get beyond that but there are people that have this deep world view that it's medicalization and will object." [768]

The media release on 27th June, 2018, pointed out the verdict that fluoridation was not unlawful, with the Chief Justice disagreeing:

> "[New Health New Zealand Inc (New Health)] claimed, among other things, that the addition of fluoride was unlawful both because it was outside the statutory powers of the Council under the Local Government Act 2002 and the Health Act 1956 and because it was in breach of the right everyone has under s 11 of the New Zealand Bill of Rights Act 1990 to refuse to undergo any medical treatment. New Health was unsuccessful in these contentions in the High Court and its appeal to the Court of Appeal was dismissed."

> …

> "On the question of whether the Council had the legal authority to fluoridate water, the majority Judges held that it did. This was based on the Council's general power of competence in s 12 of the Local Government Act and in light of its duty under the Health Act to protect, promote and improve public health in its region. The relevant provisions had to be interpreted against the background that fluoridation had been lawful in New Zealand for decades prior to enactment."

> "The Chief Justice disagreed. She concluded that the Council had no statutory authority to fluoridate water supplies."

Four of the five judges believed addition of fluoride constituted medical treatment:

> "On the question of whether the addition of fluoride to the water supply engaged the right to refuse to undergo medical treatment under s 11 of the Bill of Rights Act, the Chief Justice, Glazebrook, O'Regan and Ellen France JJ held that it did. Even having regard to the genesis of s 11, there was no basis to read down its text so as to exclude medical treatment which occurs outside of a therapeutic relationship."

> "William Young J disagreed, holding that a person who ingests fluoridated water does not thereby undergo medical treatment."

> …

> "The Supreme Court has unanimously dismissed New Health's appeal against both aspects of the Court of Appeal decision." [769]

I don't believe the media mentioned that the Chief Justice disagreed. Reading the entire decision is hard going for the legal layman such as myself, but different views were shared. People opposed to fluoridation took delight in some views, a couple of paragraphs are quoted in Appendix 7. I will quote some sections from the Supreme

Court judgement that I think are relevant to a nutritional or medicative role. The Court consisted of Elias CJ, William Young, Glazebrook, O'Regan and Ellen France JJ.

While there is much I found interesting in the document, I will quote here from William Young J. Any footnotes not stating an expert witness's title are their words. Young looked at the work of Dr. Robin Whyman[174], Associate Professor David Menkes[175], and Professor Martin Ferguson[176]. In the judgement I have underlined their words to avoid confusion. Underlined words here are the court's, not mine. This is a very small section of Young's words:

> Fluoridating water/"undergo medical treatment": general considerations
>
> [188] The argument against the view that those who drink fluoridated water thereby undergo medical treatment is as follows. Fluoride occurs naturally in drinking water at varying levels. In areas where the drinking water is fluoridated, those levels are adjusted so that the fluoride content is around one part per million. At this level, fluoride has beneficial effects on tooth enamel without significant health disbenefits.[177] Fluoride added to water is therefore properly to be seen as a supplement, rather as iodine in salt and folic acid in bread are supplements. Further, and in any event, fluoridated water which is supplied to consumers is not in the nature of a medicine as the primary purpose of supply is to provide drinking water rather than to protect dental health. "Medical treatment" characteristically involves treatment solely for therapeutic purposes. It also characteristically involves a one-on-one relationship between a health professional and a patient. In areas of the world in which fluoride occurs naturally in water, the supply of such (naturally) fluoridated water to those without water could not sensibly be regarded as medical treatment. This being so, why should supply of water which is materially identical in chemical constitution be differently regarded?[178] (footnote in original)
>
> [189] These aspects of the case were developed by Dr Robin Whyman in his evidence:
>
> Fluoridation of water, is in my view, a supplement rather than medication:
>
> (a) Fluoride ions already exist naturally, both in the human body, primarily in bone and enamel, and in drinking water. Water fluoridation increases the quantity of these ions present in water – and therefore the body – by a small amount. The additional fluoride added to New Zealand drinking water supplies recreates naturally occurring levels in other areas of the world and is therefore in my view a supplement rather than a form of medication.
>
> (b) The situation is analogous to adding iodine to salt to prevent thyroid difficulties. Like fluoride, iodine and salt have associated nutrient reference values derived by the New Zealand Ministry of Health and the Australian National Health and Research Medical Council.
>
> Water fluoridation is not in my view "medical treatment":

---

[174] Clinical Director, Oral Health Services, Hawkes Bay District Health Board.

[175] School of Medicine, Faculty of Medical and Health Sciences, University of Auckland.

[176] Emeritus Professor of Oral Medicine and Oral Surgery at the University of Otago's School of Dentistry.

[177] Peter Gluckman and David Skegg *Health effects of water fluoridation: A review of the scientific evidence* (Office of the Prime Minister's Chief Science Advisor and the Royal Society of New Zealand, August 2014).

[178] "Where the natural water supply contains levels of fluoride which are inimical to health, the water supplier will reduce the fluoride content. Is the resulting supply of water medical treatment if the reduction is to an optimal therapeutic level which is beneficial but not if it is sub-optimal? And what if the water supplier has a choice of two natural supplies, one naturally fluoridated and one not? Is it medical treatment if the water supplier uses the water supply which is naturally fluoridated?"

(a) Water fluoridation is a population health, or public health, measure that works in a prophylactic, or preventive way.

(b) Water fluoridation increases the community's environmental exposure to fluoride in a way that replicates normal environmental exposure levels in some parts of the world.

(footnotes omitted in original)

[190] Those who oppose fluoridation have a number of arguments in response. Thus Associate Professor David Menkes, a witness for the appellant, observed:

... there is no physiological reaction in the human body that requires fluoride. Nor is fluoride required for any aspect of human growth, development, or reproduction.

On this basis, he asserted that "fluoride cannot be considered a nutrient or dietary supplement". And Professor Martin Ferguson made what seems to me to be the same point when he said:

While topical or systemic fluoride has been shown to have some effect in reducing dental caries, there is no disorder recognised that is due to a deficiency of fluoride. Therefore it cannot be classified as a supplement.

The Commission of Inquiry into fluoridation

[191] Water fluoridation was the subject of a 1957 report of a Commission of Inquiry in which the Commission specifically addressed the question whether fluoridation of water was in the nature of mass medication. Its conclusions (and the associated reasons) were as follows:[179]

223. ... Supporters of fluoridation have stated that the term "mass medication" is a misnomer. They pointed out that fluoride is not used to treat dental decay but to reduce the incidence of the disease. This fact was not disputed. According to them, the process consists of adding to water, which no one has disputed is itself a food, a sufficient amount of another food substance (fluoride ions) already naturally present in it to raise the total concentration to the optimum nutritional level. On this reasoning, they have argued that the process is food fortification completely analogous to examples mentioned in the evidence of Professor Gregory and Dr Muriel Bell and referred to in the following paragraph.

224. Well recognised examples of food fortification are the addition of calcium carbonate to "national flour" in Great Britain, the compulsory addition of vitamins A and D to margarine in Great Britain, the compulsory nutritional enrichment of bread and flour with B-group vitamins in some parts of the United States, the addition to some salt of iodide and the addition of synthetic vitamin C to a lemon-flavoured powder used by the New Zealand Navy. The addition of trace elements to the soil for the benefit of animals (e.g., the addition of cobalt to deficient pasture to combat bush sickness in sheep or cattle) or of plants (e.g., the addition of boron, manganese, molybdenum, or zinc to deficient soils) are examples of the way in which food deficiencies are supplemented in these cases for animals or for plants.

225. At the concentrations under discussion, fluoride is not a poison and is either a drug on the one hand or a food on the other. There is no doubt that it is beneficial to the human body just as the substances mentioned by Professor Gregory and Dr [Muriel] Bell are beneficial. It is certain, however, that it neither "counteracts the effects of disease nor reinforces the tissues in their struggle to maintain their functions when these are rendered abnormal". It does not counteract the effects of dental decay nor does it assist the teeth to maintain their functions after they are decayed.

---

[179] WF Stilwell, NL Edson and PVE Stainton "Report of the Commission of Inquiry on the Fluoridation of Public Water Supplies" [1957] V AJHR H47.

226. We are satisfied that the process by which fluoride achieves its beneficial result is that a trace of the substance is utilised by the active tissues of the tooth germ as a foodstuff while they are forming the mineral substance of the tooth. Any effect subsequent to eruption of the tooth is an incidental ion-exchange at the surface exposed to drinking water.

227. Some authorities (see for example the evidence of Mr Needham (9J 3)) regard fluorine as an indispensable trace element in the diet, whereas others question its indispensability but do not categorically deny that it is a food. (Mitchell & Edman, 1953; McLester & Darby, 1952). None, however, questions the usefulness of dietary fluorine to civilised man in reducing susceptibility to dental decay, and the evidence has shown that the usefulness of fluoride arises from its incorporation into the organised structure of tooth enamel (para. 74). In this regard, therefore, we consider that whatever academic discussion may revolve around the question of indispensability, it is certainly no less than common sense to make use of the beneficial properties of this trace element. If the intake is insufficient the deficiency should be made up in imitation of nature by fortification of the drinking water (cf. Waldbott, 1955 a).

228. For the foregoing reasons we express our conclusion that fluoride is not a drug but a nutrient and that fluoridation is a process of food fortification. As a process it is quite analogous to the compulsory addition of fat soluble vitamins to margarine, of vitamin B1 (thiamine) to bread, or the non-compulsory addition of potassium iodide to salt. For this reason there are no valid grounds for calling the process "mass medication", a term which has acquired a certain emotional content in the course of controversy. In reaching this decision, we believe we are applying to the word medication the meaning most people attach to it.

[192] It will be observed that this discussion records the conflicting positions in similar terms to those proposed by Associate Professor Menkes and Professor Ferguson, on the one hand, and Dr Whyman on the other, with the Commission coming down on the same side as Dr Whyman. [770]

In paragraph 208, William Young J justified his inclusion of the Commission of Inquiry:

"The question whether fluoridation is in the nature of mass medication was addressed by the Commission of Inquiry in 1957. It concluded that it was not. The reasons for this conclusion do not seem to me to have been undermined by subsequent developments."

After spending so much time in the Health Department archives looking through the 1950s files, I was quite surprised to see the Commssion of Inquiry mentioned in 2018, yet after reading Young's words above I can appreciate the reason for its use, appearing no doubt as common sense.

Incidentally, the word "sugar" appeared once, in dentist Dr. Stan Litras' discussion. In the recent Supreme Court judgement, Elias C J had this to say about the 1957 Commission of Inquiry:

[241] The Council in its submissions suggested that the acceptability of the addition of fluoride in New Zealand had been addressed by a Commission of Inquiry into fluoride in 1957 and a report of the Human Rights Commission in 1980.[180] Both reports, however, preceded enactment of the New Zealand Bill of Rights Act. Indeed, in considering "personal rights in relation to fluoridation", the 1957 Commission of Inquiry proceeded on the basis that "the subject does not possess guaranteed rights".[181] These reports therefore are not

---

[180] WF Stilwell, NL Edson and PVE Stainton "Report of the Commission of Inquiry on the Fluoridation of Public Water Supplies" [1957] V AJHR H47; and Human Rights Commission *Report on Representations on Fluoridation of Water Supplies* (August 1980).
[181] At *[496]–[500]*, citing *Halsbury's Laws of England* (3rd ed, 1954) vol 7 Constitutional Law at *[416]*.

<u>concerned with the purpose of s 11, which derives from more recent insights into the values of human dignity and autonomy.</u>

<u>*[243]* For these reasons I conclude that the addition of fluoride to the water supplied by the Council is medical treatment within the meaning of s 11 of the New Zealand Bill of Rights Act. (footnotes in original)</u>

A few statements of the 1957 Commission of Inquiry have been discussed already. It was in this year that the Maurer and Day experiment was published [17].

I have been unable to obtain the 1952 edition of the McLester and Darby work, but the 1954 edition claimed fluorine to be an essential element for teeth, claiming research (unspecified) from the University of Rochester had shown sound teeth contained more fluorine than decayed teeth. Such claims did not take fluorine accumulation over time into account and have since been disregarded. I addressed this in Chapter 1.2, yet the 1938 research I cited was from the University of Minnesota. McLester and Darby claimed fluorine was thought to be harmful prior to this research.

Following is a letter written by one of the three authors of the 1957 Commission of Inquiry, Dr. Edson, a biochemist of Otago University (**Figure 98**). It is available in the Health Department archives. Edson wrote this letter in response to being asked by Dr. Maclean, Director of the Division of Public Hygiene, if he (Edson) would serve on the Commission[182]. The letter is not shown here to offend or belittle those experts who have done time-consuming, sincere research on this topic. The only place I've seen it mentioned is John Colquhoun's PhD thesis [329] (Chapter 11). Edson was described as "one of the world's most distinguished biochemists and the editor of the journal **The Annual Review of Biochemistry**" in a letter authored by Dr. Muriel Bell's stepson and published in New Zealand's **The Listener** in 2013 [771].

Like seeing so many Jaycees, and the odd public relations company promoting CWF without their qualifications or understanding of the topic even vaguely discussed, this letter tells us how high the bar is set for those who would write CWF policy, and be among the experts.

---

[182] John Colquhoun pointed out that of the three commissioners appointed, Edson was the only scientist (though many scientists presented evidence *to* the Commission), the other two being a businessman and a judge. Colquhoun said of Otago "… where the Dean, Charles Hercus, and the nutrition researcher, Muriel Bell, were strong advocates of fluoridation."

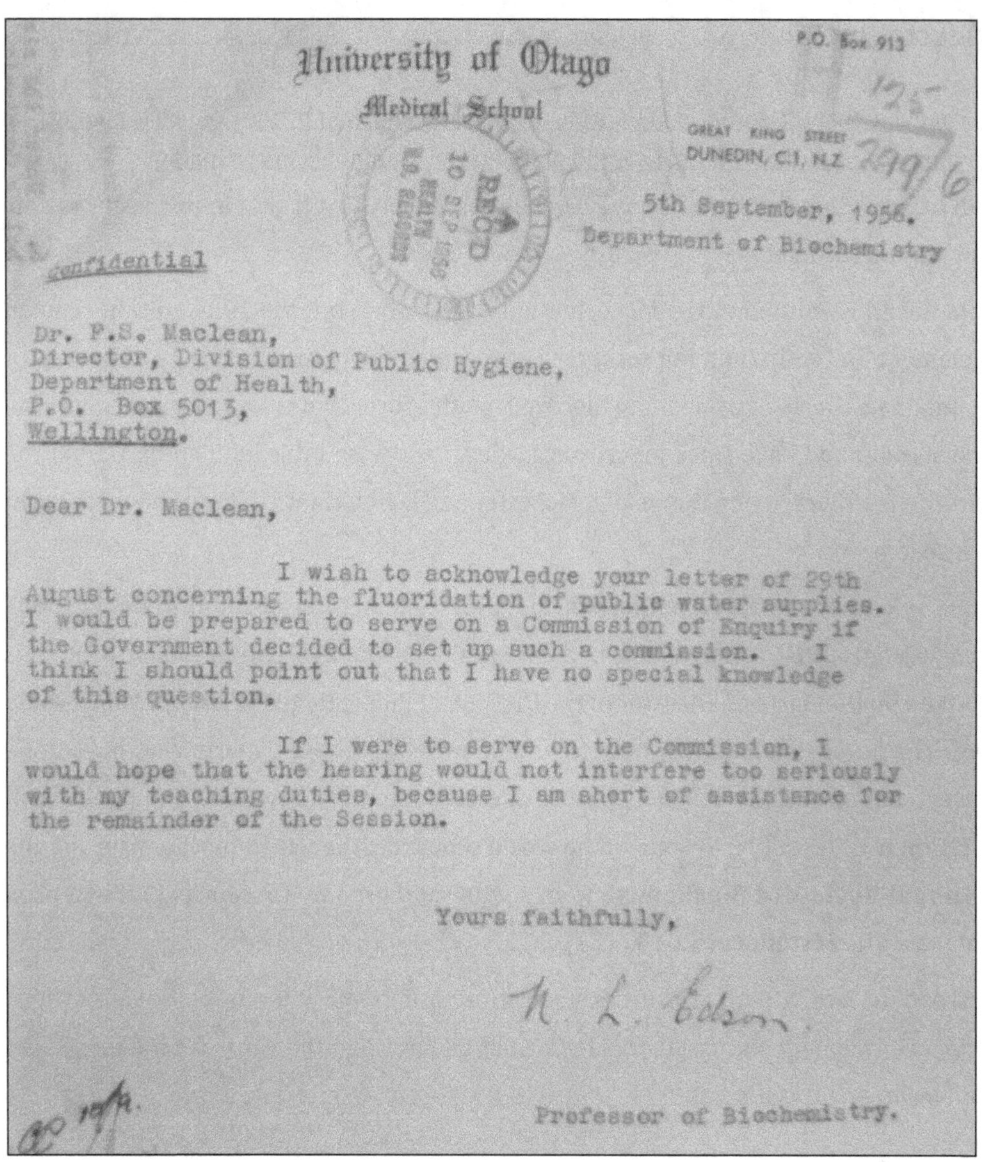

University of Otago
Medical School

P.O. Box 913

GREAT KING STREET
DUNEDIN, C.1, N.Z.

5th September, 1956.
Department of Biochemistry

Confidential

Dr. P.S. Maclean,
Director, Division of Public Hygiene,
Department of Health,
P.O. Box 5013,
Wellington.

Dear Dr. Maclean,

I wish to acknowledge your letter of 29th August concerning the fluoridation of public water supplies. I would be prepared to serve on a Commission of Enquiry if the Government decided to set up such a commission. I think I should point out that I have no special knowledge of this question.

If I were to serve on the Commission, I would hope that the hearing would not interfere too seriously with my teaching duties, because I am short of assistance for the remainder of the Session.

Yours faithfully,

N. L. Edson.

Professor of Biochemistry.

Figure 98. Letter from Edson to Maclean. Source: HD 125/299/6 H1 1674, 1956-1957.

I believe my work raises very important questions about the insular nature of scientists and researchers, and of the way they can be used to bring about claims favourable to powerful groups. It brings a couple of other factors relating to public participation into play. Does the public have the right to know that the experts have exaggerated, and do experts have an obligation to tell the public about their exaggeration? It also helps us to see that divisive issues can lead to distortions in research, especially when convenient claims are easily accessible and made with repetition. Too often we echo each other's opinions without clarification, without investigation, without feeling for the strength of the underlying foundation. It's only fair that we trust others and their research; if we didn't we would have nothing, but we seem to like the conclusions of people who agree with us a little too much.

The competitive nature of people involved with fluoridation has had a large influence on this topic of a nutritional or non-nutritional role. It has marginalized the journalists and councilors who cared little for taking sides and simply wanted to get as close to the truth as they could. The importance of this topic fluctuates depending on who is winning the argument. Such dynamics are more about reinforcing power structures than impartial science.

I am largely uninterested in future work on this question of a nutritional role for fluorine, unless the biases and use of words discussed in this book are brought to the public's eyes. Two things we need to study are biases in experts' work and the monitoring of fluoride levels in diets and people.

Can we really have a functioning democracy (assuming democracy means the public participates with full knowledge) in a society that is increasingly run by businesses? Business requires secrecy, which means that public participation (voting, referenda, etc) *must* be made on *minimal* public knowledge.

In New Zealand and Australia we have been heavily influenced by America, and I don't mean the American citizenry. We may want to reconsider how closely we follow, as our own inequalities spiral even further out of control.

Life expectancy in America is now in decline. While deaths from cancer had declined 2014-2015, other causes had increased; heart, respiratory, kidney and Alzheimer's disease, diabetes, suicide and others. It appears "'despair deaths' – alcoholism, drugs, suicide" have become more frequent as well as "obesity, poverty, and social isolation." [772] The rates of early death increased for white men and women, and for black men. Research from the Kaiser Family Foundation claims the USA now has the lowest life expectancy at birth among eleven comparable countries and slower growth in life expectancy than comparable countries [773].

Work published in the **Journal of the American Medical Association** has pointed to poverty, income inequality and declining economic prospects for the poor as a powerful cause of these problems [774]. According to the World Health Organization, depression rates increased 18% between 2005 and 2015 [775].

I include this not to condemn the United States or the people within it, but to suggest we rethink some of the fundamental aspects of our economic and social policies. I believe American policy has been subverted by corporate interests, and I do not think we are following traditional American virtues [776]. Given that these impact our health so heavily such a thing does not feel out of place to suggest. Why should we follow someone else's ideals anyway? Are our own unworthy? We have a rugby team that is famous around the world for performing a traditional Māori dance unique to our country before a game. Can we not be original and free in the creation and customizing of our own social policies?

I am not totally set in stone in my scepticism regarding a nutritional role for fluorine. Nor am I totally set in stone regarding benefits, harm and wastefulness of CWF. What offends me most about CWF is the way in which it is promoted. One thing this investigation has developed within me is a confidence in my conclusion of expert bias historically, another is a humility for all of the numerous things I don't understand.

Given fluorine's abundance I don't believe CWF is really needed in modern public health. That deficiency states of fluorine were researched at all after the 1930s seems wasteful. Nevertheless, I am sceptical of using "benefit as a criterion for essentiality" because it seems a little too easy, a little unearned – especially when contrasted to the strictness promoters apply to activists' claims.

I was quite surprised by the rescinding of the 1991 Australian report, and by the fact that the NHMRC would not send me a pdf. One understands such things in light of Professor Huntington's work on elites not desiring a "crisis of democracy".

In 2017, the NAS wrote about CWF harming teeth (fluorosis) to make them harder. No such thing could have been said in the 1950s, without one being cast as antifluoridationist, so times are changing.

In the examples given in this book, the bias of the experts becomes quite clear – there is information that is simply unacceptable in media, in public dialogue. It eventually finds its way onto the internet, where concerned parties can discuss it, spin it, turn it into whatever they want. Their work is not perfect, they do not have large research labs to pursue their questions, they receive little feedback from experienced scientists, and many of their hypotheses are probably untestable given prevailing ideologies on research direction, and lack of money. Experts and media share a partial responsibility for this. In 1997, the Brisbane Lord Mayor's Taskforce wrote:

> "The majority of the Taskforce found it surprising that the concern about the lack of research in Australia expressed in the 1991 NHMRC Report (Section 8), and the call for an effective monitoring and research program in relation to Australia's water fluoridation policy, appeared to have gone largely unheeded." [610] (page 47)

One of the most dissonant features of the promotion of Community Water Fluoridation is that the experts encourage us to use our heads not our hearts – to make scientific arguments instead of emotional arguments.

Yet what is more emotional than caring for children? But we should not do such a thing emotionally, we should do it technologically. The experts tell us to use technology, which employs experts. Is that biased? The purpose of CWF is primarily to help children. This leads us to the conclusion that we are supposed to care (emotion) for children with logic, science, technology and calculations.

In this way the scientific community have inadvertently expropriated our freedom to care for our children. One will note something becoming obvious now – the complete lack of concern from corporations over environmental problems such as plastic pollution and global warming [373]. They only desire to sell, sell, sell. The emphasis is on short-term profits, not the long-term survival of the human race. The call to use a scientific approach in our concern for children is intended as a call to common sense and reality. This should not conflict with changing our economic system to something fairer.

In 1978 the journal **Iron Age** claimed business was spending about a billion dollars a year on communications, not including the advertising of consumer products, toward the American public [777]. According to sociologist Alex Carey,

"This expenditure was aimed at persuading the American public that their interests were the same as business's interests." [342]

Carey points out that there was no discussion on the consequences for democracy.

Experts want us to keep off the internet when we get our information on fluorides. They complain that people have a lack of trust in science [767, 778, 779].

In 2007, Trevor Sheldon, Chair of the Advisory Board of the York Review, suggested:

"Against this backdrop of one sided handling of the evidence, the public distrust in the information it receives is understandable" [605]

Why are people sceptical of the science involved with CWF? Personally I think it is not so much *science* that people mistrust, it is the *simplification of science* – something most of us probably remember from high school as quite technical – reduced to clichés and catchphrases by people claiming to be so much smarter than us. For others, mistrust is due to decades of dishonesty, favouritism and double standards, some in areas and industries totally unrelated to CWF. Some people just expect such things from human endeavor. Others are sceptical of the incredibly confident, having been disappointed before. Another aspect has been pointed out in much sociological work, and acknowledged now by media – people approach issues with fundamentally different underlying assumptions, questions and ideas. That the experts agree in public is a source of celebration and machismo for them. That they disagree when the long string of scientific documents are placed upon a timeline and compared is a source of exasperation to the experts when pointed out by antifluoridationists. The occasional newspaper journalist dips their toe in this garble; Varney and Bryson dived in – their work largely ignored by the mainstream.

Many of us, while applauding the experts' concern for children, simultaneously want what is best for *us*. Focus on population-level work ignores the subtleties and nuances of the individual. Fluoridation's effect, however grand or slight, is not *obvious* to *most* individuals.

We blame poor people for eating badly, but our economic model of power and wealth to the rich necessitates pricing them out of good health. Yet there are changes. A recent article in the **Dominion Post** gave something close to an apology to an Australian man who had been recommending natural food [780].

My personal feeling is that much science and research is escapism and distraction. We spend enormous amounts of money to study one aspect or variable for one small moment in time. This is like taking a photograph of a rushing river. By the time the picture is studied and publicized, the situation has changed. Scientists have a vested interest in doing more research because it not only keeps them employed and helps them to feel useful, it allows them to avoid being the target of scorn from the business community. There are exceptions to this. If politicians will not stand up and regulate the behaviour of the business community, the few scientists who do take a brave stand will take the brunt of the smear tactics and name-calling.

The "freedom of choice" argument in fluoridation normally refers to the people who oppose CWF, and their freedom to not have added fluoride in their water; quite often this argument is voiced hand in hand with the "mass medication" argument. Yet there is a counterpart to the normal "freedom of choice" argument that is never discussed, which is the freedom of the experts to experiment on populations. The experts want to use the rest of us in their experiments, and they'll swear black and blue that it's for purely altruistic reasons, yet this is in denial to the fact that they get something out of it – the most obvious being employment and a sense of social purpose. What about bragging rights to a study published in a prestigious journal? Another collection of experiences to put into a CV? A specialist study type that will yield experience to help get a foot in the door at a prestigious research institute? A book published, or an extension on a contract in an uncertain work future?

Another aspect of this whole study is the fact that dentists and fluoridation supporters in many instances have cast the guidelines of basic biochemistry aside in order to make their incredibly emphatic claim that fluorine is a nutritional essential. Their statements on the matter are in many instances:

- Simple.

- When precise, only willing to include experiments that conclude essentiality.

- Defiant of conclusions of non-essentiality, from lack of caring [38], to a point of total ignorance.

- Unaware or unwilling to acknowledge standard procedures of biochemistry to investigate essentiality, even when these are mentioned in literature supportive of fluoridation (for instance the 2005 textbook *Essentials of Medical Geology*).

- Lack an appreciation of the scepticism of the public.

Consider what's really going on here: to incorporate the basic standards of protein biochemistry (replicable creation of deficiency to demonstrate need, etc) in one's investigation, is considered extremism. The benefits of fluoridation surpass these basic standards with their grandiose percentages in reduction, so to *ignore* these basic standards is seen as a *good* thing. This is not openly stated most of the time, it is implied.

It is also considered perfectly acceptable if experts don't publicly discuss this. This fits in with fluoridation's relationship with democracy – it is a matter for experts, not the public.

An argument can be made for taking research direction almost completely out of the hands of self-serving corporations. Our advances in dental science over the last century have been vast, but tying our food to our economic system has led to obvious deficiencies in elements that are *definitely* essential.

This calls into question the experts' ability not only to self-regulate, but to openly disagree with the work of other experts. One problem is the constant citing of authorities. Experts are treated as though they cannot misrepresent authorities or make mistakes, yet we can see from this investigation they are very content to disagree with authorities and experimental conclusions without exploration or discussion.

In the issue of CWF, media yield freely to experts and have virtually withdrawn from investigation beyond quoting experts almost completely. This is probably for fear of being labelled 'unscientific' – one of the great exclusions of the modern world.

7.   Conclusion

"...more courage is needed to admit a mistake than to persist in it. ..."

-     Javier Cercas, *Outlaws*, 2012. English translation by Anne Maclean 2014.

The understanding of a nutritional role has suffered because of a lack of definition regarding terms and words used; this has helped the promotion of CWF. Somehow fluoride is simultaneously an essential nutrient [121, 125], a micronutrient [106], a trace element [158], and a non-essential beneficial element [120, 146]. It is the chameleon of elements. Apparently we're all deficient in it [Appendix 1], though its abundance is legendary to the point of lawsuits [Appendix 4]. Activists and people sceptical of experts may not have seen the wordplay in many instances. Such work is time-consuming and difficult; one must work through many dead ends in research to see a full picture before behavioural tendencies become apparent.

It is not a big deal that experts and media disagree with claims of non-essentiality made by presitigious bodies those same experts and media suggest we follow, yet it *is* a big deal that these disagreements are not discussed in any depth. Such lack of depth allows discussions to become knee-jerk clichés and catchphrases.

Various aspects of the element fluorine have been focussed on and other aspects ignored, because of the biases involved in a polarized struggle.

The fact that experts in New Zealand and Australia did not publicly mention the work of Armstrong *et al.* and Schwarz in the early 1970s demonstrates that experts in this part of the world were ignorant even of studies that *did* support their point of view.

There is no such thing as fluorine deficiency, and the idea that people are at risk of "not getting enough fluoride" is quite laughable, considering the abundance of the element. It is often claimed that when fluoridation began, fluoridated water was the only source of fluoride. This is not true, as can be evidenced from research presented in Chapter 4.

The claim that fluorine is essential functions as a foundation for experts to introduce other concepts into their arguments, for instance "we don't have enough".

One may think a lack of public mention of the McClendon studies was due to their being performed on rats, yet there are 3 more realistic explanations: one is that the studies were performed for the express purpose of helping ALCOA fight lawsuits against fluoride pollution; that the experts simply did not know about them because of the group mentality; and that there was a flood of experts and literature claiming CWF a necessity, and calling natural water "fluoride-deficient" even *without* the McClendon studies.

The experts in the United States Public Health Service had no problem using rat experiments to claim fluorine essential in the 1970s, even after those experiments had been criticized or refuted by scientists, a few of whom *agreed* CWF was beneficial.

Fluorine's interactions are complex. I have found almost nothing written on the similarities and differences between human and rodent teeth; no doubt researchers around the world will be aware of such work somewhere. Most deficiency experiments have focussed on rodents.

Experts who have supported Community Water Fluoridation (CWF) have claimed a nutritional role for fluorine while disregarding research that concluded otherwise. Experts in positions of leadership made claims, other experts followed without publicly questioning.

The claim of a nutritional role has also been of political use in refuting claims of "mass medication" made by people opposed to CWF. This argument became useful to experts who cared more about convenience, reputation and winning a competition they felt would influence oral health rates, instead of keeping abreast of complicated, obscure research. This is particularly important if the American Federal Drug Administration considers fluoride a drug, which appears true as of 2013, at least according to the expert source quoted previously.

New Zealand is a country in which animals outnumber humans many times over, yet animals have no need of fluorine supplementation, even with New Zealand's soil and water.

Many pre-European societies such as the Māori had near-perfect teeth and jaw structure, as well as excellent physiques on a diet without Community Water Fluoridation and refined food influenced by technology.

Poor quality food including refined sugars and flours are large contributors to dental decay rates, not non-existent "deficient" levels of fluorides. It has been impossible for researchers to create diets without fluorine due to the abundance of the element, and the difficulties in preventing the removal of necessary nutritional factors. If there is any need for fluorine in the human body it is probably so insignificant as to be not worth concern. It becomes obvious why so many believe and have believed fluorine to be essential in the face of conflicting evidence: without this belief, one is less justified in supporting Community Water Fluoridation programs.

Abusive arguments over fluoridation led to journalists stepping away from the subject. This had a detrimental effect on the quality of discussion. When people speak or write on the matter to oppose or promote it, journalists and editors are seldom capable of correcting them.

Journalists and experts have a symbiotic relationship; they need each other. If experts are shown to be mistaken journalists suffer because they often invoke and use experts and their arguments to challenge people and ideologies.

Journalists and New Zealand's entire scientific community publicly ignored the analyses of Hastings' water during the first fluoridation trial in the Health Department Archives, even though these have been available since 1982, and were discussed in John Colquhoun's PhD thesis in 1987.

The New Zealand Health Department has used the word "propaganda" to describe their own communications to the public in some instances.

Experts may be accurate in their claim that the scientific method is ideally objective, yet even the World Health Organization can be influenced by political and financial pressure exerted by the business community.

A logical hypothesis that follows from the observation that fluorine's *essentiality* has been exaggerated for decades by experts, is that the *benefits* of CWF have also been exaggerated. In conjunction with this is the hypothesis that the benefits or necessities of other elements involved in dental health have been downplayed. It follows as logical that any harm or *potential* harm associated with CWF will also have been downplayed and denied.

The focus on population-level work ignores the subtleties and nuances of the individual. The 1991 Australian document pointed out that toothpaste use had "almost certainly" added to the amount of fluoride accumulating in the bodies of Australians. The authors suggested cases of skeletal fluorosis in Australians with thirst disorders or compromised renal function would not be surprising, however this had not been examined.

Conflicts of interest do not only have to do with money. Fear of exclusion and/or loss of reputation, a competitive nature and self-righteousness can also dissuade one from asking certain questions, thereby determining research conclusions even before a study has begun. A lack of studies on conflicts of interest within researchers studying CWF is a demonstration of a bias, and a glaring abnormality in the biological sciences.

Judging by this topic of a nutritional role for fluorine, any work that concluded CWF less beneficial than experts had claimed publicly would probably be much less discussed publicly, and is demonstrated by the rescinding of the 1991 NHMRC document. This is one area where researchers may want to look to examine potential biases.

Blame for children having poor teeth is given to parents, not shared with businessmen whose advertising undermines parents' authority and whose food pricing undermines healthy food affordability, politicians who allow advertising through many mediums, and finally the public relations industry who attempt to frame issues as "us normal people" vs "those extremists".

The food industry and their unfair pricing of natural food has led many citizens to compromised health in the name of financial benefits for industry. There are sometimes unseen costs and consequences for convenience, quick fixes and shortcuts. A most important part of putting such sincerity into action is a firm hand holding those predatory business communities at bay.

If we are ever to have real honesty in the CWF issue, the public relations industry *must* face strict regulation. Media *must* differentiate between public relations paid for by industry and actual journalism. It is very difficult to know how influential the public relations industry has been on CWF, how distorting its messages, who cheerleads to earn its money, as almost nobody studies it. Most experts barely know it exists – if one judges by how little publicity it gets.

The insistence that fluorine is a nutritional essential, even in the face of conflicting evidence, represents part of a refusal to acknowledge wrongness in our own assumptions. It also reflects our desire to solve our issues in dental health with a one-size-fits-all solution, without disturbing the power and technological structure of our current economic and social model. Experts have an obvious bias against being wrong, and against contradicting other experts in public. Biologically, we have claimed so many of our dental problems to be fluorine-related when caries, as any dentist can tell us, is a multifactorial disease.

Healthy children cannot exist without reverence and concern for our environment, oceans, and soils.

To such ends this book is written.

Respectfully Submitted,

Guy Armstrong, September, 2018.

Shortly after the publication of this book I contacted various organizations to ask if they had official definitions of the term "Trace Element". I realise this is inconveniently late, but in my defence it was not a subject discussed in most of what I read. The International Union of Pure and Applied Chemistry (IUPAC) replied, providing the following:

"Any element having an average concentration of less than about 100 parts per million atoms (ppma) or less than 100 µg/g." (https://goldbook.iupac.org/terms/view/T06421)

By this definition, fluorine *would* be considered a trace element in most foods and waters, but note that this definition does not specify essentiality or non-essentiality.

March, 2021 update: there have been a few recent claims of fluoride's essentiality in the New Zealand media. One in an article called *It's all down to the dose* by Keith Davis published in the journal **Water**, issue 206, September/October 2018; and the other by Professor of Chemistry Allan Blackman (Auckland University of Technology) in an interview called *Fluorine - the non-stick element*, 20th May 2019 on Radio New Zealand (https://www.rnz.co.nz/programmes/elemental/story/2018694328/fluorine-the-non-stick-element).

A third from dentist Dr. Adam Durning in the **Whanganui Chronicle** (21st March, 2021), who claimed: "There are only two components that make up your teeth – fluoride and calcium. That's it." And that fluoride is "… very, very necessary for our teeth." Neither of these gentlemen provided any citation or reference to support their claim, or mentioned any of the statements made in technical literature claiming the opposite.

I must thank Lisa and Karen from Vic Books (Pipitea, Wellington) for allowing me to present some of my work at their store, October 2020.

8.   References

Chapter 1

1. http://www.waikato.ac.nz/events/hangout/fluoride.shtml.
2. Gerald F. Combs, *Essentials of Medical Geology*, pp. 115-6, 125, 2005.
3. *Fluorides and Human Health*, World Health Organization Monograph Series, p. 163, 1970.
4. H. H. Messer, *et al.*, *Influence of Fluoride Intake on Reproduction in Mice*, **Journal of Nutrition**, Vol. 103, pp. 1319-1326, 1973. I will refer to the set of four experiments in the early 1970s by this group as either Messer *et al.* or Armstrong *et al.*
5. P. C. Jeans (Chairman), C. A. Elvehiem, C.G. King, G. Toverud, G. J. Cox, S. B. Finn, C. F. Bodecker, J. H. Shaw, Committee on Dental Health, **A Survey of the Literature of Dental Caries**, National Research Council, National Academies Press, p. 325-414 (essentiality discussed on pp. 390-394), 1952. Willard and Winter discussed on p. 327. For a mid-century appraisal of methods regarding quantifying amounts of fluorine, see James G. Weart of the Bureau of Sanitary Bacteriology, Department of Public Health, Springfield, Illinois, Determination of Fluorides in Water, in *Fluoridation as a Public Health Measure*, edited by James H. Shaw, of the Harvard School of Dental Medicine, pp. 203-214, Published by the American Association for the Advancement of Science, 1954. Consider this in relation to the precision of pre-1930s experiments.

Chapter 1.1

6. G. R. Sharpless, and E. V. McCollum, *Is Fluorine an Indispensable Element in the Diet?* **Journal of Nutrition**, 1933 Vol. 6, No. 2, pp. 163-178.
7. Floyd DeEds, 1933, *Chronic Fluorine Intoxication*, **Medicine**, Vol. 12, No. 1, pp. 1-60. Also see A. Gautier, **C. R. de l'Ac. Des Sc.**, 158: 159.
8. P. H. Phillips, E. B. Hart, and G. Bohstedt, *The Influence of Fluorine Ingestion Upon the Nutritional Qualities of Milk*, **Journal of Biological Chemistry**, Vol. 105, pp. 123-134, 1934.
9. R. J. Evans and P. H. Phillips, *A Low Fluorine Diet and Its Effect Upon the Rat*, **Journal of Nutrition**, Vol. 18, No. 4, pp. 353-360, 1939.
10. H. H. Mitchell and Marjorie Edman, *Fluorine in Soils, Plants, and Animals*, **Soil Science**, Vol. 60, pp. 81-90, 1945. Lawrenz's unpublished data cited in this article.
11. J. F. McClendon and W. C. Foster, *The Necessity of Fluorine in the Diet of the Rat*, **American Journal of Medical Science**, Vol. 210, p. 131, 1945. Abstract: J. F. McClendon, *Fluorine is necessary in the diet of the rat*, **Federation Proceedings**, American Institute of Nutrition, Vol. 3, pp. 94-95, 1944.
12. J. F. McClendon and J. Gershon-Cohen, *Water-Culture Crops Designed to Study Deficiencies in Animals*, **Journal of Agricultural and Food Chemistry**, Vol. 1, No. 6, pp. 464-466, 10th June, 1953. Named "Albert Einstein" laboratory because Einstein was asked if his name could be used; he did not have anything to do with the laboratory. https://web.archive.org/web/20110527042247/http://www.einsteinnewsroom.com:80/index.php/About-Us/history-of-albert-einstein-healthcare-network.html.
13. J. F. McClendon, Ph.D., and J. Gershon-Cohen, M.D., *The Effect of Fluorine-Free Food on Dental and Periodontal Structures as Revealed by Roentgen Studies*, **The American Journal of Roentgenology, Radium Therapy and Nuclear Medicine**, Vol. 71, No. 6, pp. 1017-1020, June, 1954.
14. Joseph C. Muhler, *Fluorine in Relation to Specific Problems of Medicine and Biology*, Ph.D. Thesis, Indiana University, 1951. I asked the New Zealand Ministry of Health to get a copy for their library, but as a result of limited space, they only focus on core collection areas. Joseph Muhler did a huge amount of research on fluorine. Indiana University has a hoard – boxes and boxes, I believe – of

his research archived. His work (underwritten by Proctor & Gamble from 1949) led to a patent of stannous (tin) fluoride in toothpaste. An almost full-page ad in the **Wausau Daily Herald**, Wisconsin, p. 13, 19th August, 1960, uses three articles from other newspapers to tell readers that Crest toothpaste was the first toothpaste the American Dental Association (ADA) recognised as a decay-preventing dentrifice marketed to the public. The same advertisement also appeared in **The Lincoln Star** (Nebraska), **Lebanon Daily News** and **The Titusville Herald** (Pennsylvania), **The Bridgeport Post** (Connecticut), **The Anderson Daily Bulletin** (Indiana), and many more in 1960. I counted the same ad a hundred times in a database search that yielded over eight hundred hits (I'm unsure what percentage of total American newspapers the database, newspapers.com, has archived). That Crest could afford full-page newspaper ads was evidenced by their happiness (every ad mentioned it) in breaking into the $300 Million per year dentifrice market (by 1970 it was $350 Million, see Leroy Pope, *Toothpaste War Catches I.U. Scientists in Middle*, **Journal and Courier**, Lafayette, Indiana, 21st November 1970. The first sentence gives us a feel of what's at stake:

"The giants of the toothpaste business, Colgate-Palmolive and Proctor and Gamble, are slugging it out in a new round of a marketing war that makes the pro football Super Bowl seem like a Sunday School picnic."

That they're still at it is perhaps evidenced by an article in the *Pharmacy Times* website: *The Role of Stannous Fluoride in Oral Health*, dated August 17th, 2014. http://www.pharmacytimes.com/publications/issue/2014/august2014/r648_august2014. The article reads like an advert for scientists, and I'm happy to report it claims "This article was sponsored by Procter and Gamble" under the headline). The 1960 ad proudly shouted that "Toothpastes containing chlorophyll, ammonia, penicillin, detergents, germ-killers, sugar-blocking enzymes and others failed to win the much-sought ADA approval." Crest of course, went on to sell very well.

Also see **New Zealand Dental Journal**, *ADA Council Approves Crest Toothpaste*, Vol. 56, p. 203, October, 1960. Claimed seven clinical studies demonstrated a reduction of dental caries when Crest was used, yet this depended upon which test was used.

15. *Joseph Muhler, 73, Dies; Made Crest Formula,* 5th Jan 1997, **The New York Times**. He investigated about 150 fluoride compounds before determining the tin compound to be most beneficial. According to the *Biographical Note* on *Archives Online at Indiana University* "Beyond his association with Indiana University, Dr. Muhler held numerous consultant positions with major companies such as Coca-Cola and S.C. Johnson and Sons (currently Johnson & Johnson, an advertisement reads "proud to support the Workshop that will alleviate the burden of dental decay among Asians", see *The Workshop on "Effective Use of Fluoride in Asia"*, edited by Piya Siriphant and Sirivimol Srisawasdi, March 22-24, 2011, available from the WHO website), as well as with the various branches of the United States military. Muhler claimed to hold over 800 patents nationally and internationally." See *Joseph Charles Muhler papers, 1919-1997, bulk 1955-1977.*

16. Joseph C. Muhler, *Retention of Fluorine in the Skeleton of the Rat Receiving Different Levels of Fluorine in the Diet*, **Journal of Nutrition**, Vol. 54, pp. 481-490, 1954.

17. Richard L. Maurer and Harry G. Day, *The Non-Essentiality of Fluorine in Nutrition*, **Journal of Nutrition**, Vol. 62, pp. 561-573, 1957.

18. R. E. Wuthier and Paul. H. Phillips, *The Effects of Long-Time Administration of Small Amounts of Fluoride in Food or Water on Caries-Susceptible Rats*, **Journal of Nutrition**, Vol. 67, No. 4, pp. 581-588, 1959. The only places I have ever seen this experiment mentioned are a 1974 National Academy of Sciences publication, *Effects of Fluorides in Animals*, p. 11, and Eric Underwood's textbook *Trace Elements in Human and Animal Nutrition.*

19. A. R. Doberenz, A. A. Kurnick, E. B. Kurtz, A. R. Kemmerer, B. L. Reid, *Effect of a Minimal Fluoride Diet on Rats*, **Journal of Experimental Biology and Medicine**, pp. 689–693, December 1964. Abstract: A. R. Doberenz, *et. al.*, *Minimal Fluoride Diet and Effect on Rats*, **Federation Proceedings**, Vol. 22, p. 554, 1963.

20. Klaus Schwarz and David Milne, *Fluorine Requirement for Growth in the Rat*, **Bioinorganic Chemistry**, Vol. 1, pp. 331-338, 1972. Schwarz and Milne claimed that "This method has recently led to the discovery of the essentiality of tin and vanadium" and cited three of their own works. In 1977, Eric Underwood would write in the 4th edition of *Trace Elements in Human and Animal Nutrition* that

Schwarz had shown a near-60% increase in the growth rate of rats given 1-2ppm additions of stannic sulfate ("stannic" means tin). Schwarz found that tin was lost "readily" in the "drying and ashing of samples due to volatility, particularly when present as organic derivatives." This no doubt led some to believe that there was more tin in biological materials than was suggested. In 1988 McKenzie and Smythe, writing in their textbook *Quantitative Trace Analysis of Biological Materials*, would only cite Schwarz as claiming tin essential. Both textbooks included the element in their chapter on 'other elements' and 'selected other trace elements'. Clearly it didn't *quite* cut the mustard. Underwood claimed tin was poorly absorbed; probably an indicator of its lack of necessity. In 2005, the European Food Safety Authority wrote that "Tin has not been shown to be nutritionally essential for humans" citing the EGVM, Expert Group on Vitamins and Minerals work from 2002. See *Opinion of the Scientific Panel on Dietetic Products, Nutrition and Allergies on a request from the Commission related to the Tolerable Upper Intake Level of Tin*, **The EFSA Journal** (2005) 254, 1-25.

In 1977 Underwood pointed to four experiments demonstrating impaired growth and reproduction, and disturbed lipid metabolism in chicks and rats experiencing vanadium deficiency (less than 10 ppb). Underwood also pointed to experiments claiming "highly divergent results" regarding vanadium's preventive and/or causative function in dental caries. McKenzie and Smythe did not include vanadium in their 1988 book mentioned here. In 2004 the European Food Safety Authority wrote:

"Vanadium has not been shown to be essential for humans... The intake of vanadium from normal food is estimated to be of the order of 10-20 µg/day. This daily intake is at least three orders of magnitude below the lowest doses reported to cause adverse effects. In the case of supplements used by athletes and body builders, however, the intake can be similar to the doses causing adverse effects in rats and humans. Therefore, a risk can be expected to result from the prolonged ingestion of such supplements." *See Opinion of the Scientific Panel on Dietetic Products, Nutrition and Allergies on a request from the Commission related to the Tolerable Upper Intake Level of Vanadium*, **The EFSA Journal** (2004) 33, 1-22. In 2009 they wrote: "The NDA Panel also concluded that vanadium has not been shown to be essential for humans." *Assessment of the safety of vanadium-enriched yeasts added for nutritional purposes as a source of vanadium in food supplements and the bioavailability of vanadium from vanadium-enriched yeasts Scientific Statement of the Panel on Food Additives and Nutrient Sources added to Food (ANS)*, **The EFSA Journal** (2009)1084, 1-7.

A little more research on vanadium and dental caries appears in Chapter 1.2.

21. Harold C. Hodge, Frank A. Smith and Phillip S. Chen (University of Rochester, School of Medicine and Dentistry, Rochester, New York), edited by J. J. Simons, *Fluorine Chemistry Volume III*, Biological Effects of Organic Fluorides, 1963. Published by Academic Press Inc., New York. Carbon-containing fluorine compounds were a focus due to the expanding use of fluorine in plastics, elastomers, resins, dyes, fire extinguishing fluids and medicine (anesthetics, tranquilizers).

22. Harold C. Hodge and Frank Smith (Departments of Pharmacology, and Radiation Biology and Biophysics, University of Rochester, School of Medicine and Dentistry, Rochester, New York), edited by J. J. Simons, *Fluorine Chemistry Volume IV*, pp. 119-123, (bone fluoride on p. 517), 1965. The study on human infants was by Smith, Hodge and D. E. Gardner, published in **Federation Proceedings**, Vol. 12, p. 368, 1953.

23. F. A. Smith, *Pharmacology of Fluorides: Handbook of Experimental Pharmacology XX/1*, p. 131, 1966. Smith's credentials are: Professor Dr., University of Rochester, School of Medicine and Dentistry, Department of Radiation Biology and Biophysics, Rochester, New York, USA.

24. Eds. J. C. Muhler and M. K. Hine, *Is Fluorine a Dietary Essential?* In *Fluorine and Dental Health: The Pharmacology and Toxicology of Fluorine*, Indiana University Press, Bloomington, p. 167, 1960. Maynard K. Hine was Past-President of the American Dental Association and Chancellor of Indiana University-Purdue University at Indianapolis, according to an article in the September 1969 **Journal of Periodontology** (Vol. 40, No. 9, pp. 554-556). Hine was awarded The Gold Medal Award in 1969. This award was made to honour distinguished men of dental science. He had served as Editor of this journal for eighteen years and was a co-author of textbooks on oral pathology, among other things.

25. Eric J. Underwood, *Trace Elements in Human and Animal Nutrition*, 2nd Edition, pp. 260-261, 1962, 3rd Edition, pp. 370-371, 449, 1971.

26.   Klaus Schwarz, *Recent Dietary Trace Element Research, Exemplified by Tin, Fluorine, and Silicon*, **Federation Proceedings**, Newer Candidates for Essential Trace Elements, Vol. 33, pp. 1748-1757, 1974.

27.   F. H. Nielsen, and H. H. Sandstead, *Are Nickel, Vanadium, Silicon, Fluorine and Tin essential for man? A review*, **The American Journal of Clinical Nutrition**, Vol. 27, May, pp. 515-520, 1974. Presented in part at the 33rd Annual Meeting of the Institute of Food Technologists, Miami, Florida, June 10-13, 1973. From the USDA, ARS. Human Nutrition Laboratory. Both of these scientists have done abundant work in the field of nutrition, many experiments are cited in **Mineral Tolerance of Domestic Animals** by the National Research Council (of the United States National Academy of Sciences), *Handbook on the Toxicology of Metals* by Gunnar F. Nordberg, Bruce A. Fowler and Monica Nordberg; as well as *Trace Elements in Human and Animal Nutrition* by E. Underwood, first published in 1956 (cited by Schwarz, among others – I have seen this book mentioned frequently).

28.   H. H. Messer, W. D. Armstrong, and L. Singer, *Fertility Impairment in Mice on a Low Fluoride Intake*, Vol. 177, No. 4052, pp. 893-894, **Science**, 1972.

29.   H. H. Messer, K. Wong, M. Wegner, L. Singer, and W. D. Armstrong, *Effect of Reduced Fluoride Intake by Mice on Haematocrit Values*, **Nature New Biology**, Vol. 240, pp. 218-219, 1972.

30.   Henry A. Schroeder, Marian Mitchener, Joseph J. Balassa, Masayoshi Kanisawa and Alexis P. Nason, *Zirconium, Niobium, Antimony and Fluorine in Mice: Effects on Growth, Survival and Tissue Levels*, **Journal of Nutrition**, Vol. 95, pp. 95-101, 1968.

31.   H. H. Messer, W. D. Armstrong and L. Singer, *Essentiality and Function of Fluoride*, in **Trace Element Metabolism in Animals-2**, University Park Press, Baltimore, pp. 425-437, 1974. Proceedings of the Second International Symposium on Trace Element Metabolism in Animals, Held in Madison, Wisconsin. Edited by W. G. Hoekstra, J. W. Suttie, H. E. Ganther (all PhDs from the University of Wisconsin) and Walter Mertz M.D., from the United States Department of Agriculture. The Weber and Reid experiment (reference No. 35, below) was also published in this document.

32.   G. A. Hall and J. McC. Howell, Department of Veterinary Pathology, University of Liverpool, *The Effect of Copper Deficiency on Reproduction in the Female Rat*, Vol. 23, pp. 41-45, **British Journal of Nutrition**, 1969. "These results clearly indicate that copper is essential for the maintenance of pregnancy in the rat."

33.   S. Tao and J. W. Suttie, *Evidence for a Lack of an Effect of Dietary Fluoride Level on Reproduction in Mice*, **Journal of Nutrition**, Vol. 106, pp. 1115-1122, 1976.

34.   M. E. Wegner, Leon Singer, R. H. Ophaug, and S. G. Magil, *The Interrelation of Fluoride and Iron in Anemia*, **Proceedings of the Society for Experimental Biology and Medicine**, Vol. 153, No. 1, pp. 414-418, 1976.

      "… it can be assumed that the fluoride content of rodent's milk under the conditions of this study is extremely low. If any difference in fluoride intake occurs between the young animals of the two groups during the first 10 days of life, it is insignificant."

35.   C.W. Weber and B. L. Reid, *Effect of Low-Fluoride Diets Fed to Mice for Six Generations*, **Trace Element Metabolism in Animals-2**, University Park Press (Baltimore), pp. 707-709, 1974.

Chapter 1.2

36.   Muriel Bell M.D. and Marion Harrison M.H.Sc., *Nutritional Factors Affecting the Teeth*, **New Zealand Dental Journal**, Vol. 43, pp. 5-34, 1947. The other experiments in that section of their paper discussed dental effects of lard, glucose, saccharine and other items. *Te Ara*, "The Encyclopedia of New Zealand" (www.teara.govt.nz) is managed and updated by the Research & Publishing Group at Manatū Taonga Ministry for Culture and Heritage in Wellington. It claims Muriel Bell obtained a public health bursary in 1921 and MD in 1926 from the University of Otago. Her research contributed to the introduction of iodised salt. In 1929 she was awarded the William Gibson Research Scholarship for Medical Women of the British Empire. She was a foundation member of the Medical Research Council (MRC) in 1937, and served for twenty years. Her CV is exhaustive. The list of committees, councils and activities is worthy of respect. I admire her dedication and effort. She chaired the MRC's nutrition committee, and was appointed Government Nutrition Officer around the Second World War. She wrote over 100 articles for

The Listener and other journals, and gave radio talks. She believed milk was 'our best single food', once it was pasteurised and kept from sunlight. She worked hard to have it used in schools. This was around 1940, after a survey showed only 0.7 pints were used per person each day, she thought this not enough. According to *Te Ara*, she butted heads with fluoridation opponent Sir Dove-Myer Robinson, Mayor of Auckland in the 1950s, after a sabbatical to study fluoridation at Harvard, where she interviewed many American experts who supported the practice. The fluoridation campaign "prompted her to describe herself as 'Battle-axe Bell' because of the struggle" with the Mayor. She won the battle, and in 1958 onward was a member of the Fluoridation Committee of the Department of Health. She died in May of 1974, still working, an article on karaka berry in her typewriter.

37. *Fluorine: Essential Nutrient?* **Nutrition Reviews**, May 1954, pp. 156-158.

38. *Dr. Wessman Replies to Dr. Kintner*, **Argus-Leader** (Sioux Falls, South Dakota), p.4, 8th April, 1963.

39. H. H. Messer, W. D. Armstrong, and L. Singer, *Fertility Impairment in Mice on a Low Fluoride Intake*, Vol. 177, No. 4052, pp. 893-894, **Science**, 1972. "… manganese deficiency has been ascribed to a delayed onset of sexual maturity."

"Infertility is a relatively common manifestation of deficiency in trace elements, including deficiencies of copper, zinc, manganese, iodine, and selenium." Organisms seem to regard self-preservation as most important, more important than bearing young, which is taxing of nutrition (also see Chapter 7 on this). Again, I'm unsure if this applies to plants, but it makes sense to me. Please also consider length of time taken for nutritional deficiencies to become apparent, as pointed out by Armstrong *et al*. This point is also very relevant regarding potential toxicity, of anything in the food chain.

A reasonably modern biology textbook, *Biology*, Seventh edition, by Campbell and Reece, contains some information on mineral deficiencies in animals (pp. 849-852) and plants (pp. 756 – 767). Incidentally, the section on animals lists fluorine as a nutritional essential with "higher frequency of tooth decay" as an effect of deficiency, but does not go into detail.

40. A summary and introduction to research on the topic of micro- and macronutrients in DNA replication and repair is by Arigony *et al.*, *The Influence of Micronutrients in Cell Culture: A Reflection on Viability and Genomic Stability*, **Biomedical Research International**, Published online 2013, May 27. doi: 10.1155/2013/597282. Discusses problems of inadequacy and excess. Magnesium is highly necessary in DNA function. These authors claim deficiency of magnesium not only promotes tumours in humans, it is a risk factor in premature aging.

41. http://ricepedia.org/rice-as-a-plant/growth-phases.

42. Elsa Orent-Keiles and E. V. McCollum, *Potassium in Animal Nutrition*, **Journal of Biological Chemistry**, Vol. 140, pp. 337-352, 1941. Funded by the Rockefeller foundation.

43. This is discussed in Frank J. McClure, *Water Fluoridation: The Search and the Victory*, Chapter 1, 1970.

44. O. Rygh, *Causes of Dental Caries*, **Research: A Journal of Science and its Applications**, Vol. 3, No. 4, pp. 193-194, 1950. The lack of usual detail is perhaps explained by the fact it was published in a section called *Research Correspondence*.

45. H. H. Mitchell, Ph.D. and M. Edman, *Fluorine in Human Nutrition*, **Journal of the American Dietetic Association**, Vol. 29, pp. 24-29, 1953.

46. O. Rygh, *Importance of Trace Elements in Nutrition*, **Research: A Journal of Science and its Applications**, Vol. 2, No. 7, pp. 340-341, 1949.

47. Frank J. McClure, *Water Fluoridation: The Search and the Victory*, 1970.

48. J. C. Muhler, *Is Fluorine a Dietary Essential?* **Journal of the American College of Dentists**, Vol. 25, pp. 287-288, 1958.

49. J. C. Muhler and M. K. Hine, *Is Fluorine a Dietary Essential?* In *Fluorine and Dental Health*, Indiana University Press, Bloomington, pp. 166-190, quotes from p. 167 and 168, 1960.

50. J. A. Schulz and A. R. Lamb, *The Effect of Fluorine as Sodium Fluoride on the Growth and Reproduction of Albino Rats*, **Science**, Vol. 61, p. 93, 1925. Quoted in Muhler and Hine, above.

51. S. Marcovitch, G. A. Shuey and W. W. Stanley, *Cryolite Spray Residue and Human Health*, **Tennessee Agricultural Experimental Station Bulletin**, No. 162, p. 20, 1937. Cited in Charles Weber's Ph.D. thesis.

52. P. Maze, *Influence du flour et de l'iode sur les fonctions de reproduction chez les rats et sur la croissance des jeunes*, **Comptes Rendus Chimie**, 180:1683, 1925. Cited in Charles Weber's Ph.D. thesis.

53. Charles Weber, *Fluoride in the Nutrition and Metabolism of Experimental Animals*, Published by The University of Arizona, Ph.D., 1966. Chemistry, Biological.

54. J. Chaneles, *Fluoride Intoxication in White Rats*, **Revista De La Sociedad Argentina De Biologia**, Vol. 5, p. 317, 1929. Cited in Charles Weber's PhD thesis.

55. E. V. McCollum, N. Simmonds, J. E. Becker, and R. W. Bunting, *The Effect of Additions of Fluorine to the Diet of the Rat on the Quality of the Teeth*, **Journal of Biological Chemistry**, Vol. 63, p. 556, 1925.

56. W. D. Armstrong and P. J. Brekhus, *Possible Relationship Between the Fluorine Content of Enamel and Resistance to Dental Caries*, **Journal of Dental Research**, Vol. 17, pp. 393-399, 1938.

57. W. D. Armstrong and L. Singer, *Fluoride Contents of Enamel of Sound and Carious Human Teeth: A Reinvestigation*, **Journal of Dental Research**, Vol. 42, No. 1, pp. 133-136, 1963. In his original 1938 investigation, he claimed there was a one in five million chance that his hypothesis was incorrect. This reinvestigation demonstrated that his original theory was incorrect, his previous results were influenced by the fact that fluoride content of teeth increased over time.

58. This information on EFAs taken from *Fats that Heal, Fats that Kill* by Udo Erasmus, a re-working of his earlier book *Fats and Oils: The Complete Guide to Fats and Oils in Health and Nutrition*.

59. Wallace D. Armstrong, *Chemical Differences of Caries-Susceptible and Immune Teeth and a Consideration of Food Sources of Fluorine*, published by the American Association for the Advancement of Science in **Dental Caries and Fluorine**, edited by Forest Ray Moulton, pp. 47-52, 1946.

60. Wallace D. Armstrong and P. J. Brekhus, *Chemical Composition of Enamel and Dentin. II. Fluorine Content*, **Journal of Dental Research**, Vol. 17, No. 1, pp. 27-30, 1938.

61. Floyd DeEds, Ph.D., *Factors in the Etiology of Mottled Enamel*, **Journal of the American Dental Association**, Vol. 28, pp. 1804-1814, November, 1941. For a recent experiment on cadmium poisoning, see Kakei *et al.*, *Mechanism of cadmium induced crystal defects in developing rat tooth enamel*, **Proceedings of the Japan Academy, Series B, Physical and Biological Sciences**, Vol. 85, No. 10, December, 2009, doi: 10.2183/pjab.85.500. This experiment also has some interesting things to say about fluorine.

62. It has been suggested that Vitamin D (along with Vitamin C and calcium) may play a "prophylactic" role in reversing reproductive problems caused by excess fluorine ("excess" being 5.8 ppm in the following experiment). See *Amelioration of Fluoride Toxicity in Rats Through Vitamins (C, D) and Calcium*, **Toxicology International**, Vol. 15, No. 2, pp. 111-116, 2008. "Fluoride water ingestion to rats for 60 days resulted in significant reduction of seminal vesicle weight, sperm motility and sperm density of cauda epididymis and testis as compared to control values. The level of testosterone diminished significantly..."

63. D. M. Hegsted, Ph.D., *The Beneficial and Detrimental Effects of Fluoride in the Environment*, **Proceedings of the University of Missouri's First Annual Conference on Trace Substances in Environmental Health**, Columbia, Missouri, pp. 105-111, 10th and 11th July, 1967. Incidentally, I don't recommend this study. Perhaps by the time I obtained it I had read too many of these similar statements, it was disappointing to find a reiteration of so many things I had heard before. The only thing of interest was the definition. Hegsted performed some of the early work on osteoporosis treatment with fluoride, a practice I know little about, but believe has changed over the years.

64. *D. Mark Hegsted 1914-2009 A Biographical Memoir* by Nevin S. Scrimshaw, National Academy of Sciences, 2014. In 1982, he worked as Associate Director for Research at the Harvard Medical School's New England Regional Primate Research Center.

    "Mark's experimental work covered nearly all of the major nutrition questions of diet and health of the late 20th century. As an educator and research scientist for nearly five decades at the Harvard School of Public Health, he influenced hundreds of students and colleagues."

    This biography provides two examples wherein scientists have been "disappointed" and "frustrated" to learn that requirements for calcium and protein have been less than desired.

65. Takao Suzuki, *Effects of Low Fluoride Feeding Through Successive Generations on Rats*, **Japanese Journal of Dental Health**, Vol. 19, pp. 51-70, 1969. I've only ever found this study cited once.

Chapter1.3

66. Donald R. McNeil, *The Fight for Fluoridation*, pp. 58 and 79, 1957. Wisconsin promoters Doctors Bull, Frisch and Hardgrove feature throughout the book.

Chapter 2

67. Anna Bradley-Smith, *'Outlier' dentist challenges plan to add fluoride to Nelson's water supply*, **The Nelson Mail**, 16th May, 2015. The statement in full is given:

"At the end of the day we're guided by the experts. You can pick people out, it's the same with vaccinations and chem trails, but if you look at the totality of evidence, which is what we have to base our beliefs on, then it's overwhelmingly stacked in our favour."

http://www.stuff.co.nz/nelson-mail/news/68514096/Nelson-dentists-support-fluoridation-Wellington-dentist-challenges-it.

Chapter 2.1

68. www.nasonline.org.

69. *Is Fluorine an Essential Element?* **Fluorides, Biological Properties of Atmospheric Pollutants**, National Academy of Sciences, Washington, D.C., pp. 66-68, 1971. While the chapter on essentiality is barely two pages with only eight references, this is an extensive document, in other places. In 1977 the NAS pointed out in **Drinking Water and Health** that this 1971 document looked at "fluoride as an atmospheric pollutant both in the work place and in the ambient air." With regard to essentiality, the experiments cited were many of those I have shown in Chapter 1.

70. **Effects of Fluorides on Animals**, Subcommittee on Fluorosis, Committee on Animal Nutrition, Board on Agriculture and Renewable Resources, National Research Council, NAS, Washington, D.C., p. 11, 1974. Study supported by the US Dept. of Agriculture.

71. **Dietary Reference Intakes for Calcium, Phosphorous, Magnesium, Vitamin D and Fluoride**, Standing Committee on the Scientific, Evaluation of Dietary Reference Intakes, Food and Nutrition Board, Institute of Medicine, National Academy of Sciences, p. 2, and see Chapters 8 and 9, 1997. Adequate intake for adults, p. 303.

72. National Academy of Sciences, **Guiding Principles for Developing DRIs Based on Chronic Disease**, pp. 60 and 63, 2017.

73. Cited in Frank J. McClure, *Water Fluoridation: The Search and the Victory*, p. 254, 1970.

74. *The National Research Council Fluoridation Report*, 29th November, 1951. Available from the **Journal of Public Health Dentistry**, Vol. 12, No. 1, pp. 24-33, 1952 and the **Journal of the American Water Works Association**, Vol 44, No. 1, pp. 1–8, January, 1952.

75. Wilson, G., *On the solubility of fluoride of calcium in water and its relation to the occurrence of fluorine in minerals, and in recent and fossil plants and animals*, **Trans. Roy. Soc. Edinburgh**, Vol.16, pp. 145-164, 1846.

76. P. C. Jeans (Chairman), C. A. Elvehiem, C.G. King, G. Toverud, G. J. Cox, S. B. Finn, C. F. Bodecker, J. H. Shaw, Committee on Dental Health, **A Survey of the Literature of Dental Caries**, National Research Council, p. 325-414 (essentiality discussed on pp. 390-394), 1952. Wilson quoted on p. 390.

77. **Nutrient Requirements of Swine: Eighth revised edition**, Subcommittee on Swine Nutrition, Committee on Animal Nutrition, Board on Agriculture and Renewable Resources, National Research Council, 1979.

78. Walter E. Brown, Ph.D., Crystal Growth of Bone Mineral, **Clinical Orthopaedics & Related Research**, Vol. 44, pp. 205-220, 1966. Cited in H. H. Messer, W. D. Armstrong and L. Singer, *Essentiality and Function of Fluoride*, **Trace Element Metabolism in Animals-2**, University Park Press, Baltimore, p. 428, 1974.

79. **Drinking Water and Health Volume 3**, Safe Drinking Water Committee Board on Toxicology and Environmental Health Hazards National Research Council, p. 4, 266, 281-282, 1983.

80. **Diet and Health: Implications for Reducing Chronic Disease Risk** Committee on Diet and Health, National Research Council, p. 373, 1989.

81. **Recommended Dietary Allowances: 10th edition**, Report of the Subcommittee on the Tenth Edition of the RDAs, Food and Nutrition Board, Commission on Life Sciences. National Research Council, National Academy Press, Washington, D.C. p. 235, 1989. "These contradictory results do not justify a classification of fluorine as an essential element, according to accepted standards." The 1974 Milne and Schwarz study was *Effect of different fluorine compounds on growth and bone fluoride levels in rats*, pp. 710-714 in W. G. Hoekstra, J. W. Suttie, H. E. Ganther, and W. Mertz, eds. **Trace Element Metabolism in Animals-2**. University Park Press, Baltimore.

82. **Nutrition During Lactation**, Committee on Nutritional Status During Pregnancy and Lactation, Food and Nutrition Board, Institute of Medicine, National Academy of Sciences, pp. 160-161, 1991.

83. **Health Effects of Ingested Fluorides**, Subcommittee on Health Effects of Ingested Fluoride, Committee on Toxicology, Board on Environmental Studies and Toxicology, Commission on Life Sciences, National Research Council, p. 30, 1993.

84. **Nutrient Requirements of Dairy Cattle: 7th Revised Edition**, pp. 148-149, 2001.

85. **Dietary Reference Intakes: The Essential Guide to Nutrient Requirements**, Institute of Medicine of the National Academies, pp. 315-316, 2006. Note that this is one of at least two documents on fluorine that were published in 2006 by the NAS; I think the other one has gained more notoriety.

86. **Earth Materials and Health: Research Priorities for Earth Science and Public Health**, Committee on Research Priorities for Earth Science and Public Health, National Research Council, p. 37, 2007. The study cited in support of the NRC's claim of essentiality for fluorine is E. J. Moynahan and M. J. Jackson, *Trace Elements in Man*, **Philosophical Transactions of the Royal Society of London**, Series B, Biological Sciences, B288, pp. 65-79, 1979.

87. Gerald F. Combs, *Essentials of Medical Geology*, Chapters 6, 7, and 12, 2005. Only pages 161-177 were cited by the NAS document. Quotes from pages 115-6, 125, 161-177, 301-3 and 325.

88. L. C. Chow was/is from the American Dental Association Health Foundation, Paffenbarger Research Center, National Institute of Standards and Technology, Gaithersburg, Maryland. The study is *Tooth-bound Fluoride and Dental Caries*, **Journal of Dental Research**, Vol. 69, No. 2 (Supplement), pp. 595-600, 1990.

89. Boyd O'Dell and Roger Sunde, *Handbook of Nutritionally Essential Mineral Elements* by pp. 1-5, 1997.

90. Campbell and Reece, *Biology*, 7th Edition, 2005, and *Molecular Cell Biology* by Lodish *et al.*, 4th Edition, 2000.

91. F. J. Maier, *Fluoridation of Public Water Supplies*, **Journal of the American Water Works Association**, Vol. 42, pp. 1120-1132, 1950.

92. *Guidelines for drinking-water quality, third edition*. WHO, 2004. Available from http://www.who.int/water_sanitation_health/publications/gdwq3/en/

93. http://www.bgs.ac.uk/research/groundwater/health/fluoride.html Accessed 25th January, 2018.

94. *Guidelines for drinking-water quality: Fourth edition incorporating the first addendum*. WHO, 2017. Available from http://www.who.int/water_sanitation_health/publications/drinking-water-quality-guidelines-4-including-1st-addendum/en/

95. Marla Sheffer and Christine Lewis Taylor, *Rapporteurs*, **The Development of DRIs: 1994-2004, Lessons Learned and New Challenges, Workshop Summary**, Food and Nutrition Board, Institute of Medicine of the National Academies, quotes from pp. 13, 149-150, 2008. Chaired by Dr. John Suttie. Paul Coates, Ph.D. was from the Office of Dietary Supplements, National Institutes of Health, Rockville, Maryland. Sanford Miller, Ph.D. was from the Center for Food, Nutrition, and Agriculture Policy, University of Maryland, College Park, MD.

96. https://www.bmj.com/about-bmj/resources-readers/publications/epidemiology-uninitiated/7-longitudinal-studies.

Chapter 2.2

97. Dr. Norman Jolliffe of the New York City Health Dept. *Nutrition Statement on Water Fluoridation*, Tuesday, November 13th, 1956. In the NZ Health Dept. archives, HD 125/299 H1 Box 1683.

98. *Review of Fluoride – Benefits and Risks – Report of the Ad Hoc Subcommittee on Fluoride of the Committee to Coordinate Environmental Health and Related Programs*. Dept. of Health and Human Services, USA. Public Health Service, February 1991. Available from quackwatch.org.

"This report is a comprehensive review and evaluation of the public health benefits and risks of fluoride in drinking water and other sources. It was prompted by a study of the National Toxicology Program which found "equivocal evidence" of carcinogenicity based on the occurrence of a small number of malignant bone tumors (osteosarcomas) in male rats.

"Extensive studies over the past 50 years have established that individuals whose drinking water is fluoridated have fewer dental caries. Although the comparative degree of measurable benefit has been reduced recently as other fluoride sources have become available, the benefits of water fluoridation are still clearly evident."

"Both animal studies and human epidemiology studies are used to identify potential hazards. Taken together, the only two methodologically acceptable animal studies available at this time fail to establish an association between fluoride and cancer."

The McIvor reference was looking at hyperkalemia (excess potassium in the blood) found in fluoride-toxic patients. McIvor ME, Cummings CC, *et al.*, *The Manipulation of Potassium Efflux During Fluoride Intoxication: Implications for Therapy*, 1985, **Toxicology** 37(3-4):233-40.

From the abstract: "Using fluoridated human erythrocytes as an in vitro model, it was confirmed that fluoride produced a marked potassium efflux from intact cells. Further, neither glucose and insulin in pharmacologic doses, nor various buffers could halt the efflux by shifting the potassium intracellularly."

The following is from the USPHS study.

Page 67: "Early studies provided somewhat conflicting evidence for the possibility that fluoride is an essential element for normal fertility. It has been suggested that fluoride promotes a more efficient dietary utilization of iron and other trace minerals (Messer *et al.*, 1973; Tao and Suttie, 1976). Further reports of avian and bovine studies have provided evidence consistent with the concept that fertility impairment occurs when animals are exposed to levels either higher or lower than normally occur in the diet (Guenter and Hahn, 1986; Carriere *et al.*, 1987; Hoffman, 1985; Patee, 1988; Van Rensburg and De Vos, 1966)."

W. Guenter and P. H. B. Hahn, *Fluorine Toxicity and Laying Hen Performance*, **Poultry Science**, Vol. 65, No. 4, pp. 769-778, 1 April 1986:

"The two highest levels of fluoride resulted in significant (P<.05) depression of feed intake, body weight gain, hen-day production, feed efficiency, and egg quality."

The two highest levels were 1,000 and 1,300 ppm. Lower levels (0 ppm added to diet) did not seem to inhibit breeding.

D. Carriere and D. M. Bird, *Influence of a diet of flouride-fed Cockerels on reproductive performance of captive American kestrels*, **Environmental Pollution**, Vol. 46 No. 2, pp. 151-160, 1987:

"Clutch sizes tended to be smaller as more fluoride was added to the diet, but not significantly so, due to an increase of the variance in the treatment group. Per cent fertility and per cent hatchability were not significantly affected by treatment."

D. J. Hoffman, O. H. Pattee, *et al.*, *Effects of fluoride on screech owl reproduction: Teratological evaluation, growth, and blood chemistry in hatchlings*, **Toxicology Letters**, Vol. 26 No. 1, pp. 19-24, 1985:

"Fluoride at 40 ppm resulted in a significantly smaller egg volume, while 200 ppm also resulted in lower egg weights and lengths." Tibiotarsus (the middle bone in the leg of a bird) appeared permanently shortened in the 200 ppm group.

O. H. Panee, S. N. Wiemeyer, et al., *Effects of Dietary Fluoride on Reproduction in Eastern Screech-Owls*, **Archives of Environmental Contamination and Toxicology**, Vol. 17, No. 2, pp. 213-218, 1988:

"Hatching success was adversely affected at the 200 ppm (mg/kg) level, suggesting potential detrimental impacts to wild populations exposed to fluoride pollution."

S. W. J. Van Rensburg and W. H. De Vos, *The Influence of Excess Fluorine Intake in the Drinking Water on Reproductive Efficiency in Bovines* **Onderstepoort J Vet Res**, Vol. 33, No. 1, pp. 185-194, 1966. These researchers observed the breeding performance in calving percentage and number of services per conception in 50 heifers given 5, 8, and 12 ppm in the drinking water.

"The third season revealed an appreciable decline in fertility, notably in the animals receiving over 5 ppm fluorine."

It is interesting to see the results graphed, as the 8 and 12 ppm cows have a downward trend when "percentage of cows calving" (y axis) is graphed against the breeding season on the x axis. The cows fed 5 ppm have an increase in the amount they breed, in the second season. Perhaps this resembles other experiments wherein fluoride can act as a drug, with an excitement of activity, followed by a depression of activity. Please note I *don't* claim or believe that fluorine *always* acts as a drug, nor do I think hyper-then hypoactivity should be the only criterion involved.

Another experiment that looked at essentiality of fluorine using necessity in reproduction as a criterion was published in the journal **Reproductive Toxicology** in 1989, performed by Nilouper J. Chinoy and Eveline Seqeira from the Department of Zoology at Gujarat University in Ahmedabad, India. It began by looking at the contradictory results of Schwarz and Milne (1972), Messer *et al.* (1972, 1973 and 1974), and Tao and Suttie (1976). The experiment lasted 30 days for four groups and 60 days for one group of 6 to 8-week-old mice. Concentrations of 230 ppm and 400 ppm per animal per day were used for two groups (this is 10 and 20 milligrams per kilo of body weight per mouse per day).

The reason such a high amount is used has to do with getting the experiment done quickly, and seeing how much is needed to cause harm. Another reason is probably that commercial rodent food used in laboratories has a fluorine content of around 40 ppm, give or take. The researchers also looked at the possibility of reversibility, with two groups of mice receiving treatment also undergoing a withdrawal of treatment for a month or two.

"The present study revealed that NaF treatment of male mice resulted in alterations in the histoarchitecture of the testis. The germinal epithelial cell height of the seminiferous tubule was significantly reduced in treated animals in comparison to controls."

"However, since a number of androgen-sensitive parameters in target organs were found to be altered by NaF, as reported by Chinoy and Sequeira, it is probable that the structure and functions of the epididymides and other accessory sex organs are changed."

99. *Toxicological Profile for Fluorides, Hydrogen Fluoride, and Fluorine*, U.S. Department of Health and Human Services, Public Health Service, Agency for Toxic Substances and Disease Registry, September 2003.

Chapter 2.3

100. www.who.int/about.

101. K. C. Kanwar, Parminderjit S. Vig and N. R. Kalla, *In Vitro inhibition of testosterone synthesis in the presence of fluoride ions*, **IRCS Medical Science**, Vol. 11, pp. 813-814, 1983.

102. *Fluorides and Human Health*, World Health Organization Monograph Series, 1970. (Quoting Introduction pp. 13-16; Chapter 2, pp. 38-40; Chapter 6, pp. 183-185.)

103. T. W. Cutress, *Book Reviews: Fluorides and Human Health*, **New Zealand Dental Journal**, Vol. 67, p. 194, July, 1971.

104. WHO. 2002. *Fluorides*. Geneva, Switzerland: World Health Organization. Environmental Health Criteria Number. 227, p. 44, 2002. "This report contains the collective views of an international group of experts and does not necessarily represent the decisions or the stated policy of the United Nations Environment Programme, the International Labour Organization or the World Health Organization." First draft prepared by Dr R. Liteplo and Ms R. Gomes, Health Canada, Ottawa, Canada and Mr P. Howe and Mr H. Malcolm, Centre for Ecology and Hydrology, Cambridgeshire, United Kingdom. http://www.inchem.org/pages/ehc.html. The 1996 document referenced here is *Trace elements in human nutrition and health*. Geneva, World Health Organization.

105. WHO. 1996. *Trace Elements in Human Nutrition and Health*, p. 187-193.

106. Charles Eason, PhD, MIBiol, J. Mark Elwood, DSc, MD, MBA, SM, MB, BSc; FRCPC, FAFPHM, Gregory Seymour, BDS, MDSc, PhD, FRCPath, FFOP(RCPA), FRACDS, FICD, FADI, FRSNZ, W. Murray Thomson, BSc, BDS, MA, MComDent, PhD, Nick Wilson, MB ChB, DIH, MPH, *Health effects of water fluoridation: A*

review of the scientific evidence. A report on behalf of the Royal Society of New Zealand and the Office of the Prime Minister's Chief Science Advisor, August 2014. Report commissioned at the Auckland Council's request. The report was reviewed by four people. Quoting from pp. 8 and 35.

107. Institute of Medicine (U.S.). Committee on Examination of the Evolving Science for Dietary Supplements and Institute of Medicine (U.S.). Food and Nutrition Board., **Evolution of evidence for selected nutrient and disease relationships**. The compass series. 2002, Washington, D.C.: National Academy Press.

108. https://www.fitday.com/fitness-articles/nutrition/vitamins-minerals/nutrients-101-essential-and-non-essential-nutrients-explained.html. You'll note fluorine is not in the list.

109. *Inadequate or Excess Fluoride: A Major Public Health Concern*, in Preventing disease through healthy environments: 2010, Public Health and Environment. World Health Organization: Geneva.

110. WHO (2000). Fluorides. In: *Air quality guidelines for Europe*, 2nd ed. Copenhagen, World Health Organization Regional Office for Europe, pp. 143–146.

111. Poul Erik Petersen, and M. A. Lennon (2004). *Effective use of fluorides for the prevention of dental caries in the 21st century: The WHO approach.* **Community Dentistry and Oral Epidemiology**, 32:319–321 (http://www.who.int/oral_health/media/en/orh_cdoe_319to321.pdf).

112. Poul Erik Petersen, *The World Oral Health Report 2003, Continuous improvement of oral health in the 21st century - the approach of the WHO Global Oral Health Programme.*

113. Marthaler T, Petersen PE (2005). *Salt fluoridation—an alternative in automatic prevention of dental caries.* International Dental Journal, 55:351–358 (http://www.who.int/entity/oral_health/publications/orh_IDJ_salt_fluoration.pdf).

114. WHO (2008). *Guidelines for drinking-water quality*, 3rd edition incorporating 1st and 2nd addenda. Vol. 1. Recommendations. Geneva, World Health Organization, pp. 375–377b (http://www.who.int/water_sanitation_health/dwq/GDW12rev1and2.pdf).

115. J. Fawell, K. Bailey, J. Chilton, E. Dahi, L. Fewtrell and Y. Magara, *Fluoride in Drinking-water*, World Health Organizaton, 2006.

116. SCHER *pre-consultation opinion on Critical review of any new evidence on the hazard profile, health effects, and human exposure to fluoride and the fluoridating agents of drinking water – 18 May 2010.* **Critical review of any new evidence on the hazard profile, health effects, and human exposure to fluoride and the fluoridating agents of drinking water**, European Commission. Written by five professors and two doctors, it appears like none from American universities.
Page 4: "Fluoride is not an essential element for human growth and development, and for most organisms in the environment."
Page 32: "Fluorides are not essential for most organisms. That said, there is evidence that at low concentrations fluorides can enhance the population growth rates of some aquatic algal species (Camargo, 2003). Some algae are able to tolerate fluoride levels as high as 200 mg F-/L."

117. SCHER, *Opinion on critical review of any new evidence on the hazard profile, health effects, and human exposure to fluoride and the fluoridating agents of drinking water – 16 May 2011.*

118. *Scientific Opinion on Dietary Reference Values for Fluoride*, **European Food Safety Authority Journal**, Vol. 192, p. 4, 2005. The first paragraph of the summary, page 1:
"Fluoride is not essential for human growth and development but is beneficial in the prevention of dental caries (tooth decay) when ingested in amounts of about 0.05 mg/kg body weight per day and when applied topically with dental products such as toothpaste. Dental enamel which contains fluoride is less likely to develop caries, because of greater resistance to ingested acids or to acids generated from ingested sugars by the oral bacteria. In addition, fluoride inhibits sugar metabolism by oral bacteria."

119. This document was created in response to a request from the European Commission, who wanted DRVs for fluoride. *Scientific Opinion on Dietary Reference Values for Fluoride*, **European Food Safety Authority Journal**, Vol. 11, No. 8, 3332, p. 10, 2013. Citing Bergmann RL, 1994. *Fluorid in der Ernährung des Menschen.* **Biologische Bedeutung für den wachsenden Organismus**. Habilitationsschrift, Free University Berlin, Berlin, Germany, 133 pp. I don't speak German. The EFSA is funded by the European Union.

Page 10: "No signs of fluoride deficiency have been identified in humans."

"A lack of fluoride intake during development will not alter tooth development but may result in increased susceptibility of enamel to acid attacks after eruption. However, caries is not a fluoride deficiency disease."

"Fluoride is not an essential nutrient. Therefore, no Average Requirement for the performance of essential physiological functions can be defined. Nevertheless, the Panel considered that the setting of an AI is appropriate because of the beneficial effects of dietary fluoride on prevention of dental caries. The AI is based on epidemiological studies (performed before the 1970s) showing an inverse relationship between the fluoride concentration of water and caries prevalence. As the basis for defining the AI, estimates of mean fluoride intakes of children via diet and drinking water with fluoride concentrations at which the caries preventive effect approached its maximum whilst the risk of dental fluorosis approached its minimum were chosen. Except for one confirmatory longitudinal study in US children, more recent studies were not taken into account as they did not provide information on total dietary fluoride intake, were potentially confounded by the use of fluoride-containing dental hygiene products, and did not permit a conclusion to be drawn on a dose-response relationship between fluoride intake and caries risk."

120.   WHO, (2017). *Guidelines for Drinking Water Quality*, p. 372.

Chapter 2.4

121.   Mr HAMER (Premier), *MINISTERIAL STATEMENT Inquiry into fluoridation of Victorian water supplies*, **Victoria Parliamentary Debates**, Session 1980-1981, Vol. 352, pp. 63-68.

122.   Update 1.1, Revision of Fluoride (2017), https://www.nhmrc.gov.au/guidelinespublications/n35-n36-n37.

"An AI has not been established for infants less than six months of age: The review of evidence did not find a preventive effect (reduction in dental caries) with fluoride intake in the first six months of life. This is in line with the view expressed by the Institute of Medicine (IOM) in 1997 and supported by the American Dental Association's Council on Scientific Affairs statement in 2011 that the preventive effect of fluoride in the first six months of life has not been established." See reference [71] above. No reference was given for the ADA statement.

123.   **Daily Independent Journal**, (San Rafael, California), p. 1 and 5, 11th September, 1959. "The San Francisco health officer [Dr. Ellis Sox] said fluoridated water is essential to children during the formation of permanent teeth." "… drinking of treated water is important during pregnancy…"

Chapter 2.5

124.   Carl C. Pfeiffer, Ph.D., M.D, *Mental and Elemental Nutrients*, p. 298, 1975.

125.   Jim Mann (Professor of Human Nutrition, University of Otago, New Zealand) and A. Stewart Truswell (Professor of Human Nutrition, University of Sydney, Australia), *Essentials of Human Nutrition*, Second Edition, Oxford University Press, p. 181- 2002. The section on Fluoride is by Truswell and Marion Robinson.

Chapter 2.6

126.   A. P. Black, *The Chemist Looks at Fluoridation*, **Journal of the American Dental Association**, Vol. 44, No. 2, pp. 137-144, 1952.

127.   *Four statements adopted by the Inter-Association Committee on Health*, **Journal of the American Dental Association**, Vol. 44, No. 3, pp. 331-333, 1952.

128.   *Fluoridation Facts: Answers to Criticisms Against Fluoridation*, published by the American Dental Association, April, 1956.

129.   Benjamin D. Paul, *Fluoridation and the Social Scientist: A Review*, **Journal of Social Issues**, Vol. XVII, No. 4, p. 1, 1961.

130.   Dr. David Ast and Bernadette Fitzgerald, *Effectiveness of Water Fluoridation*, **Journal of the American Dental Association**, Vol. 65, No. 5, pp. 581-589, 1962. I count seven uses of the term "fluoride-deficient" in this article.

131. Harold R. Englander, D.D.S., M.P.H., (NIDR, Bethesda, Md.); Rudolph de Palma, D.D.S. (College of Dentistry, Illinois), and Robert G . Kesel D.D.S., M.S. (College of Dentistry, Illinois), *The Aurora-Rockford, III., study I. Effects of water having naturally occurring fluoride on dental health of young adults*, **Journal of the American Dental Association**, Vol. 65, No. 5, pp. 614-621, 1962. Study supported in part by a USPHS grant. "… differences between communities with fluoride-bearing and fluoride-deficient water…"

132. Bruce L. Douglas, Donald A. Wallace, Monroe Lerner, Sylvia B. Coppersmith, *Impact of water fluoridation on dental practice and dental manpower*, **Journal of the American Dental Association**, Vol. 84, pp. 355-367, February, 1972. I count just over 110 uses of the term "fluoride-deficient" (using community as subject) in this article.

133. Rhys B. Jones, DDS, MS, Douglas N. Mormann, MS, and Timothy B. Durtsche, DDS, *Commentary. Fluoridation Referendum in La Crosse, Wisconsin: Contributing Factors to Success*, **American Journal of Public Health**, Vol. 79, No. 10, 1989. I have not obtained the newspaper cited. Anon: *Fluoridated water biting issue in La Crosse*. **Wisconsin State Journal** April 4, 1988; p4.

134. A. B. Morrison, Ph.D. and J. A Campbell, Ph. D., *Review Article: Trace Elements in Human Nutrition*, **Journal of the Canadian Medical Association**, Vol. 88, 9th March, 1963.

135. Elia, Marinos, *Changing concepts of nutrient requirements in disease: Implications for artificial nutritional Support*, **The Lancet**, Vol. 345, Issue 8960, pp. 1279-1285, 20th May, 1995.

136. Yaqiu Jiang, Xiujuan Guo, Qiuyan Sun, Zhongyan Shan, Weiping Teng, *Effects of Excess Fluoride and Iodide on Thyroid Function and Morphology*, **Biological Trace Element Research**, Vol. 170, No. 2, pp. 382–389, April 2016. Department of Endocrinology and Metabolism, Institute of Endocrinology, Liaoning Provincial Key Laboratory of Endocrine Diseases, The First Affiliated Hospital of China Medical University, Shenyang, People's Republic of China.

137. Zheng-hui Wang, Xiao-li Li, Zhuang-qun Yang and Min Xu, *Fluorine-Induced Apoptosis and Lipid Peroxidation in Human Hair Follicles In Vitro*, **Biological Trace Element Research**, Vol. 137, pp. 280–288, 2010.

138. Bhavtosh Sharma, Prashant Singh, Rajendra Dobhal, V.K. Saini, Manju Sundriyal, Shashank Sharma, S.K. Khanna. *Occurrence, Detection and Defluoridation of Fresh Waters*. **American Journal of Water Resources**. 2017; 5(1):5-12. doi: 10.12691/ajwr-5-1-2.

139. Anna L. Choi, Ying Zhang, Guifan Sun, David C. Bellinger, Kanglin Wang, Xiao Jing Yang, Jin Shu Li, Quanmei Zheng, Yuanli Fu and Philippe Grandjean, *Association of lifetime exposure to fluoride and cognitive functions in Chinese children: A pilot study*, **Neurotoxicology and Teratology**, Vol. 47, pp. 96-101, 2015.

Chapter 2.7

140. Donald R. McNeil, *The Fight for Fluoridation*, p. 48, 1957.

141. *The Fluoride Saga*, **Science**, Vol. 169, pp. 1301-1302, 25th September 1970.

142. Food and Nutrition Board of the National Research Council, 1968. Cited in McClure, *Water Fluoridation - The Search and The Victory*, p. 254, 1970.

143. Grace Noda, *The Controversy over Community Water Fluoridation : an Analysis of its Effects and Reasons Behind the Arguments*, University Honors Theses, Portland State University, 2016

144. *Handbook of Nutrition: A Symposium*, Second Edition, Chapter 7, pp. 137-161 (Fluorine on pp. 137-148). Prepared under the auspices of the Council on Foods and Nutrition of the American Medical Association, 1951.

145. *Abuse of the Scientific Literature in an Antifluoridation Pamphlet*, Second Edition, 1988.

146. These statements are taken from Paul Connett and Ken Perrott, *The Fluoride Debate*, available from https://openparachute.wordpress.com/fluoride-debate/ as pieces with comments from interested parties, or available as a pdf without comments from https://www.researchgate.net/publication/298124881_The_fluoride_debate. The title suggests a "gladiatorial sense" but this was, according to the introduction, "not about 'winners' and 'losers'." The document states they both have PhDs in chemistry. Quotes from Pages 4, 10 (Dr. Perrott's first

response), 43, 47, 60, 85, 204 and 210. SCHER document quoted on p. 202 of this debate, referenced on p. 212.

147. https://openparachute.wordpress.com/2013/10/29/the-fluoride-debate-introduction/

148. https://openparachute.wordpress.com/2013/10/30/fluoride-debate-part-1-connett/.

149. Beck, Connett, and Micklem, *The Case Against Fluoride: How Hazardous Waste Ended Up in Our Drinking Water and The Bad Science and Powerful Politics That Keep It There*, Chelsea Green Publishing, 2010. See pages 6-7 and 292.

150. *The Fluoride Debate*, p. 63, see above.

151. Nowhere in the debate did Dr. Perrott address this letter, the NAS' 1989 conclusion, or any of the experiments upon which it rested. Perhaps this illustrates how unimportant the question of necessity is – safety and effectiveness being of course more so. I've wondered what could be said against the 1989 conclusion expressed by the NAS. This is getting into potentials and hypotheticals, but I think it interesting:

Perhaps the argument of the NAS' 1989 conclusion could have been considered lacking for only using animal experiments, similar to what Joseph Muhler had said in 1959 (in the book with M. K. Hine, *Fluorine and Dental Health* cited in Chapter 1.2) that the results of human studies in cities and towns should also be included. "Contradictory evidence" suggests we don't really know for sure whether it's essential or not. However, it has been pointed out that evidence claiming essentiality has been either criticized heavily or outright refuted, and evidence claiming non-essentiality has been mostly ignored. I must point out Dr. Perrott cited a study that looked at hip fracture rates in humans (discussed below). A detractor from the NAS' point of view would had to have addressed whether experimenting on humans was appropriate, and how much can be learned from animal and human experiments related specifically to deficiency – and maybe why the USPHS, probably the biggest fluoridation-supporting agency in the world, had commissioned animal experiments, and why experts in the NAS and WHO had cited them).

One could point out that this letter was written in 1989, and since that time research on fluorine's essentiality had been updated. One would have to supply updates, looking beyond what I've shown here [109, 116, 117, 118] - because none of these groups had done any original research on the matter of fluorine's necessity. If they had, it went unmentioned in the documents I've found.

Or one could show more recent NAS work that had claimed fluorine essential – for instance the 2007 document… but this didn't really elaborate on *why* fluorine's category had changed. And if one follows *that* reference through, one must ask how fluorine becomes essential with no biochemical function.

Perrott didn't discuss Connett's reference, or the studies it was founded upon, before claiming the two could not agree. This is interesting to me considering a website called thestandard.org reproduced one of Dr. Perrott's articles, noting that "he tends to actually read the papers cited by others." See https://thestandard.org.nz/fluoridation-it-does-reduce-tooth-decay/.

152. You can also see Dr. Perrott's article on fluoride's essentiality on his website here: https://openparachute.wordpress.com/2013/06/16/is-fluoride-an-essential-dietary-mineral/.

153. The study regarding hip fractures is Li *et al.*, *Effect of Long-Term Exposure to Fluoride in Drinking Water on Risks of Bone Fractures*, **Journal of Bone and Mineral Research**, Vol. 16, No. 5, 2001. Dr. Perrott used this Chinese study which claimed that overall fracture rates were lowest in people who had been drinking water with between 1 and 1.06 ppm fluoride. However, the purpose of this study had almost nothing to do with testing if fluorine was an essential nutrient:

"The purpose of this study was to determine the prevalence of bone fracture, including hip fracture, in six Chinese populations with water fluoride concentrations ranging from 0.25 to 7.97 parts per million (ppm)."

I can appreciate the logic in applying one of the study's tables to the U-shaped curve. How well can Dr. Messer's first criterion be applied to humans? In this study, the authors wrote:

"In addition, a 3-day dietary survey and analysis for dietary intake of calcium, protein, and fluoride were conducted in a randomly selected 10% of subjects to ensure that all study populations had adequate nutrition and to determine fluoride exposure from diet." It appears this survey occurred only once, read the study and see what you think. The authors also wrote:

"A major factor that may have caused controversial findings on water fluoridation and bone fracture is the difficulty in locating study populations with definable fluoride exposure." Consider this along with Chapter 3.

They discussed how an increase in the usage of fluoridated toothpaste, mouthwashes, gums and the like since the 1970s has occurred. Population mobility also helps to weaken the ability to determine individual exposure.

"Thus, it is erroneous to use the community water fluoride level as the sole indicator for long-term fluoride exposure."

Consider here the importance of studying exposure over many generations, difficult in human populations. They discussed the differences in Chinese and American populations, and claimed that Chinese were more suited for this kind of study, due to factors like a lack of residential mobility and less variation in diet. The researchers managed the study more from a safety perspective than a dietary one, not mentioning once if they believed their study proved or disproved any necessity for fluorine. They mentioned a "beneficial window" of 1 ppm, lower or higher levels impacted overall fracture rates.

"Water fluoride levels of 1.00–1.06 ppm decrease the risk of overall fractures relative to negligible fluoride in water; however, there does not appear to be a similar protective benefit for the risk of hip fractures."

"The prevalence of overall fractures was lowest in subjects with 1.00–1.06 ppm of fluoride in water; however, it was not significantly different from the values for the groups in which water contained 0.58–0.73 ppm, 1.45–2.19 ppm, and 2.62–3.56 ppm of fluoride."

154. https://openparachute.wordpress.com/2013/09/15/when-politicians-and-bureaucrats-decide-the-science/. Quote from SCHER at Point 4.

155. https://openparachute.wordpress.com/2014/01/23/fluoride-debate-final-article-ken-perrott/. Under the sub-heading 'Breast feeding and the naturalistic fallacy'.

156. https://www.britannica.com/science/trace-element. Accessed 18th October, 2017.

157. W. G. Hale, BSc, PhD, DSc, FIBiol, V. A. Saunders, BSc, PhD, and J. P. Margham, BSc, DepAnGen, MIBiol, CBiol, *Collins Dictionary of Biology*, p. 316, 2003. At the time of publication Hale was Emeritus Professor of Animal Biology, Saunders was Professor of Microbial Genetics, and Margham was a principal lecturer and programme leader for biological degrees, all three at Liverpool John Moores University.

158. Comments section, 17th July, 2013, water supplies deficient:
https://openparachute.wordpress.com/2013/07/10/fluoridation-topical-confusion/
Comments section, 3rd July, 2013, twice, 7th July, says trace element:
https://openparachute.wordpress.com/2013/07/03/fluoridation-the-violation-of-rights-argument/
Comments section, likens to calcium and iodine, talks about correcting deficiency, discussed in same paragraph as other nutrients, November 11, 2016, 12:51 pm:
https://openparachute.wordpress.com/2016/11/06/anti-fluoride-claims-often-not-relevant-to-new-zealand/
Correcting mineral deficiency, likened to iodine, 19th February, 2018:
http://healthcentral.nz/opinion-ken-perrott-fluoridation-critics-tour-is-scaremongering-with-irrelevant-research/

159. https://openparachute.wordpress.com/2015/10/13/responding-to-tracey-brown-on-fluoridation/.

160. *Misrepresenting fluoride science – an open letter to Paul Connett*, posted on July 14, 2016.
https://openparachute.wordpress.com/2016/07/14/misrepresenting-fluoride-science-an-open-letter-to-paul-connett/

161. https://openparachute.wordpress.com/2017/01/01/december-16-nz-blogs-sitemeter-ranking/

162. https://en.wikipedia.org/wiki/Mineral_(nutrient). Accessed 24th October, 2017. (This appeared on Perrott's website as well, but worded a little differently).

163. John E. Dodes, D.D.S., F.I.S.M. and Michael E. Easley, D.D.S., M.P.H., F.I.S.M., *White Paper: The Anti-Fluoridationist Threat to Public Health*, Institute of Medicine (IOM), April 2012, p. 1. Available from https://www.scienceinmedicine.org/fellows/Easley.html.

164. https://www.dentalwatch.org/usphs/index.html.

165. *Classification and Appraisal of Objections to Fluoridation*, Kenneth R. Elwell, B.S.D., D.D.S., M.P.H and Kenneth A. Easlick, A.M., D.D.S, University of Ann Arbor, Michigan, 1960. Available from Dentalwatch.org. Quote on p. 66. Also in the November, 1962 issue of the **Journal of the American Dental Association** (p.128/690). The 1953 document referenced is National Research Council. Committee on Dental Health. *The problem of providing optimum fluoride intake for prevention of dental caries.* Washington, Division of Biology and Agriculture, National Research Council, 1953. 15 p. (NRC publication 294).

166. cpb-15, Available from https://www.dentalwatch.org/usphs/index.html. Department of Health, Education and Welfare, Public Health Service, National Institutes of Health, *Adults Benefit from Fluorides*, May, 1970. Quoting National Research Council, Food and Nutrition Board: **Recommended Dietary Allowances**, Seventh Revised Edition, National Academy of Sciences, Washington, D.C., 1968 (Publication No. 1694).

   The DHEW also quoted a study from the **Journal of the American Medical Association**: "The time may not be far distant when fluoride will be recognized as essential to health and when, in addition to being added to the water supply, it will be prescribed for older persons to prevent senile osteoporosis and frequent fractures." See Shambaugh, G. E., Jr., and Petrovic, Alexander: *Effects of Sodium Fluoride on Bone; Application to Otosclerosis and Other Decalcifying Bone Diseases*, Vol. 204, pp. 969-73, 10th June, 1968.

167. ppb-33, Available from https://www.dentalwatch.org/usphs/index.html. United States Department of Health, Education and Welfare, Public Health Service, National Institutes of Health, *Essentiality of Fluorine*, January, 1972.

168. ppb-48, United States Department of Health, Education and Welfare, Public Health Service, National Institutes of Health, *Nutritionist Emphasizes Need for Fluoride*, November, 1978.

169. ppb-66, Available from https://www.dentalwatch.org/usphs/index.html. United States Department of Health, Education and Welfare, Public Health Service, Health Resources Administration, *Misrepresentations of National Research Council's: Fluorides*.

170. ppb-67, Available from https://www.dentalwatch.org/usphs/index.html. *Fluoride: An Essential Mineral Nutrient*, U.S. Department of Health, Education and Welfare, Public Health Service, Health Resources Administration, June 1974.

171. *Safe Drinking Water Act of 1973*, Hearings before the Subcomittee on Environment of the Committee on Commerce, United States Senate, Ninety-Third Congress, May 31, 1973.

172. fl-91, Available from https://www.dentalwatch.org/usphs/index.html. United States Department of Health, Education and Welfare, Center for Disease Control, Atlanta, Georgia, *National Nutrition Consortium Endorses Fluoridation*, March 1977.

173. Stephen Barrett M.D., *Should You Believe Paul Connett?* https://www.dentalwatch.org/fl/connett/01.html, April 10th, 2013.

Chapter 2.8

174. *Book Review*, Margaret Ashwell, Ed., *McCance and Widdowson: A Scientific Partnership of 60 Years*, Published by the British Nutrition Foundation, **Asia Pacific Journal of Clinical Nutrition**, Vol. 2, p. 101, 1993. According to this review, Professor Robinson had worked with McCance and Widdowson in the 1970s and 1980s. This book "provides windows on many key developments in nutrition science".

Chapter 2.9

175. *Report of the Commission of Inquiry on the Fluoridation of Public Water Supplies*, Presented in the House of Representatives by Command of His Excellency, 1957. Paragraph 150, p. 51.

176. Unknown newspaper, 3rd April 1963. found in New Zealand Health Department archives HD 125/299/9 H1 202, 1961-1965. The letter was written in response to a talk given by K. E. Swann, the Secretary of the Fluoridation Committee of the Department of Health, "… in his address to the Kaitaia Borough Council, has failed to mention the main reasons for much of the opposition to fluoridation of water supplies."

177. Mike Berridge, *The Edge of Life, Controversies and Challenges in Human Health*, published by Bridget Williams Books, p. 80, 2015. He cites the US NRC (National Research Council – a subgroup of the NAS).

178. http://www.naturalmedicine.net.nz/childrens-health-and-development/fluoride-debate-coming-nz-tv/. Dr. Berridge spoke on soil and water deficiencies about four minutes in.

Chapter 3.1

179. HD 125/299 H1 Box 1635. Available at the archive in Wellington, see http://archives.govt.nz/.

180. HD 125/299/6 H1 Box 1679.

181. HD 125/299/4 H1 Box 1828.

182. HD 125/299 H1 Box 1667.

183. HD 125/299/1 H1 Box 1674.

184. HD 125/299 H1 Box 1714.

Chapter 3.2

185. Muriel E. Bell, *Nutrition in New Zealand : forty years history, 1920-60*, p. 9, 1962.

186. Diana Brown, *The Unconventional Career of Dr. Muriel Bell*, p. 93 (citation 21 is McCollum's 1925 experiment), 2018, Otago University Press.

187. Kaj Roholm, *Fluorine Intoxication: A Clinical-Hygiene Study. With a Review of the Literature and some Experimental Investigations*, pp. 92-93, 1937. Colquhoun pointed out that: "Roholm wrote his interpretation before acceptance, while Bell recalled hers following acceptance, of the fluoridation paradigm." See Colquhoun, *Education and Fluoridation in New Zealand: an Historical Study*, pp. 178-201, 1987. Submitted for the degree of Doctor of Philosophy, University of Auckland. Available online from the National Library of New Zealand. These statements may help us understand why two opposing points of view may exist.

Of Dr. Bell, Colquhoun also wrote:

"She clearly believed that the United States researchers were the most informed and up-to-date, and the only ones worth consulting or quoting. Her long years of influence in medical and dental education in New Zealand could be one reason for the ready acceptance of the fluoridation paradigm by health professionals in New Zealand." (page 220)

188. Dr. Muriel Bell, *Soils and Our Food Supply*, 7th July. This and the following five articles from **The Listener**, 1944.

189. *Soil Fertility*, 14th July.

190. *Miscellaneous Minerals*, 4th August.

191. *Fluorine and Teeth*, 11th August.

192. *Fluorine and Teeth II*, 18th August.

193. *Fluorine and Teeth III*, 25th August.

194. *Medical and Nutritional Aspects of Fluoridation.* Available in HD 125/299/4 H1 Box 1716. On the first page she talks about a lecture in London taken by J. B. S. Haldane, who swallowed a dose of cyanide, with no problem, no drama. He said "that was a sub-lethal dose of cyanide." Haldane explained that the body is capable of dealing with these things "by its many detoxication mechanisms." Bell claims to have "regularly demonstrated this idea of a sub-lethal dose of cyanide" to pharmacology students.

195. *Tea May Help Protect Teeth* (22nd April, year and paper unknown) and *Report of Tea's Value to Teeth Discounted*, Press Cuttings and Letters to the Editor, James Fuller Papers, General Files – MS Papers – 6167-09 –National Library, Wellington, New Zealand.

196. HD 125/299/4 H1 1716, Letter from Muriel Bell to Mr. D. L. Darley, Managing Director of Thames Valley Newspapers Ltd., Head Office, Paeroa. She did not mention degrees of fluorosis severity in this letter.

197. *U.S. Researcher Here To Solve Caries Mystery*, **The Evening Post** (Wellington, New Zealand), 23rd May, 1958.

198. *Fluoridation Benefits Older Folk*, **The Evening Post**, 21st February, 1967.

Chapter 4

199. *Jonathan Broadbent: For Fluoride*, **The New Zealand Herald** (Hamilton, New Zealand), 7th June, 2013, https://www.nzherald.co.nz/opinion/news/article.cfm?c_id=466&objectid=10888925.

Chapter 4.1

200. G. R. Sharpless, and E. V. McCollum, *Is Fluorine an Indispensable Element in the Diet?* **Journal of Nutrition**, Vol. 6, No. 2, p. 163, 1933. Incidentally, the 1925 experiment by McCollum and co-workers cited eleven studies that examined fluorine's presence in a variety of foods and other substances, which by today's standards are probably imprecise. However, the abundance was noted. McCollum *et al.* concluded that "fluorine is found in nearly all food materials…" see E. V. McCollum, N. Simmonds, J. E. Becker, and R. W. Bunting, *The Effect of Additions of Fluorine to the Diet of the Rat on the Quality of the Teeth*, **Journal of Biological Chemistry**, Vol. 63, p. 556, 1925. This study was discussed in Chapter 3.

201. Klaus Schwarz and David Milne, *Fluorine Requirement for Growth in the Rat*, **Bioinorganic Chemistry**, Vol. 1, p. 336, 1972. In support of the first part of their statement on food fluoride, they cite five experiments: **Fluorides and Human Health, WHO Monograph**, No. 59, World Health Organization: Geneva, 1970, *Pharmacology of Fluorides* edited by F. A. Smith, Vol. XX/1 of *Handbook of Experimental Pharmacology*, Springer, New York, 1966, *Fluorine Chemistry, 3 & 4*, edited by J. J. Simons, Academic, New York, 1965, F. J. McClure, **Public Health Reports**, Vol. 64, pp. 1061-1074, 1949, and G. L. Waldbott, **American Journal of Clinical Nutrition**, Vol. l2, p.455, 1963. The "careful balance studies" belong to H. Spencer, I. Lewin, J. Fowler, and J. Samachson, **American Journal of Clinical Nutrition,** Vol. 22 (though there is a typographical error in the Schwarz and Milne experiment, they put Vol. 23), p. 381, 1969, and H. Spencer, D. Osis, E. Wiatrowski, and J. Samachson, **Journal of Nutrition**, Vol. 100, p. 1415, 1970.

Chapter 4.2

202. F. J. McClure, **Public Health Rep** Vol. 64, pp.1061-1074, (1949).

203. *Ibid*, p. 1071. The two citations are W. D. Armstrong, and M. Knowlton, *Fluorine derived from food*, **Journal of Dental Research**, Vol. 21, pp. 326, 1942, and W. Machle, E. W. Scott, and E. J. Largent, *Absorption and Excretion of Fluorides. Part I. The normal fluoride balance*, **Journal of Industrial Hygiene and Toxicology**, Vol. 24, p. 199, 1942.

204. *Scientists Heavily in Favor of Adding Fluoride to Water*, **The Lincoln Star**, Nebraska, March 25th, 1961. This headline may be slightly amusing to some. A thoughtful person might ask why it would be required added to water when already in such a wide variety of food, that creating a deficiency of fluoride for a control group would be "almost impossible".

205. S. M. Levy, M. C. Kiritsy and J. J. Warren, *Sources of Fluoride Intake in Children*, **Journal of Public Health Dentistry**, Vol. 55, No. 1, pp. 39-52, 1995.

Chapter 4.3

206. *Inorganic Solutes,* **Drinking Water and Health Volume 1**, Safe Drinking Water Committee, National Research Council, National Academy of Sciences, Washington, D.C., both quotes from p. 371, 1977. In support of this statement they cited H. Spencer, D. Osis, E. Wiatrowski, and J. Samachson, **Journal of Nutrition**, Vol. 100, pp. 1415-1424, 1970. (The NAS also claimed on the same page that bone retention was as high as 2.0 mg per day, instead of 0.2 mg [sic] per day, as previously thought. The Spencer study was also cited by Schwarz and Milne, above.)

207. **Diet and Health Implications for Reducing Disease Risk**, Committee on Diet and Health, National Academy of Sciences, Washington, D.C., p. 367, 1989.

208. **Health Effects of Ingested Fluorides**, Subcommittee on Health Effects of Ingested Fluoride, National Research Council, National Academy of Sciences, Washington, D.C., pp. 125-127, 1993.

Chapter 4.4

209. Dan Milne, Wellington Bureau Editor, *Fluoridation Furore Capital Report*, **Sunday Herald**, 7th October 1973. "Dr. Ludwig bolsters his arguments with a massive and detailed study by the World Health Organization, published in 1970…"

210. *WHO Expert Committee on Oral Health Status and Fluoride Use*, **Fluorides and Oral Health**, WHO Technical Report Series, No. 846, 1994.

211. P. E. Petersen and H. Ogawa, *Prevention of Dental Caries Through the Use of Fluoride – the WHO Approach*, **Community Dental Health**, Vol 33, pp. 66-68, 2016. "The Technical Report Series 846 (TRS 846) on 'Fluorides and Oral Health' (WHO, 1994) is the existing authoritative WHO publication offering advice and technical support to countries."

212. WHO Technical Report Series, No. 846, 1994, p. 5. For detrimental environmental consequences of desalination plants, see Steve Davidson, *Making Water – Hold the Salt*, **Ecos**, Issue 124, p23-26, 2005. A desalination plant in Western Australia was said to produce 100,000 tonnes of CO_2 via its electricity consumption per 45 gigalitres of water. See Brett Koontz, DPA, REHS and Thomas Hatfield, DrPH, REHS, DAAS, from California State University, Northridge, *The Permitting of Desalination Facilities: A Sustainability Perspective*, **Journal of Environmental Health**, Vol. 79, No. 4, pp. 28-32, 2016.

213. See Petersen and Ogawa, above [211], p. 67. "Experience has shown that it may not be possible to achieve effective fluoride-based caries prevention without some degree of mild enamel fluorosis, regardless of which methods are chosen to maintain a low level fluoride in the mouth. Public health administrators must therefore seek to maximize caries reduction while minimizing enamel fluorosis."

214. World Health Organization Oral Health Programme, Geneva, R. J. Baez, P. E. Petersen, and T. M. Marthaler, *Basic Methods for Assessment of Renal Fluoride Excretion in Community Prevention Programmes for Oral Health*, p. 7, 2014.

Chapter 4.5

215. **On Tap** 2014; (10): 4-6. **On Tap** is a publication of the National (New Zealand) Fluoridation Information Service.

216. J. Ferris Fuller, O.B.E., E.D., B.D.S., F.D.S.R.C.S. (Edin.), Q.H.D.S., *Should We Fluoridate Our Water Supplies?* **New Zealand Dental Journal**, Vol. 52, January, 1956.

217. Sharon Beder, co-written with Richard Gosden (PhD in psychiatry) and Wendy Varney (journalist), *This Little Kiddy Went to Market: The Corporate Capture of Childhood*, p. 20, 2009. Beder is an honorary professor in the Faculty of Arts at the University of Wollongong in New South Wales, Australia.

"Coca-Cola's Beverage Institute for Health and Wellness emphasises the importance of drinking enough fluids so as not to become dehydrated and argues that any drink suits this purpose, so 'there's no need to stick to plain water if it bores you'." (Beder is quoting a 2007 document, 'The Wellness Beverage Guide'.

The Motherhood Project Institute for American Values, *Watch Out for Children: A Mothers' Statement to Advertisers* is written with an acceptance of responsibility on behalf of mothers, while expressing indignation that advertisers have avoided their own share of responsibility for so long. Both of these documents have sections on manipulative tactics used by advertisers to sell junk food to children.

218. Examples can be found in old newspaper articles and letters. *Fluoridation*, **Taihape Times**, 1st October, 1956: "The astounding feature of Dr. Turbott's address is that he made no mention of the cause of dental decay – our refined, processed foods, our eating habits of sugars, cakes, ice cream etc." *Our Society*, **The Evening Post**, 5th February, 1972: "Fluoride is added to our drinking water in an effort to reduce tooth decay yet advertising encourages the consumption of soft drinks, sweets and ice cream." **Wanganui Chronicle**, 14th August, 1957. *Use of Fluorine*, **Marlborough Express**, 27th August 1953: "… it is not lack of fluorine in water which is the major cause of dental decay, but faulty diet and food produced in soils exhausted…" S. P. Abraham, *Flaws in Fluoride Fight*, **The Dominion** (Wellington), 5th April, 1990. "… our hierarchy are content to exploit the best that nature provides, and to exploit the bounty of our seas for the benefit of our overseas customers, while denying a major proportion of our population, the economically deprived, the whole gamut of cheap seafood… We are bombarded with propaganda urging us to consume more and more junk foods, a major cause of dental caries… as a retired medical practitioner I am appalled by the myopic view… what is needed is a wholesome approach and the provision of the best of nature's food at affordable prices to halt our decline into a sick society…" (Ms) Helen Ledger, (letter to) **Dunedin Star Midweek**, 2nd May, 1990. "May I inquire why these zealous advocates of fluoridation are not equally zealous in demanding that the Government

ban all refined sugars? There appears to be some doubt over whether fluoride actually does prevent caries and cavities, but little doubt that an excess of sugar produces them."

An editorial in the **New Zealand Dental Journal** (Vol. 54, No. 257, p. 95, July, 1958) claimed: "We have recently observed that many people who oppose fluoridation are also exponents or followers of the Back to Nature cult. Some of them drink unpasteurised milk, avoid iodised salt, eat or compost potato skins, and save their cabbage water. And, be it said to their credit, they advise the nation, as we have done without effect for fifty years, to abstain from eating sweets."

In the 2016 Berridge/Connett debate (cited at the end of Chapter 2.9), both men agreed that junk food was a cause for real concern. Dr. Rob Beaglehole of the New Zealand Dental Association has been speaking publicly about sugar intake for many years now.

219.   The National Party are "investing in primary care, screening and early interventions…" (https://www.national.org.nz/health). Annette King from the Labour party says "In Government, we will provide a clear time-frame for industry to reduce sugar content in all processed food." (http://www.labour.org.nz/annette_king_speech_to_2015_nzlp_conference.) Key Principle One from The Green Party "Everyone should have access to healthy, nutritious and affordable food." (https://www.greens.org.nz/sites/default/files/food_20170503.pdf). NZ First didn't respond when I asked through facebook, their website was down. Current (posted September, 2016) NZ Ministry of Health policy can be seen here, https://www.health.govt.nz/publication/national-healthy-food-and-drink-policy

About 20% of the NZ population didn't vote at all in 2017 (http://www.elections.org.nz/events/2017-general-election/2017-general-election-results/voter-turnout-statistics). The party that suggested a 20% tax on all junk food that it estimated would raise about $1b from (http://www.top.org.nz/top15), to be spent on subsidizing whole foods, received about 2.2% of the vote.

220.   Author unknown, *Why We Need Fluoride*, **The Dominion Post**, p. A10, 7th June, 2017. Also see Appendix 1 for a complete list of media examples, some recent.

221.   Likened to iodine: Victoria White, *Oral Health Expert Robin Whyman Slams Claims made by Fluoride Critic Paul Connett*, **New Zealand Herald**, 16th February, 2018. Dr. Whyman is the Hawke's Bay District Health Board clinical director for oral health. "The question turns on whether I want this done for me versus the wider interests of the whole population's health. This is a population, or public health measure, it's alongside the same things as we iodise our salt, we put folate in bread. We take those measures in the interest of the wider population's health."

Compared to Vitamin K on the Hamilton City Council 2013 Fluoride Tribunal, Day One, Part Two, a little after one hour and fifty minutes. Compared to cobalt and iodine, Day One, Part Three, a little after 45 minutes.

222.   Stephen Peckham and Niyi Awofeso, Review Article. *Water Fluoridation: A Critical Review of the Physiological Effects of Ingested Fluoride as a Public Health Intervention*, **The Scientific World Journal**, Volume 2014, Article ID 293019, http://dx.doi.org/10.1155/2014/293019. published 26th February, 2014. Peckham is from the University of Kent, Awefoso is from the e-School of Health and Environmental Studies, Hamdan Bin Mohammed e-University.

"A change in the ideological approach to fluoride use for dental caries prevention is essential in the global public health community. An important change would be for the World Health Organization to repudiate its assertion that fluoride is an essential nutrient or trace element…"

223.   David Stuckler, Aaron Reeves, Rachel Loopstra and Martin McKee, *Textual analysis of sugar industry influence on the World Health Organization's 2015 sugars intake guideline*, 2015, http://www.who.int/bulletin/volumes/94/8/15-165852/en/. The document claims WHO's policies are often formed with less conflicts of interest than other bodies, largely due to WHO being able to prioritize health exclusively. Historically, organizations linked to the sugar industry have attacked WHO's recommendations on limiting sugar consumption.

224.   Dated 25th November, 2017. The video was shared on Dame Helen Clark's facebook page on 20th November 2017, and was originally posted by the page Breakfast. "We are seeing the sugar-related industry using the same tactics as tobacco did by trying to influence research and discourse." The post began: "I am increasingly concerned about the deterioration in New Zealanders' dental health."

Chapter 5.1

225. Available on https://www.dawn.com/news/160693. Accessed 25th January, 2018.

226. Hamilton City Council, *Extraordinary Council Open Agenda*, 5th June, 2013. Number of letters on p. 10. http://www.hamilton.govt.nz/our-council/Council_meetings_and_public_information/meetings-and-minutes/Pages/default.aspx.

227. An example of following the leader in the Australian media? Here are the words of Dr. Bruce Noble, the Australian Dental Association of South Australia President, appearing in 2006:

    "'Fluoride in drinking water is essential to ensuring healthy teeth,' Dr Noble said. 'It has been rated by the US Centres for Disease Control as one of the top 10 public health achievements of the 20th century.'"

    (*Bottled water a dental disaster* By: Verity Edwards. **The Australian**, 02/08/2006.)

    Compare Dr. Noble's statement above with a statement made by Dr. Derek Lewis, chairman of the Australian Dental Association's Oral Health Committee, reported in the **Geelong News**, on the *same day*:

    "'Fluoride in drinking water is essential to ensuring healthy teeth,' Dr Lewis said. 'It has been rated by the US Centres for Disease Control as one of the top 10 public health achievements of the 20th Century.'"

    (*Drink warning on teeth*, **Geelong News**, Section: Advertising feature, pg. 29, 02/08/2006.)

228. H. A. McKenzie, *Situation Hard to Resolve Unequivocally*, **Canberra Times**, p. 8, 2nd October, 1989.

229. Edited by Hugh A. McKenzie and Lloyd E. Smythe, *Quantitative Trace Analysis of Biological Materials*, Elsevier, 1988. Quotes from pages *XII*, 9 and 503.

230. *Fluoride in waters, effluents, sludges, plants and soils 1982: methods for the examination of waters and associated materials*, Her Majesty's Stationary Office, London, 1982.

231. D. Raubenheimer, K. P. Lee and S. J. Simpson, *Does Bertrand's rule apply to macronutrients?* **Proceedings of the Royal Society of Biology**, (2005) 272, 2429–2434 doi:10.1098/rspb.2005.3271.

232. Eric J. Underwood, *Trace Elements in Human and Animal Nutrition*, 4th Edition, pp. 347-374 (quotes from pp. 355-356), 1977.

233. *Ibid*, p. 472.

234. *Fluoride Findings*, **The Advocate** (Coffs Harbour, Queensland), p. 13, 24th July, 2013.

235. *Anti-Fluoride Group Present their Case*, **Taupo Times**, 21st July, 1964. Other claims of the article were that children up to age 12 would benefit from fluoridation but adults would not, that fluorine is stored in the aorta, adrenal and pituitary glands (this claim attributed to Dr. G. L. Waldbott without specific work cited), that not all medical and dental experts were in favour of fluoridation, that no research into "long-term effects of life-time dosing" were done, that fluoridation was illegal in Norway, France and Denmark, and not adopted in Austria, Finland, Sweden and Germany, that over 2,000 cities in the USA had rejected it including New York, and that fluoride tablets were cheaper and "far more accurate", and that parents could stop their use if mottling occurred.

236. *Anti-Fluoride Questions and Answers Rebutted by Ex-World Health Officer*, **Taupo Times**, 23rd July, 1964. Dr. Rice's claims are summarized: Children receive greatest benefit but this continues into adulthood, "of course fluoride is stored in vital organs... so is calcium, phosphorus..." the body regulates and rejects surpluses, Waldbott's views have been refuted by the American Medical Association, fluoridation is safe, most European countries have pilot programs in place, American cities only rejected fluoridation after groups using 'scare headlines far removed from scientific fact' were campaigning heavily, Mayor Wagner 'forecast' that New York would fluoridate, and that fluoride tablets only worked half as well as fluoridated water.

    It is very important to point the reader toward the example given in Chapter 5.2 regarding Stephen Barrett and Sheldon Rovin's publication *The Tooth Robbers*. Their claim, along with Dr. Rice's here regarding fluorine being similar to calcium is actually contradicted by claims made in World Health Organization research.

Why was New York mentioned when Washington is the capital? This is one of those times we need to venture into the literature opposing CWF; I haven't seen this discussed elsewhere. According to journalist Christopher Bryson, author of the book *The Fluoride Deception* (page 160), propagandist and public relations industry leader Edward Bernays said in an interview "If New York accepts an idea, the other states will accept the idea too." Bernays apparently claimed that both sides understood the importance of victory in New York, at a time when public opinion seemed to favour those opposed to fluoridation (presumably the mid 1960s, when New York's water was fluoridated). Bryson's work is discussed *a little* in Chapter 5.6, to provide context to some statements made by experts.

237. *Answers to Some Questions Asked About Fluoride*, **Taupo Times**, 14th July, 1964.

Chapter 5.2

238. *Letters from Argus-Leader Readers, Dr. Wessman Replies to Dr. Kintner*, **Argus-Leader** (Sioux Falls, South Dakota), p. 4, 8th April, 1963 and, 11th April, same paper, page number and year.

239. *Dentist Talks for Fluorides*, **The Daily Chronicle** (Centralia, Washington), p. 1, 22nd Feb, 1955. McClendon's work was not mentioned.

240. *Water Fluoridation Supplements Diet; Medication Claim Disputed*, **The Post-Standard** (Syracuse, New York), p. 39, 18th March, 1956.

241. *Third Round of Fluoridation Bout Slated Tuesday*, **The Raleigh Register** (Beckley, West Virginia), p. 9, 22nd February, 1960.

242. *Council Gets Fluoridation Ordinance*, **The Decatur Daily Review**, (Illinois), p. 28, 30th April, 1956. Dr. Weatherbee claimed there was a 55 to 70 percent reduction in tooth decay in children affected. Points 7 and 8 are also of interest: "No responsible medical group is against fluoridation" and "There should be no referendum – laymen should not decide about health." Perhaps pre-empting this point of view, no opponents of fluoridation attended the meeting. "Dr. Wray S. Monroe, dentist, was the master of ceremonies today."

243. *Fluoride as a Nutriment*, **The Honolulu Advertiser** (Hawai'i), p. 4, 25th January, 1957.

244. Food and Drug Research, *Other Editors' Views: Science on the Lay Front*, **The Evening Times** (Sayre, Pennsylvania), 24th April, 1958. "The evidence that this element is needed to build decay-resistant teeth is overwhelming." Note the word 'needed'.

245. *Tin Fluoride Best for Tooth Decay*, **The Republic** (Columbus, Indiana), p. 7, 19th November, 1955.

246. All from 1960: F. Stare and Mary B. McCann, M.P.H. (also Harvard), *Food and Your Health: Tooth Decay Reduced By Fluoridated Water*, **The Indianapolis Star** (Indiana), p. 59, 24th July, *Food and Your Health: Board Lists Fluorine As Necessary Nutrient*, **Tucson Daily Citizen** (Arizona), p. 28, 25th July, *Dr. Stare Lists Advantages of Fluoride*, **Press and Sun-Bulletin** (Birmingham, New York), p. 16, 26th July, *Fluoridation Fears Don't Hold Water*, **The Baltimore Sun** (Maryland), 14th August, *How Long, Oh Barron, How Long?* **Beckley Post-Herald** (West Virginia), p. 4, 23rd August, F. Stare, *Food and Your Health: Fluorine is Needed as Nutrient*, **The Courier-Journal** (Louisville, Kentucky), p. 12, 26th July. There are probably more.

247. *Readers' Views*, **The Cincinnati Enquirer** (Ohio, Kentucky Edition – this is the letter in which Stare addressed research financing), p. 10, 27th August, 1960. Is he saying that fluoridation is greater than the polio vaccine?

248. **Recommended Dietary Allowances**, National Research Council, National Academy of Sciences, p. 22 and p. 34, 1958.

249. Book Reviews, *The Biochemistry and Physiology of Bone*, **Archives of Disease in Childhood** Vol. 31, No. 160, p. 529, 1956.

250. *Books, Articles not Doing Food Industry any Good*, **The Daily Times** (Salisbury, Marlyand), p. 21, 6th November, 1962.

251. **The Ithaca Journal** (Ithaca, New York), p. 6, 7th March, 1963. This letter opened with the editor claiming arguments had become repetitive.

252. **Recommended Dietary Allowances**, 6th Revised Edition, p. 37, 1964.

253. National Academy of Sciences, National Research Council publication 294, *The Problem of Providing Optimum Fluoride Intake for Prevention of Dental Caries*, Washington, 1953.

254. British Ministry of Health, *Report on the Five Year Fluoridation Studies in the United Kingdom*, 3rd July, 1962, **Roy. Soc. Health J**. 82: 173, 1962.

255. *Fluoridation*, **Journal of the American Dental Association**, Vol. 65, pp. 578-580, and Frank Smith, *Safety of Water Fluoridation*, pp. 598-602, 1962.

256. *Harvard Receives Gift of $500,000*, **The Salt Lake Tribune** (Utah), p.12, 26th December, 1935, a "Christmas present" from J. P. Morgan and Co. for the establishment of a new political economy chair. "He stipulated that there was no restriction whatsoever to his gift, but since the university ordinarily follows a donor's suggestions in such matters, it appeared like the $500,000 would be used for a professorship in political economy."

257. *Harvard Receives Gift of $50,000*, **Portland Press Herald** (Maine), p. 56, 20th November, 1949.

258. *$1 Million Given Harvard for Study*, **Poughkeepsie Journal** (Poughkeepsie, New York), p. 5C, 14th February, 1960.

259. *School Gets Record Charitable Gift*, **The Baltimore Sun** (Maryland), p. A1 and A11, 9th November, 1979.

260. *Harvard Receives Gift*, **The News Leader** (Staunton, Virginia), p. 8, 26th April, 1994.

261. Jennifer Washburn, *University Inc. The Corporate Corruption of Higher Education*, pp. 81-82, 2005. Washburn gives many examples. Enron is one, Harvard produced thirty-one studies promoting energy market deregulation in California, while receiving funding from Enron, who would have benefited from this policy.

    Sheldon Krimsky, Professor of Public Policy at Tufts University, found a little over a third of lead authors based at research institutions in Massachusetts had "a significant financial interest" in the reports they had written. This was in the form of patents, an "executive, advisory or major equity position in a company with a stake in the research." The study referenced is S. Krimsky, L. S. Rothenberg, *et al.*, *Financial Interests of Authors in Scientific Journals: A Pilot Study of 14 Publications*, **Science and Engineering Ethics**, Vol. 2, No. 4, 1996. The study concluded that science may reach a point where readers of articles expect conflicts of interest, and that it would be "less burdensome" to point out when they *don't* occur, instead of when they do, though this may be harmful to the prestige of universities.

    Many of Washburn's articles are available online here: https://www.theatlantic.com/feed/author/jennifer-washburn/.

262. *Fredrick Stare*, **The Telegraph**, 26th April, 2002, http://www.telegraph.co.uk/news/obituaries/1392213/Frederick-Stare.html.

263. Kevin Myron, *Fredrick Stare*, **The Economist**, 18th April, 2002, http://www.economist.com/node/1086689.

264. Stare was criticized in some literature opposed to fluoridation for claiming fluorine essential, and for apparently (I haven't investigated much) claiming sugary snacks cause no problems. See Gladys Caldwell's *Fluoridation and Truth Decay*, pp. 10-11, and Phillip Zanfagna M.D., F.A.C.A., p. 244-245 (these two books are together as one book). Also see Beck, Connett and Micklem, *The Case Against Fluoride*, pp. 262-265, 2010.

265. National Academy of Sciences, **Oral Health Literacy**, 2013. In 1962, **The Evening Post** (Wellington, New Zealand) reported that "Fluoridation in Philadelphia had reduced decay in the permanent teeth of six-year-old children by 77 percent", according to Director of Health Education, Dr. Derek Taylor. *Thinks Well of Fluoridation*, 4th August, 1962, held in Wellington Public Library's Archive under Health/National/Fluoridation. If you wonder how much reduction in decay other age groups experienced, he didn't say.

266. John L. Hess, *Harvard's Sugar-Pushing Nutritionist*, **Saturday Review**, p. 10-18, 1978. Available from Industry Documents Library, https://www.industrydocumentslibrary.ucsf.edu/about/overview/. Readers may be interested in the work of Kristin Kearns, who has amassed a collection of about 2000 internal documents, regarding the sugar industry, she claims they influenced nutrition research heavily in America. See Melissa Bailey, *Sugar industry secretly paid for favorable Harvard research*, 12th Septmeber, 2016, https://www.statnews.com/2016/09/12/sugar-industry-harvard-research/.

267. The answer is aspartame. Is it better or worse than sugar? Breanna Barraclough, *Coca-Cola unveils new sugar-free product No Sugar it promises tastes just like original*, http://www.newshub.co.nz/home/money/2017/06/new-coca-cola-no-sugar-sugar-free-without-costing-flavour.html, 8/6/2017, accessed 19th January, 2018.

268. Fredrick Stare M.D., *It's Not A Drug At All*, **The Honolulu Advertiser** (Honolulu, Hawaii), p. 16, 3rd March, 1962.

269. *Gives Ruling by Courts on Fluoridation Issue*, **The Times Herald** (Port Huron, Michigan), p. 2, 28th April, 1966.

270. Incidentally, Joseph Muhler may be a bit of a wacky outlier as far as experts go. He openly disagreed with another expert about fluoride tablets (Tomi Knaefler, *Effectiveness of Fluoride Tablets Said Not Proven*, **Honolulu Star-Bulletin**, p. 4, 12th February, 1964), saying there was no evidence they worked ("There's nothing in the literature to indicate that they're effective. Your guess is as good as mine"), yet he went on to use this as a reason to endorse Community Water Fluoridation.

271. I believe Newspapers.com is in the process of digitizing more and more American newspapers every day. They also have a few British and Australian papers. They didn't have the **New York Times**, Charleston's **Post and Courier**, **The Washington Post** or the **Pontiac Press** while I was a member. Sometimes simple searches yielded many hundreds of results, quite impractical for a researcher with time limits. It is a very good website.

272. *Fluorine Held Vital for Survival, Growth*, **Independent** (Long Beach, California), p. 25 and 28, 29th December, 1971. Currently our NZ newspapers have seven columns of type across, this paper had eight. This headline was three columns wide.

273. *Official Records of the World Health Organization*, No. 176, Twenty-Second World Health Assembly, Boston, Massachusetts, 8th – 25th July, 1969.

274. *Three state plants still shy of compliance with Clean Air Act*, **Great Falls Tribune**, (Montana), p. 29, 3rd May, 1973. With sulfur, the environment was the loser. Obviously taller stacks just spread fumes further.

"ASARCO (American Smelting and Refining Co.) makes no attempt to capture sulfur fumes. It has relied on a 400-foot smoke stack to disperse the pollution into the air. 'From our point of view,' says [manager Stan] Lane, 'a taller stack is the answer' (rather than retaining emissions)… ASARCO has 'no plans at all to go to the [preventing] 90 percent [of fumes] standard,' says Lane. 'It's economically impossible.'"

275. Dr. Suttie *was* mentioned as an organizer of the second biochemistry symposium where Dr. Messer shared the experiments his team had done in the early 1970s, see *Steenbock Symposium Held at UW-Madison*, **The Sheboygan Press** (Sheboygan, Wisconsin), 20th Jun, 1973. Suttie and Paul Phillips were also mentioned in a letter against fluoridation; neither of them wrote it. See **The Central New Jersey Home News** (New Brunswick, New Jersey), p. 58, 12th Dec, 1974.

276. Fredrick J. Stare, M.D., and George R. Kerr, M.D., Department of Nutrition, Harvard University, *Variety aids nutrition, eating pleasure: food and health*, **The Morning News** (Wilmington, Delaware), p. 52, 12th July, 1973. This article mentioned the Messer *et al.* experiment published in the journal **Science**.

277. A letter in the New Zealand Health Department archives provides one example specific to Community Water Fluoridation. Fred L. Garland to the Fluoridation Commission, 7th December, 1956, HD 125/299/6 H1 1674. The language used demonstrates the class difference between supporters and objectors: "Gents – Re this fluoride stunt: if I can make it, I would like to present my objection… Being short-handed at work, it may be very difficult for me to spare the time…" The handwriting is easier to read than many.

278. *Study says mice need fluoride in their diets*, **Star Tribune** (Minneapolis, Minnesota), p. 6, 11th September, 1972, *Scientists suspect fluoride needed in diet*, **Montana Standard** (Butte), p. 27, 17th September, 1972, *Fluoride Called Vital for the Diets of Mice*, **Arizona Republic** (Phoenix, Arizona), p. 38, 7th October, 1972.

279. *Importance of Mineral Nutrient Fluoride Stressed*, **The Times** (Shreveport, Louisiana), p. 64, 13th February, 1972.

280. *Stare Endorses Use of Fluoridated Water*, **The Times** (Shreveport, Louisiana), p. 18, 20th Oct, 1973, Boyce Rensberger, *Evidence Found That Fluoride Is Vital Element in Diet of Mice*, **New York Times**, p. 78, 10th September, 1972.

281. *Mice Found to Need Fluoride*, **The Cincinnati Enquirer** (Cincinnati, Ohio), p. 10, 10th September, 1972, *Study Shows Mice Need Fluorides*, **The Montgomery Advertiser** (Montgomery, Alabama), p. 16, 17th September, 1972, *Study finds evidence fluorides are essential part of diet*, **Arizona Republic** (Phoenix, Arizona), p. 39, 22nd February, 1973.

282. *Editorial*, **Fredericksburg Standard** (Fredericksburg, Texas), p. 10, 23rd June, 1971, *Water Fluoridation Widely Debated Health Issue*, **The Deer Park Progress** (Deer Park, Texas), p. 2, 4th November, 1971, *Opposition fading: Water supplies with fluorides gain popularity*, **Tucson Daily Citizen** (Tucson, Arizona), p. 14, 12th March, 1973 (Among the claims of bone strength and money saving, this article also claimed that "[fluoridation] has been shown to be beneficial in preventing one type of ear disease which leads to deafness..."), Dr. Jean Mayer, Harvard Nutritionist, *Fluoride Essential to Health*, **The Cincinnati Enquirer** (Ohio), p. 58, 12th September, 1973, *Fluoridation's Pros and Cons: Two Opposing Views... A Few Answers* (by Ithaca dentist James Orcutt, President of the Tompkins County Dental Association), **The Ithaca Journal** (New York), p. 9, 26th July, 1974,

Fluoridation may be required, **The Daily News** (Port Angeles, Washington), p. 1, 20th September, 1974, (Vincent L. Shoemaker, assistant supervisor for the dental health unit of the state Department of Social and Health Services was definite about his claim of a nutritional role). The word 'required' in the article's title actually refers to mandatory fluoridation wherein a law is passed to enforce it. The word 'mandatory' was discouraged in voting ballots in a 1981 article by Robert Isman, DDS, MPH, *Fluoridation: Strategies for Success*, **American Journal of Public Health**, Vol. 71, No. 7, pp. 718:

"... the use of the term "mandatory" may have generated some antifluoridation votes, because it is a value-laden and inflammatory term: it gives the impression that freedom of choice is being lost."

Isman also recommends using celebrities to endorse fluoridation. He agrees with three other authors who suggest avoiding debates. Interestingly, one of the articles he cites is called *How to lose a fluoridation referendum*. Perhaps this is one factor that lead to what one supporter of the practice has called 'tiptoe' fluoridation – meaning it gets done without the public knowing. You can read about this in **Oral Health Literacy**, National Academy of Sciences, pp. 49-52, 2013:

"Such an approach might involve quietly approaching a sympathetic city council member or a county commissioner to see if they would float a proposal to fluoridate the public water system. Next, a paediatrician or a dentist would be called on to testify. The goal was to bring the measure to a vote of the council or commission without the kind of loud, contentious public debate that could delay action for months or even years. According to [Matt] Jacob [Director of Communications and Outreach at the Children's Dental Health Project (CDHP) in Washington D.C], this 'tiptoe' approach was quite successful."

283. Angelyn Nelson, Tribune Medical Editor, *Fluoride Backers Outnumber Foes at Slim Hearing in S.L.*, **The Salt Lake Tribune** (Salt Lake City, Utah), p. 44, 9th July, 1976, *Fluoridation Controversy Still Lives Across U.S.*, **The Sheboygan Press** (Sheboygan, Wisconsin), p. 11, 12th July, 1977, Vivian Brown, AP Newsfeatures, *Here's How: Don't Let Lightning Strike*, **The Lawton Constitution** (Lawton, Oklahoma), p. 19, 15th July, 1977, Sherman R. Dickman, Ph.D. (professor of biochemistry and lecturer in nutrition at the University of Utah), *Common Carrier: Fluoride Use Safe, Essential for Utah*, **The Salt Lake Tribune**, p. 181, 11th September, 1977, *Fluoridation best way to fight dental caries*, **Chillicothe Gazette** (Chillicothe, Ohio), p. 7, 7th February, 1980. "Fluoride is not a medication – it is a nutrient – just as iodine for the thyroid gland is a nutrient." Dr. Joe Forgey, (a copyright to the American Dental Association appears, but this may simply refer to the cartoon used, I'm unsure), *Captain Wondertooth says: SMILE AMERICA*, **The Noblesville Ledger** (Noblesville, Indiana), p. 12, 17th February, 1982.

284. Fredrick Stare, M.D., *Food and Your Health: Body Needs Minerals Daily to Perform Vital Roles*, **The Hartford Courant**, p. 15, 20th January, 1976.

285. *Fluoride Issue is Still Live*, **The Gettysburg Times** (Pennsylvania), p. 18, 13th July, 1977.

286. F. J. Stare M.D. and E. M. Whelan, SC. D., *Seniors Need No Special Foods But Enough of the Right Ones*, **The Tampa Tribune** (Florida), p. 13-E, 25th May, 1978.

287. Neil Solomon, M.D., *Is fluoridation really safe?* **News Herald**, p. 11, 2nd October, 1979.

288. *Fluorides and Human Health*, World Health Organization Monograph Series, p. 185, 1970.

289. Victor Cohn, Staff Writer, *'U' Professor Plays Part in Giving Irish Children Good Teeth*, **Minneapolis Tribune**, p. 14-B, 13th December, 1964. People opposed to fluoridation may be interested to know Armstrong referred to fluoride as a drug:

"'Medically, of course, it is safe and effective.' In fact, he told the Irish Court, 'I know of no other drug that has had the same degree of clinical trial involving so many people over such a long time.'"

He also claimed CWF was a controlled process.

290. *Nutritionists Consider Anti-Fluoridation Actions Criminal*, **The Tampa Tribune** (Florida), p. 91, 1st October, 1981.

291. Stephen J. Barrett, M.D. and Sheldon Rovin, D.D.S., M.S., *The Tooth Robbers: A Pro Fluoridation Handbook*. I'm unsure what year this small booklet was published, but Benjamin Spock's introduction is dated June, 1980. It contains a lot of arguments for fluoridation, and addresses a lot of arguments against it.

292. Consumers Union, *A Report on Fluoridation* in *The Tooth Robbers*, p. 23.

293. Stephen Barrett, M.D., *Don't Let the Poisonmongers Scare You!* In *The Tooth Robbers*, pp. 103-104. The article notes that Barrett has "become the nation's most vigorous opponent of health fraud and quackery." Consider this with the example given at the end of Chapter 2.7.

294. Stephen J. Barrett, M.D. and Sheldon Rovin, D.D.S., M.S., *The Tooth Robbers: A Pro Fluoridation Handbook*, pp. 118-125. The ads were made by New York agency Ogilvy & Mather, Inc.

295. Jean Mayer and Johanna Dwyer, *Taste Nutrition: Cancer-Fluoride Myth Dispelled*, **The Minneapolis Star**, p. 48, 23rd August 1978, "Fluoride is an essential nutrient that everyone needs." This article mentioned the WHO's work from the 1960s as proving fluoridation safe and effective, but did not suggest where the assertion of essentiality came from. Dr. Frank Falkner, *Fluoride is Judged Essential*, **The Philadelphia Inquirer**, p. 28, 4th December, 1979, "Fluoride is now known to be an essential nutrient." Jane E. Brody, *Personal Health*, **New York Times**, 10th January, 1979. "Small amounts of fluorine, starting before birth and continuing throughout life, are essential for the formation of strong, decay-resistant teeth. This element may also help to prevent the breakdown of bone that is common with aging."

All from **The Tampa Tribune** (Florida):

F. J. Stare, M.D. and E. M. Whelan, Sc.D., *Dieters Can Continue Eating Cheese – Sparingly*, p. 14-E, 12th March, 1981, "Fluoride is a tasteless, odourless, colorless chemical, and an essential mineral nutrient, which if added to the drinking water in small amounts from infancy on, reduces tooth decay in children by 60 percent or more."

Stare and Whelan, *Elderly Need Variety of Foods, Not Special Ones*, p. 15-E, 16th July, 1981, "One important nutrient, which is available at low cost and which in the proper amount can help prevent bone deterioration in the elderly, is fluoride."

Stare and Whelan, *Water: Essential Nutrient*, p. 17-E, 28th January, 1982, "Fluoride is an essential mineral nutrient and the most important single factor, from a practical and economic viewpoint, in reducing tooth decay."

F. J. Stare, M.D. and Diane H. Morris, Ph.D., *Food and Your Health: Opponents Kill Health Measure*, **The Tampa Tribune** (Florida), p. 118, 17th April, 1988, "Health food fanatics fear that fluoride is an unnatural "poison," despite the fact that fluoride is an essential nutrient."

All from the **Charleston Evening Post** (South Carolina):

J. R. Paul JR., M.D., Professor of Pediatrics, Medical College of South Carolina, Charleston, *The Reader's Forum: Fluorine Benefits*, p. 4-A, 13th June, 1964, "There continues to appear in medical literature, with increasing frequency, clear-cut clinical and basic science research evidence supporting the tremendous value and need for fluorine as a nutrient which is essential to the proper hardening of the crystals in dental enamel." "... I am a paediatrician and not an internist, but Dr. David S. Bernstein, who heads a National Institute of Health study on the incidence of osteoporosis (poorly mineralized bones subject to fracture – i.e., of hip) in high and low fluoride areas, states that 'fluorine is a nutrient necessary for healthy bone growth, which has demonstrated it's ability to build strong bones and prevent crippling bone diseases in the elderly'." An editor's note after this letter claimed that on 11th June the previous year, voters in Charleston rejected fluoridation 4,425 to 2,723.

Michael A. Bergevin (American Medical Student Assn.), *For Fluoridation*, 13th March, 1977, "The use of this system to provide an essential nutrient, fluoride, to the diets of children susceptible to dental caries, who otherwise would have no fluoride, is a most laudable public health development."

Dr. Jean Mayer, *Let's Talk About Food*, p. 2-C, 14th March, 1979, "Fluoride is an essential nutrient that everyone needs. And in the recommended amounts in drinking water, it is the best single way we know for preventing cavities, especially in young children."

Jane E. Brody, *Fluoride Faces Up To Claims*, p. 10-C, 5th March, 1980, "In evaluating fluoridation, it pays to know the facts about its effectiveness and safety. Fluoride is considered an essential nutrient. It protects the teeth by increasing the formation of crystals of the mineral hydroxyapatite in the tooth enamel.

296.	World Health Organization, Geneva, J. J. Murray (editor), *Appropriate Use of Fluorides for Human Health*, p. 12, 1986. Murray was Professor of Child Dental Health, and Dental Postrgraduate Sub-Dean at the University of Newcastle upon Tyne, England.

297.	John E. Mueller (University of Rochester, New York), *The Politics of Fluoridation in Seven California Cities*, **Western Political Quarterly**, Vol. 19, No.1, March 1966, p. 66.

Chapter 5.3

298.	Shiloh Lindsey, DDS, Fort Collins, *Fluoride is a nutrient*, **Fort Collins Coloradoan**, p. 9, 2nd April, 2005. Dr. Lindsey also claims to have heard of a 50-year-old study that concluded that people who kept most of their natural teeth lived about ten years longer than people who had lost many. This letter was written in response to a 'soapbox' piece by Roger Billica, M.D., (FAAFP), President of Tri-Life Health, PC. The piece was called *Fluoride cannot be called a nutrient*. Dr. Lindsey recommended readers go to www.healthysmile.org for more information.

299.	*Dental Abstracts, A Journal Every Dentist Should Read,* **Journal of the American Dental Society of Anesthesiology**, Vol. 8, No. 1, p. 10, January, 1961. "Every reader of the **JADSA** has the same problem of too much to read. Probably most of us also suffer some degree of guilt that we cannot find the time to maintain contact with the scientific literature that relates to our work."

300.	Also see Dan Milne, *Fluoridation Furore*, **The Sunday Herald** (New Zealand), 7th October, 1973. Dr. Ludwig and Mr. Milne claim the 1970 WHO monograph No. 59 looked at all the relevant research. Some of Dr. Ken Perrott's statements will substantiate this claim to objectivity and the belief that (CWF-supporting) experts are not selective, not playing favourites, not 'cherry-picking' only the research that suits them, see *The Fluoride Debate*, pp. 17, 60, 61, 110, 136, 143, 209. Available from https://www.researchgate.net/publication/298124881_The_fluoride_debate.

301.	See **Oral Health Literacy** by the National Academy of Sciences, p. 52, 2013. "When a mother of a 3-year-old hears the word 'chemical,' she does not feel reassured."

Chapter 5.4

302.	Alex Carey, *Taking the Risk out of Democracy*, 1995.

303.	Howard Zinn, interviewed on C-Span. *In-Depth: Howard Zinn*, BookTV. He made this statement about 21 minutes in. https://www.c-span.org/video/?171876-1/depth-howard-zinn. Zinn was discussing World War II and the 'good guys vs bad guys' mentality.

304.	Anna Salleh, *Science and the Media: The Good, the Bad and the Ugly*, **Australian Science Teachers Journal**, Vol. 47, No. 4, pp. 28-37, November, 2001.

305.	*Proceedings of the Fourth Annual Conference of State Dental Directors with the Public Health Service and the Children's Bureau*, p. 34, June 6-8, 1951. If there is any doubt as to the existence of this document, it is mentioned in fluoridation-supporting literature like *The Tooth Robbers* by Doctors Stephen Barrett and Sheldon Rovin (page 2, Mary Bernhardt and Bob Sprague's article), and in the **Journal of the American Dental Association** (Vol 44, No. 3, p. 368, March 1952). Also see Mark Diesendorf's article *Science Under Social and Political Pressures* in David Oldroyd's 1980 collection *Science and Ethics.*

306.	*Proceedings of the Fourth Annual Conference of State Dental Directors with the Public Health Service and the Children's Bureau*, op. cit., p. 37.

307. Frank Bull, D.D.S., M.S.P.H., *A Public Health Dentist's Viewpoint*, **Journal of the American Dental Association**, Vol. 44, No. 2, pp. 147-151 (quoting p. 149), 1952.

308. Milton E. Nicholson, *The Practicing Dentist's Viewpoint*, **Journal of the American Dental Association**, Vol. 44, No. 2, pp. 144-147, 1952.

309. Pearce Roberts (Chairman), T. E. Sikes, Jr., W. Stewart Peery, Fred Hunt, E. D. Baker, *Fluoridation Committee*, **Journal of the North Carolina Dental Assocation**, p. 185-187, Vol. 38, No. 4, August, 1955. The article begins:

"During the 1954 meeting of the North Carolina Dental Society, Dr. John C. Brauer, Chairman of the Fluoridation and Public Relations Committee brought to the members attention the formation of a corporation 'The Fluoridation Educational Society of the Carolinas, Inc.' At that time we knew that this corporation with substantial financial backing had as its objective a campaign for the removal of Fluorides from communal water supplies in North Carolina. During the past year we have watched this organization at work noting how effective its campaign was in Greensboro by influencing the people to vote in November 1954 the discontinuance of Fluoridation after two years successful operation. We also observed how effectively the dental society members of Charlotte prevented a similar occurrence in their city."

There was no elaboration on "substantial financial backing" for the 'antis'. The Fluoridation Committee who authored this article claimed their own budget was $1,000.

310. Dr. Carl Weatherbee, quoted in *Council Gets Fluoridation Ordinance*, **The Decatur Daily Review**, (Illinois), p. 28, 30th April, 1956.

311. *Dental Association's Attitude Criticised*, **Dunedin Evening Star**, 4th Feb, 1958.

312. **Northland Age**, 10th October, 1963 quoted in *Compulsory Fluoridation*, **South Auckland Courier**, 9th September, 1964.

313. Dr. Frederick Stare, *Finding Out About Fluoridation* **The Detroit Free Press**, p. 34, 8th May, 1964.

314. Appleby, *Capitalism and a New Social Order* (NYU, 1984, 73). Quoted in Noam Chomsky's *Necessary Illusions*, p. 27.

315. *The Crisis of Democracy. Report on the Governability of Democracies to the Trilateral Commission*, New York University Press, 1975. Quoting from pp. 87-88, 113 and 114.

316. HD 125/299/1 H1 Box 1634, 6th April 1954.

317. HD 125/299/1 H1 Box 1634, 5th May 1954.

318. *Hastings Jaycees' Fluoridation Campaign*, **Hawke's Bay Herald Tribune**, 4th May, 1954.

319. HD 125/299 H1 Box 1667, 3rd February 1956.

320. 125/299/10 H1 Box 1734, 31st August 1959.

321. HD 125/299/10 H1 Box 1734. *Fluoridation Referendum – Masterton – November 1959*, p. 1.

322. 125/299/10 H1 Box 1734, 4th February 1960.

323. For instance, in discussing the **National Fluoridation News** (a newspaper dedicated to ending fluoridation, published I believe quarterly or monthly from the USA), G. R. Jensen, the Medical Officer of Health, wrote in a letter dated 4th October 1962, to K. E. Swann, the Secretary of the Fluoridation Committee that "it impresses me as excellent health propaganda and I think it admirably complies with the sub-title you have given it 'Fact versus Fancy'." HD 125/299/4 H1 Box 1828.

An example from 'the other side' is given in a letter from a member of the public to the Minister of Health dated 7th March 1958, that contained the question: "Is it fair or just that the taxpayer should have to pay the cost of all this propaganda being issued by the Health Dept., advocating fluoridation?" HD 125/299 H1 Box 1714.

324. *Fluoridation Wanted by Masterton*, **The Evening Post**, 23rd October, 1957.

325. Dr. John Knutson, D.D.S., Dr.P.H., *Water fluoridation after 25 years*, **Journal of the American Dental Association**, Vol. 80, No. 4, pp. 765-769, 1970. Don't confuse this article with the editorial, page 697, that has a similar title.

326. John E. Mueller, Ph.D., *Reply by Dr. Mueller*, **American Journal of Public Health**, Vol. 58, No. 10, pp. 1881-1882, October, 1968.

327. Robert Isman, D.D.S., M.P.H., *Fluoridation: Strategies for Success*, **American Journal of Public Health**, Vol. 71, No. 7, p. 717-721 (quote from p. 721), 1981.

328. John E. Mueller, Ph.D., *Fluoridation Attitude Change*, **American Journal of Public Health**, Vol. 58, No. 10, pp. 1876-1880 (quoted p. 1879), October, 1968.

329. John Colquhoun, B.D.S., *Education and Fluoridation in New Zealand: An Historical Study*. A thesis submitted for the degree of Doctor of Philosophy, University of Auckland, 1987. Available through the Alexander Turnbull Library.

330. Brian Martin Ph.D., *Strip the Experts*, Chapter 1, p. 11, 1991. Martin is currently Professor Emeritus, University of Wollongong.

331. Robert Isman, *op. cit.*, p. 717, 1981.

332. The Wisconsin State Dental Society announced on December 29th that it had accomplished its goal of introducing fluoridation to 50 Wisconsin cities by the year 1950. According to the article, Dr John Frisch, the Dane County Society Chairman, Wisconsin was in the lead with more cities fluorinated than any other state. See *State Leads in Fluorination of Water for Dental Health*, **Eau Claire Leader**, Wisconsin, 31st Dec, 1949. **Chemical Week**, p. 14, 17th July, 1951, claims 174 American (not only Wisconsin) communities fluoridating or had ordered equipment to do so. The 1953 Mitchell and Edman review (see Chapter 1.2) claims that by June 1952, 233 communities were partaking in fluoridation. According to **The Greenville News** (North Carolina, p. 8, *Public Health Service Worried About Fluoridation Foes, Says Militant Minority Perpetuates Tooth Decay*, 18th Oct, 1959), 1953 was a peak year with 378 communities fluoridating. However a year earlier in 1952, according to **The Courier-Journal** (Louisville, Kentucky), Dr. H. Trendley Dean, Director of the National Institute of Dental Research, told the lawyers at the 17th annual conference of the National Institute of Municipal Law Officers, that 461 cities were using fluoridation. See *Fluoridated Water Called Boon to Future Dental Care*, p. 17, 2nd December, 1952. America's a big place and fluctuations in numbers were probably difficult to keep track of. On the 17th December, 1955, **The Courier-News** (page 6, Bridgewater, New Jersey), reported that 1,115 communities were using fluoridation, this according to Dr. Herman E. Hilleboe, New York State Health Commissioner.

333. Dr. Molly L.R. Melbye, DDS, MPH, Dr. Jason M. Armfield, PhD, *The dentist's role in promoting community water fluoridation: A call to action for dentists and educators*, **Journal of the American Dental Association**, Vol. 144, No. 1, pp. 65-75, January, 2013.

334. Edward Herman and Noam Chomsky, *Manufacturing Consent*, Introduction to the 2002 Edition, p. xi, 2008.

335. Alex Carey, *Taking the Risk out of Democracy*, Reshaping the Truth, p. 79, 1995.

336. Michael Easley D.D.S., M.P.H., *Community Water Fluoridation in America: The Unprincipled Opposition*, p. 10, 1999.

337. Children's Dental Health Project, July, 2015 report *Fluoridation Advocacy: Pew's Contributions and Lessons that Emerge*, p. 24.

338. R. C. Faine, D.D.S., J. J. Collins, M.P.H., J. Daniel D.M.D., B. Isman, D.D.S., J. Boriskin, D.D.S., K. L. Young, D.D.S., and C.M. Fitzgerald, D.D.S., *The 1980 Fluoridation Campaigns: A Discussion of Results*, **Journal of Public Health Dentistry**, Vol. 41, No. 3, pp. 138-143, September, 1981.

339. This ad can be viewed on the Fluoride Free New Zealand website: http://fluoridefree.org.nz/. You can read their summary of events on their website: http://fluoridefree.org.nz/fluoride-free-nz-wins-advertising-complaints/.

340. The Radio New Zealand interview is available on the RNZ website, http://www.radionz.co.nz/national/programmes/afternoons/audio/201811759/complaints-over-anti-fluoride-ads, 11th August, 2016.

341. You can read about Griffin on the Science Media Centre website: https://www.sciencemediacentre.co.nz/about/board-staff/.

342. Alex Carey, *Taking the Risk out of Democracy*, Exporting Free-Enterprise Persuasion: Grassroots and Treetops Propaganda, p. 89, 1995.

343. *Toxic Sludge is Good for You*, p. xii, Introduction to the UK Edition, 2004.

344. https://www.pressassociation.com/pr-industry-monitoring/. Accessed 28th May, 2018. Regarding 'publicity crises' and how agencies deal with them, some good examples are given in *Secrets and Lies* by Bob Burton and Nicky Hager, as well as *Toxic Sludge is Good for You*, Chapter 12 and Appendix B: The Clorox PR Crisis Plan, pp. 197-212. "… the PR industry is constantly vigilant about its own image…"

345. Virgil Dickson, *CDC awards $12m in work before end of fiscal year*, **PRWeek**, 11th September, 2012. I believe this was reported by FAN (Fluoride Action Network) on their website, claiming $6.5m was spent. They cited Capitol Communicator as the source, a website similar to PR Week that keeps up to date with the PR industry. I could not find it as I searched in late 2017. I wrote to request it but they claimed their archive did not go back far enough. In October of 2017 when I looked, Capitol Communicator reported that the CDC and Hager Sharp received the Thoth Best of Show award for their work on cancer prevention.

346. In *Doubt is their Product* (Chapter 15), David Michaels gives a couple of examples of the CDC putting political and perhaps even the Bush and Clinton Administration's religious ideologies before science, on the issues of abstinence vs condom use, and needle exchanges as a way of preventing AIDS.

    Michaels expressed his view on the 'committee stacking' of the Bush Administration: "Regulatory paralysis appears to be the goal here, rather than the application of honest balanced science." This is a quote from an editorial he co-authored with E. Bingham, L. Boden, et al., *Advice without Dissent*, **Science**, 2002; 298 (5594): 703.

    Of more relevance to us is an example of the CDC's advisory committee on childhood lead poisoning. The CDC was asked by a Senator to lower the amount of lead defined as "elevated" in children from 10 to 5 micrograms per decilitre of blood. The CDC said it would probably occur, yet then proceeded to instigate changes on the advisory committee related to childhood lead poisoning. One of the researchers who was disqualified from serving had carried out research supporting levels of less than 10 micrograms lead as harmful, another was disqualified who had been on the committee for five years. A replacement scientist had had work funded by Asarco, "a leading metals smelter facing large clean-up costs that would be reduced substantially if lead were deemed to be less hazardous" (the work had been done at product defence firm Exponent). The doctor withdrew after her corporate ties became known. Also nominated were a member of a New York medical centre who had called the 1991 committee "well-meaning fanatics" and a pediatric toxicologist from the University of Oklahoma Health Sciences Center, who had believed lead levels less than 70 microgram were harmless, and "dismisses all conclusions to the contrary".

347. *Science Should Decide on Fluoride*, **The Dominion Post**, 7th of October, 2013.

348. In Hamilton in the October 2013 referendum the "pros" spent $47,000 (of District Health Board money, $8,000 of which was on billboards and banners). See *Anti-fluoride campaigners dealt triple blow* by Tony Wall, **Waikato Times**, 13th October 2013.

    The "antis" spent "a few thousand" dollars of their own money, see *Fluoride back on the Hamilton menu* by Daniel Adams, **Waikato Times**, 10th October 2013. The vote to return fluoride to water in Hamilton was 68 to 32%.

    The Waikato DHB said fluoridation saved $1M in dental costs for the $40,000 spent on it. See *Editorial: Vote to ditch fluoridation defies all logic*, **New Zealand Herald**, 7th June 2013.

Chapter 5.5

349. John E. Mueller (Political Scientist, University of Rochester, New York), *The Politics of Fluoridation in Seven California Cities*, **Western Political Quarterly**, Vol. 19, No.1, p. 61, March 1966. The word "pros" refers to supporters of fluoridation, the word "authorities" refers to the more medically inclined and qualified opponents of fluoridation.

350. Sean Plunket, *Fluoride nutters may be biting off more than they can chew*, **The Dominion Post** 8 June, 2013, http://www.stuff.co.nz/dominion-post/comment/columnists/sean-plunket/8770145/Fluoride-nutters-bite-off-too-much.

351. Michael Easley D.D.S., M.P.H., *Community Water Fluoridation in America: The Unprincipled Opposition*, p. 9, 1999.

352. *Fluoride Gets a Kick in the Teeth*, **Dominion Sunday Times** (Wellington, New Zealand), 1st April, 1990.

353. https://www.sciencemediacentre.co.nz/2013/06/07/hamiltons-fluoride-furore-makes-a-splash/

354. Hamilton City Council, *Extraordinary Council Open Agenda*, points 8 and 12, p. 5-6 of 28, Wednesday 5th June 2013.

355. Harry Pearl and Elton Smallman, *'Absolutely gutless': Judith Collins slams Hamilton over fluoride*, **Waikato Times**, 7th June, 2013.

356. According to the Health Quality and Safety Commission New Zealand website, "Dr. Felicity Dumble grew up and trained in Medicine in Auckland and completed her house surgeon years in Auckland and Palmerston North. After moving to Hamilton, Dr Dumble was the senior medical staff member in charge of the Waikato Hospital Emergency Department medical team for two years. Becoming frustrated with the number of preventable injuries and admissions, Dr Dumble commuted to Auckland to train in Public Health Medicine and undertook advanced training with ACC, Midland Regional Health Authority and the Public Health Unit of the Waikato DHB."

This is about half of the accomplishments listed. She is chair of the Child & Youth Mortality Review Committee. See https://www.hqsc.govt.nz/our-programmes/mrc/cymrc/about-us/members/.

Julie Hardaker spent two terms as Mayor of Hamilton from 2010-2016, currently working in her own law firm, *Julie Hardaker Lawyers*. According to this website, "Julie was the top graduating student in her law degree at the University of Waikato and was a partner in long established Hamilton law firm McCaw Lewis. From 2010 – 2016, Julie served two terms as Mayor of Hamilton and in 2017 was a Principal in leading New Zealand public law and employment firm Chen Palmer. Julie was a finalist in the New Zealand Law Awards Employment Team in 2008 and in 2016, she was one of the first recipients of Order of Te Arikinui Queen Te Atairangikaahu (Waikato Tainui) for services to Maori. She is a commentator in the media and a regular presenter at conferences."

Her qualifications are listed as LLB (Hons 1st class), 1994 | MMS (Hons 1st class), 2017. Roles in governance are many.

357. Michael Easley D.D.S., M.P.H., *Community Water Fluoridation in America: The Unprincipled Opposition*, pp. 8-9, 1999. "… debates give the illusion that a scientific controversy exists…"

358. *Councillor Dave Mcpherson talks about Water Fluoridation*. I must apologize to those who want their citations from peer-reviewed journals or legitimate media publications that this talk is on Youtube. Perhaps this is because Cr. McPherson was critical of media's attitude, participation, and knowledge of the issue. If any readers find his comments in a peer-reviewed journal, or in media, I'm happy to substitute that in place of this.

"Like a lot of people beforehand, I was slightly sceptical about the tribunal process because I hadn't been through it before but following our experience with it I thought it was great because it allowed each side of the argument to bring out all the points that they wanted and to have us question them on them and to have us go into any detail that we wanted, so … I don't think anyone, from either the council's side, or the submitters' side, thought that there hadn't been a fair hearing of the issues." https://www.youtube.com/watch?v=Zcu7XIIZyt4.

359. Denise Irvine, *Fluoride vote doesn't wash with me*, **Waikato Times**, p. B-5, 15th June, 2013. According to her LinkedIn profile, Irvine is Telehealth Facilitator at Waikato DHB since May 2013, CEO at e3health since January 2006.

360. USA: Robert A. Downs, D.D.S., M.S.P.H, *The Dentist's Responsibility in Community Water Fluoridation Programs*, **American Journal of Public Health**, Vol. 42, pp. 575-576, 1952. "Due to excellent publicity in lay publications such as **Reader's Digest** and **The American Magazine**, and to the energetic activities of organizations such as the Junior Chambers of Commerce, as well as to the professional efforts of the dental profession and health departments, the number of communities that are actively interested in fluoridation at the present time is growing by leaps and bounds." Also see letter from A. Taxpayer, *In Connection with the Jaycees*, **Journal Gazette** (Mattoon, Illinois), p. 4, 12th October, 1962.

New Zealand: Letter from J. R. Grant, Chairman, Jaycee Fluoridation Education Committee, Hastings, to **Hawke's Bay Herald-Tribune**, 30th April 1954. *Jaycee "Saved" Fluoridation In Hastings*, **Hawke's Bay Herald-Tribune**, 22nd January, 1957. Also see the letters dated 5th of May from C. N. D. Taylor to F. S. Maclean, and 6th of April, cited in Chapter 5.4.

The only time I ever saw it mentioned that the Jaycees had listened to the arguments was in J. Ferris Fuller's *Should We Fluoridate Our Water Supplies?* **New Zealand Dental Journal**, Vol. 52, January, 1956 (cited in Chapter 4): "At Hastings another turning point was the help given by the Junior Chamber of Commerce. Consisting significantly of men under forty with children of an age who would benefit by fluoridation, they heard both sides of the subject, voted unanimously in its favour, and from then on campaigned most actively for it." These words are interesting because in the previous paragraph he spoke of "... a matter as scientifically complex as fluoridation... even though the average citizen has insufficient scientific understanding to judge the matter." It appears to me that the Jaycees in the USA and NZ were a sort of relaxed fraternity with some obvious prestige associated. I have not found much information about what proportion or percentage of them were scientifically educated or not. This demonstrates how infrequently this is considered.

The second instance is found in J. Ferris Fuller's *Dreams Pursued* available at the National Library of New Zealand, MS-Papers-6275-06, p. 31. Claims the Jaycees "... studied it themselves for two or three years and finally made it their prime project..." after NZ Dental Association President Amos McKegg asked Fuller to address a meeting in Palmerston North. Fuller concludes; "The point to be made is that the successful project was handled by a community group ably assisted and guided where required by the local doctors and dentists." Cited in my Chapter 5.8.

361. John E. Mueller (University of Rochester, New York), *The Politics of Fluoridation in Seven California Cities*, **Western Political Quarterly**, Vol. 19, No.1, March 1966, p. 64. "When there is an adequate opposition, however, the pros can win only if they are able to overwhelm it. This was the case in Palo Alto where the pros spent four to six times as much money as did the antis and organized through the PTA and the Junior Chamber of Commerce what was probably the largest political volunteer group in Palo Alto history. The antis for their part campaigned actively and got out a mailing to all voters, but they were unable, because of deficiencies in money and in number of workers, to buy many ads or to do any door-to-door campaigning."

    (Also remember that the people opposed to fluoridation were historically not given much space to write in academic literature.)

    "... Even with the massive pro campaign and limited anti response, the pros were able to get only 55.5 percent of the vote."

362. Richard Smith, *The Trouble with Medical Journals*, pp. 125-126, 2007. Chapter 11, *How Money Clouds Objectivity*, contains many examples that pertain specifically to editorial positions and therefore are not frequently discussed in articles regarding conflicts of interest.

363. *Fluoridation of Water a Trampling of our Rights*, **The Timaru Courier**, Views, 26th May, 2016. "Tom O'Connor is a retired journalist, political commentator, president of Grey Power for New Zealand and vice-president of Grey Power Timaru." O'Connor invokes the New Zealand Bill of Rights Act 1990, Part 2, Clause 11.

364. One example can be given in *The Fluoride Issue – Conclusion. Children, Adults Can Benefit*, **The Sedalia Democrat**, Missouri, 31st Mar, 1972: "Like many in his profession, Dr. Shackles cannot understand the reasoning of those opposed to fluoridation. '... Why is it that fluoridation becomes so involved with politics? I really don't understand it,' he said."

365. *Dentists Urged to Fight Foes of Fluoridation*, **Stevens Point Journal** (Stevens Point, Wisconsin), p. 12, 26th October, 1959.

366. http://msof.nz/2015/04/the-loose-change-range-a-bunch-of-fallacies-an-anecdote-and-a-fluoridated-drink/#comments. In the comments section from Daniel Ryan.

367. John E. Chrietzberg, D.D.S., M.P.H., *Georgia's water fluoridation program*, **Journal of the American Dental Association**, Vol. 65, No. 5, pp. 81-85, November, 1962.

368. Walter C. Kraatz, *Fluoridation Foes Ignore Facts*, **The Akron Beacon Journal** (Akron, Ohio), p. 6, 23rd September, 1961.

369. *Harold Hillenbrand, Leader In U.S. Dentistry*, **Chicago Tribune**, June 03, 1986 and *Harold Hillenbrand, 74; Ex-Dental Assn. Director*, **Los Angeles Times**, June 05, 1986.

370. Brian Martin, *Analyzing the Fluoridation Controversy: Resources and Structures*, **Social Studies of Science**, Vol. 18, pp. 331-363, 1988.

371. **On Tap** 2014;(10):4-6. **On Tap** is a publication of the National Fluoridation Information Service. See https://www.health.govt.nz/our-work/preventative-health-wellness/fluoride-and-oral-health/water-fluoridation/national-fluoridation-information-service. "The service was delivered by a consortium including the Hutt Valley DHB Community Dental Service, Regional Public Health, ESR, the Massey University Centre for Public Health Research, and the National Poisons Centre."

372. *Fluoride back on the Hamilton menu* by Daniel Adams, **Waikato Times**, 10th October 2013.

373. *A million bottles a minute: world's plastic binge 'as dangerous as climate change'*, **The Guardian**, 28th June, 2017.

374. A good book on this is Eli Pariser's *The Filter Bubble*, published in 2011.

Chapter 5.6

375. Ben H. Bagdikian, *The Media Monopoly*, Acknowledgements, p. v, 18th November 1982.

376. *Ibid.*, p. 135.

377. *Ibid.*, p. 159.

378. Robert McChesney and Edward Herman, *The Global Media.*, pp. 182-183, and 189, 1997.

379. Alex Carey, *Taking the Risk out of Democracy*, Exporting Persuasion, p. 111, 1995.

380. One of which (discussed in Dr. Smith's book) is the Committee for Publication Ethics (COPE), whose writings are found online, https://publicationethics.org/. This group began in 1997 as an advisory group for editors of medical journals who were uncertain of what to do with cases of research misconduct.

381. One is the World Association of Medical Editors (WAME). To quote Iain Chalmers, director of the UK Cochrane Centre, "Medical editors are important people because they control the primary means for communicating the results of billions of dollars of publicly funded research. Yet we see deficiencies in standards of medical editing, and we are understanding better that most of the world's medical editors work with limited support, no training, and inadequate contacts with other editors. These editors need support, training, information, and help to raise their standards…" See *World Association of Medical Editors (WAME) launched*, **British Medical Journal**, 1995;310:761.

382. *Business is Still in Trouble*, **Fortune**, Vol. 39, No. 5, May 1949.

383. V. O. Key, *Politics, Parties and Pressure Groups*, 5th Edition, pp. 84 and 91, 1964.

384. *Water Boom for Fluorides*, **Chemical Week**, page 14, 7th July, 1951. As of early 2018, physical copies of this journal are available at the Alexander Turnbull Library in Wellington, New Zealand.

385. https://www.chemweek.com/CW/about-us.

386. Donald R. McNeil, *The Fight for Fluoridation*, pp. 58 and 79, 1957. Wisconsin promoters Doctors Bull, Frisch and Hardgrove feature throughout the book.

387. As I say, I have not *once* seen the **Chemical Week** article *Water Boom for Fluorides* cited by a single supporter of fluoridation. One anti-fluoride pamphlet from Ohio found in the New Zealand Health Department archives does mention it: C. T. Betts, D.D.S., *Poisoning City Water with Fluorine*, undated (the author of this pamphlet claimed it was reprinted from the **Journal of Medico-Physical Research**, August 1952).

The following articles, all opposed to fluoridation, mention it: A. C. Palmer, *Tribune Readers Express Their Opinions: An Intolerable Infringement*, **Des Moines Tribune**, 24th January, 1952,

Fluorides Boom to Chemical Firms, **The Post-Standard** (Syracuse, New York) p. 4, 28th April, 1952,

WATER FLUORIDATION, **Journal Gazette** (Mattoon, Illinois), p. 4, 11th August, 1952. "The haste to push fluoridation also has critics suspicious. They point out the magazine **Chemical Week**…" quotes follow. This article also claimed that the **Hastings Law Journal** of Hastings College of Law, University of California, says "water fluoridation is mass medication and cites grounds to prove that fluoridation of water has no legal standing" McNeil mentioned this in *The Fight for Fluoridation* (p. 191, 1957) and claimed the **LaCrosse Tribune** (1st, 2nd and 3rd of April, 1954) printed this and counter arguments. It doesn't look like McNeil obtained the original articles. I share this for American activists. UK activists may be interested in a paper with semi-similar claims in the journal **Medical Law International**: David

Shaw, University of Glasgow, UK, *Weeping and Wailing and Gnashing of Teeth: The Legal Fiction of Water Fluoridation*, Vol. 12, No. 1, pp. 11-27, 2012. I don't know enough about the law to tell you if these papers are accurate or not, or if the Hastings one even exists; David Shaw's paper does. This one is quite critical of fluorosis; at the end we see a probable reason why: under 'conflicts of interest' the author admits he *has* fluorosis. He cites Lord Jauncey, who oversaw the infamous McColl case, where a 69-year-old grandmother with no teeth won a courtcase against fluoridation in 1983: "While the addition of extra fluoride might indeed reduce caries rates, it was quite possible that people might obtain enough fluoride from other sources, and it would therefore be wrong to state that water fluoridation corrected a deficiency in the water." It's interesting to us that he talks about "enough fluoride".

The following newspaper articles also mention the July, 1951 **Chemical Week** document: Citizen's Medical Reference Bureau, *Fluoridation, Pro and Con – Part Two; What is Real Purpose of this Plan? Con: Federal Government's Hand Seen; Chemical Industry Gets Aid*, **Daily Independent Journal** (San Rafael, California), p. 7, 19th August, 1952,

The Ogden Nutrition Club, **Ogden Standard-Examiner** (Ogden, Utah), p. 7, 10th October, 1952,

M. D. Bieth, *The People's Forum: Cost of Fluoridation Overwhelms its Benefits*, **Hartford Courant** (Connecticut), p. 16, 21st November, 1952,

Go Slow on Fluoridation, **Orem-Geneva Times** (Orem, Utah), p. 4, 16th July, 1953,

Anti Fluoridation League, *Why You Should Oppose Fluoridation, VII: Because Fluoridation is a Boom for Chemical Companies, but not for the Health of the People of Council Bluffs* (Advertisement), **Council Bluffs Nonpareil** (Council Bluffs, Iowa), p. 7, 12th September, 1953,

A.P.M., **The La Crosse Tribune** (Wisconsin), p. 10, 2nd April, 1954,

Fluoridation – Why Not An Election? **Monroe Morning World** (Monroe, Louisiana), p. 4, 8th August, 1954,

Last five paragraphs of Radio Broadcast over KWK, St. Louis, by Dr. W. J. Schrenk, Chairman of Dept. of Chemical Engineering, University of Missouri (Advertisement paid for by Kalispel Citizen's Committee), **The Daily Inter Lake** (Kalispell, Montana), p. 7, 1st April, 1955,

B. C. Holland, Committee on Fluoridation, Springfield Property Owners Association, *The People's Forum: Springfield Looks at Fluoridation*, **Hartford Courant** (Connecticut), p. 12, 12th April, 1955

Milford R. Van Houtan, *Against Fluoridation*, **Albany Democrat-Herald** (Oregon), p. 8, 3rd March, 1956.

Maxine Hill, *Not Sound Business*, **Medford Mail Tribune** (Medford, Oregon), p. 4, 7th March, 1956,

Lancaster Eagle-Gazette (Ohio), 26th March, p. 6, 1956,

John Sprunt Hill, **Asheville Citizen-Times** (North Carolina), p. 8, 20th May, 1956,

Christina Berham, *Opposes Fluoridation of Water*, **Asbury Park Press** (New Jersey), p. 6, 8th October, 1956.

388. *By the Public, El Paso Man Hits Water Fluoridation*, **The Pantagraph** (Bloomington, Illinois), p. 4, 13th March, 1958,

C. M. Van Stone, **Great Falls Tribune** (Great Falls, Montana), p. 6, 14th December, 1961

A TAXPAYER, **Journal Gazette** (Mattoon, Illinois), p. 4, 12th October, 1962.

D. L. Carter, *Antis Continue Writing Attack on Fluoridation*, **Pensacola News Journal** (Pensacola, Florida), p. 17, 16th February, 1964.

Open Letter Sponsored by Citizens for Safe Water, *Citizens Protest: Ask Council to Rescind Fluoridation Ordinance*, (Kansas) **Telescope**, 4th January, 1968.

Gladys Caldwell, *Critic Answers Fluorides Article*, **Independent Press-Telegram** (Long Beach, California), p. 35, 28th September, 1969 (Caldwell authored a book called *Fluoridation and Truth Decay*).

Willard E. Edwards, Honolulu Engineer, *Fluoridation: Benefit, Blunder, Fraud?* **The Honolulu Advertiser** (Honolulu, Hawaii), p. 27, 8th December, 1972.

389. Earl Brooks, *He's Amazed*, **The Morning News** (Wilmington, Delaware), p. 16, 9th November, 1956.

390. *Fluoridation Facts: Answers to Criticisms Against Fluoridation*, published by the American Dental Association, paragraphs 8, 10, 12, 33, 36 and 40, April, 1956. "Fluoride-deficient" waters mentioned on p. 16 (citing[127]).

391. Smith, F. A. *An Annotated Bibliography of the Literature on the Pharmacology and Toxicology of Fluorine and its Compounds*, University of Rochester, Atomic Energy Project, 29th January, 1951.

392. *ALCOA Answers Lake Letter on F*, **Press Democrat** (Santa Rosa, California), 27th Feb, p. 10, 1967. This letter was written in response to an anonymous letter to the editor dated 9th January, 1967, appearing on page 8, that claimed ALCOA was making money off water fluoridation. *Letters to Editor on Fluoridation*, **The Morning Call**, 28th Jun, p. 36, 1970. *Alcoa and fluoride*, **The Journal News** (White Plains, New York), 5th November, p. 14, 1974.

393. *Fluoridation Facts*, American Dental Association, p. 31 and 32, 2005.

394. *Ibid*, p. 43.

395. H. B. Turbott, *Answers to Allegations About Fluoridation*, available in the Wellington Central Public Library, **The Evening Post** Health/National/Fluoridation archives. I'm sure I saw a copy in the Health Department archives somewhere. Turbott was appointed to this position in 1947, making Director-General in 1959. I find no date on the document, but it quotes the 1957 Commission of Inquiry heavily, so it is easy to place its date within a few years. On Turbott's biographical page on Te Ara, the following is written (retrieved 2nd September, 2017): "Reviewing New Zealand's health system in 1937 on behalf of the Labour government, S. M. Lambert of the Rockefeller Foundation noted it was hard to attract good staff other than those possessed of a 'certain missionary fanaticism'. He may well have had Turbott – one of his principal informants – in mind. Within months of his appointment to Gisborne Turbott had initiated a comparison of the health of Maori and Pakeha children, the results of which helped to allay pessimism among senior departmental officers regarding the future of the Maori people." The website citation is Derek A. Dow, **Dictionary of New Zealand Biography**, Vol. 5, 2000, updated January, 2012. Another potentially interesting insight into the mentality of one of the experts is apparent when McClure writes (*Water Fluoridation: The Search and the Victory*, p. 111): "This is, therefore, a beneficial physiological effect of fluoride which merits unquestionable authority and acceptance."

396. Letter dated 20th May, 1958. HD 125/299/4 H1 Box 1716. One of the brochures reads "While sound teeth are one of man's most prized possessions, much of the food and drink he uses contributes either directly or indirectly to tooth decay." Wallace & Tiernan Fluoridation, Publication No. TA–1016–C-2. HD 125/299 H1 Box 1615.

397. *Fluoride Relief*, **Chemical Week**, pp. 39-40, 8th September 1951.

398. *Tests Completed On New Water Fluoridation Agent*, **The McIntosh County Democrat**, p. 7, 20th March, 1952.

399. *Only 1 Fluorine Compound Reported As Satisfactory*, **Palladium-Item** (Richmond, Indiana) Fri, Jan 18, p. 2, 1952. The report was published in the **American Journal of Public Health**, *Choice of Fluoridating Agents in the Control of Dental Caries* by C. L. Howell, D.D.S., L. E. Burney, M.D., M.P.H., F.A.P.H.A., Harry G. Day, Sc.D., AND Joseph C. Muhler, D.D.S., pp. 44-48, January, 1952. The "except for study purposes" quote looks to me like a loophole in public health. By saying this, it appears you can use whatever you want if it's for study purposes. The logic in this study is quite detailed however, and Muhler *et al.* express caution about using just anything. Again I'm impressed by the intelligence and depth of the team from Indiana. The reader is also encouraged here to read Chapters 3 and 4 of Donald McNeil's book *The Fight For Fluoridation* regarding the efforts of men like Dr. John Frisch and Dr. Frank Bull to get the ADA and USPHS to publicly endorse CWF as quickly as possible. One can understand that making CWF into a black-and-white or good-and-bad strict sort of polarity does no favours to scientific understanding when Muhler *et al.* write comments like "… the evidence indicates that some importance should be attached to the cation as well as to the anion."

Harry G. Day died in 2007. He co-authored a book with Elmer McCollum on nutrition, published in 1939, *The Newer Knowledge of Nutrition*. "Day mentored hundreds of students and often provided financial support to enable them to continue their education. Day was interested in wherever he thought he could be of service not only professionally, but locally through civic organizations such as Kiwanis and Bloomington Hospital, where he was the first male to serve on the Women's Board." Publicly, (see the two references from Chapter 1) it looks to me like Joseph Muhler received a lot of the accolades regarding Crest toothpaste, but it appears Day, his mentor, also contributed a lot to the research. Presumably the entire department at IU would be responsible.

See https://honorsandawards.iu.edu/search-awards/honoree.shtml?honoreeID=885 and https://www.jhsph.edu/about/history/heroes-of-public-health/harry-g-day.html. In 1991, another book by Day, on the history of his department, was published;, *Development of Chemistry at Indiana University in Bloomington*. "Joseph Muhler and William Nebergall were also an integral part of the development team, and Harry, with undue but characteristic modesty, gave them most of the credit for this triumph." See *Harry G. Day — A Century of Life*, by Rupert Wentworth, available online.

400. Jesse Francis McClendon, *Physiological Chemistry*, 7th edition, C. V. Mosby Company, 1946.

401. *Huge Sum Spent To Stop Fumes of Plant*, **Corvallis Gazette-Times** (Oregon), 9th October, p. 1, 1948.

402. *Counteraction Sought Of Chemicals At Alcoa*, **Kingsport News** (Tennessee), 3rd Jan, p. 7, 1948. The Tao and Suttie experiment in 1976 boasted a large amount of funders, many of which were metals corporations (see end of Chapter 1.1). Also see the NAS publication **Nutrient Requirements of Dairy Cattle**, pp. 148-149, 2001: "Fluorine is generally regarded as a toxic element with regards to domestic livestock because in large amounts fluorine will accumulate in bone to an extent that actually weakens bone, increasing lameness and increasing wear of teeth. The teeth of cattle intoxicated with fluorine become mottled and stained, and are eroded or pitted." "Soluble forms of fluoride, such as NaF, are rapidly and nearly completely absorbed by cattle. About 50 percent of fluorine in undefluorinated phosphates of bone meal is absorbed. Dietary calcium, aluminium, sodium chloride, and fat can reduce fluorine absorption (in support of this, they cite a report from the NRC, **Mineral Tolerance of Domestic Animals**, 1980)." "Fluorine in the form of hydrofluoric acid, silicon tetrafluoride, or fluoride containing particulates can be released from industrial sites associated with aluminium or phosphate processing. These emissions can contaminate water, soil, and plants near these sites, resulting in fluorine intoxicosis in animals grazing in the areas."

403. *Alcoa Tries To Stop Fumes*, **Eugene Guard** (Oregon), 10th Oct, p. 2, 1948.

404. *$900,000 Suit Is Filed Against Aluminum Co.*, **The News-Review** (Roseburg, Oregon), 11th Jan, p. 11, 1950. The farmers claimed damages of $300,000 and were asking treble.

405. *Reynolds Metals v. Lampert*, 324 F.2d 465 (9th Cir. 1963), cited in William Rodgers, *Corporate Country: A State Shaped to Suit Technology*, Chapter 7, pp. 161-188, 1973.

406. Donald R. McNeil, *The Fight for Fluoridation*, p. 48, 1957.

407. Benjamin D. Paul, *Fluoridation and the Social Scientist: A Review*, **Journal of Social Issues**, Vol. XVII, No. 4, p. 1, 1961.

408. Dr. David Ast and Bernadette Fitzgerald, *Effectiveness of Water Fluoridation*, **Journal of the American Dental Association**, Vol. 65, No. 5, pp. 581-589, 1962.

409. Harold R. Englander, D.D.S., M.P.H., (NIDR, Bethesda, Md.); Rudolph de Palma, D.D.S. (College of Dentistry, Illinois), and Robert G . Kesel D.D.S., M.S. (College of Dentistry, Illinois), *The Aurora-Rockford, Ill., study I. Effects of water having naturally occurring fluoride on dental health of young adults*, **Journal of the American Dental Association**, Vol. 65, No. 5, pp. 614-621, 1962. Study supported in part by a USPHS grant.

410. Donald McNeil, *The Fight for Fluoridation*, p. 187 and 225-226, 1957.

411. *City Urged to Get Fluoridated Water*, 27th August, 1954, *Health Unit Asks for Fluoridation*, 14th September, 1954, *Fluoridation Endorsed: Question of Safety was Adequately Considered, it is Said*, 27th January, 1956, *Fluoridation Put to Estimate Body*, 26th July 1956. All from the **New York Times**, cited in Chapter 10 of McNeil's *The Fight for Fluoridation*, 1957.

    Hearing Divided on Fluoridation: State Aid Bill Gets Official Support at Albany but Most Citizens Oppose it, **New York Times**, 1st March, 1956.

    Mayor Says Officials Get Much Anti-Fluoride Mail, **New York Times**, 26th July, 1963. **Journal of the American Dental Association** Vol. 52, p. 97, January 1956. Board of Health of the City of New York, *Report to the Mayor on Fluoridation for New York City*, pp. 1-52, 24th October, 1955.

    Of these, I have obtained the **New York Times** articles and another two: the journal of the ADA article and the 1955 Report for the Mayor of New York. Neither of these mention the journal **Chemical Week**.

A 1956 article cited by McNeil discussed the Newburgh study's impression on the agricultural chemist H.V. Smith of Arizona University. Smith had written a letter claiming he was very pleased with the results of fluoridation in Newburgh, and Arizona University became one of fluoridation's endorsers.

The August 27th article discussed a recommendation from the New York City Health Department that the city commence with fluoridation. It claimed that fluorine was a "trace element", that it was not stored in the body if a concentration of 1 ppm was used. Fluoridation of milk was said to be too expensive, and fluoride tablets and toothpastes were said to not "assure that the necessary fluoride intake will be achieved." Spokesmen for the Health Department claimed that "virtually every major health agency" had endorsed CWF.

The September 14th article discussed how the New York City Board of Health "strongly" urged CWF as soon as possible. The Board apparently listened to estimates from engineers of $1,000,000 to install equipment then a yearly cost of between $680,000 to $800,000 for the compounds. They claimed that the costs "do not appear to be excessive in view of the benefits…"

A Bronx Democrat, Councilman Louis Peck, had introduced a resolution calling for CWF on August 24th. I found no article dated 30th August, 1954 on the **New York Times** website.

The January 27th issue contained an article by reporter Charles Bennett, and a letter written by N. H. Cooper, M. D. The article discussed a public hearing featuring federal and state officials, and an audience of 250. Opponents outnumbered proponents by two to one. Of fifty-nine speakers, sixteen favoured CWF and one was neutral.

The letter from Dr. Cooper expressed his gratitude for the fact that "not all of those opposed to fluoridation of community water supplies approach the subject in an emotional way". He was referring to a previous letter (18th January) by Dr. Ludwik Gross. However, Cooper claimed Gross still could not refrain from using "exaggerated, biased and illogical tactics…" by referring to so many of the endorsing groups as "pressure groups".

The July 26th article discussed how the Mayor, Mr. Wagner, had been visited by "a group of medical, dental and civic leaders who called on him at his office in City Hall." The Mayor also said that the Board of Estimate would hold a public hearing on the topic. This article potentially highlights some of the difficulty of governance: Mayor Wagner was firmly on the side of the Board of Health which wanted CWF, but was also dealing with the Water Department, which opposed it.

The Mayor also put rumours of a referendum to rest in this election year. This may have been because (as the article pointed out) 172 communities out of 284 had rejected CWF when it had been put to referendum. The article did not state whether this was the Mayor's reason or not.

A couple of other articles in the **New York Times** around this time claimed similar feelings among the public. In March of 1956, a small headline read *State Aid Bill Gets Official Support at Albany but Most Citizens Oppose it*. The article mentioned a four-hour debate. Discussed was a bill that would allow half a million dollars to be appropriated for state aid to communities setting up approved CWF programs with the state and locality halving the cost equally. Clearly the public relations aspects of the issue needed work. In July of 1963, it was reported that the Mayor had received 4,994 letters against fluoridation and only 968 for it since the beginning of January. In 1965, he went ahead with fluoridation.

412. *Report to the Honorable J. T. Tonkin, M.L.A., Premier of Western Australia, On the Fluoridation of Public Water Supplies.* By A. F. Cant, WA Government Printer, Perth, 1972. "The research began with a study of the existing Premier's Department files (which had been compiled since December 1961) books and documents loaned by the Deputy Commissioner for Public Health, and the minutes of the Advisory Committee on Fluoridation. Particular attention was given to the Report of the Tasmanian Royal Commission (1968), and the W.H.O. Monograph 'Fluorides and Human Health' (1970)." I believe Cant's document is to be credited with making popular the statement that Sweden had banned fluoridation (discussed on page 14). Few details were given, but there was a citation: National Board of Health and Welfare, Sweden – *Paper on Water Fluoridation*, 1972.

413. *Fluoridophobe*, **Chemical Week**, p. 4, 12th June, 1954.

414. *More Facts, Less Bias*, **Chemical Week**, pp. 7-8, 21st August, 1954.

415. Anna Bradley-Smith, *'Outlier' dentist challenges plan to add fluoride to Nelson's water supply*, **The Nelson Mail**, 16th May, 2015. Also cited at the beginning of Chapter 2.

Quoting: "[Beaglehole said] 'But it's just outrageous that these [anti-fluoride] people are causing unnecessary pain and suffering.' Litras said much of the evidence, including the review conducted by the Government's chief science advisor, Sir Peter Gluckman, that groups such as the Dental Association used was invalid because objective standards of analyses weren't followed.

'They need to have a committee that is balanced and the Gluckman review chose pro-fluoridation people which means they limited their literature search solely to evidence that supported their position. Plus they've overstated the benefits and understated the health risks quite largely.'

Beaglehole said the claim was 'outrageous' and Gluckman's review went through 'every single argument that an anti-fluoridationist has ever come up from and picks up the details' and concluded water fluoridation had no proven negative effects."

416. Christopher Bryson, *The Fluoride Deception*, Seven Stories Press, New York, 2004.

417. *Health effects of water fluoridation: A review of the scientific evidence.* Cited fully in Chapter 2.3. A report on behalf of the Royal Society of New Zealand and the Office of the Prime Minister's Chief Science Advisor, August 2014. Report commissioned at the Auckland Council's request. Bryson mentioned on page 15.

418. Professor Jason M. Armfield, Debate: When public action undermines public health: a critical examination of antifluoridationist literature, **Australia and New Zealand Health Policy**, 2007, 4: 25, page 8.

419. http://www.doctoryourself.com/news/v4n18.html. Twentieth of August, 2004. Accessed April, 2018.

420. IS: Review of *The Fluoride Deception*, https://www.publishersweekly.com/978-1-58322-526-4.

421. Katherine Hartley, *The Toxic Compound with a Polished Image*, **The Environmental Magazine**, Vol. 15, No. 4, p. 61, 2004.

422. James Clark, *A Chemical Conspiracy?* **Nature**, Vol. 434, p. 275, March 2005.

423. Clementine Norton, *Fluoride decision for greater minds*, **Fraser Coast Chronicle**. 15th February, 2013.

424. Ralph Blumenthal, *New York's Fluoridation Fuss, 50 Years Later*, **New York Times**, 23rd February, 2015.

425. IS: *Sinking His Teeth Into… Fluoridation*, posted February 5, 2015 by rblumenthal, https://blogs.baruch.cuny.edu/ipaprocessing/2015/02/sinking-his-teeth-into-fluoridation/. Search 'fluoridation' on the library website.

426. Jason M. Armfield, *op. cit.*, p. 11.

427. See Varney's book *Fluoridation: A Case to Answer*, p. 72, 1986. See *Who's Who in Australia*, 1983. See Michael Collins Persse, *A fine fit in an illustrious family*, **The Sydney Morning Herald**, 21st August, 2012. In WWII, Alan worked on neutralizing carbon monoxide in bombers. In the 1970s, he worked in Consolm Fertilizers Ltd., Australian Fertilizers Ltd., and Fibremakers. In the 1980s he worked in EZ Industries, Tubemakers of Australia Ltd. (who were members of the Dental Health Education Research Foundation in 1979), and Reckitt and Colman Australia. Also see Stephen Cauchi, *A city toasts its 'fluoride heroes'*, **The Age** (Sydney), 21st March 2002.

"Health Minister John Thwaites and former Liberal premier Dick Hamer will host a party at a Carlton restaurant honouring the 'Fluoride Heroes' - the dentists and doctors who lobbied hard in the 1970s for fluoride to pour from the city's taps.

The benefits of fluoridation are overwhelming, say the government and the Australian Dental Association. Tooth decay rates in Melbourne have halved since its introduction, with cavities almost a thing of the past."

428. *Indiana Board Of Health Makes Report Of Benefits Derived From Adding Fluoride To Water Systems*, **Rushville Republican**, (Rushville, Indiana), p. 4, 26th Dec, 1953.

429. Leroy Pope, *Toothpaste War Catches I.U. Scientists in Middle*, **Journal and Courier**, Lafayette, Indiana, 21st November 1970.

430. Examples can be found in Sheldon Rampton and John Stauber's work, *Trust Us We're Experts: How Industry Manipulates Science and Gambles with Your Future* and the aptly titled *Toxic Sludge is Good for You: Lies, Damn Lies, and the Public Relations Industry*. Also see *Merchants of Doubt: How a Handful of*

Scientists Obscured the Truth on Issues from Tobacco Smoke to Global Warming by Naomi Oreskes and Eric. M. Conway. An excellent book on public relations and science is *Doubt is Their Product* by David Michaels. Nicky Hager and Bob Burton's book *Secrets and Lies* gives a very interesting insight into how media and PR firms frame issues: By definition, actions that make corporate profits go upward are progressive, sensible, intelligent, and people who do things that inhibit corporate profits going upward are extremists.

431. Corey Hannah Basch, Ed.D., M.P.H., C.H.E.S.; Sonali Rajan, Ed.D., M.S., *Marketing Strategies and Warning Labels on Children's Toothpaste*, **Journal of Dental Hygiene**, Vol. 88, No. 5, pp. 316-319, October, 2014.

432. CFR - Code of Federal Regulations Title 21, c.1. "For all fluoride dentifrice (gel, paste, and powder) products."

    "Keep out of reach of children under 6 years of age. [highlighted in bold type] If more than used for brushing is accidentally swallowed, get medical help or contact a Poison Control Center right away."

    https://www.accessdata.fda.gov/scripts/cdrh/cfdocs/cfcfr/CFRSearch.cfm?fr=355.50&SearchTerm=fluoride.

    Recently the American Dental Association (ADA) has updated their products with the ADA's "Seal of Acceptance", https://www.ada.org/en/science-research/ada-seal-of-acceptance/ada-seal-products/product-category?supercategory=Toothpastes.

433. *Much Ado about Nothing*, **Journal of the American Dental Association**, Vol. 128, pp. 1347-1348, 1997.

434. Dana Canedy, *Toothpaste a Hazard? Just Ask the F.D.A.*, **New York Times**, 24th March, 1998.

435. Corey Hannah Basch, Ed.D., M.P.H., C.H.E.S.; Sonali Rajan, Ed.D., M.S., *Marketing Strategies and Warning Labels on Children's Toothpaste*, **Journal of Dental Hygiene**, Vol. 88, No. 5, pp. 316-319, October, 2014.

436. Editorial, *More is not always better*, **New Zealand Dental Journal**, Vol. 79, p. 73, 1983.

437. Leslie Winston, D.D.S., Ph.D., *Building Relationships from an Industry Perspective*, **Canadian Journal of Dental Hygiene**, Vol. 43, No. 5, pp. 231-232, 2009.

438. One hour fifteen minutes into the talk. The talk is available on the RAND Corporation's YouTube channel. Specifically, RAND Corporation was concerned with people who did not believe in the safety of vaccines and GMOs, even though they claimed science had proven these technologies safe beyond all doubt.

439. *Colgate-Palmolive donates $1M to APHA*, **Nation's Restaurant News**, p. 74, 29th March, 1999.

440. Richard Brunelli and Laureen Miles, *The market makers of health & beauty; six companies drive the media markets, and drive them they do*, **MEDIAWEEK**, 12th April, 1993.

441. 20th March, 2015, https://www.prweek.com/article/1337841/global-campaign-year-2015. Also see Roo Ciambriello, *P&G Breathes New Life Into 'Thank You, Mom' Ahead of Another Olympics, Campaign champions diversity with #LoveOverBias*, **Adweek**, https://www.adweek.com/creativity/pg-breathes-new-life-into-thank-you-mom-ahead-of-another-olympics/.

442. *Jordan Brings the Heart of the Marketer to CBS-TV*, **Advertising Age**, http://adage.com/article/news/jordan-brings-heart-a-marketer-cbs-tv-ceo-parent-westinghouse-hawks-message/69342/. P. 18, 3rd February, 1997.

443. https://openparachute.wordpress.com/2013/06/07/tactics-and-common-arguments-of-the-anti-fluoridationists/. Note that of the three hundred comments, not a single commenter discussed the point on industry funding in any real detail. This demonstrates how poorly investigated this topic is, even by enthusiasts.

444. A recent critique of antifluoridationist literature, https://www.dentalwatch.org/.

445. Bruce Munro, *Screening of Fluoride TV Programme Up in the Air*, **The Star**, 22nd May, 2008. The City Council Communications Co-ordinator, Rodney Bryant, "said the City Council had not seen the interview but had concerns about whether it was fair and balanced." Mr. Bryant said, "we encourage debate." "If a programme was broadcast which was 'alarmist' or 'could cause disquiet in the community' then the City Council or Public Health South might 'feel obliged' to take some action, he [Bryant] said."

446. The debate is available here: http://www.channel39.co.nz/content/stars-f-word-debate-fluoride. Also see the following articles from **The Star**, 2008: *TV Programme Cancelled but Debate Likely to Screen*, *Freedom of Choice the Issue, Reader Says*, and *Correspondents Hope to Encourage Fluoride Debate*, 29th

May; *Fluoride a Concern, FANNZ Says*, 5th June; *Channel 9 Brings Fluoride Foes Together for Debate*, 26th June; *Fluoride Debate Available on Website*, 3rd July; *Fluoridation Briefing Plan*, 31st July.

447. V. O. Key, *Politics, Parties and Pressure Groups*, 5th Edition, p. 96, 1964.

448. *Proceedings of the Representative Board,* **British Dental Journal Supplement**, 3rd September, p. 24, 1963.

449. Simmel, *An Analysis of Opinion on Fluoridation*, New York State Department of Health, Albany, New York (September, 1961), mimeographed. Eleven out of 188 people gave this argument. Simmel claims "some rare arguments not naturally falling into any of the given categories were excluded." Cited in John E Mueller, *The Politics of Fluoridation in Seven California Cities*, **Western Political Quarterly**, Vol. 19, No. 1 pp. 62-63, 1966.

450. Discussed *a little* recently in **The Guardian**. "Fluoride is not medication. If anything, it's a supplement." "Anti-fluoride activists may keep on coming back like zombies, but their line of argument remains brain-dead." Michael Vagg, *Anti-fluoride activists should put their tinfoil hat theories to rest*, https://www.theguardian.com/commentisfree/2013/sep/19/anti-fluoride-science-australia. Ben H. Bagdikian points out in *The Media Monopoly* (p. 51) that in 1961, when twenty-nine corporations were convicted of conspiracy, one lawyer's argument was that "everybody's doing it" so the executives should be let off. "Everyone" of course, was a slight exaggeration. The U.S. Department of Justice found in 1979, only about sixty percent of the largest 582 corporations were engaged in some kind of criminality, including "evasion of taxes, unfair labor practices, dangerous working conditions, price fixing, pollution, and illegal kickbacks."

451. John Maher, *Introducing Chomsky: A Graphic Guide*, Icon Books Ltd, 2012.

452. **Chemical Week**, 8th September, p. 8, 1st December, p. 28, 29th December, p. 3, 1951; 7th November, p. 20, 5th December, p. 73, 1953; 16th October, p. 83, 1954.

453. *U.S. Steel and Du Pont Sued Over Pollution*, **The Los Angeles Times**, p. 5, 20th February, 1971; Nathaniel Rich, *The Lawyer Who Became DuPont's Worst Nightmare*, **New York Times**, 9th January, 2016, discusses DuPont's "decades-long history of chemical pollution."

454. Ben H. Bagdikian, *The Media Monopoly*, p. 25, 1983.

455. William Rodgers, *Corporate Country: A State Shaped to Suit Technology*, pp. 176-177, 1973. "Protection of Proprietary and Confidential Information" is the name of the clause, according to Rodgers, in a grant contract from Kaiser Aluminum and Chemical Corp., on file at the University of Washington, Office of Grants and Contract Research. The clause was "inoperative" at Washington University due to university regulations.

456. *PR Field is not for the Faint of Heart*, **Reno Gazette-Journal** (Nevada), p. 29, 23rd August, 1999.

457. Ben Bagdikian, *The Media Monopoly*, pp. 51-53 and 25, 1983.

458. Kenneth Reich, Times Staff Writer, *Hearing Told Polluters Control Water Boards*, **L. A. Times**, p.4, 4th February, 1969.

459. Kate Zernike, *In New Jersey, a Battle Over a Fluoridation Bill, and the Facts*, **New York Times**, 2nd March, 2012.

460. http://www.tampabay.com/opinion/editorials/reverse-the-decay-of-common-sense/1220395. 1st June, 2018.

461. John Troan, *Typhoid Victory Put Chemistry on Top Here*, **The Pittsburgh Press** (Pennsylvania), 13th September, p. 24, 1953. Incidentally, this was mentioned in the February, 1952 (Vol. 44, p. 135) issue of the **Journal of the American Dental Association**, wherein it was stated: "This study in Bauxite led directly to the discovery of fluoride, an unexpected constituent of domestic water supplies. This was announced in a personal letter from the discoverer, H. V. Churchill, chief chemist of the Aluminum Company of America, dated January 20, 1931. The letter gave the fluoride content of the deep well water at Bauxite as 14 ppm. This extremely high content was reflected in the general severity of the enamel lesion." This may have been where Dr. Muriel Bell got her claim that 14 ppm was harmless in her letter dated 1958 that was discussed at the end of Chapter 3.2.

462. Frederick S. McKay, D.D.S., *The Study of Mottled Enamel (Dental Fluorosis)*, **Journal of the American Dental Association**, Vol. 44, No. 2, pp. 133-137, February, 1952; and A. P. Black, Ph.D., *Facts in*

refutation of claims by opponents of fluoridation, Vol. 655-664 (though Black's article did not mention Churchill worked for ALCOA).

463. William Rodgers, *Corporate Country: A State Shaped to Suit Technology*, 1973.

464. Rodgers, *op. cit.*, citing *Quest: Annual Report Issue*, October, 1971, pp. 14-15, Washington State University College of Engineering.

465. Rodgers *op. cit.*, citing *Meyer v. Harvey Aluminum, Inc.*, No. 6402, R. on Appeal, Vol. 8, pp. 1535-36 (Or. Hood River Cir. Ct. 1970).

466. https://btiscience.org/explore-bti/history/, 1980-2000.

467. **Fluorides: Biological Properties of Atmospheric Pollutants**, National Academy of Sciences, Washington, D.C., p. 134, 1971.

468. John Suttie, *Air Quality Criteria to Protect Livestock from Fluoride Toxicity*, Aluminum Association, New York, 1969; *Air Quality Standards for the Protection of Farm Animals from Fluorides*, Vol. 19, No. 4, pp. 239-242, 1969; *Effects of Inorganic Fluorides on Animals*, Vol. 14, No. 3, pp. 461-480, 1964 (both **Journal of the Air Pollution Control Association**).

469. *The Fluoride Debate*, pp. 28-30, cited in Chapter 2.7.

470. *Ibid.*, p. 40.

471. https://www.floridaphosphatecce.com/.

472. Letter from John Place, chairman of the board, Anaconda Copper Co., to Peter M. Flanigan, Assistant to the President, Dec. 29, 1971. See Rodgers, *op. cit.*, p. 53.

473. University of Sydney, *Dental Health Education Research Foundation Annual Report 1979*.

474. Creators of Meridol toothpaste, 1400 ppm fluoride. Incidentally, Colgate were sued for £1,000 in 1996, see Linda Jackson, **The Sunday Telegraph**, 24th November.

"A leading toothpaste manufacturer has paid £1,000 to a child whose teeth appear to have been damaged by fluoride. In what is believed to be the first such case, Colgate-Palmolive made a 'goodwill' payment after an independent specialist diagnosed the boy as suffering from a condition linked with fluoride."

"Colgate-Palmolive has denied liability and refused to discuss the case."

"More than 200 parents are attempting to claim damages…"

Their website uses the phrase "Colgate-Palmolive World of Care", https://www.colgatepalmolive.com/en-us/brands, accessed April, 2018.

475. Johnson & Johnson have some videos and figures about their societal impact available on their website. See https://www.jnj.com/global-environmental-health/product-stewardship-earthwards and https://www.jnj.com/global-environmental-health/product-end-of-life. These corporations claim such virtues and values on their websites yet create such incredible mess in the form of plastics. One can see something quite awful here: if one company withdraws from using plastic or some other harmful substance in its packaging to focus on the creation of something more ecosystem-friendly, they will have to compromise their focus on short-term profits, leading to a loss of market share. Then they will lose consumer loyalty and the other corporations will receive the short-term profits. This means that a corporation that prioritizes environmental health above profits will potentially go out of business, while a less responsible corporation is rewarded with a larger slice of the market.

476. An eyewear company.

477. Creators of Sensodyne toothpaste and oral health products, Louis Marcel body care products, Nytol sleep aid, Piriton anti-allergy medication, Polident denture adhesives.

478. Parent organization Mars Incorporated. "Celebrate diversity with Maltesers…" See http://www.mars.com/global/brands/confectionery, accessed April, 2018. "Mars Wrigley Confectionery is the world's leading manufacturer of chocolate, chewing gum, mints, and fruity confections. Once the planned worldwide integration of the Mars Chocolate and Wrigley businesses is complete, Mars Wrigley Confectionery will employ over 34,000 Associates globally and have operations in approximately 70 countries." Brands include M&M's®, Snickers®, Twix®, Skittles® and Orbit®.

479. **Canberra Times**, p. 9, 21st March, 1972.

480. Mark Diesendorf, *Fluoridation: Breaking the Silence Barrier*, Published in Brian Martin (editor), *Confronting the Experts*, (Albany, NY: State University of New York Press, 1996), pp. 45-75, on the last page he discusses the funders – Arnott's, Schweppes, Cadbury, etc. Also mentioned in (by Diesendorf) *Science under Social and Political Pressures*, in *Science and Ethics: Papers presented at a symposium held under the aegis of the Australian Academy of Science University of New South Wales 7th November, 1980*, pp. 48-73, DHERF mentioned on p. 67.

481. Wendy Varney, *Fluoridation: A Case to Answer*, p. 57, 1986.

482. William Rodgers, *The National Industrial Pollution Control Council: Advise or Collude?* 13 B.C. Indus. & Com. L. Rev. 719 (1972), https://digitalcommons.law.uw.edu/faculty-articles/274.

483. Alex Carey, *Taking the Risk out of Democracy*, Exporting Persuasion, p. 130, 1995.

484. Alex Carey, *op. cit.,* Grassroots and Treetops Propaganda, p. 98.

485. John Yudkin, *Pure White and Deadly*, pp. 159-162.

486. *Over Half Your News is Spin*, https://www.crikey.com.au/2010/03/15/over-half-your-news-is-spin/.

Chapter 5.7

487. The PLoS Medicine Editors, **PLoS Medicine** *Series on Big Food: The Food Industry Is Ripe for Scrutiny*, Published: June 19, 2012, https://doi.org/10.1371/journal.pmed.1001246.

    The authors' individual competing interests are at http://journals.plos.org/plosmedicine/s/staff-editors. PLoS is funded partly through manuscript publication charges, but the *PLoS Medicine* Editors are paid a fixed salary (their salary is not linked to the number of papers published in the journal). The entire series can be viewed here: http://collections.plos.org/big-food.

488. *Playing the policy game: a review of the barriers to and enablers of nutrition policy change*, **Public Health Nutrition**, Vol. 19, No. 14, pp. 2643-2653, 1st April, 2016.

489. *Sweeter for Industry*, **Chemical Week**, pp. 35-36, 19th July, 1952.

490. *Tempest in a Pop Bottle*, **Chemical Week**, pp. 73-74, 15th August, 1953.

491. Benjamin Rosenthal (New York Democratic Representative), Michael Jacobson, and Marcy Bohm, (both CSPI), *Professors on the Take*, **The Progressive**, pp. 42-47, November, 1976.

492. Richard Smith, *The Trouble with Medical Journals*, pp. 125-137, 2007. Chapter 11, *How Money Clouds Objectivity*, contains many examples that pertain specifically to editorial positions and are therefore not normally discussed in academic literature regarding conflicts of interest. He does make the point that "Academia and industry are becoming increasingly entangled." The later sections of the book look at solutions that medical journals are able to apply but as they are only one sector of power and influence in science, even if the behaviour of journals was perfect, their behaviour alone should not be considered a fix-all.

493. Robert L. Glass and Sylvia Fleisch, *Diet and dental caries: dental caries incidence and the consumption of ready-to-eat cereals*, **Journal of the American Dental Association**, Vol. 88, pp. 807-813, April, 1974.

494. Herschel Horowitz and Howard Greene, *Caries and cereals*, **Journal of the American Dental Association**, Vol. 89, pp. 30-31, July, 1974.

495. Dr. Fredrick Stare, *Diet Histories Taken*, **Journal of the American Dental Association**, Vol. 89, No. 3, September, 1974.

496. **Public Policy Options for Better Dental Health: Report of a Study**, National Academy of Sciences, p. 37, 1980.

497. Gustafsson, B. E., Quensel, C. E., and Lanke, L. S. *The Vipeholm Dental Caries Study: The Effect of Different Levels of Carbohydrate Intake on Caries Activity in 436 Individuals Observed for 5 years*. **Acta Odont Scand** 11:232-364, 1954. This study is notorious. It concluded the risk of caries from sugar was from eating it in between meals. A review of the study was published 50 years after, claiming it was unethical, but accurate. Bo Krasse, *The Vipeholm Dental Caries Study: Recollections and Reflections 50 Years Later*, **Journal of Dental Research**, Vol. 80, p. 1785, 2001. DOI: 10.1177/00220345010800090201.

498. Kate MacArthur and David Goetzl, *Coke, Turner ink $200 mil pact*, **Advertising Age**, Vol. 71, No. 22, pp. 82-83, 22nd May, 2000.

499. *Global Campaign Protests Coca-Cola's Use of 'Harry Potter' to Market Junk Food*. Save Harry Potter, 11th October, 2001, https://cspinet.org/new/saveharry.html. Philip Nel, Assistant Professor of English at Kansas State University, argues that this kind of deal is influenced possibly as a result of trademark law in the US lasting as long as a product exists; as opposed to copyright law that lasts for a set time. See *Is There a Text in This Advertising Campaign?: Literature, Marketing, and Harry Potter*, **The Lion and the Unicorn**, Vol. 29, pp. 236–267, 2005, Johns Hopkins University Press.

500. Tom Leonard, Media Correspondent, *£95m Harry Potter deal with Coca-Cola*, **The Telegraph**, 21st Feb 2001.

501. Lindsey Tanner, *Some Decry Dental Group's Coca-Cola Deal*, My Plainview, 3rd March 3, 2003, https://www.myplainview.com/news/article/Some-Decry-Dental-Group-s-Coca-Cola-Deal-8763298.php.

502. Jonathan D. Shenkin, *Corporate Versus Personal Responsibility*, **Journal of Public Health Dentistry**, Vol. 63, No. 3, pp. 139-140, 2003. Also see Lindsey Tanner (AP Medical Writer), Some Decry Dental Group's Coca-Cola Deal, 3rd March, 2003, https://www.myplainview.com/news/article/Some-Decry-Dental-Group-s-Coca-Cola-Deal-8763298.php.

503. Center for Science in the Public Interest, *Pediatric Dentists Accused of Selling Out to Coke*, 4th March, 2003, https://cspinet.org/new/200303041.html and https://cspinet.org/resource/letter-aapd-re-coca-cola-partnership.

504. Allen D. Kanner and Joshua Golin, *Does Coke Money Corrupt Kids' Dentistry?* **Mothering**, March/April 2005.

505. *Nation's Dentists Get Behind Fluoride Awareness Campaign for Kids*, **PR Newswire**, 1st February, 2006.

506. Mark Gleason, *Dannon Water Springs into U.S.; Evian Parent Puts $10 Mil Ad Budget Behind Low-Price Segment Entry*, **Ad Age**, 15th January, 1996, http://adage.com/article/news/dannon-water-springs-u-s-evian-parent-puts-10-mil-ad-budget-low-price-segment-entry/80518/. Accessed 6th July, 2018.

507. *$5m hard to swallow - Costly healthy eating blitz panned as waste* By: Clare Masters, **The Daily Telegraph** (Sydney), 3rd April, 2007.

508. Julian Lee, Marketing Reporter, *TV fast food advertising ban rejected*, **Sydney Morning Herald**, 14th September, 2005:

    "According to sources at a closed meeting of food industry executives in Canberra yesterday, the Federal Government's leading health bureaucrat told the meeting responsibility for reducing obesity lay with parents rather than the companies that spend an estimated $200 million a year advertising junk food."

    Selina Powell, *Call for sugar to be treated like alcohol and tobacco*, **Marlborough Express** (New Zealand), 1st July, 2015:

    "Earlier this month Health Minister Jonathan Coleman ruled out a tax on sugar-laden products, saying exercise and education should be the focus in efforts to reduce obesity."

    Paula Oliver, *TV heads oppose ban on fast-food ads*, **New Zealand Herald**, 6th March, 2003, https://www.nzherald.co.nz/nz/news/article.cfm?c_id=1&objectid=3199281:

    "Banning fast-food advertising during children's television programmes could spell the end of the shows, television chiefs warn… Television advertising was not to blame for the problem of child obesity. 'If we were seriously harming New Zealand's children by broadcasting food commercials, I would be in the sales offices at TVNZ tomorrow morning saying, 'Take them off air'. We are not,' [TVNZ chief executive Ian Fraser] said. 'It is not open slather.'

    "Parents needed to start a change."

    "Mr Fraser's words, which were spoken as a member of the NZ Television Broadcasters' Council, were largely supported by other speakers. Massey University researcher Lynn Eagle said three years of independent research had shown that advertising bans did not work."

    Diego Cevallos, *Latin America: Parents and Lawmakers Attack Junk Food Ads*, **Global Information Network**, New York, 25th April, 2007 (ProQuest document ID: 457560609):

"Upholding the discourse of snack food and beverage manufacturers in other countries, Ignacio Lastra, spokesman of the Mexican National Chamber of Industry, declared that a law will not resolve the obesity problem. Lastra believes that families should instruct their children about adequate nutrition."

Kaare R. Norum (2005) *World Health Organization's Global Strategy on diet, physical activity and health: the process behind the scenes*, **Scandinavian Journal of Nutrition**, 49:2, 83-88, DOI: 10.1080/11026480510037147:

"[The food industry] claimed that there are no bad foods, only bad diets, and these were due to personal choices."

509. K. D. Brownell and K. E. Warner, *The perils of ignoring history: Big Tobacco played dirty and millions died. How similar is Big Food?* **Milbank Q**, Vol. 87, No. 1, 259–294, 2009. Discussed in App. 6. In 1954, the tobacco industry publicized statements that claimed public health was "industry's concern above all others."

510. https://www.coca-colacompany.com/press-center/press-releases/healthy-fun-in-the-summer-sun-coca-cola-heats-up-support-of-active-healthy-lifestyles-and-military-heroes. This article claims people drink 1.8 billion servings of Coke beverages daily (this includes juices and pre-made coffees).

511. https://www.coca-colacompany.com/transparency/our-commitment-transparency.

512. Cristin E. Kearns, Stanton A. Glantz, Laura A. Schmidt, *Sugar Industry Influence on the Scientific Agenda of the National Institute of Dental Research's 1971 National Caries Program: A Historical Analysis of Internal Documents*, **PLoS Med** 12(3): e1001798. doi:10.1371/journal.pmed.1001798. Their work also appeared in the **Journal of the American Medical Association** supplement, **Internal Medicine**, *Sugar Industry and Coronary Heart Disease ResearchA Historical Analysis of Internal Industry Documents*, 2016; 176(11): 1680-1685. doi:10.1001/jamainternmed.2016.5394.

513. All **New York Times**: Anahad O'Connor, *How the Sugar Industry Shifted Blame to Fat*, 12th September, 2016, *Study Tied to Food Industry Tries to Discredit Sugar Guidelines*, 19th December, 2016. David Singerman, Op-Ed contributor, *The Shady History of Big Sugar*, 16th September, 2016. Mark Bittman, *The Right to Sell Kids Junk*, 27th March, 2012. Bittman is an author of many books on food, http://markbittman.com/.

514. Sugar Research Foundation, *Progress and prospects, scientific research in physiology, nutrition and special uses of sugar: seventh annual report*, 1950. New York: Sugar Research Foundation.

515. Gary Taubes and Cristin Kearns Couzens, *Big Sugar's Sweet Little Lies. How the industry kept scientists from asking: Does sugar kill?* **Mother Jones**, November/December 2012 Issue. https://www.motherjones.com/environment/2012/10/sugar-industry-lies-campaign/. They also claim Stare tried to obtain industry funding for a study aiming at exonerating tobacco as a cause of heart disease. The Silver Anvil awards can be seen on the Public Relations Society of America's website, https://apps.prsa.org/Awards/SilverAnvil/Search?sayear=1976&pg=3&sacategory=&sakeyword=&saindustry=&saoutcome=.

516. *Universities Should Not Lend Names to Coca-Cola "Energy Balance" Network*, Statement of CSPI President Michael F. Jacobson, 9th August, 2015. Jacobson, Ph.D. (microbiology), is a Co-founder and long-time Executive Director of CSPI. He is now serving as Senior Scientist at CSPI. https://cspinet.org/new/201508191.html.

517. Anahad O'Connor, *Coca-Cola Funds Scientists Who Shift Blame for Obesity Away From Bad Diets*, **New York Times**, 9th August, 2015.

518. THE PRAXIS PROJECT, a non-profit corporation, Plaintiff, v. THE COCA-COLA COMPANY and AMERICAN BEVERAGE ASSOCIATION, Defendants. available on the CSPI's website, 4th January, 2017, *Coca-Cola, American Beverage Association are Targets of Lawsuit Charging Deceptive Sugary Drink Marketing*.

519. https://www.gizmodo.com.au/2017/01/5-of-the-most-egregious-health-claims-from-the-new-us-coca-cola-lawsuit/

520. http://journals.plos.org/plosone/article?id=10.1371/journal.pone.0163463.

521. https://www.coca-colacompany.com/content/dam/journey/us/en/private/fileassets/pdf/unknown/unknown/2009_annual_review_Year_in_Review.pdf. José Octavio Reyes, the President, Latin America Group, said: "... when we reached a per capita of 426 in 1999, no one thought we could continue to grow, and yet we did." By

2014, Argentina, America and Chile had outdone Mexico in soda drinking, Marc Silver, 19th July, 2015, https://www.npr.org/sections/goatsandsoda/2015/06/19/415223346/guess-which-country-has-the-biggest-increase-in-soda-drinking.

522. https://www.bottledwater.org/public/2011%20BMC%20Bottled%20Water%20Stats_2.pdf#overlay-context=economics/industry-statistics.

523. Julie Turkewitz, *In Denver, Persuading Latino Immigrants to Trust the Tap Water*, **New York Times**, 31st March, 2016.

524. Mexico: WHO Statistical Profile, http://www.who.int/gho/countries/mex.pdf?ua=1.

525. CSPI, *Raw Deal: School Beverage Contracts Less Lucrative Than They Seem*, pp. 8 and 12, 2006.

526. J. McNeal, *Tapping the Three Kids' Markets*. **American Demographics**, p. 36, April 1998.

527. Anthony Winson, *School Food Environments and the Obesity Issue: Content, Structural Determinants, and Agency in Canadian High Schools*, **Agricultural Human Values**, Vol. 25, pp. 499-511, 2008. Also examines U.S. schools. "Canadian society today, as for most developed countries, faces a looming health crisis related to the characteristics of diets and lifestyles as they have evolved over the twentieth century."

528. Center for Science in the Public Interest, *Anticipated National School Nutrition Standards Should Have Negligible Financial Impact on Schools and Beverage Industry*, 28th May, 2013, https://cspinet.org/new/201305281.html.

529. Juliet Schor, *Born to Buy*, pp. 91-96, 2003; and see https://consumersunion.org/news/captive-kids-a-report-on-commercial-pressures-on-kids-at-schools-part-one/.

530. S. Beder, W. Varney and R. Gosden, *This Little Kiddy Went to Market*, Chapter 8. p. 103, 2009. Page 107: "A 1989 Ford Foundation report … suggested that the inability of those who had jobs to support a family on low wages was a consequence of their low education, rather than of the poor wages being offered by employers."

531. J. S. Beresford, B.D.SS (NZ), H.D.D. (Edinburgh), D.Orth.R.C.S. (England), *London Newsletter*, **New Zealand Dental Journal**, Vol. 56, p. 93, 1960.

532. *Damages for Decay*, **The Evening Post** (Wellington), 15th November, 1991.

533. Shelov *et al.*, *Children, Adolescents, and Advertising*, **Pediatrics**, Vol. 95, No. 2, February, 1995. This article summarizes the reasons behind the recommendations of the Committee on Communications – eight MDs (Shelov was Chairman). See Appendix 6.

534. *Are Commercials Making You a Junk-Food Freak?* **Scholastic Scope**, Vol. 57, No. 9, pp. 14-15, 13th December, 2010.

535. Jennifer L. Harris, PhD, MBA, and Samantha K. Graff, JD, *Protecting Young People From Junk Food Advertising: Implications of Psychological Research for First Amendment Law*, **American Journal of Public Health**, Vol. 102, No. 2, pp. 214-222, February, 2012. The figure of thirteen ads daily comes from L. M. Powell, G. Szczpka, F. J. Chaloupka, *Trends in Exposure to Television Food Advertisements among Children and Adolescents in the United States*, **Archives of Pediatrics and Adolescent Medicine**, Vol. 164, No. 9, pp. 794-802, 2010.

536. *Kids exposed to 'enormous amounts of junk food advertising'*, Checkpoint, 9th October, 2017, http://www.radionz.co.nz/national/programmes/checkpoint/audio/201861738/kids-exposed-to-enormous-amounts-of-junk-food-advertising.

537. *Rich Media, Poor Democracy* (2003). A documentary featuring Bob McChesney, in which he argues that corporate mergers of media ownership cause firms to conglomerate, leading to more wealth and power for the wealthy and powerful. Larger media simply drown out smaller media because smaller media cannot compete. Argues that capitalism is based on "smashing competition" – not competition.

538. https://www.stuff.co.nz/national/health/101920079/dr-eric-crampton-theres-no-good-reason-for-a-sugar-tax-in-new-zealand. Dr. Crampton was responding to another op-ed piece by Otago University's Dr. Simon Thornley, advocating a tax: https://www.stuff.co.nz/national/health/101921052/dr-simon-thornley-a-sugar-tax-would-be-a-fence-at-the-top-of-a-cliff.

539. Duff Wilson, Janet Roberts, *Special Report: How Washington went soft on childhood obesity*, 27th April, 2012, https://www.reuters.com/article/us-usa-foodlobby/special-report-how-washington-went-soft-on-childhood-obesity-idUSBRE83Q0ED20120427.

540. *Unhealthy foods get chop from tuck shops*, **New Zealand Herald**, 22nd September, 2006.

541. Eleanor Black, *Unhealthy 'lunch packs' costing $2 marketed to children*, 29th September, 2017, https://www.stuff.co.nz/life-style/well-good/97305941/Unhealthy-lunch-packs-costing-2-marketed-to-children. Also see Rob Stock: *Can you do a $2 lunch for the kids?* https://www.stuff.co.nz/business/money/97491965/rob-stock-can-you-do-a-2-lunch-for-the-kids.

542. Kaare R. Norum (2005) *World Health Organization's Global Strategy on diet, physical activity and health: the process behind the scenes*, **Scandinavian Journal of Nutrition**, 49:2, 83-88, DOI: 10.1080/11026480510037147.

543. *Diet, Nutrition, and the Prevention of Chronic Diseases*, Technical Report Series 916 (TRS 916), World Health Organization, Report of a joint WHO/FAO consultation, Geneva 2003.

544. https://www.sugar.org/search/world+health+organization.

545. Just consider in 2018 the Labour Party announced their Child Poverty Reduction Bill. It was the only thing I've seen them do that the National Party did not oppose. https://www.national.org.nz/national_supports_bipartisan_child_poverty_approach.

546. Editorial, *Ions in the Water*, **New Zealand Dental Journal**, Vol. 52, No. 247, January, 1956.

547. *Why does he have to wait*, **The Dominion Post**, Letters, p. B6, 6th June, 2005.

548. *Fight over fluoride reignited*, **Sunday Star Times**, 26th January, 2014.

549. Jared Nicoll, *Porirua's Pasifika children suffering high levels of tooth decay*, 3rd May, 2017, https://www.stuff.co.nz/national/health/92169692/poriruas-pasifika-children-suffering-high-levels-of-tooth-decay.

550. The Right Honorable Simon Bridges, *Helping New Zealand businesses succeed*, 3rd July, 2018, https://www.facebook.com/simonjbridges/videos/1990435000988659/.

551. https://www.stuff.co.nz/national/politics/81194202/Public-health-researchers-fighting-back-against-lobbyists.

552. John Dewey, *Later Works, 1925-1953*, p. 163.

553. Gretchen Reynolds, *Parents Aren't Good Judges of Their Kids' Sugar Intake*, **New York Times**, 19th July, 2018. Mattea Dallacker, Ralph Hertwig and Jutta Mata, *Parents' considerable underestimation of sugar and their child's risk of overweight*, **International Journal of Obesity**, Vol. 42, pp. 1097-1100, 2018.

554. Serge H. Ahmed; Karine Guillem; Youna Vandaele, *Sugar addiction: pushing the drug-sugar analogy to the limit*, **Current Opinion in Clinical Nutrition and Metabolic Care**. 16(4):434–439, JUL 2013, DOI: 10.1097/MCO.0b013e328361c8b8. Argues for a similarity between sugar and cocaine in rats.

Jacki M. Rorabaugh, Jennifer M. Stratford, and Nancy R. Zahniser, *Differences in bingeing behavior and cocaine reward following intermittent access to sucrose, glucose or fructose solutions*, **Neuroscience**, 2015 Aug 20; 301: 213–220.

James J DiNicolantonio, James H O'Keefe, William L Wilson, *Sugar addiction: is it real? A narrative review*, **British Journal of Sports Medicine**, 23rd August, 2017.

Is sugar really as addictive as cocaine? Scientists row over effect on body and brain, **The Guardian**, 25th August, 2017. Looks at the opinion of some experts, regarding the paper published two days previous (DiNicolantonio *et al.*). They agree that there are no physical withdrawals – e.g. tremors, cold sweats, etc. Suggests that the general idea of sugar being as addictive as cocaine is an exaggeration.

A review that claims no conflicts of interest or research funding is available: Margaret L. Westwater, Paul C. Fletcher, Hisham Ziauddeen, *Sugar addiction: the state of the science*, **European Journal of Nutrition**, (2016) 55 (Suppl 2):S55–S69 DOI 10.1007/s00394-016-1229-6. Claims sugar should not be considered an addictive drug.

Chapter 5.8

555. T. G. Ludwig, B.D.S., M.S., *The Hastings Fluoridation Project I. Dental Effects Between 1954 and 1957*, **New Zealand Dental Journal**, Vol. 54, pp. 165-172, October 1958.

556. P. B. Hunter and E. Storey, *The Hastings Experiment Confirmed* (1987). Held in the National Library of New Zealand in Wellington with the title *Reply to the Health Department by Colquhoun & Mann* (1988).

557. John Colquhoun, *Education and Fluoridation in New Zealand: an Historical Study*. Thesis submitted for the degree of Doctor of Philosphy, University of Auckland, New Zealand, 1987. Available through the National Library of New Zealand. Hastings is discussed in the final chapter. Colquhoun referred to fluorine's status as "essential nutrient" (his speech marks) as part of a foundation of the fluoridation paradigm, pp. 61-62.

558. https://www.health.govt.nz/our-work/preventative-health-wellness/fluoride-and-oral-health/water-fluoridation.

559. HD 125/299/1 H1 Box 1634, 5th May, 1954.

560. *Experts on Water Fluoridation to Speak in Hastings*, Unknown paper (marked "Times") 12th May, clipping found in 125/299/1 H1 Box 1634.

561. P. T. Gifford, Member Jaycee of the Fluoride Education Committee, **Hawke's Bay Herald-Tribune**, 7th May, 1954.

562. **The Daily Telegraph**, 15th May, 1954.

563. HD 125/299/1 H1 Box 1634, 18th May, 1954.

564. *VISITING AUTHORITIES UPHOLD FLUORIDE*, **Hawke's Bay Herald-Tribune**, 19th of May, 1954. *American Experts Term Fluorine Harmless*, **Daily Telegraph** (Napier), same date. A sub-heading in this article described England as "not asleep" by Dr. Parfitt, who went on to say that England was following the example set by America. Here we see the association of fluoridation with intelligence.

565. HD 125/299/1 H1 Box 1634, 20th May, 1954.

566. HD 125/299/1 H1 Box 1634, 4th June, 1954.

567. HD 125/299/1 H1 Box 1634, 25th June, 1954.

568. *Why Water Fluoridation is Being Continued: Opponents Entirely Mistaken, Assert Mayors. Controversy Surveyed*, **Hawke's Bay Herald-Tribune**, 26th June, 1954.

569. *Notes on Meeting Regarding Fluoridation*, Held in Borough Engineer's Office, Hastings, 30th June, 1954, HD 125/299/1 H1 Box 1634.

570. HD 125/299/1 H1 Box 1634, 2nd July, 1954.

571. HD 125/299/1 H1 Box 1704, *Objections Raised by Dr. Eva Hill*, p. 4.

572. HD 125/299/1 H1 Box 1634, 16th December, 1954.

573. HD 125/299/3 H1 Box 1835, 19th January, 1954.

574. HD 125/299/3 H1 Box 1835, 20th – 27th February.

575. **The Daily Telegraph**, 26th June, 1956.

576. HD 125/299/1 H1 Box 1704, *Letter from Dr. Cairney*, 22nd June, 1956.

577. IS: HD 125/299 H1 Box 1725, 16th June, 1959.

578. *Report of the Commission of Inquiry on the Fluoridation of Public Water Supplies*, paragraph 382, 1957.

579. *Ibid*, chapter 24, 1957. Also see *Hastings Fluoridation Petition "Received" – Town Clerk to Give Signatures "Strict Scrutiny"*, **Hawke's Bay Herald-Tribune**, 28th May, 1954; *Anti-Fluoridation Petition Lodged with Council*, 17th May, 1954; and by Alan Lerner, *N.Z's Battle of Hastings: Is Good Drinking Water Being Poisoned?* **The New Zealand Observer**, 30th June, 1954, all in 125/299/1 H1 1634.

580. *Report of the Commission of Inquiry on the Fluoridation of Public Water Supplies*, paragraph 472, 1957.

581. Fuller, James Ferris (Brigadier), 1913-2001: Papers. MS-Papers-6275-06. *Dreams Pursued, or, The Saga of Fluoridation*, p. 12. Available at the National Library, Wellington, New Zealand.

582. Letter from J. Ferris Fuller to H. Brown, 19th September, 1997. MS-Papers-6275-06.

583. *Manufacturing Consent*, citation 134, Introduction to the 2002 Edition. Herman and Chomsky cite Andrew Pollack, **New York Times**, *Talks on Biotech Food Turn on a Safety Principle*, 28th January, 2000.

"But European countries and the developing countries, which have been pitted against the United States and a handful of its allies all week, say precaution is justified because not enough is known about the environmental effects of genetic engineering. And if a 'superweed' or dangerous bacteria were to get loose in the environment, it could not be recalled like a defective car."

"Washington wants to make sure any agreement on biosafety does not take precedence over the World Trade Organization rules. That is because under W.T.O. rules an import can be banned only on the basis of scientific evidence."

Therefore a country must give scientific justification to corporations in order to refuse imports. The country is not supposed to use their own free will, their opinion of common sense, or look to history's track record.

Also see same author and paper, *130 Nations Agree on Safety Rules for Biotech Food*, 30th January, 2000.

"The biosafety talks themselves broke down a year ago in Cartagena, Colombia, when the United States and a handful of other big agricultural exporters blocked a treaty agreed to by virtually all the other countries."

The attitude of business to democracy is apparent here. Often when activists are represented politically, people are frustrated about a "militant minority" – yet we see a more powerful version in the business community.

"Still, early this morning, it appeared that history might repeat itself. The United States and Canada refused to agree to a requirement -- supported by virtually all the other countries -- that shipments of genetically altered commodities like corn or soybeans identify the specific variety."

"A tense standoff ensued for hours. Finally, frowning and grumbling, the Europeans backed down, and the treaty requires stating only that the shipment 'may contain' genetically modified organisms."

The treaty did not look at whether GMOs should be labelled on shelves in stores, only that they should be labelled vaguely ("*may* contain GMOs" vs names of specific strains) on international shipments – so consumers would not know for certain whether they were eating GMOs or not. Industry "cheered" when the treaty no longer applied to human pharmaceuticals.

Also very relevant here is the exceptionally detailed book *Doubt is their Product* by Professor David Michaels. If there is one book I could inspire you to read regarding business's influence on science, make it this one.

584. John Colquhoun and Robert Mann, *The Hastings Fluoridation Experiment: Science or Swindle?* **The Ecologist**, Vol. 16, No. 6, pp. 243-248, 1986.

585. HD 125/299/1, H1 Box 1634, 2nd August, 1954. From H. W. Carter, Director, Division of Public Hygiene to the Medical Officer of Health, Palmerston North.

586. Peter Hunter, *Evidence Supports Fluoride Benefits*, **The Evening Post**, 17th April, 1990.

587. John Colquhoun and Bill Wilson, *The Lost Control*, **Accountability in Research**, pp. 373-394, 1999. Claim of media publicity on p. 374. Claim of overdosing on p. 380 and in the "Discussion" section.

588. *Mr. Nash Comments on Dentists and Fluoridation*, **The Evening Post**, 18th September, 1957.

Chapter 6

589. Despina S. Koussoulakou, Lukas H. Margaritis, Stauros L. Koussoulakos, *A Curriculum Vitae of Teeth: Evolution, Generation, Regeneration*, **International Journal of Biological Sciences**, Vol. 5, No. 3, pp. 226-243, 2009.

590. World Health Organization, *Fluoride and Dental Health*, p. 163, 1970.

591. Denes V. Agoston, *How to Translate Time? The Temporal Aspect of Human and Rodent Biology*, **Frontiers of Neurology**, Vol. 8, Article 92, March 2017, doi: 10.3389/feur.2017.00092.

592. Richard A. Smith, D.D.S., M.S.D., *The Effect of Roentgen Rays on the Developing Teeth of Rats*, **Journal of the American Dental Association**, Vol. 18, No. 1., pp. 111-118, 1931.

593. *The world's favourite lab animal has been found wanting, but there are new twists in the mouse's tale*, **The Economist**, 24th December, 2016, https://www.economist.com/christmas-specials/2016/12/24/the-worlds-favourite-lab-animal-has-been-found-wanting-but-there-are-new-twists-in-the-mouses-tale. Erika Check Hayden, *Misleading mouse studies waste medical resources*, Nature, 26th March 2014, https://www.nature.com/news/misleading-mouse-studies-waste-medical-resources-1.14938.

594. Alla Katsnelson, *Male researchers stress out rodents*, Nature, 28th April, 2014, https://www.nature.com/news/male-researchers-stress-out-rodents-1.15106.

595. Bronwen Martin, Sunggoan Ji, Stuart Maudsley, and Mark P. Mattson, *"Control" laboratory rodents are metabolically morbid: Why it matters*, (Proceedings of the National Academy of Sciences (PNAS), 6th April, 2010. 107 (14) 6127-6133; https://doi.org/10.1073/pnas.0912955107. This study was discussed in *Fat rats skew research results* by Daniel Cressey, **Nature**, 2nd March, 2010, Vol. 464, 19 (2010), doi:10.1038/464019a.

596. Day, C. D. M., *Nutritional Deficiencies and Dental Caries in Northern India*. **British Dental Journal**, Vol. 76, No. 5, pp. 115-122, 3rd March, 1944. Second part printed in issue dated 17th March, 1944.

597. Josef Warkany, M.D. and Frederick M. Deuschle, D.D.S., *Congenital malformations induced in rats by maternal riboflavin deficiency: dentofacial changes*, **Journal of the American Dental Association**, Vol. 51, No. 2, pp. 139-154, August, 1955.

Chapter 6.1

598. Henry F. Helmholz, M.D., *Views of the National Congress of Parents and Teachers in Regard to Fluoridation*, **American Journal of Public Health**, p. 884, July, 1954.

599. *Tempest in a Reservoir*, **Chemical Week**, pp. 18-19, 14th February, 1953.

600. *Grand Rapids Death Rate Data Analyzed*, **Stevens Point Journal** (Stevens Point, Wisconsin), p. 3, 20th February, 1956.

601. Samuel L. Andelman, M.D., M.P.H., *Chicago's experience with fluoridation*, **Journal of the American Dental Association**, Vol. 65, No. 5, p. 613, 1962.

602. *Fluoridation may be Required*, **The Daily News** (Port Angeles, Washington), p. 1, 20th September, 1974.

603. Under the headline *Evidence: effectiveness of water fluoridation*, https://www.health.govt.nz/our-work/preventative-health-wellness/fluoride-and-oral-health/water-fluoridation/effective-and-safe.

604. *I Think You'll Find it's a Bit More Complicated Than That*, pp. 22-25, 2014.

605. *Adding fluoride to water supplies*, **British Medical Journal**, Vol. 335, pp. 699-702, 6th October, 2007.

606. NHS Centre for Reviews and Dissemination. *A systematic review of public water fluoridation*. York: NHS CRD, 2000, p. x.

607. *Health effects of water fluoridation: A review of the scientific evidence*, p. 34, 2014. A report on behalf of the Royal Society of New Zealand and the Office of the Prime Minister's Chief Science Advisor.

608. E. T. Treasure, I. G. Chestnutt, P. Whiting, M. McDonagh, P. Wilson and J. Kleijnen, *The York Review – A systematic review of public water fluoridation: a commentary*, **British Dental Journal**, Vol. 192, No. 9, 11th May, 2002.

609. http://www.radionz.co.nz/news/regional/136913/hamilton-to-end-water-fluoridation.

610. Brisbane Lord Mayor's Taskforce, Australia, 1997.

611. http://www.cochrane.org/about-us.

612. Iheozor-Ejiofor Z, Worthington HV, Walsh T, O'Malley L, Clarkson JE, Macey R, Alam R, Tugwell P, Welch V, Glenny A, *Water fluoridation to prevent tooth decay*, 18th June, 2015, http://www.cochrane.org/CD010856/ORAL_water-fluoridation-prevent-tooth-decay. The quotes here are from the "plain language summary". A fully detailed version of the study exists here: http://cochranelibrary-wiley.com/doi/10.1002/14651858.CD010856.pub2/full.

613. http://oralhealth.cochrane.org/news/impact-story-water-fluoridation-prevention-dental-caries.

614. Maryanne Demasi, PhD, *Cochrane – A sinking ship?* https://blogs.bmj.com/bmjebmspotlight/2018/09/16/cochrane-a-sinking-ship/. Ray Moynihan: *Let's stop the burning and the bleeding at Cochrane—there's too much at stake*, https://blogs.bmj.com/bmj/2018/09/17/ray-moynihan-lets-stop-the-burning-and-the-bleeding-at-cochrane-theres-too-much-at-stake/. Trish Greenhalgh: *The Cochrane Collaboration—what crisis?* https://blogs.bmj.com/bmj/2018/09/17/trish-greenhalgh-the-cochrane-collaboration-what-crisis/. https://blogs.bmj.com/bmjebmspotlight/files/2018/09/Why-we-resigned.pdf.

615. A. J. Rugg-Gunn, A. J. Spencer, H. P. Whelton, C. Jones, J. F. Beal, P. Castle, P. V. Cooney, J. Johnson, M. P. Kelly, M. A. Lennon, J. McGinley, D. O'Mullane, H. D. Sgan-Cohen, P. P. Sharma, W. M. Thomson, S. M.

Woodward and S. P. Zusman, *Critique of the review of 'Water fluoridation for the prevention of dental caries' published by the Cochrane Collaboration in 2015*, **British Dental Journal**, Vol. 220, pp. 335-340, 8th April, 2016, https://www.nature.com/articles/sj.bdj.2016.257.

616. Australian National Health and Medical Research Council, *The Effectiveness of Water Fluoridation*, pp. 28-33, 1991.

617. Arnold FA Jr, Dean HT, Jay P, Knutson JW. *Effect of fluoridated public water supplies on dental caries prevalence. 10th year of the Grand Rapids-Muskegon Study.* **Public Health Reports** 1956;71:652-8.

618. WHO, Poul Erik. Petersen and Michael A. Lennon, *Effective use of fluorides for the prevention of dental caries in the 21st century: the WHO approach*, **Community Dent Oral Epidemiol**, 2004; 32: 319–321. "Despite great improvements in the oral health of populations across the world, problems still persist particularly among poor and disadvantaged groups in both developed and developing countries." (Page 319.)

Also claimed in the 2014 report commissioned by Sirs Gluckman and Skegg of New Zealand: "The burden of tooth decay is highest among the most deprived socioeconomic groups, and this is the segment of the population for which the benefits of CWF appear to be greatest." (Page 6.)

619. Personal communication from Australian NHMRC to author, 10th June 2018.

620. *Dental Service Held Matter of Teamwork*, **Daily Telegraph**, 14th May, 1954.

621. John Colquhoun MS-Papers-6670-81 Department of Health Research Papers, available at the National Library, Wellington, New Zealand. Marked "NZDA files. Box 2. File 34. Fluoridation."

622. Julian D. Boyd, M.D., and Kenneth E. Wessels, D.D.S. *Epidemiologic Studies in Dental Caries, III: The Interpretation of Clinical Data Relating to Caries Advance*, **American Journal of Public Health**, Vol. 41, pp. 976-985, 1954.

623. Joe Mullen, *History of Water Fluoridation*, **British Dental Journal**, Vol. 199, pp. 1-4, 2005.

624. *SCIENTIFIC REPORT submitted to EFSA: Literature search and review related to specific preparatory work in the establishment of Dietary Reference Values Preparation of an evidence report identifying health outcomes upon which Dietary Reference Values could potentially be based for Fluoride*, p. 168, 2012. Prepared by Tracey Brown, Dr Amy Mullee, Rachel Collings, Dr Linda Harvey, Dr Lee Hooper and Prof Susan Fairweather-Tait, Department of Nutrition, Norwich Medical School, Faculty of Medicine and Health Sciences, University of East Anglia, Norwich.

625. Bronwyn Torrie, *Dental woes putting kids in hospital*, **The Dominion Post**, 7th November, 2012. Professor Thomson's profile: https://www.otago.ac.nz/healthsciences/expertise/Profile/?id=196.

626. *The Untold Benefits of Fluoridation*, **The Dominion**, 8th April 1965. "Thousands of dental cavities – soon it will be millions – are being prevented…". Also see New Zealand Fluoridated Zones 20 June 2006, https://www.parliament.nz/resource/0000069144, https://wellingtonwater.co.nz/your-water/drinking-water/whats-in-your-water/fluoride/.

Chapter 6.2

627. Jean Mayer , Ph.D., D.Sc. (EDITOR) & D. M. Hegsted , PH.D., *Osteoporosis and Fluoride Deficiency*, **Journal of Postgraduate Medicine**, pp. A 49-A 53, January, 1967.

628. *How to Live Five Years Longer: A Prominent Physician Gives you Useful Advice on Diet, Exercise and Danger Signals*, **Nation's Business**, pp. 78-81, December, 1967. Regarding the prevention of hardening of the arteries, he was discussing the work of Dr. Mark Hegsted, at the time also working for Harvard. Hegsted compared two cities, and claimed collapsed vertebrae and calcification of the aorta was higher in the city with lower fluoride. This was discussed in the article *Harvard Researcher Tells of Study: Fluorides said to Reduce Hardening of the Arteries*, **Asheville Citizen-Times** (Asheville, North Carolina), p. 1, 18th April, 1967.

629. Robert Van Reen, Ph.D., *Review of biochemistry of the calcified tissues*, **Journal of the American Dental Association**, Vol. 76, No. 6, pp. 1340-1349, 1968.

630. Gordon SL, Corbin SB. *Summary of workshop on drinking water fluoridation influence on hip fracture on bone health.* **Osteoporosis Int** 1992;2:109-17. This was cited in the email I received from Harvard.

631. Personal communication from Harvard University Dean's Office to author, 20th July, 2018.

632. https://hollis.harvard.edu/primo-explore/fulldisplay?docid=01HVD_ALMA211768338010003941&context=L&vid=HVD2&lang=en_US&search_scope=default_scope&adaptor=Local%20Search%20Engine&tab=books&query=any,contains,hegsted%201967.

633. A. Catharine Ross, Benjamin Caballero, Robert J. Cousins, Katherine L. Tucker, Thomas R. Ziegler editors, *Modern Nutrition in Health and Disease*, eleventh edition, (2014), p. 171, 646, 1221, 1380.

634. *Ibid.*, p. 1232. This chapter authored by Katherine L. Tucker, Professor of Nutritional Epidemiology at Northeastern University; and Clifford J. Rosen, Center for Clinical and Translational Research, Maine Medical Center Research Institute.

635. *Ibid.*, p. 766. This chapter authored by Douglas C. Heimburger, Professor of Medicine, Vanderbilt University School of Medicine.

636. *Ibid.*, p. 1019. This chapter authored by Riva Touger-Decker, Professor, Nutritional Sciences, New Jersey Dental School; Diane Rigassio Radler, Associate Professor, Nutritional Sciences, University of Medicine and Dentistry, New Jersey; and Dominick P. Depaola, Associate Dean, Academic Affairs, College of Dental Medicine, Nova Southeastern University, Fort Lauderdale, Florida.

637. Romina Brignardello-Petersen, DDS, MSc, PhD, *Evidence suggests a small association between malocclusions and caries in adolescents*, **Journal of the American Dental Association**, in press, 3rd July, 2018.

638. Ross *et al. op cit. Modern Nutrition*, pp. 245-246, 2014.

639. Lindsay Clark, *NZ nuclear science confirms fluoride action against decay*, **The Press**, p. 19, 27th January, 1993.

640. WHO, *Fluorides*, 2002, Chapter 8.1.3.

641. Levy, *et al.*, *Infants' Ingestion from Water, Supplements and Dentifrice*, **Journal of the American Dental Association**, Vol. 126, pp. 1625-1632, December, 1995.

642. *Report of the Commission of Inquiry on the Fluoridation of Public Water Supplies*. Dominion of New Zealand 1957, p. 149-150. Quoted in *Fluoridation Safe, Maintain International and National and Community Health Authorities*, **Journal of the American Dental Association**, Vol. 65, No. 5, pp. 603-607, 1962.

643. Kehoe, Robert A., *Safety of Fluoridation*. In *Our Children's Teeth*, New York, Committee to Protect Our Children's Teeth, Inc., 1957, p. 27. Quoted in *Fluoridation Safe, Maintain International and National and Community Health Authorities*, **Journal of the American Dental Association**, Vol. 65, No. 5, pp. 603-607, 1962.

644. Levy SM, Guha-Chowdhury N. *Total Fluoride Intake and Implications for Dietary Fluoride Supplements.* **Journal of Public Health Dentistry**, Vol 59, No. 4, pp. 211-223, December, 1999.

645. *Ibid*, p. 221.

646. **British Dental Journal**, Vol. 189, pp. 406–407, 28th October, 2000.

647. http://www.cochrane.org/CD007693/ORAL_is-the-use-of-fluoride-toothpaste-during-early-childhood-associated-with-discolourationmottling-of-teeth. This is the "plain language summary"; a full review is Wong *et al.*, *Topical fluoride as a cause of dental fluorosis in children*, http://cochranelibrary-wiley.com/doi/10.1002/14651858.CD007693.pub2/full.

648. John D. B. Featherstone, *The Science and Practice of Caries Prevention*, **Journal of the American Dental Association**, Vol. 131, pp. 887-899, July, 2000.

649. Frances B. Glenn, D.D.S. Miami, *Preeruptive Effect of Fluoride*, **Journal of the American Dental Association**, Vol. 131, pp. 1670-1671, December, 2000.

650. National Academy of Sciences, **Guiding Principles for Developing DRIs Based on Chronic Disease**, pp. 43, 46, 51, 60, 63, 281, 284, 2017.

651. Peter Cressey BSc(Hons), *Dietary fluoride intake for fully formula-fed infants in New Zealand: impact of formula and water fluoride*, **Journal of Public Health Dentistry**, Vol. 70, No. 4, 1st December, 2010.

652. Dr. John Dodes, D.D.S., Quoted in *The Tooth About Dentistry* hosted by Karen Stollznow, available from *Point of Inquiry with Paul Fidalgo*,

http://www.pointofinquiry.org/john_dodes_the_tooth_about_dentistry/ (about 6½ minutes into the interview) 5th September, 2011.

653. *Where We Stand: Fluoride Supplements*, https://www.healthychildren.org/English/ages-stages/baby/feeding-nutrition/Pages/Fluoride-Supplements.aspx, accessed July, 2018.

654. *ADA Applauds Final Announcement on Optimal Fluoride Level in Drinking Water*, 27th April, 2015, https://www.ada.org/en/press-room/news-releases/2015-archive/april/hhs-announcement-on-optimal-fluoride-level-in-drinking-water.

Chapter 6.3

655. Weston Price, *Nutrition and Physical Degeneration*, 6th Edition, pp. 138-139, 1998 (first published 1939).

656. *Ibid.*, p. 209.

657. https://price-pottenger.org/. Also see the book *Nourishing Traditions* by Sally Fallon and Mary G. Enig, Ph.D. (Second Edition published in 1999).

658. Dr. Henry Pickerill, *The Prevention of Dental Caries and Oral Sepsis*, pp. 11-12, 1914. Published by Bailliere, Tindall and Cox, London.

659. Dr. Jean Mayer, *The Bitter Truth about Sugar: It's bad for health, bad for teeth, and we all eat more of it than we think*, **New York Times**, 20th June, 1976.

660. Weston Price, *Op. Cit.*, p. 205.

661. *Ibid.*, p. 206.

662. *Ibid.*, p. 209.

663. *Ibid.*, p. 212.

664. For instance Dr. Mike Berridge's book and his statements in his 2016 debate with Professor Paul Connett, and Dr. Ken Perrott's statements in *The Fluoride Debate*.

665. *Ducks, Bulls, and a Trace Element*, by Taranaki Daily News Columnist Gordon Burnside, a guest post on the Making Sense of Fluoride Website, dated 22nd February, 2015, http://msof.nz/2015/02/ducks-bulls-and-a-trace-element/.

666. Don Weaver and Jon Hamaker, *The Survival of Civilization*, p.4.

667. Ashmead, *Chelated Mineral Nutrition*, pp. 6-7, 1989.

668. Presented by Mr. Fletcher 1st June, 1936, and Ordered to be Printed by the United States Government Printing Office Washington: 1936, During the 74th Congress, Second Session, Document No. 264.

669. Weston Price, *Op. Cit.*, p. 275. Incidentally, Dr. Price was a little critical of NZ regarding the application of his recommendations to Maori children. He claimed the doctors provided high energy food but did not emphasize the mineral aspect (page 298-299).

670. P. T. Gifford, Member Jaycee Fluoride Committee, Hastings, *Reader's Opinions*, **Hawke's Bay Herald-Tribune**, 30th April, 1954.

671. Weston Price, *Op. Cit.*, p. 201.

672. Dr. Henry Pickerill, *The Prevention of Dental Caries and Oral Sepsis*, pp. 309-310, 1914. Published by Bailliere, Tindall and Cox, London.

673. *Ibid.*, p. 329.

674. *Ibid.*, pp. 312-313.

675. R. M. S. Taylor, B.D.S., *Maori Foods and Methods of Preparation*, pp. 1 and 9, 1934. Originally printed in the **New Zealand Dental Journal**, November, 1934.

676. Rebecca Malcolm, *The case for fluoridated water*, **Rotorua Daily Post**, 23rd Jun, 2014. https://www.nzherald.co.nz/rotorua-daily-post/lifestyle/news/article.cfm?c_id=1503432&objectid=11279829. This article contains a suggestion of fluorine's nutritional role. It is written in a Q&A fashion, like many:

"Can a person have too much fluoride in their body? Yes, like vitamins and other dietary supplements. In countries where there are extremely high levels of fluoride, it can cause skeletal fluorosis but this requires taking in much more fluoride than anyone in New Zealand would be exposed to."

677. These muscular relationships are taken from *Gray's Anatomy*, 1994.

678. Dr. Henry Pickerill, *Op. Cit.*, p. 333.

679. *Ibid.*, p. 334.

680. *Ibid.*, p. 35.

681. Harold M. Schmeck Jr., *To Conquer Tooth Decay*, **New York Times**, p. 12, 9th June, 1968.

682. Weston Price, *Op. Cit.*, p. 164.

683. *Ibid.*, p. 167.

684. *Ibid.*, p. 174.

685. *Ibid.*, pp. 178-179.

686. *Ibid.*, p. 182.

687. *Ibid.*, p. 186.

688. Personal communication, TVNZ OnDemand Support, 16th January, 2018. There exists the possibility TVNZ has shown it since I inquired. John Pilger has spent much time on native Australian issues, in documentaries like *The Secret Country* and *The Last Dream*. See his website, http://johnpilger.com/videos.

689. Weston Price, *Op. Cit.*, pp. 198-200.

690. See Jerry Mander's work *In the Absence of the Sacred*, Chapter 14.

691. Free trade agreement NAFTA was blamed for water contamination in Mexico in 2016. They faced dental and possibly skeletal fluorosis, and excess arsenic. See Elisabeth Malkin, *Prosperous Mexican Farms Suck Up Water, Leaving Villages High and Dry*, **New York Times**, 19th May, 2016.

    The journal **Adbusters** looked at British children in No. 71, Vol. 15, May/June 2007. *Generation F*cked* by Maria Hampton. "The UN's first ever report on the state of childhood in the industrialized West made unpleasant reading for many of the world's richest nations."

    It appears that the situation of British children has improved recently a little, see UNICEF's 2013 report, *Child Well-Being in Rich Countries: A Comparative Overview* (Report Card 11).

    Also see *Children in the UK feel more disempowered than those in India*, **The Guardian**, 20th November, 2017.

692. See Noam Chomsky's *Understanding Power: The Indispensable Chomsky*, Edited by Peter R. Mitchell and John Schoeffel, p. 376, 2002. More of the story is discussed in the 2009 **Milbank Quarterly** study cited in Chapter 5.7 and Appendix 6. The US delegation led the opposition to a WHO treaty that would abolish most tobacco advertising and fight cigarette smuggling. The authors write that "the Bush administration did not even forward the treaty to the Senate for its consideration." Also see Thomas H. Maugh II; Times Medical Writer, *Worldwide Study Finds Big Shift in Causes of Death*, **Los Angeles Times**, September 16, 1996, Home Edition, p. 1. "... within 25 years smoking will become the single largest cause of death and disability in the world."

693. National Academy of Sciences, **Diet and Health: Implications for Reducing Chronic Disease Risk**, pp. 637-638, 1989.

694. *Tooth Decay is By-Product of World's Modern Living*, **Pensacola News** (Pensacola, Florida), 26th December, 1964.

695. *Decay Reductions*, **The Evening Post** (Wellington, New Zealand), 27th December, 1969.

696. **Wall Street Journal**, 12th October, 1984, quoted in *Fluoride the Aging Factor*, p. 112, 1993.

697. Robin McKie, *Infertility Crisis Sperm Counts Halved*, **The Guardian,** 29th July, 2017, https://www.theguardian.com/science/2017/jul/29/infertility-crisis-sperm-counts-halved.

698. Weston Price, *Op. Cit.*, p. 487.

699. Ryota Hosomi, Munehiro Yoshida & Kenji Fukunaga, *Seafood Consumption and Components for Health*, **Global Journal of Health Science**, Vol. 4, No. 3, 2012. Quoting pages 72 and 77. To support the statement, the authors cite Food and Agriculture Organization of the United Nations, World Health Organization. (2010). *Report of the Joint FAO/WHO Expert Consultation on the Risks and Benefits of Fish Consumption*. FAO Fisheries and Aquaculture Report No. 978.

700. P. Hujoel, *Dietary Carbohydrates and Dental-Systemic Diseases*, **Journal of Dental Research**, Vol. 88 No. 6, 490-502, 2009.

701. Marion Nestle, *Soda Politics: Taking on Big Soda (And Winning)*, p. 84, 2015.

702. Sigmund W. A. Franken, D.D.S., Bureau of Dental Health Education, *Treatment of Sensitive Cervices of Teeth*, **Official Bulletin of the National Dental Association**, Vol. 18, No. 1, pp. 156-163, January, 1931.

703. Franklin C. Bing, Ph.D., *Council on Dental Therapeutics: Diet and the Teeth*, **Official Bulletin of the National Dental Association**, Vol. 19, No. 10, October, pp. 1843-1850, 1932.

704. Craig D. Butler, *Nutritional Factors in Dental Development*, **Official Bulletin of the National Dental Association**, Vol. 25, No. 10, pp. 1599-1605, 1938.

705. Philip Jay, D.D.S., M.S., *The Role of sugar in the Etiology of Dental Caries*, **Journal of the American Dental Association**, Vol. 27, No. 3, pp. 393-396, March, 1940.

706. *The Michigan Workshop on the Evaluation of Dental Caries Control Technics*, **Journal of the American Dental Association**, pp. 3-22, Vol. 36, January, 1948.

707. A. Catharine Ross, Benjamin Caballero, Robert J. Cousins, Katherine L. Tucker, Thomas R. Ziegler editors, *Modern Nutrition in Health and Disease*, eleventh edition, p. 1380, 2014.

708. *Ibid.,* p. 766.

709. *Nourishing Traditions*, 2nd edition, by Sally Fallon and Mary G. Enig, Ph.D. (Second Edition published in 1999), p. 16 and 39. Also see Weston A. Price, D.D.S., M.S., F.A.C.D., *Control of Dental Caries and Some Associated Degenerative Processes through Reinforcement of the Diet with Special Activators*, **Journal of the American Dental Association**, pp. 1339-1369, 1932 and Dr. Price's book, *Nutrition and Physical Degeneration*.

710. https://jada.ada.org/action/doSearch?occurrences=all&searchText=maori&code=adaj-site&searchType=quick&searchScope=fullSite&journalCode=adaj. The study was T. G. Ludwig, M. R. Kean, and E. I. Pearce, *The Dental Condition of a Rural Maori Population*, **New Zealand Dental Journal**, Vol. 60, pp. 106-114, 1964, cited in J. David Erickson, DDS, PhD, *An Unusual Pattern of Caries Occurrence*, **Journal of the American Dental Association**, Vol. 103, pp. 30-31, July, 1981.

711. Hamilton B. G. Robinson, D.D.S., M.S., *The Metabolism of Minerals and Vitamins and the Effect of Systemic Conditions on Dental Caries*, **Journal of the American Dental Association**, Vol. 39, July, 1949.

712. https://www.ada.org/en/about-the-ada/ada-positions-policies-and-statements/policies-and-recommendations-on-diet-and-nutrition.

713. Timothy II, 3:7, *The Companion Bible*, E. W. Bullinger.

Chapter 6.4

714. *Chronic Fluorine Intoxication*, **Journal of the American Medical Association**, pp. 151-152, 18th September, 1943.

715. *Medical and Nutritional Aspects of Fluoridation.* Available in HD 125/299/4 H1 Box 1716. 14 ppm in Bauxite, Arkansas, discussed on p. 20. McCollum discussed on p.7.

716. **Journal of the American Dental Association**, Vol. 31, p. 1362, 1st October, 1944.

717. Margaret and H. V. Smith, **American Journal of Public Health**, Vol. 30, No. 9, pp. 1050-1052, September, 1940.

718. Anne-Lise Gotzche, *The Fluoride Question: Panacea or Poison*, 1975.

719. **New Scientist**, 29th May, 1975 and FL-82, Book reviews: *Fluoridation and Truth Decay* and *The Fluoride Question*, available from https://www.dentalwatch.org/usphs/index.html. Another review, dated 1st April 1975, is available, https://www.kirkusreviews.com/book-reviews/anne-lise-gotzsche/the-fluoride-question-panacea-or-poison/.

720. Maury Massler, D.D.D., M.S., and Isaac Schour, D.D.S., Ph.D., *Relation of endemic dental fluorosis to malnutrition*, **Journal of the American Dental Association**, Vol. 44, No. 2, pp. 156-165, 1952. Quoting pages 164 and 165. The study was "under the auspices of the Italian Medical Nutrition Mission. Massler was Professor of pedodontics, University of Illinois Dept. of Dentistry." This study was also cited by NZ fluoridation promoter Colonel Fuller (see Chapter 4.5).

721. Editorial, *Ten cent arguments against fluoridation*, **Journal of the American Dental Association**, Vol. 44, No. 5, pp. 563-564, 1952.

722. *A Study of the Anti-Scientific Attitude*, **Scientific American**, Vol. 192, No. 2, pp. 35-39, February, 1955.

723. *Report of the Commission of Inquiry on the Fluoridation of Public Water Supplies*, paragraph 244, 1957.

724. National Academy of Sciences, **Recommended Dietary Allowances**, p. 238, 1989.

725. WHO, *Fluorides*, Chapter 1.9, 2002.

726. *What are the Facts About Fluoridation?* **The News Journal** (Wilmington, Delaware), p. 4, 26th February, 1953. "… the third in a series of articles prepared by the Delaware State Dental Society prepared at the request of the journal…" The article claimed there was no such thing as artificial fluoridation. Fluorides were added by nature, the difference being that if added by people, they were certain to be harmless because the amount was controlled.

727. *Nutrition and Disease*, **Journal of Nutrition Education**, Vol. 12, No. 2, p. 65, 1980.

728. Doug Struck, *Fluoride spill may be cause of Annapolis death*, **Baltimore Sun**, p. 32, 28th November, 1979.

729. Anderson, Beard and Sorbey, *Fluoride Intoxication in a Dialysis Unit – Maryland*, **Morbidity Mortality Weekly Report**, Vol. 29, pp. 134-136, 1980.

730. *Annapolis is ruled liable in fluoride-death lawsuit, 30th September, **Baltimore Sun**, p. 26, 1980 and Fluoride-spill suit settled out of court, 3rd April, p. 33, 1983.*

731. *Fluoridation Facts: Answers to Criticisms Against Fluoridation*, published by the American Dental Association, paragraph 26, April, 1956.

732. Rugg-Gunn *et al.*, *Critique of the review of 'Water fluoridation for the prevention of dental caries' published by the Cochrane Collaboration in 2015*, **British Dental Journal**, Vol. 220, pp. 335-340, 8th April, 2016. As of July, 2018, this study is available online, freely.

733. NHS Centre for Reviews and Dissemination. *A systematic review of public water fluoridation*. York: NHS CRD, 2000, p. xi and xiv.

734. Letter from J. R. Grant, Chairman, Jaycee Fluoridation Education Committee, Hastings, to **Hawke's Bay Herald-Tribune**, 30th April 1954.

735. Eric J. Underwood, *Trace Elements in Human and Animal Nutrition*, 3rd Edition, p. 388, 1971.

736. P. F. Foote, President, Hawke's Bay Branch, N.Z. Dental Association, Hastings, *Fluoridation*, **Hawke's Bay Herald-Tribune**, 30th April, 1954. "There is no difference between natural and artificial fluoridation; the salt used is immaterial; only the fluorine ion is active. Authority: The report of the United Kingdom Mission on Fluoridation of Water Supplies in North America."

Deputation asks Council to Fluoridate Water, **Manawatu Daily Times** (New Zealand), 20th June, 1961. "Fluoride is no more artificial or unnatural than phosphorous [sic], copper, cobalt, zinc, molybdenum or selenium – other trace elements which are deficient in some of our farmlands."

8 S. D. Cities Add Fluoride to Water Supplies, **Argus-Leader** (Sioux Falls, South Dakota), 27th March, p. 28, 1963. "There is no difference. The fluoride ion found in the water is exactly the same whether placed in water by nature or by man."

Alan L. Proud (Secretary, Australian Dental Association, Victorian Branch) and A. W. Burton (Deputy Medical Secretary, Australian Medical Association, Victorian Branch) of *Benefits of Fluoridation*, **The Age** (Melbourne), p. 2, 15th April, 1964. "[fluoridation]… does not claim to treat an existing disease…" Compare this with the IOM statements about the 'nutrient-disease' relationship cited by Sirs Gluckman and Skegg's 2014 report. The letter in **The Age** continued: "Fluoridation is not the introduction of a foreign chemical to a water supply, but merely the adjustment to a desirable level of a trace element…"

The Fluoride Issue – Conclusion: Children, Adults Can Benefit, **The Sedalia Democrat** (Sedalia, Missouri), p. 1, 31st March, 1972.

Editorial… Fluoridation Foes Stir, **The Leavenworth Times** (Leavenworth, Kansas), p. 4, 16th May, 1974. "When all of the unfounded scare words are stripped away, fluoridation remains as nature's way to prevent tooth decay. Certainly we owe that much to our children."

Misusing the Term 'Artificial Fluoridation', **American Journal of Public Health**, Vol. 87, No. 7, pp. 1235-1236, July 1997.

Chapter 6.5

737. WHO, *Fluorides*, Chapter 10.1.2, 2002.

738. *Fluorides and Human Health*, World Health Organization Monograph Series, p. 194, 1970.

739. http://healthcentral.nz/opinion-ken-perrott-fluoridation-critics-tour-is-scaremongering-with-irrelevant-research/, 19th February, 2018.

740. 24th January, 2016, http://www.crescentcitytimes.com/beware-of-newly-formed-the-american-fluoridation-society/.

741. Gordon Burnside, *Guest Post: Ducks, bulls and a trace element*, Making Sense of Fluoride website, http://msof.nz/2015/02/ducks-bulls-and-a-trace-element/.

742. http://msof.nz/2015/04/dr-paul-connett-gets-schooled/, 26th April, 2015.

743. *Dentists Resent "False Statements" on Fluoridation*, date and newspaper unknown, but possibly **Hawke's Bay Herald-Tribune**, found in Health Department archives HD 125/299 H1 1635 (years 1954-1955). The article continues: "If this were not, how do the millions of people in the world who have been living on water containing one part per million of fluoride and more, have just the same health and longevity as other peoples living on a non-fluoride supply?"

744. E. V. McCollum and Cornelia Kennedy, *The Dietary Factors Operating in the Production of Polyneuritis*, **Journal of Biological Chemistry**, Vol. 24, pp. 491-502, 1916.

745. E. V. McCollum and Marguerite Davis, *The Necessity of Certain Lipins in the Diet During Growth*, **Journal of Biological Chemistry**, Vol. 15, pp. 167-175, 1913.

746. Xin Wen and Michael L. Paine, *Iron Deposition and Ferritin Heavy Chain (Fth) Localization in Rodent Teeth*, **BioMed Central Research Notes**, Vol. 6, p. 1, 2013.

747. Taina Pihlajaniemi, Raili Myllylä, Kari I. Kivirikko, *Prolyl 4-hydroxylase and its role in collagen synthesis*, **Journal of Hepatology**, Vol. 13, Supplement 3, pp. S2-S7, 1991.

748. S. S. Prime, D. G. MacDonald, H. W. Noble, J. S. Rennie, *Effect of prolonged iron deficiency on enamel pigmentation and tooth structure in rat incisors*, **Archives of Oral Biology**, Vol. 29, No. 11, pp. 905-909, 1984.

749. Mummery, *Microscopic Anatomy of the Teeth*, p. 47, 1919.

750. Michael J. Hubbard, B.D.S., Ph.D., *Guest Editorial. Molar hypomineralization: What is the US experience?* **Journal of the American Dental Association**, Vol. 149, Nol 5, pp. 329-330, 2018.

751. http://www.thed3group.org/the-basics-4.html. See their concerns about sugar here: http://www.thed3group.org/plaque-bugs.html.

752. http://www.thed3group.org/mission-origins.html.

753. Franklin García-Godoy, DDS, MS; M. John Hicks, DDS, MS, PhD, MD, *Maintaining the integrity of the enamel surface: The role of dental biofilm, saliva and preventive agents in enamel demineralization and remineralization*, **Journal of the American Dental Association**, Vol. 139 (Supplement), pp. 25-34, 2008.

754. *Modern Nutrition*, pp. 142, 221, 2014.

755. Te Ara, Carl Walrond, *Story: Salt*, https://teara.govt.nz/en/salt.

756. Venkatesh Babu NS, Purna B. Patel, *Oral health status of children suffering from thyroid disorders*, **Journal of Indian Society of Pedodontics and Preventive Denistry**, Vol. 34, No. 2, pp. 139-144, April-June, 2016.

757. Dr. Henry Pickerill, *The Prevention of Dental Caries and Oral Sepsis*, pp. 232 and 236, Chapter 13, 1914. Published by Bailliere, Tindall and Cox, London.

758. Lowe *et al.*, *Equine Hypothyroidism: The Long Term Effects of Thyroidectomy on Metabolism and Growth in Mares and Stallions*, **Cornell Veterinarian**, Vol. 64, pp. 276-294, 1973.

759. A. C. Acevedo, H. Chardin, J. F. Staub, D. Septier, M. Goldberg, *Effects of thyro-parathyroidectomy and parathyroidectomy upon dentinogenesis: Part I: Light microscopy*, **Connective Tissue Research**, Vol. 32, pp. 261-267, 1995.

452

760. A. C. Acevedo, H. Chardin, J. F. Staub, D. Septier, M. Goldberg, *Morphological study of amelogenesis in the rat lower incisor after thyro-parathyroidectomy, parathyroidectomy and thyroidectomy*, **Cell Tissue Research**, Vol. 283, No. 1, pp. 151-157, 1996.

761. Andres Pinto D.M.D., Michael Glick D.M.D., *Management of patients with thyroid disease: Oral health considerations*, **Journal of the American Dental Association**, Vol. 133, July, 2002.

762. Imran Farooq, Imran A. Moheet, Zonera Imran, and Umer Farooq, *A review of novel dental caries preventive material: Casein phosphopeptide–amorphous calcium phosphate (CPP–ACP) complex*, **King Saud University Journal of Dental Sciences**, Vol. 4, No. 2, pp. 47-51, July 2013.

763. National Academy of Sciences, **Guiding Principles for Developing DRIs Based on Chronic Disease**, p. 284, 2017.

764. Jonathan Forman, M.D. and A. Allen Londond, D.D.S., *A Statement on the Fluoridation of Public Water Supplies*, 20th February, 1957.

765. Steve Slott, D.D.S., comment left on 22nd September, 2013, https://www.theguardian.com/commentisfree/2013/sep/19/anti-fluoride-science-australia#comment-27123738. Michael Vagg, *Anti-fluoride activists should put their tinfoil hat theories to rest*, **The Guardian**, 19th September, 2013.

766. Supreme Court Decisions 2018, http://www.courtsofnz.govt.nz/the-courts/supreme-court/judgments-supreme.

767. New Zealand Environmental Protection Authority, *Annual Report for the year ended 30th June*, Report from the Chair, p. 5, 2017.

768. https://www.tvnz.co.nz/shows/q-and-a/episodes/s2018-e16.

769. http://www.courtsofnz.govt.nz/cases/new-health-new-zealand-incorporated-v-south-taranaki-district-council-2/@@images/fileMediaNotes?r=240.841120575.

770. http://www.courtsofnz.govt.nz/cases/new-health-new-zealand-incorporated-v-south-taranaki-district-council-1/@@images/fileDecision?r=275.125761855.

771. Jim Hefford, *Fluoride Debate*, **The Listener**, 3rd August, 2013.

772. Olga Khazan, *Why Are So Many Americans Dying Young?* **The Atlantic**, 13th December, 2016.

773. https://www.healthsystemtracker.org/chart-collection/u-s-life-expectancy-compare-countries/#item-disparity-life-expectancy-u-s-comparable-countries-continues-older-ages.

774. Laura Dwyer-Lindgren, MPH; Amelia Bertozzi-Villa, MPH; Rebecca W. Stubbs, BA; *et al., Inequalities in Life Expectancy Among US Counties, 1980 to 2014: Temporal Trends and Key Drivers*, **Journal of the American Medical Association**, July, 2017.

775. *"Depression: let's talk" says WHO, as depression tops list of causes of ill health*, June 2, 2018. http://www.who.int/news-room/headlines/30-03-2017--depression-let-s-talk-says-who-as-depression-tops-list-of-causes-of-ill-health.

776. Elizabeth Fones-Wolf, *Selling Free Enterprise*, 1994.

777. J. D. Baxter, *Is Government Having a Chilling Effect on Business's Right to Speak?* Chilton's **Iron Age**, pp. 85-110, 23rd October, 1978.

778. Government-University-Industry Research Roundtable; Policy and Global Affairs; National Academies of Sciences, Engineering, and Medicine, National Academy of Sciences, *Examining the Mistrust of Science: Proceedings of a Workshop–in Brief*, 2017. Available from http://nap.edu/24819.

779. Michael Glick, D.M.D.; H. Austin Booth, M.A., M.I.S., *Conspiracy Ideation: A public health scourge?* **Journal of the American Dental Association**, Vol. 145, No. 5, pp. 798-799, 2014. "Conspiracy theories are easy to spread and tough to eradicate. How do we prevent conspiratorial thinking from taking hold? As oral health care professionals, how do we (or should we) engage conspiracy thinkers whose health may be at risk or who are putting the health of others at risk?"

780. *We Were Wrong about Paleo Pete*, **Dominion Post** (Wellington, New Zealand), 15th May, 2018.

Appendix 1. Media Articles from Chapter 5.1

Some articles/letters may fit into more than one category.

Australian Media articles

Claims of Essentiality:

Evening News (Sydney, NSW), Saturday 10 September 1892, p2 *"Tooth Culture"*,

Mercury (Hobart, Tas.), Tuesday 17 February 1953, p3 (This article also appeared in **Advocate** (Burnie, Tas.), Tuesday 17 February 1953, p3),

Northern Champion (Taree, NSW), Friday 3 July 1953, p1 (Mr. Haddan is quoted as making the same statements "… one of the essential elements for building decay-resistant teeth…" in **Daily Examiner** (Grafton, NSW), Thursday 9 July 1953, p6 "Decay-Resistant Teeth"),

Cairns Post (Qld. : 1909 - 1954), Tuesday 28 July 1953, page 5,

Mercury (Hobart, Tas.), Wednesday 23 September 1953, p25,

Examiner (Launceston, Tas.), Wednesday 23 September 1953, page 5,

Also in **Advocate** (Burnie, Tas.), Thursday 24 September 1953, p15,

Canberra Times (ACT), Saturday 21 September 1957, p8,

Australian Women's Weekly, Wednesday 4 September 1963, p10,

Canberra Times (ACT), Friday 24 July 1964, p3 "Fluoride need 'urgent'",

Beverley Times (WA), Friday 15 April 1966, p7 "Fluoride is Favoured",

Canberra Times (ACT), Saturday 31 August 1968, page 7 *"FLUORIDE AN 'ESSENTIAL' IN BALANCED DIET"*,

Canberra Times (ACT), Thursday 28 September 1989, page 8,

"Minerals essential in minute amounts" **Canberra Times** (ACT), Wednesday 8 December 1993, p19,

"Every drop you drink" by Woffinden, Bob. **Sydney Morning Herald** (Sydney, N.S.W) 16 August 1997 p42,

Teeth that Gleam. **Australia's Parents.** 01/04/2000, Issue 115, p58,

NEW PRODUCTS. **Australian Parents.** 01/06/2000, Issue 116, p28, FILTERED WATER THE EASY WAY (Advertisement),

Fynes-Clinton, Jane. **Northern Miner** [Charters Towers, Qld] 07 Aug 2012: 13,

Many missing out on fluoride benefits, **Newcastle Herald, The** (includes the **Central Coast Herald**). 30/01/2004,

Dehydration warning as the heat continues, **Gold Coast Bulletin, The.** 13/03/2004,

Putting bite on decay; **GP Herald** [Newcastle, N.S.W] 06/07/2004 p30, by Dr Heather Stephenson,

Qld: State should butt out of fluoride issue: LGA By: Alex Murdoch. AAP **Australian National News Wire.** 30/08/2004 (uncertain – "essential for strengthening and protecting),

DENTAL HEALTH ADVERTISING FEATURE *Dangers with sports drinks:* [1 Edition], **Townsville Bulletin** [Townsville, Qld] 12 Aug 2005: p17. Bottled water,

Turkish Delights, **Australian Table,** 01/06/2006, Vol. 7, Issue 10, p. 56,

Aged three and in need of dentures: [1 State Edition] Williams, Matt. **The Advertiser** [Adelaide, S. Aust] 20 July 2006: 24,

Daily Telegraph, The (Sydney), 01/08/2006 p37 *"Teens face growing risks - A SPECIAL ADVERTISING REPORT - BE YOUR OWN BOSS"*,

Dentists shocked at rise in tooth decay in children, **The Canberra Times** [Canberra, A.C.T] 05 Aug 2006: B4,

PARENTHOOD: [M Edition] Fine, Duncan. Sunday Telegraph [Surry Hills, N.S.W] 20 Aug 2006: 31,

Bottled water a dental disaster By: Verity Edwards. **Australian, The.** 02/08/2006 (This claim of essentiality also appeared in: **Advertiser, The** (Adelaide). 02/08/2006 p. 15, *"Dentists' warning as rot sets in"* By: XANTHE KLEINIG),

Drink warning on teeth, **Geelong News,** 02/08/2006.

Section: Advertising feature, pg. 029, *Drinks blamed for rise in decay* By: GILL VOWLES. **Sunday Tasmanian** (Hobart). 22/07/2007 p13,

Tap into benefits of fluoride By: GR. **Newcastle Herald, The** (includes the Central Coast Herald). 20/09/2007, WHAT'S NEW Courier Mail, The (Brisbane). 07/02/2007 (Advertisement),

Essential public health initiative: [1 Edition] **The Cairns Post** [Cairns, Qld] 10 Dec 2007: 13,

What's cooking? **Australian House & Garden.** 01/02/2008, Issue 2 p168 (Advertisement),

Did you know? **Rouse Hill Times.** 13.05.2009, p. 25,

Kangaroo Valley to get fluoridated water, Anonymous. **ABC Regional News** [Sydney] 08 Sep 2009.

Mythbusters --- mX Active MX Sydney. 11.10.2010, p23,

Your HANDY HINTS. **Real Living**. 01/04/2011, Issue 64, p39 (Advertisement),
Where's the fluoride? Residents find out after seven months, By: Ami Humpage. **Melton Moorabool Leader**. 03.01.2012, p. 1,
Fluoride is 'essential' **Ayr Advocate**. 18.01.2013, p6,
Top doctor in fluoride town water campaign. By Janelle Miles. **Courier Mail, The** (Brisbane), 15.01.2013, p9,
LIVERPOOL Plains Shire Council will delay discussion, Tyson, Ross. **The Northern Daily Leader** [Tamworth, N.S.W] 19 Oct 2013: 13,
Fluoride debate back on agenda [Cairns Edition] Forbes, Scott **The Cairns Post** [Cairns, Qld] 26 Feb 2015: 9.

Likened to Nutrients Definitely Essential:

Canberra Times (ACT), Wednesday 4 March 1964, p6 *"Fluoride 'Not Dangerous'"*,
"A terrible tale of teething troubles in Tasmania" By Crane, Wilfred. **Canberra Times** (ACT), Sunday 29 October 1989, p7,
"What's wrong with nutrition labeling?" (cover story) By: Hunter, Beatrice Trum. **Consumers' Research Magazine**, 01 February 1993, Vol. 76 Issue 2, p10,
Donna Aston's Guide to Stayin' Alive: [1 - FIRST Edition], Curtis, Maree, **Sunday Herald - Sun** [Melbourne, Vic] 03 Mar 2002: Z.24,
Courier Mail, The (Brisbane). 29/05/2003 p17 *"Give water extra bite"* By: Jane Fynes-Clinton,
Fluoride 'risk' on council's agenda By: GLENN ROBERTS. **Northern Times** (Brisbane). 07.12.2012, p3,
Untitled, **NewsMail**. 12/01/2013 (Dr Foley's statement here could be taken to mean fluoride is 'highly beneficial' instead of essential. He has not specified which, so it stands to reason some uninformed readers will incorrectly conclude fluoride is essential),
Vital ingredients, **Geelong Advertiser** [Geelong, Vic] 27 Sep 2016: 27. **Tharunka** (Kensington, NSW), Friday 27 September 1963, p6,
"Our water should be Fluoridated", **Vegetarian Times**. 01/01/1998, Issue 245, p66,
"Navigating the labyrinth: 30 things you need to know about..." By: Challem, Jack; Ciuccoli, Stephen.

Claims of Deficiency:

Canberra Times (ACT), Saturday 31 August 1968, page 7 *"FLUORIDE AN 'ESSENTIAL' IN BALANCED DIET"* (Professor Elsdon Storey),
Beverley Times (WA), Friday 23 May 1969, p4 *"Australians have the worst teeth in the world"*,
Osteoporosis. By: Sinclair, Mary. **Good Medicine** (Australian Consolidated Press). 01/11/2004, p1.

Claim of Mass Medication Countered by Claims of Nutritional Likeness:

Untitled, **NewsMail**. 12/01/2013 (likened to folic acid in bread).
There were nine articles in Australian media claiming fluorine non-essential, all nine were discussing, or representative of, people opposed to CWF.

Australian Letters to Editors

Claims of Essentiality:

Letters to the Editor, **Canberra Times** (ACT), Monday 2 October 1989, p8.
The Gold Coast Bulletin (Southport, Qld) 13 Dec 2004, p39.
The Gold Coast Bulletin (Southport, Qld) 15 Dec 2004, p32.
Celebs save money, plastic, **Sunday Herald Sun** (Melbourne). 09 March 2008
Opinion **Noosa Journal**. 05 March 2009, p28
The Advocate (Coffs Harbour, Qld) 24 July 2013, p13, *Fluoride Findings* (cited 2007 NAS),
Herbert, Judy. **Advocate** (Burnie, Tas) 12 July, 2014 p24, *Fluoride Levels*,
Untitled, **Melton Moorabool Leader**, 17 January, 2012, p18.

Likened to Nutrients Definitely Essential:

Canberra Times (ACT), Friday 24 April 1964, p. 2, *"8 Major Questions"*,
Central Coast Express Advocate (Gosford, N.S.W) 09 Jan 2008, p48,
The Cairns Post (Cairns, Qld) 02 Feb 2013, p25.

Claims of Deficiency:

Sun (Sydney, NSW), Monday 14 December 1953, p. 16 Letters to the Editor, *"Fluorine and Dental Decay"* (this also appeared in the **Newcastle Sun** (NSW), Monday 4 January 1954, p8 "'Sun' Letter Box"),
Canberra Times (ACT), Friday 24 April 1964, page 2
I did not find any examples of the claim of mass medication countered by fluorine's essentiality in Australian letters to editors. Twelve letters opposed fluoridation, all twelve claimed the element non-essential.

New Zealand Media Articles 1892-1992

I believe that in 1892 British researchers claimed fluorine deficiency a possibility; this was in the American media a couple of times also. The two earliest articles mentioned here are shown mainly for interest; I don't believe they're all that relevant to today's work.

Claims of Essentiality:

Otago Witness, 10th November 1892, p44, *"Tooth Culture"*,
Otago Witness, 5th January 1893, p44, *"Science Notes"*,
29th October, 1955, *WHO Authority Champions Fluoridation*, **The Evening Post**, (Dr. John Knutson),
16th September, 1957, **Auckland Star**, *Auckland Fluoridation is "Necessary and Feasible"* (headline gives the impression of essentiality),
1959, March 3rd *Fluoridation Now Matter for State*, **The Evening Post**, ("necessary medical benefit"),
21st June, 1961, *Fluoridation of Water Supply*, **Manawatu Daily Times**,
23rd May, 1962, *Value Proved of Fluoridation in Hutt Valley*, **The Evening Post** (last paragraph),
What Authorities Declare on Fluoridation of Water, **Waikato Times**, 21st March, 1964 (trace element),
Fluoridation Benefits Older Folk, 21st February, 1967, **The Evening Post** (Dr. Fredrick Stare),
Fluoridation of Water Still Safest Measure – Expert, by Paul Gorman, **Otago Daily Times**, 18th August, 1990 (Jocelyn Hampton, director of dietetic services, Waikato Health Board; "the importance of fluorine as a nutrient which is normally present in the diet... is an approach which is rarely considered in the news media.")

Likened to Nutrients Definitely Essential:

Doctor's Support for Water Fluoridation, **Hawke's Bay Herald-Tribune**, 13th March, 1954 (implied iodine),
Nutritionist Voices Support for Water Fluoridation, 29th November,1956, **Daily Telegraph** (Dr. Muriel Bell),

Claims of Deficiency:

Fluoridation Experiment "Purely Local Matter" – Minister Tells of Overwhelming Support of Authorities, **Hawke's Bay Herald-Tribune**, 8th July, 1954,
7th September, 1956, *Let's Get on with Fluoridation*, **The Dominion**,
17th April, 1957, **The Evening Post**,
28th January, 1958, *Hutt to Have Fluoridation*, **The Evening Post** ,(mentions 1957 Commission of Inquiry),
23rd May, 1958, U.S. Researcher Here to Solve Caries Mystery, **The Evening Post**, (Captain F. L. Losee),
17th September, 1958, *Fluoridation Benefits Apparent in Teeth of Children*, **The Evening Post**,
21st September, 1963, *Medical Memo: Some Simple Facts on Fluoridation*, **The Evening Post**,
1964, 14th July, **Taupo Times**, *Answers to Some Questions Asked about Fluoride*,
City and Hutt Fluoride Supply Ample, **The Evening Post**, 8th April, 1965, (Suggestive of deficiency – "no need to worry about children getting sufficient fluoride")
31st March, 1965, *Fluoride Will be Added to City Water Tomorrow*, **The Evening Post**,
Dentists Resent "False Statements" on Fluoridation, Date and newspaper unknown, but possibly **Hawke's Bay Herald-Tribune**, found in Health Department archives HD 125/299 H1 1635 (years 1954-5).

Claim of Mass Medication Countered by Claims of Nutritional Likeness:

Editorial in **The Press**, Christchurch, Monday, December 15th, 1958 (mentions 1957 Commiss. of Inquiry);
Anti-Fluoridation Attitude Draws Comment, 27th August, 1959, **The Evening Post**, (Assistant Director of the Health Department's dental hygiene division, Mr. J. Francon Williams at the State Dental Nurses' Institute Conference);
20th June, 1961, **Manawatu Daily Times**, *Deputation asks Council to fluoridate water – Half city population has tooth decay, says dentist* ("natural trace element", "vital nutrient" say Jaycee);
23rd July, 1964, *Anti-Fluoride Questions and Answers Rebutted by Ex-World Health Officer*, **Taupo Times** (Dr. F. Bruce Rice);

Rotorua Post, 26th August, 1965, *Fluoridation Urged* ("normal nutrient required… not a drug").

New Zealand Media Articles 1993-2017

Claims of Essentiality:

Dentist puts bite on fluoride bashers, by McLean, Robyn, **Taranaki Daily News**. 01/08/2000, p4,
A chance to win, **Southland Times, The**, 05/09/2009, pC4 (Advertisement),
GIVEAWAY **Dominion Post, The**, 01/10/2009, p. D3 (Advertisement),
Win a Brita health pack, Anonymous, **Bay of Plenty Times** (Tauranga) 6th October, 2009, p. A.4 (Advertisement),
New Zealand Doctor, 9th March, 2011, p. 27, *Enhanced water too sweet a treat*, by Julia Sekula,
Garth George, *Fluoride addition an essential step*, **Bay of Plenty Times** (Tauranga) 17th March, 2012, p. A17,
Time to revise fluoride theories? **Manawatu Standard** (Palmerston North) 25th June, 2013, p. 7,
Fluoridation a `nightmare', **The Daily Post** (Rotorua) 8th July, 2013, p. A6,
Put the passion aside and let the fluoride flow, say top scientists, by Michael, Daly, **Dominion Post, The**, 23/08/2014, p. A5,
Fluoride critics slam law 'rush', by Edmonds, Elesha, **Sunday Star - Times** (Wellington) 4th January, 2015, p. A6,
Fluoride essential, **Timaru Herald, The**, 27/04/2016, p. 6,
What's wrong with nutrition labeling? (cover story), by Hunter, Beatrice Trum, **Consumers' Research Magazine**, 01/02/1993, Vol. 76, Issue 2, pp. 10-15,
Why We Need Fluoride, **Dominion Post**, Wednesday, June 7, 2017, P. A10.

Claims of Deficiency:

What's the matter with milk, by Weiss, Rick, **Health** (Time Inc. Health) 01/01/1993, Vol. 7, Issue 1, p18,
How to raise a good eater, by Colino, Stacey, **Redbook**, 01/07/2002, Vol. 199, Issue 1, p152 (implied).

New Zealand Letters to Editors 1892-1992

(This section is very small because old NZ newspapers have not been digitised in a manner that allows for much searching.)

Claims of Essentiality:

27th November, 1962, **The Evening Post**.

Claims of Deficiency:

30th April, 1954, **Hawke's Bay Herald-Tribune** (found in HD 125/299/1 H1 Box 1634, year 1954).
24th September, 1990, Unknown Christchurch paper found in archive MS-Papers-6670-57 available at the National Library in Wellington (water referred to as deficient).

Claim of Mass Medication Countered by Claims of Nutritional Likeness:

19th February, 1965, **East Harbour Sun**.

New Zealand Letters to Editors 1993-2016

Claims of Essentiality:

"*Fluoridated water*", **Nelson Mail, The**, 29/04/1999, p9,
Fluoride essential, [2 Edition] **The Press** [Christchurch] 7th Sep, 2004, A; 8,
Timaru Herald, The. 19/05/2006, p4,
Timaru Herald, The. 13/06/2006, p14,
Timaru Herald, The. 05/09/2006, p4,
Waikato Times. 27/06/2009, pE6,
Taranaki Daily News. 05/02/2015, p10,
Turning a blind eye. **Herald on Sunday** [Auckland] 13 Mar 2011: A.50.

Likened to Nutrients Definitely Essential:

Timaru Herald, The. 17/10/2005, p4,

Letters: [2 Edition] *Ingesting fluoridated water* and *Rabid Fanatics*, **Waikato Times** (Hamilton) 08 Jan 2005: A; 10.
Timaru Herald, The. 13/09/2006, p4,
Essential elements, **Waikato Times** (Hamilton) 23 Apr 2011: A.14,
Waikato Times. 08/11/2012, p16,
"*Wairoa Dosage levels key*", **Hawkes Bay Today**. 26/04/2014
One man's poison . . . **The Nelson Mail** [Nelson] 28 July 2014: 9,
Flouridation, **Timaru Herald** [Timaru] 09 Apr 2016: 7 (note spelling mistake).

Claims of Deficiency:

Fluoride beneficial: [2 Edition] **The Press** [Christchurch] 26 Aug 2004: A; 8,
"*Beneficial contamination*" **Dominion Post, The** 23/08/2001, p6.

Claim of Mass Medication Countered by Claims of Nutritional Likeness:

Timaru Herald, 30 May 2006: 4,
Your View, **Wanganui Chronicle**, 29 Oct 2016: A.6,
Dominion Post, The. 19/09/2013, pA10,

Of twenty-three letters to editors claiming fluorine non-essential, all were critical of Community Water Fluoridation.

Appendix 2. Notes on Letters and Articles Defining "Essential"

This appendix deals with the inclusion of statements in the table from Chapter 5.1

When searching the two databases, *Trove* and the National Library, I used *fluoride* instead of *fluorine* because this is a more colloquially used form, it is more frequently used in contemporary news. I found in experiments and in media people used the N decades ago while the D is used much more nowadays. So there is a possibility I may have missed a few articles in recent times where the N was used.

In both of these searches I used "fluorid* essential" as a search term. The asterisk allows for differing endings of the word, this broadened the search to include "fluoridation" "fluoride" "fluoridisation" (very uncommon) and any other stragglers.

People phrase things differently – there is definitely a blurry line between a statement like "water fluoridation is essential for oral health" and "fluorine is an essential nutrient."

There are a few statements with ambiguity: does "fluoride treatments are essential" mean that fluorine/fluoride is an essential nutrient?

It does if they're *correcting a deficiency* but it does not if they're simply *adding protection*.

Consider this statement:

"… he believed adding fluoride to town drinking water supplies was essential to promoting healthy teeth…"

It isn't *necessarily* saying that fluoride is an essential nutrient, but because it could be taken to imply nutritional essentiality, I have included it (*LIVERPOOL Plains Shire Council will delay discussion*, Tyson, Ross. **The Northern Daily Leader** [Tamworth, N.S.W] 19 Oct 2013: 13).

Another:

"Given the NSW Health Department's position that fluoride is essential in fighting tooth decay, the decision was always going to be in the affirmative."

Is "fighting tooth decay" the same as correcting a nutritional deficiency? I have not included this one in my sample (*Thirty years on…* below).

This sort of nit-picking is extremely tiring to me, especially coupled with the often abusive nature and frequent arrogance of the articles and letters, so I think a different person would achieve slightly different numbers.

Of the total number of Australian and New Zealand media articles used, only six (listed below) were "close but no cigar." As I say, you may think differently.

Australia

The Courier - Mail (Brisbane, Qld) 26 July 2004, p10.

Fluoride debate still simmering: Water Debate, Anonymous. **The Observer** [Gladstone, Qld] 22 Oct 2009: 22. ("Fluoride treatments essential.")

Disappointment over closure, **Port Lincoln Times** [Port Lincoln, S. Aust], 29 Dec 2011: p6.

Thirty years on, town gets fluoride, Carswell, Andrew. **Sunday Telegraph** [Surry Hills, N.S.W] 09 Feb 2014: 41. ("FINALLY, the good folk of Lismore, home of the worst childhood tooth decay in the state, have something to smile about: their smiles. A healthy dose of fluoride is coming their way and no protester is going to stand in the way.")

LETTERBOX, **The Gold Coast Bulletin** (Southport, Qld) 11 Mar 2013, p37.

New Zealand

Timaru Herald, The. 04/03/2016, p5.

"Our world renowned late Sir John Walsh, dean of the school from 1946 to 1971, built the school's reputation, advocated of stable fluoride water supply, including fluoride medication, as completely safe, economic, and an essential health measure, giving direct improvement for life to our whole digestive system."

No Social Media

There is often little focus in social media if a topic is introduced. I have often seen the comments and responses rail further away from the initial topic – one of the professors from Victoria University advised students "read the exam question twice". If an initial post could be likened to an exam question, I think often people don't read it once. The exclusion of social media in this investigation should not be considered a criticism of the medium, but something based more on practicality.

Appendix 3. Letter from H. W. Carter Regarding Political Motives of Antifluoridationists

The letter in question was written by H. W. Carter, the Director at the Division of Public Hygiene to The Medical Officer of Health in Palmerston North. It was dated 2nd August, 1954. It described how the "political motives of those opposing fluoridation in Hastings" in the early 1950s were thought to warrant investigation by the New Zealand Police due to involvement by an "outside organization" that "joined in the controversy for no apparent reason".

Carter claimed that the Commissioner of Police stated that enquiries "do not suggest that opposition has been engineered by Communist Party members or that the Communist Party is interested in the result of the campaign."

John Colquhoun reproduced this letter in his 1987 Ph.D. thesis. The letter ended with the sentence

"The fact that enquiry was made, and its result, should of course be kept confidential."

I've never seen it mentioned outside this thesis and the **Dominion Sunday Times** article (cited in Chapter 5.5). I have no idea how the media obtained it.

Appendix 4. Fluoride Pollution Lawsuits

(This appendix contains its own reference section.)
In August of 1950, twenty farmers brought a $3,690,000 damage action suit against Reynolds Metals. This was one of

"… several other suits… pending against ALCOA and the Reynolds Metals Corporation plants at Troutdale and Longview."
[1]

Reynolds leased the plant in 1946, giving $300,000 to settle fluoride damages [2]. ALCOA operated the plant until the end of WWII. While ALCOA ran the plant, about $150,000 was paid to property owners near the plant in damages. A farmer named Paul Martin of Troutdale erected a billboard on his property criticizing Reynolds "for killing his dairy cattle".
Reynolds sued him. Professor Rodgers wrote:

"… his own damage suit against Reynolds was met by a phalanx of top attorneys from the likes of Harvey Aluminum, Alcoa, Georgia Pacific, Wyerhaeuser, and the Association of Oregon Industries." [3]

Rodgers claims Martin's widow sold out to Reynolds:

"… technology got its breathing room. While some succeed by confronting a legal system that puts a premium on high-priced lawyers, understanding experts and long waits, many do not."

In 1955, Reynolds was forced to pay Paul and Verla Martin $38,823. Toxicologist Dr. Robert A. Kehoe and air pollution expert Dr. Willard Machle testified on behalf of Reynolds, claiming that based upon their examinations, none of the plaintiffs had suffered from ingestion of fluorides.

In 1970, the Troutdale plant had 560 pots in 8 rooms producing about 100,000 tons of aluminium yearly, with fluorides being the primary contaminants. Around 1945, 7,000 pounds per day were emitted, reduced to around 3,000 by installing a spray system. The Department of Health, Education and Welfare (DHEW) claimed this was reduced to about 700 lbs/day by 1953 due to hood installations that gave a partial cover to individual pots and water towers. In the DHEW report for the U.S. Congress, we read:

> "From 1948 to 1957, an associate professor of horticulture at Oregon State University concluded that the fluoride effects were limited to the gladiolus and to pasture land. In samples of gladiolus leaves obtained in September and October 1953, he found fluoride contents of 0.01-0.114 mg/g (10-114 ppm). Grasses contained as high as 1 mg/g (1,000 ppm) and averaged above 0.03 mg/g (30 ppm)." [2]

The citation given is a letter from O. C. Compton, to the Oregon State Air Pollution Authority, 5th October, 1953 and 11th May, 1957. There is no mention of who funded his work. Rodgers claims that when questioned in a 1967 court case, Dr. Compton admitted that Harvey Aluminum had contributed financially to his work, but did not say how much. The counsel asked "give me an approximation then", to which Compton replied "I wouldn't even mention a figure" [3].

Not everybody had access to research on fluorides. In 1967 a lawyer representing Japanese-American vegetable growers wrote to Washington for help. His client was up against Harvey. The scientist recommended by the State refused to "knowingly engage our efforts for one party in a legal dispute…"

In 1968, he was rebuffed again, with the claim that surveillance of fluoride pollution would require "meteorologists, fluoride specialists, bio-chemists, agriculture and animal scientists with adequate field laboratories as well as back-up laboratories…" the figure $75,000 was suggested [4].

Rodgers was also rebuffed when he wrote to J. C. Dale of the Aluminum Association to obtain a study that was "… completed on schedule but not released. Our reason for withholding this is due to the fact that in our view the study was incomplete. We have since provided additional funds to Battelle Memorial Institute…"

Regarding the funding of experiments, Rodgers writes of a "boiler-plate clause" in a contract belonging to Kaiser regarding "Measurement of Particle Size Distribution at Tacoma Works of Kaiser Aluminum":

> "plans or data prepared by the researcher or disclosed to him are 'the property of the owner.'" [5]

The researcher is obliged to "limit access" only to Kaiser employees directly involved with the work.

Judge Learned Hand "condemned" ALCOA in 1945 as a monopolist of the aluminum ingot market [6]. In the 1940s Reynolds and Kaiser were jealous of ALCOA, charging that the company had purposefully built "mammoth" plants in remote areas for the purpose of rendering their competitors unnecessary.

After WWII, the US government disbanded many of these plants, allowing Reynolds and Kaiser to join the aluminium market with greater presence [7]. Rodgers writes:

> "The big three have learned to live together, working through international consortiums, joint ventures and sometimes plain old conspiracies." [3]

In 1940, 2.5% of electricity produced in the USA went to the aluminium industry, by 1980 it was closer to 5%. Rodgers wrote of the aluminium industry's penchant for favourable tax rates and subsidies going well into the millions, as well as plant sites. The "Intalco tax law" cost taxpayers $25 million, but brought no new industry into the state [8]. A tax write-off for Harvey Aluminum was 85% of $65 million.

The democratic mentality is blatantly obvious in the setup of plants, shown by Rodgers' work. In the 1960s, Northwest Aluminum obtained a long-range power commitment from the Bonneville Power Administration (BPA), "without the knowledge or consent of the affected states," Governor Dan Evans claimed [9].

A decade later, Northwest had sold out to American Metal Climax, which was planning another site at Warrenton, Oregon; Rodgers writes of the "quiet consummation" that occurred between the firm and BPA. Elimination of uncertainties is a powerful tool in business. BPA and its clientele "rewrote" a "dangerous" anti-pollution clause that had been included in its contracts for many years. The clause, titled "Conservation of Natural Resources" stated that BPA was "not obligated to deliver power" to a client that produced wastes which may destroy fish, aquatic life, pollute the Columbia River, or affect the scenic beauty of the area.

According to Rodgers, BPA was not about to cause concern for its customers by invoking such a law, but industry no doubt feared the possibility BPA may be swayed by the public and, as Rodgers put it, "unacceptable risks for the modern corporation are eliminated; the law conforms to the technology." [3]

The law change had its effect. Intalco Aluminum Co. owned one of the biggest plants in the world. Ian MacGregor, president of American Metal Climax and would-be member of the National Industrial Pollution Control Council, claimed Intalco had "spared no expense" with regard to pollution control. A primary treatment system installation was delayed for five years, around the time water quality was found to face challenges for about four miles around the plant. The company discharged about 800 pounds of hydrogen fluoride daily, and around 15,000 pounds of "particulates".

Complaints to BPA from a Department of the Interior Regional Representative, and the Department's Bureau of Sports Fisheries occurred when Intalco asked for a contract granting more electricity. BPA's administrator, H. R. Richmond, never got the second letter, and didn't care about the first. Intalco won its contract. When Richmond was brought to a House subcommittee in December of 1971 to justify this, he explained:

"We were not informed [by State agencies] of any official complaint having been received relative to Intalco's operations."

Rodgers writes that Richmond had ignored

"Extensive, documented damage, a dozen pending lawsuits, a notorious record of intransigency, files full of angry correspondence..." [3]

In October of 1950, the **Daily Chronicle** (Washington) reported that

"... a new damage suit of $3,000,000 was filed in federal court here yesterday against ALCOA by 48 residents of Sauvies Island in the Columbia River." [10]

The article also said that the William Fraser family, who had sought $900,000 earlier that year, had been granted "only a part of one of 11 damage counts."

These three articles quoted here did not mention fluorides, yet it can be safely assumed fluorides were one of the issues, as the next article will show. Eventually Fraser filed suit against the Vancouver, Washington plant again, for $200,000 in 1952. This was reported in the **Daily Capital Journal** (Salem, Oregon) [11]. His $900,000 suit had yielded only $60,000, but with the provision that he could

"seek additional damages in the same suit if the situation was not corrected."

"The court agreed with Fraser that the company was at fault in dumping from 1,000 to 7,000 pounds of fluorides per month in the Columbia river. The fluorides contaminated the grass and forage and resulted in injury to the internal organs and death [of cattle owned by Fraser]..."

This article claimed that during the previous Fraser suit (in 1950), ALCOA had corrected the situation, telling the court

"it had made many grants to research groups to find a cure."

There was no detail on this. Fraser claimed his farm had been "irreparably damaged." In 1953, Chancellor Byrne of Oregon University told the **Albany Democrat-Herald** of a $30,000 research grant from ALCOA to Oregon State College

"to continue a study of the effect of fluorides from the Vancouver, Washington, Alcoa plant on the animal and plant life of nearby Sauvies Island." [12]

According to one article ALCOA had spent $33,000,000 on a government-built plant in Chicago. Aluminium was necessary for production of planes and much other military hardware during WWII. The US government had spent over $20,000,000 to build four plants to produce aluminium from various clays to end American dependence on British bauxite, the supply of which they believed could be cut off by enemy submarines. ALCOA had "a virtual monopoly" on the British bauxite, as well as on the domestic source. One article alleges that I. W. Wilson, Vice President of Alcoa at the time, also the Chairman of the Committee on Aluminum Production of the Aluminum and Magnesium Advisory Committee of the Army-Navy Munitions Board, had sold three of these four government/military-owned plants to other corporations, very quickly. None of these buyers intended to pursue aluminium manufacture or production, thus allowing Alcoa to keep its strong position in the market.

The "opponents of this liquidation program" wrote Ray Tucker in the Ohio **Times Recorder**, would

"try to make the point that Mr. Wilson was chiefly responsible for the hurried disposition of prospective Alcoa competitors' plants to companies which do not intend to make aluminum. They will also contend that the munitions board, as well as the R.F.C.[183] as reorganized, serves private rather than national interests." [13]

It seems techniques to control fluoride pollution improved over time as one would expect; in 1963 Harvey Aluminum reported new control equipment had reduced emissions by half [14].

---

[183] Reconstruction Finance Corporation, an agency of the U.S. government that helped banks, and loaned to businesses large and small, during and after the Great Depression.

The Secretary of the Pico County Water District charged that the Los Angeles Regional Water Quality Control Board was "dominated six to one by pollution interests." [15]

Professor William Rodgers quotes a letter from the Chairman of the Board at Anaconda Aluminum to the Assistant to the President asking for "… any help you can give…" regarding EPA regulations for sulphuric acid pollution. Rodgers claims that of the worst air polluters in the USA, the "first half-dozen spots" would probably go to copper smelters.

Rodgers' work on the copper industry is quite amazing regarding the amount of influence the industry had. Not surprisingly, we find ALCOA's presence here too – they too wanted to stop a law that would demand reductions of sulfur dioxide emissions by 90%. The Mining and Non-Ferrous Metals Sub-Council of the National Industrial Pollution Control Council (NIPCC), was in business with the Department of Commerce in 1970, "to give top executives a direct pipeline to the administration on pollution control issues."

The sub-council chairman was Frank Milliken, Chairman of the Board for Kennecott. Other members included the executives of ASARCO, Lone Star Cement Corporation, Utah Construction & Mining Company, ALCOA, American Metal Climax, Hecla Mining Company, International Minerals & Chemical Company and "anyone else interested in killing the 90 percent standard" – who was "welcome at the meetings."

Milliken argued; "… testimony and data presented by industry have not received due consideration by government…" he complained that "… unnecessarily severe ambient air standards…" would place "… an undue economic burden on industry."

Rodgers writes:

> "It is time to recognize that the great changes in the industrial organizations that rule modern technologies have brought changes also in the political decision-making that affects these technologies.

According to a Report from the Secretary of the Department of Health, Education and Welfare (DHEW), sulfur dioxide is colourless, pungent above 3 ppm in the air, can be tasted from 0.3 to 1 ppm. SO_2 also attacks "a wide variety of building materials, protective surface coatings, textile fibres…" and of course vegetation [2].

After a judgement was placed against Harvey Aluminum from the plant at The Dalles in Oregon, the company provided data showing the fluoride emissions had dropped from 1,300 pounds daily to around 640 pounds. Lawyers pounced on the Court of Appeals in San Francisco.

This was found to be false by Joe Schulein, who taught chemical engineering at Oregon State University for 17 years. Schulein did not believe the sudden drop. He obtained charts that recorded the power usage of the plant. Sure enough, during testing times the voltage was very low, the company had turned off the power, no fluorides were emitted. The appeals were ignored [3].

Ben Bagdikian claimed in his 1983 investigation *The Media Monopoly* that when ALCOA was "found guilty of illegal damage to competitors," the company's legal defence was powerful enough that it had "delayed court action for sixteen years." He also claimed that ALCOA shared directors with CBS (Columbia Broadcasting Systems) [16].

One reason all of this pollution was able to continue is also found in Bagdikian's work. He claimed the Business Roundtable caused the "unexpected collapse" of a 1974 bill that "would have established a consumer protection agency."

> "Defense industry executives sit on the Pentagon's Industry Advisory Council, oil executives sit on the National Petroleum Council, and some of the heaviest polluting industries have executives on the National Industrial Pollution Control Council."

Bagdikian also claims that managers felt "pressured to compromise personal ethics to achieve corporate goals" – according to two 1976 surveys by Pitney Bowes and Uniroyal.

Fluoride's role continued in American Air Pollution problems in the 1960s [17]. An article appeared in Florida's newspaper **The Palm Beach Post** in August of 1961, discussing the study of fluoride emissions from phosphate works on citrus [18]. These are great examples of retroactive regulation, a policy that favours industry, wherein there is a problem, *then* a study… all the while pollution may continue. In a society where people were more important than profits, one might see regulation occur first, or earlier, *then* relax if studies found things safe.

A study of 164 employees of the phosphate industry failed to find any health problems in 1962 [19]. The study was done by Dr. Willard Machle, of Resources Research, Inc., formerly of Kettering Institute, Cincinnati. Dr. Machle and Dr. Louise C. McCabe were both "recognized as experts in air pollution control."

In 1963, The Florida State Board of Health filed charges against a phosphate company at Fort Meade, in response to a report presented by the Sanitary Engineering Director, which revealed "sources of major emission of fluoride into the atmosphere". This was reported on the 23rd of February. The firm appeared to be one of five firms in Polk County that were violating air pollution regulations.

"The Fort Meade firm is Armour Davidson Chemical Co. Bartow, American Cyanamid, Brewster. Virginia-Carolina Chemical Co. Nichols, and the Armour plant at Bartow." [20]

In November of the same year, The State Health Department said the plant was still polluting the area.

"Armour officials said that was because the new equipment installed to control pollution wasn't in use until Oct. 15." [21]

According to the Department, there had been a decrease in pollution across the country, this being independent of this particular plant. Several firms were installing pollution control equipment, also dealing with sulfur dioxide pollution [22].

Noting that many people were moving to Florida to avoid air pollution, the Fort Myers **News-Press** discussed in 1966 how the once-clean state, and the inhabitants were suffering the effects of its phosphate plants. Jacksonville air was "heavy with a faint odor of something dead and decayed."

"The gaseous atmosphere has been known to rot clothing, discolor house paint, rust metals, stunt vegetables, sicken livestock and wildlife, and make eyes water and burn."

This article focused only a little on fluorides, saying that the State Board of Health claimed the emission of fluorides was cut from 33,500 pounds/day in 1960 to 11,800 pounds in 1965. To quote:

"Eventually, unable to eat, many of the animals died of starvation, bawling in pain. The State Department of Agriculture said 25,000 acres of citrus land was damaged in Polk County and 150,000 acres of pastures abandoned."

They interviewed a resident:

"... I was working in my orchid house and through the window I saw my gardener stagger like a drunken man. I ran out to help him and he pointed to a ghostly gray haze suspended over the lake. 'It's that stuff' he said. 'It's killing me.'

"I turned into the wind, took a breath and became dizzy and vomited. I told the gardener to get into the house and went to my doctor. He found severe inflammation of the mouth, throat and respiratory tract."

"My black Angus show cattle all died and plants and trees were burned all over the place... There has seldom been a time in the last two months that the fumes have not been present part of the day or night. Our citrus has been killed. Our cattle died when their teeth fell out and they could not eat. We have lived here 28 years and have seen it develop from the beginning. We are deeply concerned about the health of our children, our grandchildren and our state as a whole." [22]

The article called it a "Curse of Progress". A courthouse tower, visible from afar, was sometimes "almost hidden" in "coffee-coloured gases". The phosphate plants were an enormous, economic boon. In 1966 alone, they created $145M in products, paid $55M in wages to 7,600 employees, and paid a little over $4M in ad valorem taxes.

The Florida Phosphate Council said that people who "voice the loudest protests today", are "living in the past." However, sulfur dioxide emissions increased from 373,500 pounds per day in March 1965, to 729,800 pounds per day in March 1966.

In 1963, Montanans began complaining of

"... fluoride-laden smoke from the [Rocky Mountain Phosphate Company] phosphate plant has caused malformations and deteriorating teeth in cattle and horses, that trees have been afflicted by cancerous growths and that people have developed symptoms akin to bronchitis, sinus trouble and heart attacks." [23]

A $123,000 award for damage to cattle was being appealed to the Montana Supreme Court. A lawyer for the company said:

"We do not constitute a threat to the health of the inhabitants of Garrison. There was no medical testimony to indicate any such threat."

Pinpointing a cause and effect relationship between smog and harm in humans was difficult, as people are not dissected until dead, may have moved from another smoggy area, or may have occupational or recreational factors that contribute to problems similar to that caused by smog.

A cattle rancher who sold some of his land to the company to build a plant on, was assured by a State Health Board official that there would be no pollution, but when operations began, sulfur dioxide and fluorides caused his cattle's milk production to drop, and a year later he was out of business. The small town of Garrison went to court five times at "great expense". Four times, there were "brief shutdowns", after which the plant was allowed to reopen, once it assured there would be no more pollution. Someone drew attention to the community by trying to blow up the smokestack with dynamite. The residents were hoping for legislation to be passed [24].

In August, 1967, a three-day conference featuring the Montana State Board of Health, and the Department of Health, Education and Welfare, recommended the plant be shut down until air pollution was controlled.

As soon as the recommendation was made, the company's attorney said,

"... the conference findings damaged the company in the public eye, deprived the firm of its constitutional rights and 'cast a shadow upon American justice.'" [24][184]

University of Montana professor, Dr. Clarence C. Gordon, said that damage to trees could be seen within a radius of 6.5 miles of the plant. Dr. Gordon claimed that "any layman can observe the damage." He testified that hydrogen fluoride was the problem, and that the phosphate plant was the source.

Another doctor, William F. Harris of Puyallup, Washington, said that fluorosis affected both large and small animals, those both wild and on ranches.

One reason some companies are relaxed about controlling pollution can be easily found in **The Orlando Sentinel**: to capture fluorides at one plant, with one installation, cost a million dollars in 1967 [25]. The cost of preventing pollution was barely going down with progress.

Discussing the draft of a new pollution code, a California newspaper claimed:

"The draft does provide for civil penalties up to $6,000 a month. But even if the maximum penalty is levied, it amounts to no more than a tolerable cost of doing business for a huge corporation." [26]

In Florida, 1969, $40 million was spent on equipment to counter pollution, and $4 million was spent annually on equipment upkeep and maintenance, said Homer Hooks, a phosphate industry official [27].

He was criticizing a **Life Magazine** article with a dramatic picture of a

"... fertilizer-producing phosphate plant which lights up the night sky burning off wastes, including fluoride compounds."

He said the picture was "phony", "dramatic but false", he "speculated" the clouds above the plant were steam. According to Hooks, the daily emission was about 1,500 pounds of fluoride, down from 18,000 pounds per day in the early 1960s, with a maximum of 5,537 pounds per day, set by the state agency. He said there was only one complaint about citrus in 1968, and that the **Life Magazine** statement that $14 million has been lost by citrus growers and cattle ranchers is outdated, "old, and discredited information".

A 1969 by-law in Texas decreed that none may emit pollutants without a variance, a sort of permission from authority. Senator A. R. Schwartz from Galveston, said:

"My experience is if it is not illegal, polluting will be done; if it is illegal, it will be done at night." [28]

A dentist from Columbia Falls, Montana, filed a $21.5 million pollution suit against Anaconda Aluminum Company in 1970. He gave up three years later, citing a lack of support from the community as his main reason. The suit was dismissed once it had been "whittled down to $6 million through successive stages of litigation" [29].

Dr. Kreck said it was "almost impossible for an individual to fight the company." He was threatened in telephone calls and poison-pen letters by workers from the company, the biggest employer in the area. The only other large employer was the timber industry.

After spending "millions of dollars" on pollution controls, the company put out 2,500 pounds of fluorides per day into the air, down from 7,500 pounds per day. This article ended by saying:

"A Forest Service study published in 1971 said more than 69,000 acres of federal, state and private lands have been damaged by fluoride pollution from the plant."

Perhaps Anaconda's success in the lawsuit can be somewhat explained by things occurring a few years before. In 1970, the Montana State Board of Health was questioned regarding a lack of enforcing pollution laws against Anaconda, when the Rocky Mountain Phosphates plant at the town of Garrison had been shut down at least six times. The reason was that there was no litigation, according to Benjamin F. Wake, the Director of the Air Pollution Control Division of the Health Department. The Board of Health had no contract with Anaconda Aluminum, but did have an agreement with Rocky Mountain Phosphate [30].

Later that year Mr. Wake said he was pleased by reduced levels of fluorides in samples of grass near the plant, but there was still work to be done.

"During the past decade, the phosphates plant has been shut down seven times by the board of health, the courts, or voluntarily. Several successful lawsuits have been brought by ranchers after their cattle developed fluorosis." [31]

In 1973, the emission standard deadline of June 30th was approaching for the Anaconda Company smelter at Anaconda, Anaconda Aluminum at Columbia Falls, and American Smelting and Refining at East Helena, Montana. Ninety percent of sulfur emissions would had to have been prevented. Fluoride emissions would had to have been limited to 864 pounds per day. In 1972, the Montana health board turned down an attempt by the companies in violation to get a three-year delay in the deadline. A variance,

---

[184] In a similar vein as 'business playing the victim' in Nicky Hager and Bob Burton's 1999 book *Secrets and Lies*, pp. 248-251.

good for one year, could have been granted after a public hearing. The **Great Falls Tribune** reported that fluoride emissions from Anaconda Aluminum had decreased from 4,500 pounds per day to 2,500, and that they were looking for more technology that would help them meet the standard [32].

One reason the environment was allowed to suffer is shown in an article that looked back on the Donora air pollution disaster, where 20 people died, just under 6,000 were sickened, including 1,440 severely ill. One person interviewed said,

"It was pretty lonely to be against air pollution in those days. The philosophy of the mill workers was 'dirty skies mean full lunchbuckets.' They equated it with prosperity." [33]

Such views may not have always originated in the workers' own minds. Elizabeth Fones-Wolf, Assistant Professor of History at West Virginia University wrote of the "Moundsville Church Plan" of a businessman called F. Steele Ernshaw, who felt he had heard too many sermons that "were on the left hand side". Ernshaw organized meetings with employers for three other plants and the nine church ministers of the community. They met monthly; by 1950 Ernshaw claimed he had convinced the ministers that both

"church steeples and smokestacks are necessary to the welfare of our community." [34]

It is the public – the farmers, the crop growers, the everyday citizens – that will be dealing with the more immediate and societal consequences of pollution, not the corporate lawyers and CEOs in plush boardrooms who justify it. One can certainly see a large motivation to give fluorine a safer appearance. I will leave the final words here to Professor William Rodgers:

"Ask whether the word conspiracy is too strong to describe the domination of economics, politics and science of those who fight under the banner of the aluminum industry. Laws do not pass, science does not come into being unless that industrial sponsor approves. Economic theories are turned upside-down by a system of favouritism that is as elusive as it is massive. The corporate aim of protecting the product and planning for its growth corrupt and overwhelm the institutions that question the inevitability of it all. Influence is not occasional but routine, not accidental but systematic, not modestly successful but thoroughly so. If a technological conspiracy exists, this is it." [3]

References for Appendix 4

1. *Alcoa Must Pay Fume Damage,* **Daily Capital Journal**, (Salem, Oregon), p. 2, 10th Aug, 1950.

2. *National Emission Standards Study*, Report of the Secretary of Health, Education, and Welfare to the U.S. Congress, U.S. Senate Document no. 91-63, pp. 2, 3, 24, Mar. 1970; Citing an Office Memorandum, Oregon State Air Pollution Authority, 11th December, 1953.

3. William Rodgers, *Corporate Country: A State Shaped to Suit Technology*, 1973. All of the work cited here from Rodgers is from Chapters 3 (copper industry, SO_2 pollution) and 7 (aluminium industry, fluoride pollution), pp. 53-84 and 161-188.

4. Rodgers, *op. cit.*, (p. 179) cites two letters here from E. W. Greenfield of Washington State's Engineering Research Division to Grant J. Saulie, 1st March, 1967, and 8th May, 1968.

5. Rodgers, *op. cit.*, "Protection of Proprietary and Confidential Information" is the name of the clause, according to Rodgers, in a grant contract from Kaiser Aluminum and Chemical Corp., on file at the University of Washington, Office of Grants and Contract Research. The clause was "inoperative" at Washington University due to university regulations.

6. Rodgers, *op. cit.*, *United States v. Aluminum Co.*, 148 F. 2d 416 (2d Cir. 1945).

7. Harold Stein, *A Casebook on Public Administration and Policy Development*, Chapter titled "The Disposal of the Aluminum Plants", p. 313, New York, Harcourt, Brace, 1952

8. Rodgers, *op. cit.*, the **Seattle Times**, 23rd January, 1969.

9. Rodgers, *op. cit.*, the **Seattle Times**, 13th November, 1970.

10. *ALCOA Facing Damage Suit,* **Daily Chronicle** (Washington) 5th Oct, p. 18, 1950.

11. Oregon newspapers were following it: see *Alcoa Sued for $200,000 Loss*, **Daily Capital Journal** (Salem), 16th Dec, p. 10, 1952 (this contained the claim about funding research); *Aluminum Firm Hit by Farmer's Suit*, **Corvallis Gazette-Times**, p. 6, same date; and *Aluminum Plant Sued for Damaging Livestock Forage*, **La Grande Observer**, p. 2, same date.

12. *State Board of Higher Education Elects President*, **Albany Democrat-Herald** (Oregon), 28th July, p. 2, 1953.

13. Ray Tucker, *Joyful Administrator*, **The Times Recorder** (Zanesville, Ohio), 27th December, p. 4, 1947.

14. *Fluoride Pollution At The Dalles Firm Reported Reduced*, **Medford Mail Tribune** (Oregon), 6th Jan, p. 2, 1963.

15. Kenneth Reich, Times Staff Writer, *Hearing Told Polluters Control Water Boards*, **L. A. Times**, p.4, 4th February, 1969.

16. Ben Bagdikian, *The Media Monopoly*, pp. 51-53 and 25, 1983.

17. *Phosphate, Pulp, Air Pollution Seen Growing Florida Problem*, **News-Press** (Fort Myers, Florida), p. 3, 1st April, 1961. *Pollution Research Plan Urged*, **The Orlando Sentinel** (Florida), p. 7, 26th August, 1961.

18. *Study on Effect of Fluoride on Citrus Urged*, **The Palm Beach Post** (West Palm Beach, Florida), p. 11, 26th August, 1961.

19. *Companies Given Clean Health Bill*, **The Orlando Sentinel** (Florida), p. 42, 13th September, 1962.

20. *Firm Facing Pollution Case*, **The Orlando Sentinel**, (Florida), p. 13, 23rd February, 1963.

21. *Pollution Case Set For Dec. 12*, **The Orlando Sentinel**, (Florida), p. 81, 24th November, 1963.

22. *Gaseous Mists Belch From Phosphate Plants,* pp. A1 and *Fair Florida Fouled By Pollution*, pp. A3, **News-Press** (Fort Myers, Florida), 18th December, 1966. This article mentioned the Florida Phosphate Council. A more modern version seems to be the Florida Phosphate Political Committee. The following is from their website, https://www.floridaphosphatecce.com/:

    > "Since November of 1979 the phosphate industry has come together as a group to educate policy leaders and promote the interests of this industry. The phosphate we mine and the fertilizer we produce is vital to our local and state economy and our nation's agriculture. As the global population grows, ensuring an adequate food supply is a challenge that the Florida phosphate industry is meeting head-on. We are quite literally helping to feed the world."

23. *Montanans Also Battle Phosphate Plant Blight*, **News-Press**, p.3, 25th December, 1966.

24. *Air Conference Asks Fluoride Pollution Halt*, **The Havre Daily News**, (Montana), p. 6, 18th August, 1967. A federal meteorologist also found high fluoride concentrations in grass near the plant. See *Garrison Phosphate Plant Major Pollution Source, Experts Declare*, **Great Falls Tribune** (Montana), p. 24, same date.

25. *Gov. Kirk To View Phosphate Industry*, **The Orlando Sentinel**, p. 56, 24th March, 1967.

26. *State, U.S. laws favor the polluters*, **Independent Press-Telegram** (Long Beach, California), p. 32, 23rd February, 1969.

27. *Phosphate Industry Pollution Report Called False*, **Florida Today** (Cocoa), p. 5C, 9th February, 1969. Hooks worked in the industry from 1965 to 1984.

28. *Houston Solon Flays Pollution Control Bills*, **The Times**, (Shreveport, Louisiana), p. 29, 12th Feb, 1969.

29. *Dentist Drops Anaconda Fluoride Suit*, **The Independent Record** (Helena, Montana), p. 6, 17th May, 1973.

30. *Pollution Control Justice Questioned*, **The Billings**, (Billings, Montana), p. 12, 18th March, 1970.

31. *Rocky Mountain Phosphates Plant Fluoride Emission Cut Significantly*, **Great Falls Tribune** (Great Falls, Montana), p. 4, 14th October, 1970.

32. *Three state plants still shy of compliance with Clean Air Act*, **Great Falls Tribune**, (Montana), p. 29, 3rd May, 1973.

33. *Donora, Pa., Recalls Night of Deadly Fog*, **The Los Angeles Times**, p. 35, 17th April, 1970. Also see *Air Pollution and Community Health* by Clarence A. Mills. Also see Christopher Bryson's book *The Fluoride Deception* (2004) and Clarence A. Mills, M.D., Ph.D., *Air Pollution and Community Health*, Chapter 4, 1954.

34. Committee on Cooperation with Community Leaders of the National Association of Manufacturers, "Proceedings," transcripts, May 17, 1950, Chicago Ill., Acc. 1411, NAM I/109, cited in *Selling Free Enterprise*, by Elizabeth Fones-Wolf, p. 221, 1994.

Appendix 5. **The Use of the "Communist plot" Accusation**

(This appendix contains its own reference section.)

One filter in Herman and Chomsky's propaganda model was anti-communism, though they were looking at the way media frames war. Meaning that people with certain views did not speak out against war for fear of appearing communist, and that people who expressed opinions outside the acceptable spectrum of debate could be called communists with minimal investigation or analysis of claims, and dismissed. Nowadays, I feel such a filter is largely redundant. Historically in fluoridation, a scientific issue, the filter worked in the opposite direction: calling someone *else* a communist put one in the "crazy" camp.

I believe people opposed to fluoridation in the 1950s called the measure communistic because calling people communists worked for Senator Joe McCarthy in removing people he disliked from positions of power. I've seen the accusation that fluoridation was part of a communist plot made many times, but no evidence ever given.

It has been difficult for me to find any information on whether Senator McCarthy supported or opposed fluoridation. Donald McNeil writes that dentist Dr. John Frisch, one of Wisconsin's biggest fluoridation promoters, asked McCarthy once for support [1]. Allan Mazur, Professor of Public Affairs at the Maxwell School of Syracuse University, writes that "conservative citizen groups in Wisconsin" who opposed the measure, championed McCarthy [2]. Mazur offers no evidence, but this is particularly ironic if it's true because McCarthy's black and white framing of issues worked in the long run against thoughtfulness and patience in politics, and presumably would have helped fluoridation, something that tended to suffer when it was given long-winded appraisals from the public. (As pointed out by Bull and Mueller, all it takes is for people to believe we don't know everything about it.) This appears to be the case until about the 1970s when the younger generation, educated in the 1950s regarding the benefits of CWF and not so sceptical, arrived at a voting age.

A biography on McCarthy published in 1953 yielded nothing on fluoridation [3], but I think McCarthy's framing of issues, and his overall effect on American thought was far-reaching. His relationship with the media was quite incredible. Alex Carey also claimed that Senator McCarthy's effect had been unappreciated by academics [4]. Carey believed millions of Vietnamese died largely as a result of such hysteria left uninhibited.

McCarthy of course became (in)famous for heavily accusing others within the American government of communism, or association with communists. He found this was not only an excellent way of getting enough mentions in the news to advance his own career, but of ridding the political landscape of those he disliked.

Alex Carey cautioned against two things; underestimating the power of McCarthy's influence even decades after his death, and regarding his techniques of 'mind control' as unique. Carey describes these as "extreme but nonetheless typical".

> "By the early 1950s corporate campaigns of persuasion, replete with their anti-American scapegoats, had become so common that there were few who saw McCarthy's anti-communist crusade as anything but a normal part of the political scene." [5]

One can see why the accusation that CWF was a communist plot was so readily voiced in much early antifluoridationist pamphlets and letters to newspaper editors. Not only was it a common accusation in the hysterical 1940s/50s, but sometimes it *worked*. The American population only needed to look at Joe McCarthy and see him throwing the accusation toward other politicians and bureaucrats, and see the subsequent castigations. The accusation *worked* for McCarthy, and it makes sense that citizens of the time opposed to CWF would use it against the huge prestige, power and money that was obviously behind fluoridation.

Carey wrote that in 1954 the American Legion[185] demanded that the Girl Scouts of America "clean up" their handbook. This demand yielded forty changes, for instance the "One World" badge became the "My World" badge. "Make up a quiz game on the UN" became "... game on the World Association of Girl Guides and Girl Scouts."[186]

Carey also claimed that President Truman's security checks ("loyalty" tests) for government employees which were brought about as a political response to Republican claims that Democrats were too soft on communism, caused a "near paralysis of liberal/imaginative political thought" in America and nearby. Truman joined in the Republican game instead of confronting it, with both parties trying to "out-accuse" each other. Against this backdrop, Joe McCarthy took to the stage.

We can learn something applicable to fluoridation from the USA's "loss of China". It has to do with the behaviour of intellectuals and bureaucrats when they think their job may be on the line. Recall John Mueller's phrase,

> "fear of ridicule helped keep 'respectable' members of the community from joining the anti forces." [6]

"Fear of ridicule" is of course a watered-down version of fear of unemployment. The 1967 reprint of the 1949 White Paper from the State Department, *United States Relations with China*, contained some of the following phrases:

> "McCarthy's charges [of Communism within the State Department] finally proved baseless, but in the meantime lives and careers were ruined and lasting harm was done to the conduct of American foreign policy. The reception of the White Paper instructed many government officials on the value of caution... Some of America's most able and best qualified China specialists were dismissed from the State Department... Others were transferred to less sensitive positions... Some were persuaded to accept early retirement... For telling unpleasant truths about the nationalists they were later called Communists." [7]

I do not think it wholly inappropriate to compare foreign policy and CWF. Propaganda is admittedly involved in both. The Democrats were forced to "ridiculous demonstrations of anti-communism" as Carey puts it. He gives the example of Dean Acheson[187] and General George Marshall[188] testifying that they would never consider "recognition of communist China or support its admission to the UN." They claimed such a thing was never even discussed. One can see how even baseless accusations can restrict the limits of free speech.

---

[185] A veterans organization formed in 1919.
[186] Here Carey cites *Reporter* 30th December, 1954:2.
[187] Truman's Secretary of State
[188] Truman's Secretary of Defense.

A 1953 biography of McCarthy, authored by two American journalists goes into great detail on not only the simplistic nature of these deceptions, but also yields a trove of information on the Senator's character. The term "power-hungry" is a vast understatement. Authors Anderson and May wrote that "dozens of McCarthy's victims" had learned a very powerful lesson:

> "... that a man can be ruined regardless of how false the charges against him, because no amount of back-page truth can offset a front-page lie." [8]

McCarthy headed a committee which looked into "un-American" activities. Carey claims the FBI were partly responsible for some of the worst of McCarthy's offences. In 1953 McCarthy had books in American Information Service libraries burnt if they were offensive to him. Carey's examples are also abundant. One of the most interesting comes from Albert Einstein in 1954:

> "If I would be a young man again... I would not try to become a scientist or scholar or teacher. I would rather choose to be a plumber or peddler in the hope to find that modest degree of independence still available under present circumstances."[189]

Regarding fluoridation, Carey cites the *Reporter*[190] as claiming that the allegation CWF was a communist plot was often successful. One can see why activists, and some scientists would make such a claim: it worked. People could read McCarthy's accusations in the news, and see the unemployment and demonization that followed. Carey described the opposition to fluoridation that came from believing it to be a communist plot as extremely paranoid. He obviously thought it was safe, effective, etc. He mentioned it in only one sentence.

There was justifiable reason, at least on behalf of biochemists to urge caution: fluorine had been demonstrated unnecessary in nutrition of rats even in tiny amounts in three experiments in the 1930s, and much of dentistry and the biological sciences had focussed on *excesses* of fluorine. The only experiment that had claimed an essential nutritional role for fluorine was funded by the Aluminum Company of America, one of many companies consistently taken to courts all over America in the 1940s and 1950s for polluting farms, rivers and the landscape with fluorides.

Carey writes,

> "Drink and ill health brought [Joe McCarthy's] death two years later. But the intolerance and paranoia his crusade embodied continued largely unabated."

There are perhaps a few lessons for journalists and media aficionados here. McCarthy used and abused the press. Quoting Anderson and May:

> "He kept a black book of all political bigshots in every city he visited; and, traveling through, he would call them and pass the time of day." [9]

There was a lot of whiskey and backslapping. McCarthy used any means he could to get votes and popularity.

> "But it was to newspapermen that he was most cordial. Some reporters kept a careful watch on the court rosters to see when their friend Joe McCarthy would arrive to pick up the tabs at the swankiest places in town."

> "He became known all over the state as the most generous, dynamic, nose-to-the-grindstone judge on the bench. And perhaps all this glare made it hard to see through the clear picture of his judicial record."

> "He built up his reputation exactly as he had in the past – quantitatively instead of qualitatively. He tried five cases for every one his colleagues tried; divorce trials were sometimes knocked off in five minutes; manslaughter trials took a little longer."

> "And when it comes to the gimmicks of modern salesmanship, Joe has gone the experts one better; he has invented the technique of calling a press conference in order to announce the calling of another press conference." [9]

Anderson and May quote Richard Rovere:

> "McCarthy will bring in the reporters in the morning by notifying their offices that he has something important to disclose. When they arrive, he will disclose that he has called them together to alert them for an afternoon press conference, at which he will have something breathless to reveal. This announcement makes the afternoon papers. The breath-taking revelations, if there are any, make the newspapers of the following morning. If, as is often the case, he has nothing of news value to announce, he has at least profited by the afternoon headlines." [10]

Whether McCarthy supported or opposed CWF is something I've never been able to discover. Anderson and May write that he joined the Junior Chamber of Commerce, who had consistently supported fluoridation so presumably he would have gone along

---

[189] The quote comes from *Reporter* 18th November 1954:8.
[190] 16th June 1955:28-30.

with this, especially considering how conscious he was of his reputation. The impression I get from Anderson and May's work is that McCarthy was obsessed with prestige. He was certainly very intelligent and ambitious in the way he went about obtaining it.

"... Joe baffled his fellow students by stopping in small towns along the way [to debates in North Wisconsin] to meet the local judges. 'Might do me good later,' he explained." [11]

Even on McCarthy's holiday during a campaign, "the handshaking and backslapping continued in between the swimming and fishing". Honesty was malleable to him.

"After dinner at a night club outside Eagle River, he collected from each member of his party the proper share of the heavy check, then walked over to the cashier with the money and announced: 'I'm Judge McCarthy, running for the Senate, you know. This dinner's on me.' He plunked the money down on the counter, shook the cashier's hand and walked out." [12]

McNeil writes that Dr. John Frisch approached McCarthy in Wisconsin for help to promote fluoridation, but McNeil did not elaborate on any public statements regarding this, or whether he even looked for any. I feel that if McCarthy did endorse the measure, he did so minimally, no examples of this have been given in any literature I have found. Nowadays, it would appear bad to CWF, and if some supporters of the measure do know of it but don't mention it this would be understandable. By the mid-1950s, McCarthy's name had become tainted.

In 1946, the Committee for Industrial Relations (CIO), a union of trade workers, voted for McCarthy, who had been very anti-communist in 1945, in the Senate. Communism had not been purged in Wisconsin by that stage. The CIO leadership managed to convince the voters that McCarthy would be better than Democrat Bob La Folette, who was, according to McCarthy, too soft on the Soviets. The CIO believed anti-communism was just on the surface, they had no way of knowing it would turn out as hysterical as it did. McCarthy helped them churn out huge amounts of anti-La Folette literature, and rallied the workers behind Joe. When the blatantly anti-communist McCarthy was asked about this by reporters, he replied:

"Communists have the same right to vote as anyone else, don't they?" [13]

McCarthy strikes me as a man who would have said anything had it made him more powerful, so I think even if he said anything about fluoridation, its relation to reality would have primarily served his own need, truth irrelevant. Aspects of intellectualism in the 1940s/50s appear quite hysterical to me. The anti-communist argument was a convenient one for those opposed to fluoridation, and it probably worked. It is this convenience, as well as the obvious out-of-place nature in modern times, and the complete lack of evidence for the claim that makes the charge largely irrelevant now, closer to an embarrassment. The secrecy and selectivity in science of these times would also have catalysed reaction against fluoridation. To anyone who had studied the biochemistry of fluorine, it was obvious that the dentists were not completely up to speed on fluorine's interactions with all tissues. The fact that there were no obvious signs of harm did not convince all of those who distrusted the obvious public relations efforts of the experts.

As evidenced in Appendix 6, the people opposed to CWF were not the only ones making accusations of communist influence. In America, the 'antis' used the argument, in New Zealand, the 'pros' suspected, and investigated it – but not in public.

I would like to end this appendix with the assertion that journalists are capable of wonderful things.

Anderson and May found an incredible amount of information not only in terms of evidence, but regarding McCarthy's personality and attitude. They wrote that McCarthy had persuaded State Senator Warren Knowles to

"... slip a secrecy bill through the Wisconsin legislature. This would have made a newsman liable for damages if he invaded the 'legal right of privacy' by asking too many questions..." [14]

Wisconsin's newspapers caught the bill in time to stop it. The authors claim such a bill would have prevented the writing of their biography.

References for Appendix 5

1. Donald McNeil, *The Fight for Fluoridation*, p. 52.
2. Allan Mazur, *A Hazardous Inquiry: The Rashomon Effect at Love Canal*, p. 47 1998.
3. Jack Anderson and Ronald W. May, 1953. *McCarthy: The Man, The Senator, The "ism"*,
4. Alex Carey, *Taking the Risk out of Democracy*, Chapter 4, The McCarthy Crusade, 1995.
5. Alex Carey, *Taking the Risk out of Democracy*, p. 64, 1995.
6. John E. Mueller (University of Rochester, New York), *The Politics of Fluoridation in Seven California Cities*, **Western Political Quarterly**, Vol. 19, No.1, March 1966, p. 64.
7. Carey, *op. cit.*, p. 68, 1995.
8. Jack Anderson and Ronald W. May, *McCarthy: the Man, The Senator, the "ism"*, Victor Gollancz Ltd, 1953.
9. *Ibid.*, pp. 44-45.

10. *Ibid.*, p. 363.
11. *Ibid.*, p. 28.
12. *Ibid.*, p. 90.
13. *Ibid.*, p. 104
14. *Ibid.*, p. 370.

Appendix 6. "Big Food" Advertising

This appendix lists studies and articles that I have found relevant regarding the effect of advertising. I think the work of Juliet Schor, and the 2008 paper by Hoek and King are of utmost importance, but all of this research is very useful. The articles are presented chronologically beginning over the past forty years until now.

Heather Morton, *Television Food Advertising: A Challenge for the New Public Health in Australia*, **Community Health Studies**, Vol. 14, No. 2, pp. 153-161, 1990. In 1981, the Australian National Health and Medical Research Council (NHMRC) urged for better self-regulation on advertisers after "strong community agitation" in the late 1970s. Levels of food advertising fell afterwards, according to this article. However, by the late 1980s, food advertising had risen beyond that of the early 1980s. The article claims most adverts were for a "narrow range of products, most of which contravene one of more of the Dietary Guidelines." The Australian Broadcasting Tribunal (ABT) did not regulate advertisers, however they stepped up, and prohibited adverts that contained "misleading or incorrect nutrition information". This sounds great until we read that very few adverts contain any information whatsoever. The article points to a survey where 72% of adults wanted government intervention to restrict food advertising to children (K. Baghurst, D. Crawford, *Attitudes of South Australians to Government Interventions to Improve Nutritional Health*, Adelaide: Human Nutrition Section CSIRO, unpublished data, 1988).

In the 45-hour sample period, there were 417 minutes of advertising, containing 851 separate advertisements (excluding station and community service). Claims there is insufficient evidence to claim there is *definite* evidence of a link between more advertising and more consumption of junk food among children; then proceeds to discuss experiments that reveal consistent trends regarding increased exposure to advertising and increased consumption of poor quality food. Coca-Cola and Pepsi spent $30 million in 1990 on advertising. This article suggests it is foolish to ignore the importance of media and discussed the "passivity" surrounding the issue. In 1990, the authors claim about a third of Australian children were overweight. Quotes a Canadian article that states, "freedom of speech for advertisers ends at a point where their manipulative sales pitches reach the impressionable minds of children." Canada was beginning to ban advertising to children.

Shelov *et al.*, *Children, Adolescents, and Advertising*, **Pediatrics**, Vol. 95, No. 2, February, 1995. This article summarizes the reasons behind the recommendations of the Committee on Communications – eight MDs (Shelov was Chairman). Claims in 1750 BC the Code of Hammurabi stated one had to obtain power of attorney to sell anything to a child. Begins by looking at two approaches to sell toys – commercials in programs unrelated to products being sold, and "program-length commercials" which are TV shows designed primarily to sell toys, though they may tell a story. Claims the "barrage" of advertising may drive a wedge between parents and children. Claims the American Academy of Pediatrics believes "advertising directed toward children is inherently deceptive and exploits children under 8 years of age."

While advertisers "insist that their intent is to promote brand selection" an obvious consequence is increased production ("good data support this conclusion"). Claims that there are often "inappropriate sexual innuendos" in advertising to children – while ads for birth control products are often illegal. The committee points to guidelines for appropriate sexual content in advertising. They claim the 1985 Guttmacher report (E. F. Jones, J. D. Forrest, N. Goldman, et al., *Teenage Pregnancy in Developed Countries: Determinants and Policy Implications*, **Family Planning Perspectives**, Vol. 17, pp. 53-63, 1985 *and* see the American Academy of Pediatrics Committee on Adolescence, Sexuality, Contraception, and the Media, **Pediatrics**, Vol. 78, pp. 535-536, 1986) found America had the highest teen pregnancy rate in the world partly due to "inappropriate depictions of sexuality in American media" and poor sex education.

The Committee's recommendations begin with an obvious statement: that "one conclusion" could be the ban of all advertising directed to under eight-year-olds, and all advertising directed to teenagers promote health. After saying this the Committee write, "However, the viewing audience cannot be accurately sequestered by age, and a ban would also infringe on the rights of free speech directed at older children." Perhaps this means the rights of corporations to advertise freely. One point: "A variety of resources should be developed to help parents teach children that commercials are designed to sell products."

Michael Crowley, *Junk Deal*, **Men's Health** (USA), Vol. 17, No. 6, pp. 136-141, July/August 2002. Claims obesity costs the USA over $100 billion annually. Claims more and more people believe junk food companies ought to be taxed for what they sell. Cites a

Men's Health survey that found 69% of people believe obesity is a matter of personal responsibility (Source: Men's Health nationwide phone survey of men and women). People who criticize junk food advertising have been called "nannies", "bullies" and "tyrants" according to this article, but examples are not given. Quotes the director of Yale University's Center on Eating and Weight Disorders, Professor Kelly Brownell, who believes the problem is that finding healthy food is so difficult, and junk food is so abundant.

Claims the food industry spends $30 billion annually on advertising, with 70% on convenience foods and only 2% on healthy foods. Calls the government's effort to educate about nutrition "shouting in a hurricane". McDonald's and Burger King spent $1 billion on advertising, the National Cancer Institute's campaign for eating five pieces of fruit or vegetables daily had a budget of only $1 million – a one thousandth of what the two burger giants spent.

This article looks at the work of Marion Nestle, author of *Food Politics*. She had worked in the U.S. Surgeon General's office in the 1980s and was disgusted by the influence the industry had over politicians and bureaucrats. "I see kids in the supermarket getting hysterical and embarrassing their parents, and I think, Advertising is designed to make that happen."

The author interviews John Banzhaf, a George Washington University Law School professor who gained notoriety by encouraging his students to think up possible law suits (license plate: SUE BAST – short for "sue the bastards"). McDonald's settled out of court for $12.4 million on a false advertising charge filed by Banzhaf; presumably they did not want a precedent set. Marion Nestle told the author of this article (Crowley) that she had received incredible amounts of abuse on her book tour.

Juliet B. Schor, *The Commodification of Childhood: Tales from the Advertising Front Lines*, **The Hedgehog Review**, Summer 2003. Previously director of women's studies at Harvard and a consultant to the United Nations, she is now Professor of Sociology at Boston College. Author of many books. Claims there has been "increased attention to children by marketers" and childhood "as a saleable cultural concept". Children are now "objects of intense marketing activity." Looks at the way in which marketers sell childhood as a concept to corporations, who manufacture what children will buy. Page 11: "The presence of controversy and debate about the entire enterprise of marketing to children also contributes to the secrecy that surrounds research on children." Page 12: "Two of the firms I tried to penetrate, Channel One and MTV Networks, were relatively closed, explicitly citing their desire to avoid criticism." Schor did not ask to see confidential material from the companies she did manage to interview. Pages 17-18: "Product seeding has also migrated out to non-celebrities. In these campaigns, companies typically identify people they consider to be 'trendsetting' individuals, give them samples of a product, and ask them to recruit friends. There are even agencies that specialize in finding these kinds of trend-setting (or 'alpha') individuals. One practice is to pay people to pose as ordinary consumers. For example, alcohol brands pay people to sit in bars and order their drinks, and then to talk to other patrons about them. Chat rooms are seeded with paid representatives to promote brands. The internet and email are full of these paid communications. Movie, book, and music reviews are increasingly written by paid representatives of marketing companies. While teens and young adults were the targets of many of the early viral campaigns, these techniques have filtered down to children." The 'Girl's Intelligence Agency' (GIA) is a peer-to-peer marketing group that organizes parties hosted by a girl (a "GIA agent") who invites a dozen or so friends over to play (for research and marketing purposes), "where they are given a sample of the product..." "The party becomes an informal, intimate sales session." Similar to Amway, or pyramid schemes in the sense of friends selling to friends, I suppose. GIA claimed to be able to reach 20 million girls in the USA, according to Schor, who wrote "I uncovered recruiting programs for children to become market consultants through Boys and Girls Clubs." A GIA leader claimed to "make contact with major organizations" (but did not want to name those involved). When Schor suggested Girl Scouts and church groups, there was no real disagreement (church groups were used to sell economic beliefs that were favourable to the business community to American citizens, including labour, in the 1940s and 1950s; discussed in Chapter 8 of Elizabeth Fones-Wolf's book *Selling Free Enterprise*). Schor suggests that peer-to-peer marketing is used because people have become more sceptical of advertising, but that this scepticism will in all likelihood be put on friends if this continues. Page 19: "Marketers are teaching children that their friends are a lucrative resource that they can exploit to gain products or money. But what we cherish most about good friendships is often their insulation from those types of pressures." This is exactly why marketers have an interest in using friendship for marketing – we trust our friends. Marketers describe modern children as savvy, intelligent and unable to be manipulated – knowledgeable about products – and there is some truth to this. Such beliefs no doubt lead to a very obvious industry-favourable conclusion: "Child advocates pushing for stricter regulations are put down as know-nothings." (Page 21) Advertisements on American children's TV "portray adults as buffoons, out of touch, or objects of ridicule" – no wonder we read that *parents* have a responsibility to regulate junk food purchases in the nutrition column of our local newspaper. The whole concept of parental duty is presented to teens as a joke. Regarding food advertising, Schor writes: "Marketers point their fingers at parents, who they fault for buying junk food, not patrolling the kitchen, and taking their children too frequently to fast food outlets. 'Just say no,' they counsel. At the same time, many of their most sophisticated approaches, they have explained to me, involve breaking down parental resistance." (Page 22) The **Community Health Studies** article cited earlier pointed to an Australian National Health and

Medical Research Council subcommittee report that claimed in 1990 "media and particularly television are more powerful in determining children's food preferences than anything else, including family example."

A **Publisher's Weekly** review of Schor's book *Born to Buy* wrote that these changes were "leading to a generation of kids with no concept of what is important and truly necessary in life." https://www.publishersweekly.com/978-0-684-87055-7. "The lesson to kids is that it's the product, not your parent, who's really on your side." (Page 55, *Born to Buy*.)

Mark Kleinman, *Marketers Must Respond to the FSA*, **Marketing**, p. 15, 2nd October, 2003. A British report gives a quite different flavour to what Dr. Schor presents. In 2002 food advertisers spent over £450 million on marketing. Kleinman claims the report simply states the obvious: that advertising works – but he is averse to using the phrase 'brainwashing' as the media did in one article by Partick McGowan. The report was written by Professor Gerard Hastings of Strathclyde University's Centre for Social Marketing. One point it makes is that differentiating between the effects of advertising and TV viewing in general is difficult (because of product placement). Claims banning advertising of junk food is not a fix-all (obviously this sort of claim is easily used by corporations to continue advertising).

Susan E. Linn, *Food Marketing to Children in the Context of a Marketing Maelstrom*, **Journal of Public Health Policy**, pp. 367-378, Vol 25, 2004. "Childhood obesity is a major public health problem in the United States, yet U.S. children are targeted as never before with marketing for foods high in sugar, fat, salt, and calories." (Citing Dalmeny K., Hanna E., Lobstein T., Bro*adcasting Bad Health: Why Food Marketing to Children Needs to be Controlled.* London: International Association of Food Consumer Food Organizations; 2003. Sponsored by the World Health Organization Consultation on a Global Strategy for Diet and Health.) Claims that "a political climate that favours deregulation" has given marketers "unprecedented access to children, including babies and toddlers." Finds the notion "promulgated by the food industry" which suggests parents "just say no" is either cynical or simplistic. Industry wants marketing viewed as familial, Linn believes it should be viewed as societal.

Changes in the 1970s caused many children to be left home unsupervised, something marketers noticed and used to their advantage. A Nickelodeon VP said "the latest European research shows that product preferences develop at a much earlier age than anyone had ever thought... As people begin to understand this, to see how brand loyalty transfers to adulthood, there is almost nothing that won't be advertised as for children." (Citing Marshall Cohen, senior VP for research at Nickeloden, quoted in: *Latchkey Kid is King in Marketing Realm Clout Carries over to Buying by Parents.* Chicago Tribune, C:3, 31st July, 1988.) Claims parents have been overwhelmed by the volume of advertising. While experts advise "pick your battles" parents have too many battles to fight. "If they are strict about food, should they also be strict about violent toys, media programs, and music? What about precociously sexualized clothing? Computer, video game, and TV time? Materialism?" Experts' advice again ignores the fact that corporations do what they can to undermine not only parental authority, but parental knowledge. Estimates $15 billion spent yearly on advertising to children in 2002 (Citing D. Barboza, *If You Pitch it, They will Eat*, **New York Times**, 3rd August, 2003). Claims Coca-Cola spent $20 million on product placement in the show American Idol, to get around the fact product placement was illegal in *children's* TV shows – Idol is a show for teens and adults. Claims the *Gilmore Girls* was created "through a consortium of corporations" called The Family Friendly Programming Forum.

David S. Ludwig and Steven L. Gortmaker, *Programming Obesity in Childhood*, **The Lancet**, Vol. 364, 17th -23rd July, pp. 226-227, 2004. Claims a causal link between advertising and obesity. Cited a study regarding the long-term consequences of TV viewing in childhood and suggested powerful impact. Claims advertising to children should be banned, not only for scientific reasons, but reasons of common sense. "In an era when childhood obesity has reached crisis proportions, the commercial food industry has no business telling toddlers to consume fast food, soft drinks, and high-calorie low-quality snacks, all products linked to excessive weight gain." Cites the **Pediatrics** article (Shelov *et al.*, 1995) claiming the American Academy of Pediatrics believes advertising to children is "inherently deceptive and exploitative." Also claims that while obesity is a condition with numerous causes, "the multifactorial nature of the problem should not be an excuse for inaction."

Diego Cevallos, *Latin America: Parents and Lawmakers Attack Junk Food Ads*, Global Information Network, New York, 25th April, 2007 (ProQuest document ID: 457560609). "The obesity epidemic is out of control. One of the most important causes is the change in eating habits and the lack of regulation of junk food advertising," claims Mexican NGO El Poder del Consumidor (Power of the Consumer). This article claims that the American Heart Association claims Latin America has the highest proportion of heart attack risk due to "high blood pressure, excess abdominal fat and permanent stress." Such a statement is interesting given the U.S. presence in the region for decades. Obesity rates in Brazil and Mexico increased significantly from the 1970s among children and teenagers. Impoverished indigenous Mexican families spent more on soft drinks ($2/week) than on milk (less than $1/week). Panama banned sales of fried food and soft drink in schools in 1997, but officials claim such a ban is difficult to enforce. Bills for labelling junk food and warnings for products have hit "legislative roadblocks" with some lawmakers "reporting threats from manufacturers." (The threats were not specified.) Food manufacturers suggested parents take responsibility for the problem.

"Upholding the discourse of snack food and beverage manufacturers in other countries, Ignacio Lastra, spokesman of the Mexican National Chamber of Industry, declared that a law will not resolve the obesity problem. Lastra believes that families should instruct their children about adequate nutrition."

I recommend the following paper. Janet Hoek (Massey University, NZ) and Bronwyn King (Canterbury District Health Board NZ), *Food advertising and self-regulation: A view from the trenches*, **Australian and New Zealand Journal of Public Health**, Vol. 32, No. 3, pp. 261-265, 2008. Begins by using the word 'epidemic' to describe obesity incidence in the civilized world. Points to the USA and Australasia as having a "self-regulatory approach" for business. This paper looks at a complaint made in May of 2005, and suggests a "use (or mis-use)" of logic can "potentially be persuasive in quasi-legal settings". The complaint was regarding an advertisement where a brother and sister have an argument with their parents, leading to the parents agreeing to serve the product, chicken nuggets, 4 nights per week and for lunch on Sundays. The complainant suggested the children "blackmailed" the parents, made an "occasional" food appear normal, and that the advertisement was contrary to the government's healthy eating guidelines.

The 4th page (264) is a must-read for understanding how industry expropriates advertising complaints. "The Television Commercials Approval Bureau (TVCAB) used hyperbole to overstate the complainant's case and undermine and belittle her argument. She did not refer to 'blatant or gross' transgressions; however, by re-casting her arguments in extreme terms, the TVCAB is better able to counter these."

The agency argued that because only 1 complaint had been made, most people had accepted the advertisement, meaning this complaint could be dismissed. By this logic an advertisement needs to receive thousands of complaints before it should be investigated. This argument also allows the reasons for the complaint to be nullified. The TVCAB argued that "suppression, repression and restriction are not the way of modern parenthood. Neither is child anarchy." The complainant had used none of these terms. The process was not "accessible, simple, and user-friendly". Industry submitted heavily, with nobody to rebut its claims.

"Our analysis does not prove that self-regulation is ineffective; however, it raises serious questions about the level of protection self-regulation affords to consumers, particularly where public health problems are concerned." This is an excellent paper and I recommend it.

K. D. Brownell and K. E. Warner, *The perils of ignoring history: Big Tobacco played dirty and millions died. How similar is Big Food?* **Milbank Q**, Vol. 87, No. 1, 259–294, 2009. In 1954, the tobacco industry publicized statements that claimed public health was "industry's concern above all others." This is one reason I think the public relations industry, along with corporate freedom of speech, need drastic regulation – such a thing simply cannot be true, and of course, was not true. The industry put its profits ahead of all other concerns. Brownell and Warner argue for some similarities in the role of the tobacco industry and the food industry. The differences are in diversity of product, including lonesome small businesses and individuals, mega corporations like McDonalds and Kraft, and everything in between. Food is necessary for human survival, tobacco is not. Claims the "restaurant industry" has sued New York City, "used its political might to weaken legislation in California, and successfully encouraged federal legislators to introduce weak national legislation that would preempt states and cities from acting more aggressively." (Page 262) "The same company making fried foods laden with saturated fat might also sell whole-grain cereal. In other ways, the industry is organized and politically powerful. It consists of massive agribusiness companies like Cargill, Archer Daniels Midland, Bunge, and Monsanto... These are represented by lobbyists, lawyers, and trade organizations that in turn represent a type of food (e.g., Snack Food Association, American Beverage Association), a segment of the industry (e.g., National Restaurant Association), a constituent of food (e.g., Sugar Association, Corn Refiners Association), or the entire industry (e.g., Grocery Manufacturers of America)." (Page 263)

Brownell and Warner cite the 2002 work of Marion Nestle (*Food Politics: How the Food Industry Influences Nutrition and Health.* Berkeley: University of California Press) which claims the "number of daily calories created for the American food supply" rose from 3,300 per person in 1970 to 3,800 by 2000. If demand for food reflected what people needed, this would result in market contraction. Yet in order for the business to survive, short term profit must be of primary concern. The "playbook" of arguments used by the food industry is similar to that of Big Tobacco:

- Personal responsibility among consumers causes problems, the industry does not recommend their product be overused;
- Government legislation, restrictions on advertising and the like remove personal freedom from citizens;
- Critics of industry are labelled as "fanatics", advocates of a "nanny state", and people who dislike freedom;
- Studies with conclusion critical of industry are "junk science";
- Physical exercise and activity is claimed to be very important;
- Stating that there are "no good or bad foods" therefore no type of food (soft drinks, confectionary, etc.) need to be changed;
- Use of strategic "doubt" through public relations and hired "experts" when there is public criticism of the food industry.

Regarding the claim that physical activity is important, this is consistently used to take away from the fact that so much of the processed food the industry sells is harmful. Regarding strategic "doubt" see the books *Taking the Risk out of Democracy* by Alex Carey, *Doubt is their Product* by Professor David Michaels and *Merchants of Doubt* by Naomi Oreskes and Eric M. Conway.

Brownell and Warner argue that in the USA the "freedom" and "personal responsibility" arguments espoused by the industry play on powerful, founding concepts of the country's collective mentality, yet the industry ignores the fact that "some of the most significant health advances have been made by population-based public health approaches in which the overall welfare of the citizenry trumps certain individual or industry freedoms." A person is inclined to ask "what about the freedom to *not* be subjected to constant advertising and public relations? What about the freedom of government to represent the wishes of people?" (The authors cite a survey from California in which residents found around two thirds of people believed advertising affected food choices, that obesity has worsened more than other issues like drugs and alcohol use, and did not want the matter left solely to parents and children.) The authors argue that it is difficult for Big Tobacco to defend half a million yearly deaths by arguing for freedom and choice. Page 266: "A great deal of influence rests in the hands of parties who control the framing of a health issue. That is, a problem framed as a matter of personal irresponsibility will be addressed differently from one for which other factors, such as corporate misbehavior, environmental toxins, or infectious agents, are responsible." Food industry front groups are aggressive in shaping public opinion with the strategies discussed above. This article quotes the president of the National Restaurant Association, Steven Anderson, as saying "Just because we have electricity doesn't mean you have to electrocute yourself" when he was asked about restaurants contributing to the obesity problem. The American Beverage Association, working with the Alliance for a Healthier Generation in 2006, guaranteed they would reduce sales of traditional carbonated soft drinks, yet completely ignored a different set of drinks with increasing sales, namely 'sports drinks' still containing large amounts of sugar. The article puts the influence of American children between $200 and $500 billion annually, so there is strong incentive in the industry to self-regulate its marketing.

Nicky Hager and Bob Burton wrote in *Secrets and Lies* that corporations will publicize 5% of their work on contributing to environmental betterment, in order to take focus from the other 95% of their work, which may be environmentally harmful. Brownell and Warner discuss the results of the conflicts of interest caused by accepting money from Big Tobacco: women's groups "buoyed by support for events like the Virginia Slims Tennis Tour," were silent on lung cancer, instead focusing on breast cancer and other problems.

The authors quote David Kessler, a former FDA commissioner: "From the White House, the pressure moved down to the Office of Management and Budget (OMB), which had the power to block our regulations. As required, we had submitted draft after draft of the final rule to OMB and often had it returned to us with industry-sought changes. More than once, OMB's wording had been taken almost verbatim from food industry comments we had already carefully considered." (Cited in Kessler, D.A. 2001. *A Question of Intent: A Great American Battle with a Deadly Industry*. New York: Public Affairs, p. 58.) Tommy Thomson, secretary of Health and Human Services (DHHS), in 2002, encouraged the Grocery Manufacturers of America (GMA) to "go on the offensive" if the industry's position on obesity was criticized. Thomson is discussed in Kaare Norum's paper regarding the sugar industry's lobbying of the World Health Organization (WHO) to ensure WHO standards were not set too low. The Sugar Association asked the US Congress to "challenge funding" of the US to the WHO - $406 million per year. Brownell and Warner point out: "This is the WHO that deals with AIDS, malnutrition, infectious disease, bioterrorism, and more, threatened because of its stance on sugar." Claims Washington's infamous revolving door is alive and well – Tommy Thomson was at the time of writing, partner with Akin Gump, a law firm that defended the tobacco industry and now food corporations.

Industry influence is pervasive and powerful (see Alex Carey's *Grassroots and Treetops Propaganda* for a history on technique); the industry pays $20,000 per fact sheet "authored by" the American Dietetic Association (ADA), actually authored by industry, yet promoted on the ADA website and in its journal. The ADA also believes there are no good or bad foods. Regarding conflicts of interest, Brownell and Warner suggest some scientists may be unaffected, but point to the simple fact that such interactions with scientists favour industry – for instance industry can claim it is searching for the truth about its products by sponsoring research endeavours. A review not funded by industry, containing studies with strong methodologies, found a link between soft drinks and poorer health outcomes. In response, the American Beverage Association funded researches to perform another review. "Two of the authors had conducted multiple industry-funded studies in the past, and one was employed by the ABA when the study was published." (Page 279) This review found no cause-effect relationship between soft drinks and poor health. Still, it seems as awareness grows around conflicts of interest, the situation improves. Consumers need to be watchful of the "script" that favours industry, even when it is mouthed by front groups with unlikely names, such as the Center for Consumer Freedom.

The paper discusses whether food is addictive, and suggests the evidence around the topic is youthful. Highlights caffeine, which has been added to "unlikely" foods like chips, jelly beans, sunflower seeds and candy. Caffiene may promote obesity when it is coupled with high-calorie drinks and the like. The paper suggests caffeine use in children could become an issue. The food industry differs from Big Tobacco in its diversity, many companies sell processed food as well as fruit and vegetables. "There are perils for both industry and the population of ignoring tobacco's history." (Page 286.) "Above all, the experience of tobacco shows how powerful profits can be as a motivator, even at the cost of millions of lives and unspeakable suffering. There is ample indication that giving industry the benefit of the doubt can be a trap. To avoid this trap, industry must meet clear expectations, complete with benchmarks and timetables and with an objective evaluation of the impact of the industry's actions. Malfeasance should be addressed swiftly, so that change is made necessary within weeks or months, not years." (Page 287.) "Because obesity is now a major global problem, the world cannot afford a repeat of the tobacco history, in which industry talks about the moral high ground but does not occupy it." (Pages 259-260) From what I can see, this is exactly what a large section of the food industry is doing.

John Hill, *SA wants more regulation for junk food ads*, Australian Associated Press General News Wire; Sydney, 16th November, 2011 (ProQuest document ID: 903989999). South Australia (SA) Health Minister John Hill claimed phone surveys showed most parents wanted the government to regulate advertising of junk food to children. In the 1990s, only a tenth of four-year-olds in SA were overweight, by 2011 this was a fifth. Hill claimed $13 million was spent in 2010 on advertising in children's TV viewing time – much more than what is generally spent on campaigns to encourage people to quit smoking. Hill said the "key problem" is "voluntary self-regulation"

Jennifer L. Harris, PhD, MBA, and Samantha K. Graff, JD, *Protecting Young People From Junk Food Advertising: Implications of Psychological Research for First Amendment Law*, **American Journal of Public Health**, Vol. 102, No. 2, pp. 214-222, February, 2012. Looked at compromises between the First Amendment rights of corporations, and the rights of children to be protected from the consequences of advertisements for unsafe food, claimed American children saw on average, thirteen junk food adverts daily on TV, this comprising about 30% of all paid TV advertising to children. Claims that advertising's effects are consistently demonstrated by research, and that advertising may have even more of an effect than previously believed. Claims a third of children and teenagers in the USA are overweight or obese, with "unprecedented" levels of diet-related disease among youth. Claims public health experts believe obesity among children "cannot be resolved without dramatic changes in the obesogenic food environment that surrounds".

Points out, as have many, that education regarding health food cannot compete with the $1.6 billion spent yearly by the industry with "continuous reminders about the rewards of consuming primarily unhealthy food". The authors believe "significant reductions" in the volume of food advertising are necessary. They point to advertising restrictions that are malleable in definition and criteria; such things obviously suit industry. Exactly what constitutes "child-targeted" advertising excludes much media that appeals to children.

Regarding the First Amendment, the authors cite a famous 1976 case, *Virginia State Board of Pharmacy v Virginia Citizens Consumer Council*, in which a statewide ban on advertisements of prescription drug prices was removed. This yielded "a new commercial speech doctrine" which made for much difficulty in government limiting advertisements for harmful products.

"The Supreme Court has held that the government's obligation to protect children from harm can be subordinated to corporations' right to express—and adults' right to receive—truthful commercial information that is not misleading." (Citing *Lorillard v Reilly*, 533 US 525, 564, (2001)). Claims no court in the USA had, at the time of writing, used their power to restrict advertising toward youth. The authors look at the "4 key premises" of commercial speech doctrine – (i) advertisers will be honest about their products "advertisers will convey concrete product information", (ii) consumers will use this information to make rational choices, (iii) misleading advertising should be distinguishable from other advertising; and (iv) disclosures should be able to cure advertising that may mislead.

One can see straight away that the fact that much advertising does not lie outright is a way around these premises. Many ads simply have the product being used in a fun-looking way by attractive people or celebrities. As Chomsky has pointed out (with Andre Vltchek, *On Western Terrorism from Hiroshima to Drone Warfare*, p. 49, 2013), this is *not* conveying "concrete product information" at all – there is absolutely no consideration in advertising of what marketers call 'externalities' – things like pollution, rubbish, stress, debt – things consumers and/or future generations are often forced to take care of.

The authors of this article state that advertising is believed to be important because it tells us who sells what, where, and for how much. If a child eats a lot of poor quality food, it is assumed that the child made the choice to eat this food, fully of its own volition, "on the basis of their calculation that the immediate gratification of consumption outweighs any negative long-term health consequences." "Advertising is indispensable because it supports rational economic decisions, which in turn ensure the stability of markets."

The Supreme Court has looked at "juveniles' lack of maturity and under-developed sense of responsibility... often result in impetuous and ill-considered actions and decisions." (Citing *Graham v Florida*, 130 SCt 2011, 2026 (2010)).

Under a sub-heading called The "Real World" of Food Advertising, the authors point out that much advertising is designed to bypass any consideration of product information, that children can still be mislead by advertisements for nutrient-poor foods, and that children have not developed the ability to consider the long-term effects adequately. In one analysis cited here, it is claimed that "the more emotions dominate over rational messaging, the bigger the business effects. The most effective advertisements of all are those with little or no rational content." (Citing Binet L, Field P. *Empirical generalizations about advertising campaign success*. **J Advert Res**. 2009;49(2):130-133.) Providing information can even make advertising less effective, reducing the impact of the message. Advertisers look for long-term brand loyalty and try to create positive emotional associations with their product. This emotional hook not only helps consumers justify unnecessary purchases of the product, it allows manufacturers to obviate scepticism about their product – if we've *always* used their product, surely it can't be harmful.

Internet games, advergames, celebrities pictured with products, product placement in movies and the like provide no real product information, yet are "often more persuasive". Coke's "Open Happiness" campaign gave no product information to consumers. Food advertising teaches children that the majority of people often eat junk food, most parents allow their children to eat abundant junk food, and that there are no consequences for eating a lot of junk food. Research cited by the authors suggests that education did not show a relationship between scepticism of advertising and reduction in purchases. This is the only article I have seen in which the topic has been studied. In one instance the children wanted more of the advertised foods that they were taught to be sceptical of (citing Chernin A. *The Relationship Between Children's Knowledge of Persuasive Intent and Persuasion: The Case of Televised Food Marketing* [PhD thesis]. Philadelphia, PA: University of Pennsylvania; 2007). Knowing intellectually that an item of junk food is not healthy or that it may cause long-term effects in many years is not a real counter to the emotional, addictive pull to eat it. Ideas on how children may learn to inculcate themselves from the advertising are given.

However, young children who do not understand persuasive intent will treat advertising as though it is another source of information – accurate. Here, the advertising could be considered misleading because the children may not understand its inherent biases, the authors argue, and not protected by the First Amendment.

The paper concludes by saying much advertising has "no intrinsic meaning, conveys no information, is inherently likely to deceive, or has proven to be misleading…", and even if these cannot be proven perfectly, potential for harm still exists in overconsumption of poor quality food (and obvious lack of good quality food). Thus, corporate advertising of junk food should not be protected under the First Amendment and should be banned.

"The commercial speech doctrine must be reconsidered. Well-tailored government actions to restrict food and beverage marketing specifically targeting children should be able to withstand First Amendment scrutiny. For the health of our children, these actions should be taken and, if necessary, tested in the courts."

Stephen A. Rauch and Bruce P. Lanphear, *Prevention of Disability in Children: Elevating the Role of Environment*, **The Future of Children**, Vol. 22, No. 1, pp. 193-217, 2012. Points out much medical treatment, while it may work and save lives, does not prevent problems. Takes the point of view that clean air and water, sanitation and the like are very important. Also claims a fifth of American children lived in poverty in 2010.

Points to the precautionary principle: "Today, however, for a variety of reasons, policy makers are reluctant to act on a hazard unless the precise way that it causes disease or disability is known." (Page 205. Citing Ernst L. Wynder, "Studies in Mechanism and Prevention," *American Journal of Epidemiology* 139, no. 6 (1994): 547–49.) "Currently, industrial chemicals are 'innocent until proven guilty'." Harmful chemicals are taken off the market only when harm is proven without doubt – a chemical "has to be proven toxic in laboratory experiments and then in a series of epidemiologic studies, which usually take decades to complete." Claims harmful effects of chemicals in children were found "at increasingly lower levels of exposure. Children are routinely exposed to thousands of man-made chemicals, most of which have not been tested for safety, from an early age, and often even before they are born." Points to a recent claim (page 209) "that a ban on fast-food advertising aimed at children and adolescents would reduce rates of overweight children by 18 percent for children aged three to eleven…" (Citing Shin-Yi Chou, Inas Rashad, and Michael Grossman, "Fast-Food Restaurant Advertising on Television and Its Influence on Childhood Obesity," *Journal of Law and Economics* 51 (2008): 599–618.)

Jerry Mander, *Privatization of Consciousness*, **Monthly Review**, Vol. 64, No. 5, pp. 18-41, 2012. This is a reprint of a section of his book published the same year, *The Capitalism Papers: Fatal Flaws of an Obsolete System*. Looks at the "power relationship" in advertising: "Some speak; others listen." Claims $450 billion is spent world-wide, annually, in getting people to behave in a way in which advertisers want. "Very few people have a similar opportunity to *speak back* through media, to make demands on the advertisers. Or to suggest some other way to find happiness besides buying things." "Life has become a process of constantly avoiding things that people are trying to sell us." Mander discussed how he organized "a small meeting" in which he asked public attorneys if they felt advertising was legal – he interpreted the First Amendment as meaning that all people have equal rights in opportunity to free speech. Advertising as a medium is confined only to the people who can afford it. Claims much of global economics rests on the expansion of selling unneeded luxuries. Claims TV does not express culture, it expresses *corporate* culture. Also looks at spending in the U.S. on advertising, claiming "tens of millions" is spent on researching advertising to children, with babies a new market for advertisers. Looks at the number of violent programs, claims children have seen thousands of simulated murders on TV by the time they have grown up, claims children's TV was very violent. In the late 1970s the Federal Trade Commission (FTC) held public hearings to look at effects of advertising on under six-year-olds. The media responded, claiming such a thing would "inhibit the free-speech rights of advertisers." President Carter had the hearings cancelled, and fired the people in charge at the FTC. "It's a primary drive of corporate globalization that every place on Earth should become like every other place on Earth." Such tendency promotes "efficiency in resource management" and creates opportunities for investment. Yet this requires a surrendering of human values to external values of monoculturalized ideals.

Mander claims corporations "seek a mental landscape that nicely matches the physical landscape of freeways, suburbs, franchises, high-rises, clear-cuts, and the sped-up physical life of the commodified world." This is an interesting article in terms of U.S. foreign policy. People all over the world watch TV from the USA that gives the message that life in the USA is better than everywhere else.

Mander worked in advertising and believes it should be outlawed. He says the problem is that because advertising is not presented as being true or false, and presented without counter argument, it can become our frame of reference. Most ads simply show style, grace, popularity, people using products happily – if they made false claims they would be easier to police. Because they saying nothing inherently false, it is hard to present any counter argument. The article points to the power of imagery over logic, particularly true in political campaign advertising. Claims some countries in Scandinavia ban paid advertising in election campaigns, and that such policy would be near impossible in the USA. Points out that in most media there is no way to 'double-check' if people are telling the truth or not. Discusses the 2006-2009 conversion from analog to digital TV sets, "that really, nobody needed". But the benefits to corporations were "stratospheric" – huge amounts of purchases made by the entire population, and "instant obsolescence" for old TVs. The shipping industry also made benefits taking the obsolete TVs to Africa and India for disposal. Mander writes, "What a vast, thoughtful undertaking, involving direct costs to every household in the country, with no public debate (or lawsuits) about the government mandate to buy, and doubtful benefit to consumers!" Mander claims Clinton promised the new law would "democratize media ownership" – yet it had the opposite effect, with a small number of companies owning almost the entire media apparatus, which nobody voted for. Mander claims it is not only media that gets privatized, it is people's minds.

He claims the way in which advertising encourages indulgence and glamourises results in the poor missing out, which is not conducive to harmony. Mander points to Zoe Gannon and Neal Lawson's 2010 book *The Advertising Effect* for seven ideas that could help reduce the problems associated with the medium. One of which is to tax advertising. Another is for ad agencies to put their names on the ads they make; presumably this would help make the public more conscious of the medium. Gannon and Lawson claim the most serious aspect is the surveillance of private lives done by companies like Google.

I also highly recommend Mander's 1978 book *Four Arguments for the Elimination of Television*. Claims that problems with TV are inherent in the medium itself, one of which is the reduction of information to clichés and slogans. Another is the way in which the same message is beamed, one-way, to entire populations.

Bronwyn Torrie, **The Dominion Post**, p. A-6, 19th April, 2013. Discusses "extremely obese four-year-olds" in the Wellington region. Quotes Children's Commissioner paediatrician Russell Wills as claiming "whole-of-family intervention" was the only way to conquer childhood obesity, similar to quitting smoking.

Swetha Sundar, *Kids in Advertisement*, **Alive**, pp. 76-78, January, 2016. Looks at advertising for children in India. Using children in advertising helps give serious products a light-hearted image. Claims obesity in under five-year-olds is increasing. Claims advertising gives children a "wrong impression… of importance to materialistic joys."

"Young consumers are special targets of the junk-food industry. The market knows that fast-food is addictive and, once young people get used to having their fat, salts and sugar-rich food, they will become their consumers for life." Youth also have the "indirect purchasing power" of family. Claims advertising is helping to shape "the attitudes and value-systems of children by making them more and more demanding."

Tomaš Karel, Marketa Lhotakova, and Květa Olšanova, *Regulate or Educate? Parental Perception of Food Advertising Targeting Children, its Regulation and Food Industry Self-Regulation in the Czech Republic*, **European Food and Feed Law Review**, pp. 94-106, January, 2016. Claims a causal link between food advertising and obesity, though still much discussed. The U.S. Institute of Medicine (IOM) claims strong, moderate and weak evidence of advertising influencing various age groups of children. Self-regulation among food companies in the Czech Republic is "relatively mild" compared to others. Food industry had a substantial influence on regulatory boards, with the Czech self-regulatory office favouring the industry. Parental awareness of parents' ability and options to influence was low. Only about 20% were aware a Code of Conduct existed, and that they could report content of adverts.

This article looks at the attitudes mothers have toward advertising, and whether they communicate with children regarding adverts. Claims a link between sugar-sweetened beverages (SSBs) and obesity. Looks at the ability of children to see "persuasive intent" in adverts, and claims it may differ child to child. Parents can mediate the influence of advertising if they participate in the viewing of adverts. One study showed Czech parents had passive attitudes to advertising, which they viewed as "a common part of our life and consequently they do not speak with children about the advertising content and do not explain its purpose and aim." Of 707 respondents in their survey, 54% answered "I do not mind advertising".

Suggests voluntary regulation of industry may not be sufficient to curb problems in childhood (this point is such an obvious understatement I was surprised to read it). Educated mothers were more likely to explain purpose of adverts to children, and to watch for nutritional content. Points out poorer, disadvantaged children with less educated parents are less likely to have discussions which may yield a more accurate, balanced view of advertising and its potential effects.

With Author and Nutritional Biochemist Dr. Libby, *Curing Teens of Junk Food Hunger*, **The Wellingtonian**, 25th February, p. 26, 2016. Written in response to "My teen seems to be consuming a lot of junk food." While Dr. Libby points out "we are surrounded by food advertisements, it's no wonder that many children/teenagers are attracted to these types of foods." There is no suggestion of regulation upon advertising in the article, all responsibility can be placed on parents, none for politicians or CEOs.

Sports Programs Expose Kids to 'Unhealthy' Messages, by Esther Han, Consumer affairs editor, **The Sydney Morning Herald**, 13th July, 2016. Claims a study shows over 1.25 million Australian children in sports programs are exposed to "unhealthy" advertising from food manufacturers that have deals with program organizers (Watson *et al.*, *Sponsorship of junior sport development programs in Australia*, **Australian and New Zealand Journal of Public Health**, Vol. 40, No. 4, pp. 326-328. August, 2016; three authors from the New South Wales Cancer Council's Cancer Programs Division, one from the Faculty of Science Medicine and Health, University of Wollongong, NSW).

Mentioned are McDonald's (11% of children) and Nestle's Milo (40% of children), involved with basketball in Victoria and swimming in Queensland. Points out what all the experts know already: that advertisers target children to create brand loyalty throughout life, influence parental decisions, and that children are unprepared mentally to critically interpret the meaning and motivation of marketing. This claimed to be the first study that looked at sponsorship of children's programs, which aimed to determine the "healthiness" of products affiliated sponsors advertised. The researchers identified 246 sponsors from 56 websites; all research was done through websites. They classified over 90% of food and beverage products from sponsors as unhealthy. Sponsorships included naming rights, branded uniforms and participant packs.

Children can also be reached through sponsorship of adult sports team. The authors said one limitation of their study was that sports are seasonal, and websites and products change; this study was a "snapshot" of one long moment, not yearly trends. The only information used in the study was that which was publicly available; "this does not give any detail about the contribution from sponsors in other ways (e.g. monetary, resources, exclusive product agreements)." The authors conclude sponsoring of children's activities should be included in food marketing regulations.

A majority of children felt they had an obligation to buy products sold by the sponsors (citing Kelly B, Baur LA, Bauman AE, King L, Chapman K, Smith BJ. *"Food company sponsors are kind, generous and cool": (Mis)conceptions of junior sports players*. **Int J Behav Nutr Phys Act**. 2011;8:95).

Adrian O'Dowd, *Clinicians underwhelmed by "watered down" childhood obesity strategy*, **British Medical Journal**, Vol. 354, 22nd August, 2016. The British Health Department described its strategy as "far reaching" when it came to cutting down the amount of sugar in food and drink, and investing millions of pounds in physical education for schools. Sugar levels would be reduced by 20%.

O'Dowd pointed to two key features that were absent in the government's policy: a ban on discounting junk foods in supermarkets, and restrictions on junk food advertising to children on TV. The plan had been delayed before. The British Medical Association's science chair, Parveen Kumar, called the plan "weak". The targets for reductions in sugar were optional, "not backed up by regulation".

The Obesity Health Alliance, a coalition of 33 British charities, royal medical colleges, and concerned groups, called obesity a "devastating burden on the health of both society and the NHS" and said the government's plan was much less than required.

One idea people opposed to advertising introduced, was that councils should have power to ban junk food advertising near school. The British Dental Association's chair, Mick Armstrong, claimed that "... watering down action on junk food advertising... sends entirely the wrong signal to business, parents, and health professionals.

In December of 2016, the **London Financial Times** (Scheherazade Daneshkhu, *UK widens ban on unhealthy food ads aimed at children*, 8th December, 2016) reported that advertising to children on Facebook and Twitter would be banned. Cancer Research UK wanted a ban on all TV advertising of junk food before 9pm, but the government believed the social media ban was enough, given that not all advertising during TV shows is aimed at children. Advertising is considered "aimed at children" if children make up at least 25% of the audience. This was seen as a loophole, because obviously information about audience composition is not always easily available or monitored; for instance *Britain's Got Talent* and *The X Factor* are popular shows among children, but not quite enough to qualify as being aimed at them.

This **Times** article claimed a third of British children were obese, and that the social media bans were enacted after "years of resisting calls for stronger measures" to limit advertising to children online.

Journalist Paul D. Thacker wrote a recent article looking at the reluctance of academics to address conflict of interest issues in the U.S. for **The Washington Post** (22nd June, 2018).

It is fascinating that we don't let the tobacco industry self-regulate its advertising and communications, yet the food industry somehow *needs* this right, even though much of what it sells has been, and still is arguably very close to tobacco in the amount of harm it causes.

Appendix 7. What do People Opposed to Community Water Fluoridation Say about Claims of Fluorine's Essentiality?

This appendix focuses on some of the more influential people who have opposed fluoridation and statements they have made regarding this issue. Please recall the claims of Connett *et al.* have been discussed in Chapter 2.7.

Benjamin C. Nesin presented a talk, in the form of a ten-page document on the 8th of February, 1956 to Maine Water Utilities Association meeting at Portland, Maine. He told them:

> "The essentiality of fluorides as an element in nutrition has not been established."[191]

In support of this statement, he cited an article called *Trace Minerals in Nutrition and Health*, published in the May, 1955 issue of the **New York State Journal of Medicine**. This article claims that fluorine "occurs regularly" in bones and teeth, between 0.02-0.05 percent (200-500 ppm).

> "This occurrence, coupled with the benefit derived from its topical application or from fluoridated water in preventing dental caries, suggests that fluorine is a dietary essential."

> "No one has been able, however, to produce experimentally any specific deficiency symptoms in animals from diets nearly devoid of the element, and there is no convincing evidence that the beneficial effect on teeth from its ingestion is the result of its metabolism following absorption from the digestive tract."

> "Thus, there is no proof that fluorine is a dietary essential."[192]

Maynard didn't say anything about McClendon's work, or the criticism from the May, 1954 issue of **Nutrition Reviews**. Maynard didn't put any citations or references in his article. It's a good article for its time, and he wasn't saying anything too controversial. His audience presumably would have known what and who he was talking about.

Two Americans, F. B. Exner, M.D. and George L. Waldbott, M.D., wrote a book called *The American Fluoridation Experiment* which claimed:

> "There is no scientific support for the official thesis that fluorine is a 'missing ingredient' which fluoridation of the water supply provides. McCollum, Maynard, Phillips, McCay, and other leading nutritionists have found no evidence to warrant the belief that fluorine in *any* quantity is essential to the human or animal organism or to the production of good teeth. Indeed, there is much evidence to refute this contention, on which the official program of 'adjusting' the fluorine intake from water to one part per million is based." [193]

Clavell P. Blount, in his book *Compulsory Mass Medication*, claimed:

> "It has never been demonstrated that fluorine, even in trace amounts, is necessary for life processes..."[194]

Quoting the infamous movie Dr. Strangelove, a 1988 article appeared in **The Tampa Tribune** which began by outlining fluoridation dramas, and introduced Dr. Joel Boriskin, Chairman of the American Dental Association Committee on Community Health (for) and Dr. John Yiamouyiannis of the (American) National Health Federation (against). The media quoted Boriskin:

---

[191] *A Water Supply Perspective of the Fluoridation Discussion*, Presented by Benjamin C. Nesin, Director of Laboratories, Department of Water Supply, Gas and Electricity, City of New York Before the Maine Water Utilities Association meeting at Portland, Maine, on 8th February, 1956.

[192] L. A. Maynard, Ph.D., *Trace Minerals in Nutrition and Health*, **New York State Journal of Medicine**, Vol. 55, No. 9, p. 1311-1312, May, 1955.

[193] F. B. Exner, M.D. and George L. Waldbott, M.D., Edited by James Rorty, *The American Fluoridation Experiment*, p. 16, 1957.

[194] Clavell P. Blount, *Compulsory Mass Medication*, p. 35, 1964, citing Edward J. Ryan, D.D.S., **Oral Hygiene**, Sept., 1954.

"'I don't think people are stupid. I think the anti-fluoridationists are very sophisticated and this is a complex issue on which it is easy to confuse people.' For example, Boriskin says, fluoride is a deadly poison in pure form, especially as fluorine gas. 'But so is sodium and chlorine, and you put those together and you have table salt. Many elements are like that. In pure form, they are poisonous, but in the minute quantities we usually find them, they are essential nutrients.'" [195]

In 1993, the third edition of Yiamouyiannis' book, *Fluoride the Aging Factor*, was published[196]. He claimed again that fluorine was non-essential. This aroused no discussion, debate or disagreement from experts in media, as far as I can tell. This will no doubt help to explain why people opposed to CWF have been irritated. I have never found an instance when journalists have asked detailed questions about this topic, which demonstrates that they do not read the work written by people opposed, or if journalists do read it they do not discuss it. Yiamouyiannis detailed some of the experiments I have discussed in Chapter 1, although he did not mention the McClendon experiments.

In Chapter 5.4 I discussed the words of Dr. John Knutson. A very similar statement is from the same article under the sub-heading *The Role of the professionals* which Yiamouyiannis quoted on page 140 of *Fluoride the Aging Factor*. He attributed the quote to the 15th September, 1970 issue of the **British Dental Journal** (page 300) so presumably the same article is published there.

The 1988 document written in response to Yiamouyiannis' work (see Chapter 2.7) claimed:

"Yiamouyiannis capitalizes on this dilemma by selectively interpreting a number of scientific articles as indicating that fluoride is not an essential nutrient. On reviewing the full texts of the reports cited in the "Lifesavers Guide" it is obvious that three of his nine citations actually confirm that fluoride is essential. Two of the references make no specific claims either way and methodological errors were obvious in another source listed."[197]

"Selectively interpreting" is a very loaded statement when we get a copy of the (CWF-supporting) National Academy of Science's 1983 **Drinking Water and Health, Volume 3** and see that Yiamouyiannis' interpretation is nearly identical to the CWF-supporting NAS[198], minus the big citywide studies (Hodge and Dean, 1941 and 1950 – hardly recent by anyone's standards).

The "three of his nine" confirming essentiality are probably the same ones that he said were refuted – Schwarz and Messer's work.

The two that "make no specific claims" are possibly the Doberenz *et al.* and the Weber and Reid study, which did not state absolutely that fluorine should or should not be considered essential based on the results presented. Nevertheless, they had been brought into the issue by the National Academies, and others such as Muhler (writing in the 1970 WHO document) and Underwood, both of whom interpreted them as concluding fluorine non-essential with no word of protest from CWF advocates.

The "errors" were probably Schwarz's or the Messer group but this is uncertain because these experts were not specific.

The University of Waikato's expert panel in 2013 could not discuss a single one of the experiments Yiamouyiannis mentioned in his book, or even knew that they had featured in NAS documents since the 1950s until the late 1980s. As advocates of fluoridation love to say, the science was settled – or extremely close to being settled, decades ago. Yet these experts didn't know about it, partly because it wasn't mentioned in promotional literature, nor discussed openly, presumably because they concluded something unhelpful in the promotion of Community Water Fluoridation.

Regarding definitions of what constitutes an essential nutrient, I am in near-total agreement with fluoridation supporter Dr. Ken Perrott, at least about "openly declared":

"But whatever definition is used should be openly declared and applied consistently." (*The Fluoride Debate*, p. 10, see Chapter 2.7.)

I agree with "openly declared" because then everyone knows what we're talking about, and when people are confused they're probably less likely to participate. "Applied consistently" is a good point as well, but must be encompassed by a willingness to change, depending on new knowledge. People who *have* been applying a definition consistently are the people who Dr. Perrott talks very poorly about, namely people who are opposed to CWF. I suppose if we dislike them, we replace the word "consistent" with "dogmatic" or "fanatic". The people who've being doing the exact *opposite* of what Dr. Perrott suggests on this aspect of CWF are the experts who advocate for CWF – publicly citing only the experiments that suit them, being as loose or as rigid with criteria as they like, and relaxing the importance of the issue when their claims are countered.

---

[195] *Scientists don't debate our need for fluoridation*, **The Tampa Tribune** (Florida), p. 125-126, 24th April, 1988.

[196] *Fluoride the aging factor*, 3rd Edition, Chapter 13, 1993. In this investigation I am ONLY looking at Chapter 13, unless otherwise discussed.

[197] *Abuse of the Scientific Literature in an Antifluoridation Pamphlet*, Second Edition, p. 16, 1988.

[198] **Drinking Water and Health Volume 3**, Safe Drinking Water Committee Board on Toxicology and Environmental Health Hazards National Research Council, p. 266, 281-282, 1983. The NAS' 1989 **Recommended Dietary Allowances**, 10th edition, went into a little more detail using some of the same studies (p. 235) – this is cited in the book by Connett *et. al.*

Regarding definitions and industrial influence, there is one claim I found relevant here: in his book *The Fluoride Deception*, journalist and author Christopher Bryson discusses interviewing Edward Bernays, the founder of the public relations industry. According to Bryson, Bernays said:

> "we would put out the definition first to the editors of important newspapers".

> "Then we would send a letter to publishers of dictionaries and encyclopedias. After six or eight months we would find the word fluoridation was published and defined in dictionaries and encyclopedias."

What have the people opposed to fluoridation said about an industrial motivation? They have provided at least one piece of evidence, a statement from United States EPA's Rebecca Hanmer:

"In regard to the use of fluosilicic (fluorosilicic) acid as a source of fluoride for fluoridation, this agency regards such use as an ideal environmental solution to a long-standing problem. By recovering by-product fluosilicic acid from fertilizer manufacturing, water and air pollution are minimized, and water utilities have a low-cost source of fluoride available to the communities."[199]

This statement has been cited in so much of the literature opposed to CWF, but I have never seen it mentioned by anyone who supports CWF. As to the veracity of the document, I have not investigated. Searching the website Open Parachute for "Hanmer", there was nothing found.

In his response to two letters in the **Canberra Times** (29th October, 1989), Dr. Diesendorf pointed out that no-one had ever been shown to have "fluoride deficiency". He also claimed that fluorine was deleted from the US Federal Register's list of "essential or probably essential" substances on the 16th March, 1979 (see Vol. 44, No. 53, p. 16180 – this is a common claim in literature opposing CWF), suggesting that some of his critics' textbooks were a decade out of date (or many decades, if we accept the 1930s experiments).

Appendix 8. Non-Essentiality/Essentiality of Fluorine and the Herman/Chomsky Propaganda Model – American and Australasian Media

"Ignorance and prejudice are the handmaidens of propaganda."

> - Kofi Annan, former United Nations Secretary General. Quoted in New Zealand's **Otago Daily Times**, 8th April, 2020.

The first-, second-, and third-order predictions of the Propaganda Model are summarized with regard to the U.S. media's treatment of three types of bloodbaths in Noam Chomsky's work *Necessary Illusions* [1].

With regard to the topic of a nutritional role for fluorine, the first-order prediction would primarily focus on experts, simply because it would be unreasonable to expect journalists to keep abreast of the more detailed aspects of experiments. However, I do not think it unreasonable to expect the occasional journalist to look at writings of the WHO and NAS to verify activist or expert statements or quotes.

The prediction would be that an experiment or official document from a prestigious body concluding or claiming a nutritional role for fluorine would be publicized or mentioned by experts, and an experiment or official document from a prestigious body concluding or claiming fluorine to be *non*-essential would *not* be publicized by experts.

This is almost *exactly* what I found, though we must remember that most of the claims in newspapers do not even cite any research or official body at all. This is probably because as soon as experiments are mentioned, people ask questions about samples sizes and methods. It's easier if "everyone knows" that the claim is true. I have mentioned occasional deviations to this ~100% but they are not in newspapers. The claims of experts in newspapers are drastically out of touch on this one topic.

The second-order prediction would be that the first-order prediction would be highly confirmed, but completely ignored by media and experts. This is confirmed when we see that experts do not disagree with each other on this topic in media. Yet if we look within scientific or official literature (WHO, NAS reports, or experiments) we find there *are* different claims (*not* acknowledging each other) of a nutritional role for fluorine among experts, even in studies and reports claiming CWF to be safe, effective, etc. It's an important point that we *don't* need to go to the work of activists or opponents of fluoridation to see these.

---

[199] Rebecca Hanmer, Deputy Administrator, Office of Water, EPA in 1983 correspondence to Dr. Leslie Russell stating EPA position on water fluoridation.

The third-order prediction would be that any study or people pointing to mistakes within media or expert mentality would be either ignored or dismissed by media and experts. Chomsky explains:

"… suppose that some study of the media escapes these bounds, and reaches unwanted conclusions. The model yields third-order predictions about this case as well: specifically, it predicts that such inquiry will be ignored or bitterly condemned, for it conflicts with the needs of the powerful and privileged."

"At this [third-order] level, the model predicts that exposure of the facts would be rather unwelcome." [1]

A further aspect of the third-order prediction is that if an experiment or official document from a prestigious body concluding or claiming fluorine to be non-essential was cited, such a thing would only be cited by activists; people labelled by experts as crazy, biased, selective, not worth listening to. Hence a justification can be given for ignoring such a statement.

I believe there is one case that can almost perfectly illustrate this third-order prediction with regard to this niche topic within CWF. A New Zealander named Pat McNair pointed out the first-order prediction:

"For 50 years [the New Zealand Dental Association] gave out incorrect information and told us fluoride was an essential nutrient." [2]

I say "almost perfectly" because like so many antifluoride letters claiming a non-essential role for fluorine, McNair did not cite any prestigious body to support her statement, though many existed. The second-order prediction would be that nobody in support of fluoridation had *also* pointed to McNair's (and my) claim. At first I thought there was no response to McNair's statement, but I was wrong. There *was* a response, from Hamilton resident M. Manley-Harris (presumably Associate Professor of Organic and Analytical Chemistry from Waikato University, though I'm not totally certain). Manley-Harris' letter to the **Waikato** Times fulfils the third-order prediction. It is reproduced here in full:

"The anti-fluoride correspondent Pat McNair, having been apparently defeated in the science field by the academics of the chemistry department, now has to resort to ad hominem arguments against the dental association. Since the internet appears to be her main source of information I reproduce the following from Wikipedia to save her the trouble of looking it up: An *ad hominem* (Latin for "to the man" or "to the person"), short for *argumentum ad hominem*, is an argument made personally against an opponent instead of against his or her argument. *Ad hominem* reasoning is normally described as an informal fallacy, more precisely an irrelevance." [3]

We must also recall what Manley-Harris (assuming this is the same person) said in the 2013 Waikato Google Hangout:

"I think there are many substances which people regard as essential which haven't actually been scientifically proven to be essential." [4]

Remember that the propaganda model says nothing about the "degree of success" of propaganda among the population.

Addressing the second-order predictions, Chomsky has written:

"My point here, once again, is not that the assumptions about U.S. policy and the media that bound discussion are false (though they are), but rather that the possibility that they are false cannot be raised; it lies beyond the conceivable." [5]

Remember that the propaganda model says nothing about the "degree of success" of propaganda among the population.

Addressing the second-order predictions, Chomsky has written:

"My point here, once again, is not that the assumptions about U.S. policy and the media that bound discussion are false (though they are), but rather that the possibility that they are false cannot be raised; it lies beyond the conceivable." [5]

My point *here* would be similar: I'm not so attached to whether the claims of a nutritional role are false, my point is also "that the possibility that they are false cannot be raised; it lies beyond the conceivable." Or at least very close to "beyond the conceivable."

References for Appendix 8

1. Noam Chomsky. *Necessary Illusions: Thought Control in Democratic Societies*, Appendix 1, pp. 212-214, 1989.

2. Pat McNair, Fluoride debate, **Waikato Times**, 27th August, 2013. See reference 743 in Chapter 6.5. *Dentists Resent "False Statements" on Fluoridation*, Date and newspaper unknown, but possibly **Hawke's Bay Herald-Tribune**, found in Health Department archives HD 125/299 H1 1635 (years 1954-1955).

3. M. Manley Harris: *Playing the man, not ball*, letter to the editor, **Waikato Times**. 28th August, p. 11, 2013.

4. http://www.waikato.ac.nz/events/hangout/fluoride.shtml.

5. Noam Chomsky. *Necessary Illusions: Thought Control in Democratic Societies*, Appendix 1, p. 229, 1989.

Appendix 9. What does the International Society for Fluoride Research Say about Claims of Fluorine's Essentiality?

Here I will share a few things from The International Society for Fluoride Research. They do not officially consider themselves to be opposed to CWF, as far as I am aware. However, individual members may be. I know their journal **Fluoride** has contained research and communications from the supporters and opponents of CWF over the years. The journal began in 1968 and is not included in the database MEDLINE[200], even though the National Research Council made over fifty citations to the journal in its 2006 publication[201]. I will include some of their work here not so much because of the positions of their large staff on CWF, whatever these may be, but because I have seen it so rarely discussed.

Dr. George Waldbott was the founder and editor. He founded the journal because:

"A group of scientists engaged in fluoride research in one department of a U.S. university was completely unaware of studies on fluoride underway in another department of the same university. In Italy, a well known scientist carrying out research on fluoride had no knowledge of fluoride research which had emanated from another university only a few miles distant. This lack of communication in fluoride research prompted the establishment of the International Society for Fluoride Research and of **Fluoride** – Quarterly Reports."

"The Reports are issued in order to establish closer rapport between scientists of various disciplines in this and other countries, and to disseminate research findings on fluoride more effectively than in the past. They will feature, particularly, research data from non-English speaking countries which, in general, are not readily accessible to the scientific community in the U.S.A."

"No advertising is contemplated as a means of financing The Reports." (Vol. 1, No. 1, p. 1, 1968.)

The requirement for essentiality that the Society has been applying is the standard biochemistry criteria for essentiality, probably best explained at the beginning of the Messer *et al.* 1973 paper (see Chapter 1.1), or the work of Ulf Lindh (*Essentials of Medical Geology*, Chapter 6, 2005). Therefore the charge of "semantics" is quite out of place. "Semantics" is what the experts have engaged in for decades in order to confound facing the reality of evidence not suited to them.

The journal of the International Society for Fluoride Research published in 1973 an editorial entitled *Is Fluoride an Essential Element?*[202] In this editorial Waldbott discussed many of the experiments I have discussed in Chapter 1.1, although he mentioned one I didn't obtain, by Devoto *et al.*[203] It appears to me that *this* paper investigates fluoride's potential toxicity, rather than necessity, so I'm not sure of its relevance to my investigation, although I'm only looking at the abstract. From the Devoto *et al.* experiment:

"The present paper deals with a possible toxic effect of sodium fluoride on placentae and foetuses of the rat."

Quoting Waldbott's article:

"No attention was given to the fluoride content of the diet nor to its accumulation in the rats' carcasses."

Devoto's experiment injected sodium fluoride peritoneally – different to other experiments that had used food and water levels, obviously less precise due to different intake. According to Waldbott, Devoto cautioned against applying experiments performed on rats, to humans.

In 1978, Waldbott's book *The Great Dilemma* was published. It included a ten-page chapter called *An Essential Nutrient?* This chapter looked at much of the work I have discussed in Chapters 1.1 and 1.2, and a lot more very obscure American work that I think someone like myself would find very difficult, expensive and time-consuming to obtain. He made an interesting point on the Schwarz and Milne experiment, that

"… the diet in this study differs so radically from a "normal" diet that fluoride effects in it simply cannot be extrapolated to a normal one."

---

[200] A. Burgstahler and B. Spittle, *Medline Again Rejects **Fluoride**, **Fluoride**, Vol. 42, No. 4, pp. 256-259, 2009; B. Spittle, *Further Medline Rejection of **Fluoride***, **Fluoride**, Vol. 47, No. 1, pp. 2-8, 2014.

[201] National Research Council of the National Academies, *Fluoride in Drinking Water: A Scientific Review of the EPA's Standards*, 2006.

[202] George Waldbott M.D., Editorial, *Is Fluoride an Essential Element?* ISFR, Vol. 6, No. 1, 1973. Waldbott has also investigated the topic in his book *The Great Dilemma*, Chapter 6, 1978, which is a little more detailed than this editorial.

[203] F. C. H. Devoto, B. M. Perrotto, B. M. Bordoni, and N. H. Arias, *Effect of Sodium Fluoride on the Placenta of the Rat*, **Archives of Oral Biology**, Vol. 17, pp. 371-374, 1972.

I would say the same of McClendon's. He also suggested that growth as a criterion is misleading, because,

"… weight gain *per se* has no necessary connection with a healthy organism, since fluoride is known to cause water retention and thus an increase in body weight."

In his 1973 editorial, he said polydipsia (excessive thirst) was

"a common manifestation associated with fluoride intake."

He didn't supply references for either of these statements, but he had gone into these topics in other work. To summarize Waldbott's ideas, he said purified diets for animals low in magnesium, calcium or iron may cause deficiency symptoms that could be "partially neutralized by fluoride supplementation."

He thought these experiments on fluoride supplementation should not be applied to humans on normal human diets. He then wrote:

"They also do *not* prove that fluoride is in any way essential for the maintenance of good health in man."

In 1974 the journal published an article by a specialist in the field of ecology of soil fungi. Here is what he said about fluorine's necessity:

"Another widespread misconception concerns the alleged 'essential' nature of fluorine or the fluoride ion. I quote from a well-known paperback on pesticides and pollution by one of our leading conservationists: (Mellanby, K,: *Pesticides and Pollution*, p. 36. Collins (Fontana), 1969)

"Fluorine occurs in minute quantities in all plants and animals and it is one of the essential elements of protoplasm. If the nature level falls below a minimum, and this occurs in nature, harmful effects may be seen." (End quote.)

"The only justification so far offered (in correspondence) for this statement has been a reference to some recent work on laboratory mice. The work with laboratory rodents on low-fluoride diets has been summarized recently in an editorial in **Fluoride**." (Citing *Is Fluoride an Essential Element?* **Fluoride**, Vol. 6, No. 1, pp. 1-3, 1973.)

"The evidence at present seems inconclusive; but if it should eventually be clearly shown that fluoride, in trace quantities, has some essential function in the laboratory rodent, this is still far from showing it is similarly essential for the natural or wild rodent; should this be so, it is still a long way from showing that it is generally essential in the mammalian, or human, metabolism; and if this should be proved, it is an even longer way from justifying the description of fluorine as an essential element of protoplasm; and finally, should this also prove to be true, it is still quite irrelevant to the 'natural level' mentioned in the quotation, since I have searched the literature in vain for evidence that, anywhere in the world, there is a natural deficiency of fluorine causing harmful effects to any organism whatever. It is notoriously difficult to produce a fluorine-free diet which is not deficient in other respects, and highly unlikely that such a situation could arise in nature, or in the human context. In fact, the whole question of the 'essentiality' of fluorine as demonstrated at experimental levels of purification is largely a matter of academic interest."[204]

"Let me now quote from *The Penguin Medical Encyclopaedia* (1972) p. 169, which states, unequivocally, under the heading fluorine:

'In most regions there is enough fluorine in drinking water, about 1 part per million.'

"It then goes on to refer to the remainder of the world's water in terms of deficiency or excess of fluorine. These terms: *optimal* (i.e. about 1 ppm fluoride) *excessive*, and *deficient*, first proposed by H. T. Dean in his '21 Cities' Study (3) related only to the diseases of caries and fluorotic mottling in the teeth of school children. Of these terms, only 'excessive' is justifiable, insofar as fluoride has been identified as the causative agent in this type of dental mottling; but there can be little doubt that the widespread use of the term 'deficient', as referring to the fluoride level in all water supplies below 1 ppm, has misled many people, including Dr. Peter Wingate, the author of this encyclopaedia, into assuming that this could refer only to a minority of water supplies, since it would not be credible that the bulk of the world's fresh water could be designated in this way." (All his emphasis.)

Likening fluoride to sulphur dioxide, a pollutant that can damage crops at a certain concentration, inhibit the growth of various fungi at a slightly lower concentration, Dobbs writes:

"I will not for a moment concede that these plant diseases are of any less importance to mankind than dental caries; for what is the use of having good teeth if there is no food to eat with them!"

"Let us suppose, therefore, that the plant pathologists, taking their cue from the dentists, designate the plant-damage level of SO_2 pollution as 'excessive', the level of fungal suppression without plant damage as 'optimal', and the entire rest of the

---

[204] C. G. Dobbs, *Fluoride and the Environment*, Vol. 07, No. 03, pp. 123-135, 1974.

earth's atmosphere as 'deficient' in SO_2. How then shall we fare in our struggle against air pollution?" (Vol. 7, No. 3, p. 125, 1974.)

The review of the National Academies' 1997 **Dietary Reference Intakes** is available in **Fluoride**, Vol. 30, No. 4, pp. 252-257. The review's author was Canadian doctor Richard Foulkes.

On the issue of whether fluorine should be considered a nutritional essential or not, two letters to the NAS can be found in **Fluoride**, Vol. 31 No. 3, pp. 153-157, 1998.

The NAS eventually replied, the discussion is found in Vol. 32, No. 3, pp. 187-192, with Yiamouyiannis' reply (pp. 192-198).

Albert Burgstahler made a point I have not, which is that if fluoride's effect on teeth is exclusively topical and not systemic ("systemic" meaning ingested through the stomach then affecting teeth from *within* or via saliva) then the phrase "Adequate Intake" is improper. I suggest that "Adequate Application" may be more appropriate.

Index